Polymeric Systems as Antimicrobial or Antifouling Agents

Polymeric Systems as Antimicrobial or Antifouling Agents

Special Issue Editors
Antonella Piozzi
Iolanda Francolini

MDPI • Basel • Beijing • Wuhan • Barcelona • Belgrade

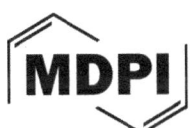

Special Issue Editors
Antonella Piozzi
University of Rome
Italy

Iolanda Francolini
University "La Sapienza"
Italy

Editorial Office
MDPI
St. Alban-Anlage 66
4052 Basel, Switzerland

This is a reprint of articles from the Special Issue published online in the open access journal *International Journal of Molecular Sciences* (ISSN 1422-0067) from 2018 to 2019 (available at: https://www.mdpi.com/journal/ijms/special_issues/antimicrobial-polymers_2018).

For citation purposes, cite each article independently as indicated on the article page online and as indicated below:

LastName, A.A.; LastName, B.B.; LastName, C.C. Article Title. *Journal Name* **Year**, *Article Number*, Page Range.

ISBN 978-3-03928-456-6 (Pbk)
ISBN 978-3-03928-457-3 (PDF)

© 2020 by the authors. Articles in this book are Open Access and distributed under the Creative Commons Attribution (CC BY) license, which allows users to download, copy and build upon published articles, as long as the author and publisher are properly credited, which ensures maximum dissemination and a wider impact of our publications.

The book as a whole is distributed by MDPI under the terms and conditions of the Creative Commons license CC BY-NC-ND.

Contents

About the Special Issue Editors ix

Iolanda Francolini and Antonella Piozzi
Polymeric Systems as Antimicrobial or Antifouling Agents
Reprinted from: *Int. J. Mol. Sci.* **2019**, *20*, 4866, doi:10.3390/ijms20194866 1

Cristina Cattò and Francesca Cappitelli
Testing Anti-Biofilm Polymeric Surfaces: Where to Start?
Reprinted from: *Int. J. Mol. Sci.* **2019**, *20*, 3794, doi:10.3390/ijms20153794 6

Carmen Mabel González-Henríquez, Mauricio A. Sarabia-Vallejos and
Juan Rodríguez Hernandez
Antimicrobial Polymers for Additive Manufacturing
Reprinted from: *Int. J. Mol. Sci.* **2019**, *20*, 1210, doi:10.3390/ijms20051210 66

Nor Fadhilah Kamaruzzaman, Li Peng Tan, Ruhil Hayati Hamdan, Siew Shean Choong,
Weng Kin Wong, Amanda Jane Gibson, Alexandru Chivu and Maria de Fatima Pina
Antimicrobial Polymers: The Potential Replacement of Existing Antibiotics?
Reprinted from: *Int. J. Mol. Sci.* **2019**, *20*, 2747, doi:10.3390/ijms20112747 93

Minghan Chi, Manlin Qi, Lan A, Ping Wang, Michael D. Weir, Mary Anne Melo,
Xiaolin Sun, Biao Dong, Chunyan Li, Junling Wu, Lin Wang and Hockin H. K. Xu
Novel Bioactive and Therapeutic Dental Polymeric Materials to Inhibit Periodontal Pathogens
and Biofilms
Reprinted from: *Int. J. Mol. Sci.* **2019**, *20*, 278, doi:10.3390/ijms20020278 124

Markéta Pazderková, Petr Maloň, Vlastimil Zíma, Kateřina Hofbauerová, Vladimír Kopecký Jr.,
Eva Kočišová, Tomáš Pazderka, VáclavČeřovský and Lucie Bednárová
Interaction of Halictine-Related Antimicrobial Peptides with Membrane Models
Reprinted from: *Int. J. Mol. Sci.* **2019**, *20*, 631, doi:10.3390/ijms20030631 153

Min Kyung Kim, Na Hee Kang, Su Jin Ko, Jonggwan Park, Eunji Park, Dong Won Shin,
Seo Hyun Kim, Seung A. Lee, Ji In Lee, Seung Hyun Lee, Eun Gi Ha, Seung Hun Jeon and
Yoonkyung Park
Antibacterial and Antibiofilm Activity and Mode of Action of Magainin 2 against Drug-
Resistant *Acinetobacter baumannii*
Reprinted from: *Int. J. Mol. Sci.* **2018**, *19*, 3041, doi:10.3390/ijms19103041 179

Malgorzata Anna Paduszynska, Magdalena Maciejewska, Katarzyna Ewa Greber,
Wieslaw Sawicki and Wojciech Kamysz
Antibacterial Activities of Lipopeptide $(C_{10})_2$-KKKK-NH_2 Applied Alone and in Combination
with Lens Liquids to Fight Biofilms Formed on Polystyrene Surfaces and Contact Lenses
Reprinted from: *Int. J. Mol. Sci.* **2019**, *20*, 393, doi:10.3390/ijms20020393 193

Bruna Agrillo, Marco Balestrieri, Marta Gogliettino, Gianna Palmieri, Rosalba Moretta,
Yolande T.R. Proroga, Ilaria Rea, Alessandra Cornacchia, Federico Capuano,
Giorgio Smaldone and Luca De Stefano
Functionalized Polymeric Materials with Bio-Derived Antimicrobial Peptides for
"Active" Packaging
Reprinted from: *Int. J. Mol. Sci.* **2019**, *20*, 601, doi:10.3390/ijms20030601 212

Olena Moshynets, Jean-François Bardeau, Oksana Tarasyuk, Stanislav Makhno, Tetiana Cherniavska, Oleg Dzhuzha, Geert Potters and Sergiy Rogalsky
Antibiofilm Activity of Polyamide 11 Modified with Thermally Stable Polymeric Biocide Polyhexamethylene Guanidine 2-Naphtalenesulfonate
Reprinted from: *Int. J. Mol. Sci.* **2019**, *20*, 348, doi:10.3390/ijms20020348 225

Marian Szkudlarek, Elisabeth Heine, Helmut Keul, Uwe Beginn and Martin Möller
Synthesis, Characterization, and Antimicrobial Properties of Peptides Mimicking Copolymers of Maleic Anhydride and 4-Methyl-1-pentene
Reprinted from: *Int. J. Mol. Sci.* **2018**, *19*, 2617, doi:10.3390/ijms19092617 244

Alexandra Muñoz-Bonilla, Daniel López and Marta Fernández-García
Providing Antibacterial Activity to Poly(2-Hydroxy Ethyl Methacrylate) by Copolymerization with a Methacrylic Thiazolium Derivative
Reprinted from: *Int. J. Mol. Sci.* **2018**, *19*, 4120, doi:10.3390/ijms19124120 266

Francesco Galiano, Raffaella Mancuso, Maria Grazia Guzzo, Fabrizio Lucente, Ephraim Gukelberger, Maria Adele Losso, Alberto Figoli, Jan Hoinkis and Bartolo Gabriele
New Polymeric Films with Antibacterial Activity Obtained by UV-induced Copolymerization of Acryloyloxyalkyltriethylammonium Salts with 2-Hydroxyethyl Methacrylate
Reprinted from: *Int. J. Mol. Sci.* **2019**, *20*, 2696, doi:10.3390/ijms20112696 279

Carolina Nascimento Galvão, Luccas Missfeldt Sanches, Beatriz Ideriha Mathiazzi, Rodrigo Tadeu Ribeiro, Denise Freitas Siqueira Petri and Ana Maria Carmona-Ribeiro
Antimicrobial Coatings from Hybrid Nanoparticles of Biocompatible and Antimicrobial Polymers
Reprinted from: *Int. J. Mol. Sci.* **2018**, *19*, 2965, doi:10.3390/ijms19102965 290

Yanna Gurianov, Faina Nakonechny, Yael Albo and Marina Nisnevitch
Antibacterial Composites of Cuprous Oxide Nanoparticles and Polyethylene
Reprinted from: *Int. J. Mol. Sci.* **2019**, *20*, 439, doi:10.3390/ijms20020439 303

Katarzyna Czarnobaj, Magdalena Prokopowicz and Katarzyna Greber
Use of Materials Based on Polymeric Silica as Bone-Targeted Drug Delivery Systems for Metronidazole
Reprinted from: *Int. J. Mol. Sci.* **2019**, *20*, 1311, doi:10.3390/ijms20061311 319

Laura Sisti, Grazia Totaro, Nicole Bozzi Cionci, Diana Di Gioia, Annamaria Celli, Vincent Verney and Fabrice Leroux
Olive Mill Wastewater Valorization in Multifunctional Biopolymer Composites for Antibacterial Packaging Application
Reprinted from: *Int. J. Mol. Sci.* **2019**, *20*, 2376, doi:10.3390/ijms20102376 331

Iolanda Francolini, Ilaria Silvestro, Valerio Di Lisio, Andrea Martinelli and Antonella Piozzi
Synthesis, Characterization, and Bacterial Fouling-Resistance Properties of Polyethylene Glycol-Grafted Polyurethane Elastomers
Reprinted from: *Int. J. Mol. Sci.* **2019**, *20*, 1001, doi:10.3390/ijms20041001 345

Cristina Cattò, Francesco Secundo, Garth James, Federica Villa and Francesca Cappitelli
α-Chymotrypsin Immobilized on a Low-Density Polyethylene Surface Successfully Weakens *Escherichia coli* Biofilm Formation
Reprinted from: *Int. J. Mol. Sci.* **2018**, *19*, 4003, doi:10.3390/ijms19124003 361

Fabienne Faÿ, Maëlle Gouessan, Isabelle Linossier and Karine Réhel
Additives for Efficient Biodegradable Antifouling Paints
Reprinted from: *Int. J. Mol. Sci.* **2019**, *20*, 361, doi:10.3390/ijms20020361 . . . . **376**

About the Special Issue Editors

Antonella Piozzi In 1987, Antonella Piozzi graduated with a degree in Industrial Chemistry at the Sapienza University of Rome. In 1987, she was awarded an E.N.I. fellowship studying biomedical polymers, synthesis, and characterization. In 1992, she obtained a Ph.D. in Chemical Science and received a fellowship for the project Chimica Fine II from the National Research Council. From 1993 to 2001, she was appointed as a researcher in the Chemistry Department of the Sapienza University of Rome. From 1997 to 2001, she lectured for the courses Macromolecular Chemistry Laboratory and Industrial Chemistry Laboratory at the Sapienza University of Rome. In 2001, Antonella Piozzi was appointed Associate Professor of Industrial Chemistry at the Sapienza University of Rome. Her research experience includes the fields of macromolecular chemistry, biomaterials, and applied enzymology, including studies on the synthesis and physico-chemical characterization of polymers in industrial and medical applications. She has authored over 90 scientific publications published in international scientific journals, 4 book chapters, and more than 60 conference proceedings. She is a member of the Editorial Board of the *International Journal of Molecular Science*, section Biomaterial Science.

Iolanda Francolini Since 2004, Iolanda Francolini has been a researcher at Sapienza University of Rome where she studies the synthesis and characterization of polymers for biomedical applications and serves as a lecturer of the science and technologies of polymers. She obtained a degree in Industrial Chemistry cum laude in 2000 from the Sapienza University of Rome. In 2001, she completed ultrastructural analysis of polymer surfaces and microbial biofilms at the Istituto Superiore di Sanità (National Institute of Health) of Rome. In 2003, she was a visiting scientist for one year at the Center for Biofilm Engineering, Montana, USA, where she worked on the development of polyacrylates releasing drugs on demand. In 2005, she obtained a Ph.D. degree at the Sapienza University of Rome in Chemical and Industrial Processes, researching antimicrobial functionalized polyurethanes. Her research interests include synthesis of antimicrobial and antifouling polymers, drug-releasing polymers, and magnetic core/shell nanocomposites for drug targeting. She has been an invited speaker at several international conferences and Guest Editor of several Special Issues of *International Journal of Molecular Science*. Currently, she is member of the Editorial Board of the *International Journal of Molecular Science*, section Biomaterial Science, and has authored 64 scientific publications in international Journals, 3 book chapters, and more than 60 conference proceedings, with an H-index of 21.

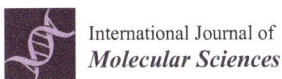

Editorial

Polymeric Systems as Antimicrobial or Antifouling Agents

Iolanda Francolini * and Antonella Piozzi *

Department of Chemistry, Sapienza University of Rome, P.le Aldo Moro, 5-00185 Rome, Italy
* Correspondence: iolanda.francolini@uniroma1.it (I.F.); antonella.piozzi@uniroma1.it (A.P.)

Received: 25 September 2019; Accepted: 29 September 2019; Published: 30 September 2019

The rapid increase in the emergence of antibiotic-resistant bacterial strains combined with a dwindling rate of discovery of novel antibiotic molecules has lately created an alarming issue worldwide [1]. Resistant genes in microorganisms may be inherited from forerunners or acquired through genetic mutations or gene exchange [2]. Although the occurrence of resistance in microbes is a natural process, the overuse of antibiotics is known to improve the rate of resistance evolution [3]. Indeed, under antibiotic treatment, susceptible bacteria inevitably die, while resistant microorganisms proliferate under reduced competition. Therefore, the out-of-control use of antibiotics causes the elimination of drug-susceptible species that would naturally limit the expansion of resistant ones. On top of that, the ability of many microbial species to grow as biofilm has further complicated the treatment of infections with conventional antibiotics. Indeed, microbial biofilms, that is microbial communities growing attached to abiotic surfaces (medical devices, surgical instruments, industrial pipelines, etc.) and tissues [4], are known to be an optimal environment to amplify both naturally occurring and induced antibiotic-resistance phenomena [5]. That together with other defense mechanisms significantly increases biofilm antibiotic tolerance.

A number of corrective measures are currently under exploration to reverse or slow down antibiotic resistance evolution, among which the development of polymer-based antimicrobial compounds has emerged as one of the most promising solutions [6,7]. Indeed, antimicrobial polymers benefit from a non-specific mode of action, primarily targeting the microbial membrane, and generally display less propensity to promote antimicrobial resistance. Most of the so far investigated polymeric biocides are able to interact with the bacterial cell membrane causing membrane disassembly and leakage of intracellular material [8,9]. Interestingly, some antimicrobial polymers have also been reported to potentiate the activity of conventional antibiotics [10].

A plethora of different polymer systems has been designed to prevent or treat biofilm formation, including: (i) cationic polymers [11,12]; (ii) antibacterial peptide-mimetic polymers [13,14]; (iii) polymers or composites able to load and release bioactive molecules [15–17]; and (iv) antifouling polymers, able to repel microbes by physical or chemical mechanisms [18]. The potential fields of application of antimicrobial polymers are numerous. They may play a predominant role in the design and fabrication of medical devices as well as in food packaging and as drug carriers.

This special issue collected nineteen papers, of which four were reviews and fifteen were original articles. All of the four reviews were essentially focused on the application of antimicrobial polymers in the biomedical field [19–22]. The review by Cattò and Cappitelli [19] provided an overview of the most common methods for testing the antibiofilm activity of polymeric surfaces. The authors underlined how there is a general lack of standardized *in vitro* methods as well as controlled *in vivo* studies, which may question the relevance of obtained results. In this regard, simplified guidelines were proposed in the review to help readers choose the most appropriate tests for their objectives.

The review by González-Henríquez and colleagues was instead focused on the manufacturing of 3D-printed objects based on antimicrobial polymers for the production of personalized devices, including implants and drug dosage forms [20]. In the first part of the review, a particular manufacturing technology to produce 3D-objects, that is "additive manufacturing", was described, and illustrative examples of fabrication of 3D-objects using natural and synthetic antimicrobial polymers were discussed.

The potentiality of antimicrobial polymers to replace existing antibiotics was reviewed by Kamaruzzaman et al. [21], who provided the latest updates in the context of ESKAPE (*Enterecoccus faecium, Staphylococcus aureus, Klebsiella pneumoniae, Acinetobacter baumannii, Pseudomonas aeruginosa*, and *Enterobacter* spp.) pathogens. Finally, the state of the art of antibacterial polymers against periodontal pathogens was reviewed by Chi et al. [22], who paid particular attention to polymeric systems for functional guided tissue regeneration (GTR) membrane, polymer composites for decay restoration, and photosensitizer (PS) modification for photodynamic therapy enhancement.

As for the 15 original articles of this special issue, they can be sketchily divided in two broad categories, namely studies focused on polymers able to kill microorganisms (*antimicrobial systems*) and studies focused on materials with fouling resistance properties (*antifouling systems*).

Among the antimicrobial systems, readers can find antimicrobial peptides [23–26], cationic polymers [27–31], and inorganic/polymer composites [32–34].

Basically, four antimicrobial peptides were investigated: (i) Halictine-1, for which the correlation between changes in primary/secondary structure and antimicrobial activity was studied through various membrane-mimicking models [23]; (ii) Magainin 2, whose antibiofilm activity was tested against *Acitenobacter baumannii* strains [24]; (iii) the lipopeptide $(C_{10})_2$-KKKK-NH_2, whose potentiality, alone and in combination with lens liquids, in the prophylaxis of contact lens-related eye infections was studied [25]; and iv) a bactenecin-derivative peptide named 1018K6, which was conjugated to polyethylene terephthalate (PET) to obtain an active packaging for the food industry [26].

As far as cationic polymers are concerned, a thermally stable cationic polymer biocide was obtained by Moshynets and colleagues [27], through polymerization of guanidine hydrochloride and hexamethylenediamine. Such polymer biocide was then incorporated into Polyamide 11 film to obtain contact-active composites. Interesting antibiofilm activities were found against two biofilm-forming model bacterial strains, *E. coli* K12 and *S. aureus* ATCC 25923 [27].

The synthesis of peptides-mimicking amphiphilic cationic copolymers based on maleic anhydride and 4-methyl-1-pentene was reported by Szkudlarek et al. [28]. The copolymers were then quaternized with either methyl iodide or dodecyl iodide to stabilize polymer cationic charges. Of particular relevance was the minimum inhibitory concentration (MIC) of quaternized copolymers, which was found to be lower than Nisin on a molar basis.

Cationic acrylic copolymers based on poly(2-hydroxy ethyl methacrylate) (HEMA), a largely employed biocompatible polymer, were investigated in 2 of the 15 studies of this special issue [29,30]. Specifically, Muñoz-Bonilla et al. [29] copolymerized HEMA with a methacrylic monomer bearing a thiazole side group susceptible to quaternization, while Galiano et al. [30] used UV-induced polymerization to copolymerize HEMA with two cationic acryloyloxyalkyltriethylammonium bromides (C-11 or C-12 alkyl chain linker). In both studies, copolymers exhibited significant activity versus Gram-positive (*S. aureus*) and Gram-negative (*P. aeruginosa* and *E. coli*) bacteria and, as expected, copolymer antimicrobial activity increased with increasing of the cationic unit content. Cationic poly(methylmethacrylate)-based nanoparticles were instead prepared by Galvão et al. [31]. The layering of such nanoparticles onto model surfaces (silicon wafers, glass, and polystyrene sheets) resulted in a significant reduction (ca. 7 logs) of the number of *E. coli* and *S. aureus* adhered onto the coated-surfaces compared to pristine surfaces.

Always in the framework of antimicrobial systems, three types of antibacterial inorganic/polymer composites were reported in this special issue [32–34]. Antibacterial cuprous oxide nanoparticles (Cu_2ONPs) were loaded into linear low-density polyethylene (LLDPE) by Gurianov et al. [32] to develop materials for tap water and wastewater disinfection. Inorganic silica materials functionalized with various types of organic groups (3-aminopropyl, 3-mercaptopropyl, or 3-glycidyloxypropyl groups) were used as bone-targeted delivery systems for metronidazole [33]. Antibacterial and antioxidant phenol molecules, extracted from olive mill wastewater, were intercalated into the host structure of ZnAl layered double hydroxide and employed for the preparation of poly(butylene succinate) composites by Sisti et al. [34]. These composites showed interesting properties for application in food packaging.

Finally, three studies of this special issue were focused on development of antifouling systems following different approaches [35–37]. Francolini and colleagues [35] functionalized segmented polyurethanes, one of the most important class of biomedical polymers, with polyethylene glycol (PEG), known to possess strong antifouling properties. Findings showed how PEG-functionalization not only positively affected polyurethane ability to resist to *Staphylococcus epidermidis* adhesion but also improved mechanical properties of the polymer with clear advantages for practical applications. Cattò et al. [36] immobilized the protease α-Chymotrypsin, supposed to degrade the biofilm matrix, on a low-density polyethylene surface. Interestingly, enzyme immobilization significantly weakened *E. coli* biofilm formation affecting thickness, roughness, and surface area coverage but not bacterial viability, thus reducing the risk of drug resistance development. Finally, Faÿ and coworkers [37] developed antifouling paints by the use of three additives (Tween 80, Span 85, and PEG-silane) as surface modifiers.

In conclusion, antimicrobial polymers may have a pivotal role in the global effort to find solutions against drug resistant infections. In the last 20 years, great scientific and technological advances have been made in this area, mainly thanks to the increased knowledge on mechanisms involved in materials/bacteria interaction as well as on the complexities of biofilm biology. Such knowledge was and still is the inspiration for biomaterials scientists to develop materials able to control biofilm formation. Despite that, a massive amount of work still remains to be done to address unsolved challenges, such as long-term stability, functionality, and biocompatibility of antimicrobial polymers. Translational research is also strongly needed in the near future, in order to make possible the transition of antimicrobial polymers from the bench to the patient bedside.

Conflicts of Interest: The authors declare no conflict of interest.

References

1. Chokshi, A.; Sifri, Z.; Cennimo, D.; Horng, H. Global Contributors to Antibiotic Resistance. *J. Glob. Infect. Dis.* **2019**, *11*, 36–42. [PubMed]
2. Blair, J.M.; Webber, M.A.; Baylay, A.J.; Ogbolu, D.O.; Piddock, L.J. Molecular mechanisms of antibiotic resistance. *Nat. Rev. Microbiol.* **2015**, *13*, 42–51. [CrossRef] [PubMed]
3. Aslam, B.; Wang, W.; Arshad, M.I.; Khurshid, M.; Muzammil, S.; Rasool, M.H.; Nisar, M.A.; Alvi, R.F.; Aslam, M.; Qamar, M.U.; et al. Antibiotic resistance: A rundown of a global crisis. *Infect. Drug Resist.* **2018**, *11*, 1645–1658. [CrossRef] [PubMed]
4. Costerton, J.W.; Lewandowski, Z.; Caldwell, D.E.; Korber, D.R.; Lappin-Scott, H.M. Microbial biofilms. *Annu. Rev. Microbiol.* **1995**, *49*, 711–745. [CrossRef] [PubMed]
5. Lewis, K. Multidrug tolerance of biofilms and persister cells. *Curr. Top. Microbiol.* **2008**, *322*, 107–131.
6. Francolini, I.; Vuotto, C.; Piozzi, A.; Donelli, G. Antifouling and antimicrobial biomaterials: An overview. *APMIS* **2017**, *125*, 392–417. [CrossRef] [PubMed]
7. Francolini, I.; Donelli, G.; Crisante, F.; Taresco, V.; Piozzi, A. Antimicrobial polymers for anti-biofilm medical devices: State-of-art and perspectives. *Adv. Exp. Med. Biol.* **2015**, *831*, 93–117. [PubMed]
8. Muñoz-Bonilla, A.; Fernández-García, M. Polymeric materials with antimicrobial activity. *Prog. Polym. Sci.* **2012**, *37*, 281–339.
9. Carmona-Ribeiro, A.M.; de Melo Carrasco, L.D. Cationic antimicrobial polymers and their assemblies. *Int. J. Mol. Sci.* **2013**, *14*, 9906–9946. [CrossRef]
10. Uppu, D.S.S.M.; Konai, M.M.; Sarkar, P.; Samaddar, S.; Fensterseifer, I.C.M.; Farias-Junior, C.; Krishnamoorthy, P.; Shome, B.R.; Franco, O.L.; Haldar, J. Membrane-active macromolecules kill antibiotic-tolerant bacteria and potentiate antibiotics towards Gram-negative bacteria. *PLoS ONE* **2017**, *12*, e0183263. [CrossRef]

11. Taresco, V.; Crisante, F.; Francolini, I.; Martinelli, A.; D'Ilario, L.; Ricci-Vitiani, L.; Buccarelli, M.; Pietrelli, L.; Piozzi, A. Antimicrobial and antioxidant amphiphilic random copolymers to address medical device-centered infections. *Acta Biomater.* **2015**, *22*, 131–140. [CrossRef] [PubMed]
12. Amato, A.; Migneco, L.M.; Martinelli, A.; Pietrelli, L.; Piozzi, A.; Francolini, I. Antimicrobial activity of catechol functionalized-chitosan versus *Staphylococcus epidermidis*. *Carbohydr. Polym.* **2018**, *179*, 273–281. [CrossRef] [PubMed]
13. Palermo, E.F.; Kuroda, K. Structural determinants of antimicrobial activity in polymers which mimic host defense peptides. *Appl. Microbiol. Biotechnol.* **2010**, *87*, 1605–1615. [CrossRef] [PubMed]
14. Takahashi, H.; Palermo, E.F.; Yasuhara, K.; Caputo, G.A.; Kuroda, K. Molecular design, structures, and activity of antimicrobial peptide-mimetic polymers. *Macromol. Biosci.* **2013**, *13*, 1285–1299. [CrossRef] [PubMed]
15. Martinelli, A.; Bakry, A.; D'Ilario, L.; Francolini, I.; Piozzi, A.; Taresco, V. Release behavior and antibiofilm activity of usnic acid-loaded carboxylated poly(L-lactide) microparticles. *Eur. J. Pharm. Biopharm.* **2014**, *88*, 415–423. [CrossRef] [PubMed]
16. Donelli, G.; Francolini, I.; Ruggeri, V.; Guaglianone, E.; D'Ilario, L.; Piozzi, A. Pore formers promoted release of an antifungal drug from functionalized polyurethanes to inhibit Candida colonization. *J. Appl. Microbiol.* **2006**, *100*, 615–622. [CrossRef] [PubMed]
17. Martinelli, A.; D'Ilario, L.; Francolini, I.; Piozzi, A. Water state effect on drug release from an antibiotic loaded polyurethane matrix containing albumin nanoparticles. *Int. J. Pharm.* **2011**, *407*, 197–206. [CrossRef]
18. Francolini, I.; Donelli, G.; Vuotto, C.; Baroncini, F.A.; Stoodley, P.; Taresco, V.; Martinelli, A.; D'Ilario, L.; Piozzi, A. Antifouling polyurethanes to fight device-related staphylococcal infections: Synthesis, characterization, and antibiofilm efficacy. *Pathog. Dis.* **2014**, *70*, 401–407. [CrossRef] [PubMed]
19. Cattò, C.; Cappitelli, F. Testing anti-biofilm polymeric surfaces: Where to start? *Int. J. Mol. Sci.* **2019**, *20*, 3794. [CrossRef]
20. González-Henríquez, C.M.; Sarabia-Vallejos, M.A.; Rodríguez Hernandez, J. Antimicrobial polymers for additive manufacturing. *Int. J. Mol. Sci.* **2019**, *20*, 1210. [CrossRef]
21. Kamaruzzaman, N.F.; Tan, L.P.; Hamdan, R.H.; Choong, S.S.; Wong, W.K.; Gibson, A.J.; Chivu, A.; Pina, M.F. Antimicrobial polymers: The potential replacement of existing antibiotics? *Int. J. Mol. Sci.* **2019**, *20*, 2747. [CrossRef] [PubMed]
22. Chi, M.; Qi, M.; Lan, A.; Wang, P.; Weir, M.D.; Melo, M.A.; Sun, X.; Dong, B.; Li, C.; Wu, J.; Wang, L.; Xu, H.H.K. Novel Bioactive and therapeutic dental polymeric materials to inhibit periodontal pathogens and biofilms. *Int. J. Mol. Sci.* **2019**, *20*, 278. [CrossRef] [PubMed]
23. Pazderková, M.; Maloň, P.; Zíma, V.; Hofbauerová, K.; Kopecký, V., Jr.; Kočišová, E.; Pazderka, T.; Čeřovský, V.; Bednárová, L. Interaction of halictine-related antimicrobial peptides with membrane models. *Int. J. Mol. Sci.* **2019**, *20*, 631. [CrossRef] [PubMed]
24. Kim, M.K.; Kang, N.; Ko, S.J.; Park, J.; Park, E.; Shin, D.W.; Kim, S.H.; Lee, S.A.; Lee, J.I.; Lee, S.H.; et al. Antibacterial and antibiofilm activity and mode of action of magainin 2 against drug-resistant *Acinetobacter baumannii*. *Int. J. Mol. Sci.* **2018**, *19*, 3041. [CrossRef] [PubMed]
25. Paduszynska, M.A.; Maciejewska, M.; Greber, K.E.; Sawicki, W.; Kamysz, W. Antibacterial activities of lipopeptide $(C(10))_2$-KKKK-NH_2 applied alone and in combination with lens liquids to fight biofilms formed on polystyrene surfaces and contact lenses. *Int. J. Mol. Sci.* **2019**, *20*, 393. [CrossRef] [PubMed]
26. Agrillo, B.; Balestrieri, M.; Gogliettino, M.; Palmieri, G.; Moretta, R.; Proroga, Y.T.R.; Rea, I.; Cornacchia, A.; Capuano, F.; Smaldone, G.; De Stefano, L. Functionalized polymeric materials with bio-derived antimicrobial peptides for "active" packaging. *Int. J. Mol. Sci.* **2019**, *20*, 601. [CrossRef] [PubMed]
27. Moshynets, O.; Bardeau, J.F.; Tarasyuk, O.; Makhno, S.; Cherniavska, T.; Dzhuzha, O.; Potters, G.; Rogalsky, S. Antibiofilm activity of polyamide 11 modified with thermally stable polymeric biocide polyhexamethylene guanidine 2-naphtalenesulfonate. *Int. J. Mol. Sci.* **2019**, *20*, 348. [CrossRef]
28. Szkudlarek, M.; Heine, E.; Keul, H.; Beginn, U.; Möller, M. Synthesis, characterization, and antimicrobial properties of peptides mimicking copolymers of maleic anhydride and 4-methyl-1-pentene. *Int. J. Mol. Sci.* **2018**, *19*, 2617. [CrossRef] [PubMed]
29. Muñoz-Bonilla, A.; López, D.; Fernández-García, M. Providing antibacterial activity to poly(2-hydroxy ethyl methacrylate) by copolymerization with a methacrylic thiazolium derivative. *Int. J. Mol. Sci.* **2018**, *19*, 4120. [CrossRef]

30. Galiano, F.; Mancuso, R.; Guzzo, M.G.; Lucente, F.; Gukelberger, E.; Losso, M.A.; Figoli, A.; Hoinkis, J.; Gabriele, B. New Polymeric films with antibacterial activity obtained by uv-induced copolymerization of acryloyloxyalkyltriethylammonium salts with 2-Hydroethyl Methacrylate. *Int. J. Mol. Sci.* **2019**, *20*, 2696. [CrossRef]
31. Galvão, C.N.; Sanches, L.M.; Mathiazzi, B.I.; Ribeiro, R.T.; Petri, D.F.S.; Carmona-Ribeiro, A.M. Antimicrobial coatings from hybrid nanoparticles of biocompatible and antimicrobial polymers. *Int. J. Mol. Sci.* **2018**, *19*, 2965.
32. Gurianov, Y.; Nakonechny, F.; Albo, Y.; Nisnevitch, M. Antibacterial composites of cuprous oxide nanoparticles and polyethylene. *Int. J. Mol. Sci.* **2019**, *20*, 439. [CrossRef] [PubMed]
33. Czarnobaj, K.; Prokopowicz, M.; Greber, K. Use of materials based on polymeric silica as bone-targeted drug delivery systems for metronidazole. *Int. J. Mol. Sci.* **2019**, *20*, 1311. [CrossRef] [PubMed]
34. Sisti, L.; Totaro, G.; Bozzi Cionci, N.; Di Gioia, D.; Celli, A.; Verney, V.; Leroux, F. Olive mill wastewater valorization in multifunctional biopolymer composites for antibacterial packaging application. *Int. J. Mol. Sci.* **2019**, *20*, 2376. [CrossRef] [PubMed]
35. Francolini, I.; Silvestro, I.; Di Lisio, V.; Martinelli, A.; Piozzi, A. Synthesis, characterization, and bacterial fouling-resistance properties of polyethylene glycol-grafted polyurethane elastomers. *Int. J. Mol. Sci.* **2019**, *20*, 1001. [CrossRef]
36. Cattò, C.; Secundo, F.; James, G.; Villa, F.; Cappitelli, F. α-Chymotrypsin immobilized on a low-density polyethylene surface successfully weakens *Escherichia coli* biofilm formation. *Int. J. Mol. Sci.* **2018**, *19*, 4003. [CrossRef]
37. Faÿ, F.; Gouessan, M.; Linossier, I.; Réhel, K. Additives for efficient biodegradable antifouling paints. *Int. J. Mol. Sci.* **2019**, *20*, 361. [CrossRef] [PubMed]

© 2019 by the authors. Licensee MDPI, Basel, Switzerland. This article is an open access article distributed under the terms and conditions of the Creative Commons Attribution (CC BY) license (http://creativecommons.org/licenses/by/4.0/).

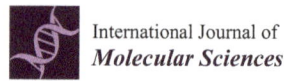

Review

Testing Anti-Biofilm Polymeric Surfaces: Where to Start?

Cristina Cattò and Francesca Cappitelli *

Department of Food Environmental and Nutritional Sciences, Università degli Studi di Milano, via Celoria 2, 20133 Milano, Italy
* Correspondence: francesca.cappitelli@unimi.it

Received: 24 July 2019; Accepted: 2 August 2019; Published: 3 August 2019

Abstract: Present day awareness of biofilm colonization on polymeric surfaces has prompted the scientific community to develop an ever-increasing number of new materials with anti-biofilm features. However, compared to the large amount of work put into discovering potent biofilm inhibitors, only a small number of papers deal with their validation, a critical step in the translation of research into practical applications. This is due to the lack of standardized testing methods and/or of well-controlled in vivo studies that show biofilm prevention on polymeric surfaces; furthermore, there has been little correlation with the reduced incidence of material deterioration. Here an overview of the most common methods for studying biofilms and for testing the anti-biofilm properties of new surfaces is provided.

Keywords: anti-biofilm surfaces; polymeric surfaces; biofilm methods; biofilm analysis; biofilm devices

1. Introduction

Polymeric materials, given their low cost, high specificity and adaptability [1], are currently used for a very broad range of applications ranging from structural materials to coatings, health care [2], packaging [3,4], communication [5], heritage [6,7], energy [8], transportation [9] and the agri-food industry [10]. Indeed, the very easy manipulation of molecular structure and chemical composition allows the production of innovative, advanced materials with specific chemical, biological, and physical features [1]. Polymer materials can be lightweight, hard, strong, and flexible, and can have peculiar thermal, electrical, and optical properties [1]. Consequently, in the last decade, material science has been experiencing an ever-growing active demand for innovative polymers of notable importance in present-day life.

Although polymeric materials play an invaluable role in providing solutions for a wide range of applications they are also easily colonized by biofilm, microorganisms that live in a self-organized, cooperative community attached to a substratum and covered by a self-produced matrix of extracellular polymeric substances (EPS) [11]. On the global scale, the impact of biofilm on present-day life is incalculable, with the spending of billions of dollars throughout the different sectors of the economy [12]. Biofilms are potentially able to contaminate all polymeric structural and infrastructural elements, systems, and devices, such as plumbing, medical implants, food processing facilities, and heating and air conditioning systems [13]. The result is a reduced industrial yield as well as the physical degradation of industrial systems such as pipe obstruction and corrosion [14]. In food-processing plants and drinking water networks, biofilm is a persistent source of microbial contamination that can affect the quality and safety of food products and water [15–17]. The worst biofilm reputation is most probably that of biofilm associated with medical implants, causing more than 60% of all microbial infection in humans [18,19]. Indeed, infection can give rise to complications, such as life-threatening systemic infections, contributing to post-operative morbidity, mortality, protracted hospitalization and re-operation rate, diagnostic tests and treatments increase, resulting in medical and financial burden [20,21]. It has been estimated that catheter-associated urinary tract infections cause approximately 40% of worldwide hospital-acquired infections, there being approximately 900,000 cases each year in the United States alone, at an annual cost ranging from 296 million to 2.3 billion dollars [22,23].

Strategies to alleviate the effects of biofilm formation on polymeric material have focused on cleaning and disinfection treatments aimed at killing microbial sessile cells already present on the surface. However, such treatments are not totally effective as biofilm microorganisms have features that provide successful conditions for microbial life, including enhanced resistance to antibiotic and biocide treatments [24,25]. Indeed, biofilm-associated resistance is due to several factors like the physiological state of the sessile cells themselves and their physical structure, as well as the presence of EPS that act as a barrier for such cells [26]. Furthermore, resistance towards many antibiotics has increased in several pathogenic microbial taxa, reducing the chances to treat effectively infections and increasing the risk of complications and fatal outcomes [27].

Consequently, in the past 20 years, studies in the field have addressed the development of preventive strategies, rather than approaches that kill microorganisms after their surface colonization. Indeed, the development of polymeric materials that can prevent microbial adhesion or weaken biofilm structure has emerged as a promising approach to overcome material-associated biofilm problems [28].

However, despite promising results, many experimental polymeric anti-biofilm surfaces reported in the literature have never been translated into real applications, nor have all newly created anti-biofilm surfaces undergone the critical step of validation of their anti-biofilm performance [29]. The in vivo testing of new anti-biofilm materials is an arduous task due to limited experimental control. It has been shown that in vivo assays can partially predict biofilm outcomes in humans, though there can be poor correlation with the clinical outcome [30,31]. Furthermore, and this is no less important, it is becoming more and more difficult to get approval for animal studies. Indeed, in most countries, the approval for animal experiments depends on convincing in vitro evidence of efficacy [29,32]. Tissue cultures have been used as a surrogate for in vivo biofilm studies, but the construction of a three-dimensional tissue culture is labour intensive and expensive. Moreover, experiments can only be conducted for short periods of time (i.e., in less than 24 hours) due to the cytotoxic effects on the cells, this cytotoxicity being due to both the biofilm itself and to the anti-biofilm surface, thus reducing the utility of these studies as biofilms generally take multiple days to reach maturity [20].

Therefore, attention here is paid to in vitro evaluation methods, which are a compromise between the reality of the in vivo ecosystem and the simplification of the system. However, a well-devised model and studies allow researchers to get relevant results [33]. Whereas there are several in vitro industrial standard tests to evaluate the antimicrobial (i.e., killing of microorganisms) efficacy of medical and non-medical products, there are no accepted standardized assays and validated methods to properly assess the activity of anti-biofilm material [34]. Indeed, current in vitro evaluation standard tests, especially tailored for specific action mechanisms that lead to cell death, are inadequate for today's different advanced anti-biofilm surface designs. Note that the surface evaluation standard tests available today are mostly intended to test the ability of the material to abate microbial viability, without taking into consideration the differences in the mechanism of action [29]. Indeed, the tests attempt to evaluate biofilm inhibition and eradication without proper investigation of the variability in biofilm architecture and the complexity of its development [34]. This deficiency in methodology has adversely affected the translation of research into practical industrial and medical applications, and to regulatory agencies that assess the real-life usefulness of anti-biofilm surfaces.

Over the last couple of decades, a variety of simplified in vitro systems have been proposed to study biofilm formation [35]. Therefore, given the lack of standardized procedures to test anti-biofilm properties of materials, the only solution to test novel anti-biofilm surfaces for clinical purposes is to adapt the lab-scale devices and procedures presently used to obtain biofilms [36].

This review provides an overview of the most commonly used in vitro methods to study biofilm formation, and the recent findings available, and methods suitable for adaptation to test anti-biofilm polymeric surfaces. After presenting a brief description of the properties of the innovative anti-biofilm polymers provided to date by the scientific community, the authors propose currently available methods for evaluating the anti-biofilm activity of new anti-biofilm surfaces, and guidelines that would help readers choose the most appropriate test according to their objectives. Notably, the experimental procedure takes into account three steps: (i) identification of the relevant model microorganisms; (ii) selection of the experimental design for growing the biofilm on the new surface and (iii) determination and execution of the appropriate analysis.

2. Anti-Biofilm Polymeric Surfaces

In the past, surface treatments aimed at killing microbial cells were proposed as valuable tools to counteract biofilm formation on polymeric materials. Indeed, the abatement of biofilm was obtained by spreading antimicrobial agents onto surfaces or by incorporating them into synthetic polymer-based products [37,38]. A number of antimicrobial-releasing surfaces have been proposed in the literature, and some of them have also reached the marketplace [38–43]. In these systems, the antimicrobial agent is actively eluted when the polymer surface comes into contact with an aqueous environment but, generally, control of the action is poor [44–47]. Indeed, smart responsive materials are designed to undergo an end-to-end chain reaction that releases the antimicrobial agent when activated by a stimulus at the terminal chain, i.e., the microbial presence [48,49].

In passive strategies, no antimicrobial agents are released into the surrounding environment. The physiochemical properties of a material surface, including composition, charge, hydrophobicity, roughness and porosity, are modified by: (i) applying to the surface, or mixing in the bulk, polymer anti-adhesive substances able to reduce the adhesion force between the microorganism and the solid surface [50–54]; and (ii) minimizing microbial attachment by providing the surface with a specific microstructure [55]. These approaches are relatively straightforward and economic. However, materials that preserve their resistance to microbial colonization are difficult to obtain by surface chemistry or surface structuring alone. Indeed, non-adhesive surfaces are often: (i) subjected to quick degradation or desorption over time [56,57]; and (ii) not always compatible with tissue cells, making them less suitable for biomaterial implants and devices requiring tissue integration [29].

In the last few years increased interest has been shown to metal nanoparticles. Nanoparticles have been successfully spread on, or incorporated into, a number of polymeric materials with versatile applications, including medical devices [58,59], marine industry paints [60] and food-contact surfaces [61]. Furthermore, nanotechnology has offered many opportunities for innovation. However, the use of nanomaterials has sometimes raised safety [62], environmental [63] and regulatory issues [64] that are still unresolved.

Nowadays, the literature reports strategies that exploit the potential of some compounds to interfere with microbial ability to develop biofilm by modalities perceived safe for human health. These approaches interfere with the following key steps that orchestrate the genesis of biofilm formation: (i) the surface sensing process to maintain the pioneering cells in a planktonic form, enabling easy removal of microorganisms before biofilm formation [65]; (ii) the disruption of biofilm physical integrity, by interfering with cell-to-cell communication or destroying the biofilm architecture by targeting the matrix [66]; and (iii) favoring biofilm dispersal by forcing the planktonic state [67,68]. In these approaches, microorganisms are still alive but deprived of their virulent properties. Thus, selection pressure decreases, limiting resistant-drug development, and potentially reinstating the efficacy of traditional antimicrobials [69]. Several natural and synthetic compounds, as well as matrix-targeting enzymes based on the previous biocide-free anti-biofilm mechanisms of action, have been coated or immobilized on polymeric surfaces, providing promising, eco-friendly, bio-inspired, anti-biofilm materials able to replace, or integrate with, presently dominating biocide-based approaches [69–74].

For example, Kim et al. [75] incorporated natural eugenol and clove oil into a biocompatible poly(D,L-lactide-coglycolide), markedly inhibiting biofilm formation and virulence of *Escherichia coli* O157:H7. Dell'Orto et al. [76] covalently grafted modified natural compounds, i.e., zosteric acid and salicylic acid, onto a low density polyethylene surface that was able to reduce *E. coli* adhesion, and thus biofilm formation, up to 73%. Sajeevan et al. [77] impregnated silicon catheter tubes with anacardic acids that efficiently inhibited *Staphylococcus aureus* colonization and biofilm formation on its surface both in vitro and in vivo. Spadoni-Andreani et al. [73] demonstrated that polypropylene surfaces coated with proteases weakened adhesion and increased the dispersion of *Candida albicans* biofilm cells and Cattò et al. [74] proved that the proteases α-chymotrypsin prevented *E. coli* biofilm formation on polyethylene materials

For further reading: recent progress in biofilm-resistant polymeric surfaces, provided by the material science community, has been extensively reviewed by Cattò et al. [36], Francolini et al. [18], Riga et al. [13] and Li et al. [49].

3. Microbial Choice

The selection of microorganisms to be included in experiments is a crucial choice. Keeping in mind the translation of the new material into real applications, the strain can be chosen ad hoc from among those existing in the natural environment where the material is to be placed. Indeed, as species vary a lot, depending on the environment, it is most important to choose and study the environment of interest.

Choices include the use of strains in microbial collections [78–80], strains isolated from the environment [81,82] or complex environmental community samples used without any cultivation steps [53,83] (Figure 1).

STEP 1: CHOOSING MICROBIAL MODEL		
	MONOSPECIES BIOFILM 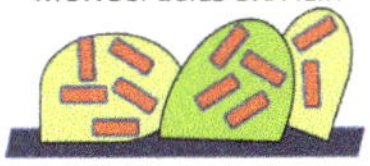	MULTISPECIES BIOFILM 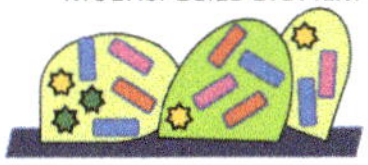
MICROBIAL COLLECTION	✓	✓
ISOLATED STRAIN	✓	✓
ENVIRONMENTAL SAMPLE	✗	✓

Figure 1. Scheme representing the first step in the experimental procedure for testing new anti-biofilm materials. The choice of the relevant model microorganisms includes the use of strains from microbial collections, strains isolated from the environment or complex environmental community samples used without any cultivation steps, in both mono- and multi-species biofilm models.

The simplest approach for studying a new material is to select a low-diversity model composed of a well-known, well-characterized, convenient and accessible laboratory strain. Such organisms should be representative of the living beings for which they are to serve as proxy. Some model microorganisms include *E. coli*, *Bacillus subtilis*, *Klebsiella pneumoniae*, *Pseudomonas* spp. and *Staphylococcus* spp. for bacteria, *Synechocystis* spp. for cyanobacteria, *C. albicans* and *Saccharomyces cerevisiea* for yeasts and *Fusarium oxysporum*, *Aspergillus* spp. and *Paenicillium* spp for filamentous fungi [78,84–87]. As these model microorganisms are frequently used, dedicated tools and resources for such organisms, e.g., databases, molecular kits, collections of techniques and methods, have been accumulated over the years, contributing to facilitate and standardize analysis [88,89].

In general, such monospecies systems have been proposed to achieve high reproducibility, short experimental timeframes and the application of widespread and well set up methodologies. They also provide several additional advantages such as low cost, easy set-up, and amenability to high throughput screens, addressing basic questions about biofilm development, physiology and architecture [90]. However, the results obtained with these systems cannot be completely translated into natural environments as the model strains were not isolated at the same time, nor at the place where the material is expected to work [91]. Indeed, as these lab strains are normally kept in laboratory stocks and have been cultured routinely, they may not exhibit the same phenotype as fresh isolates [92].

The approach based on isolated strains is better for obtaining a more representative view of biofilm behavior. Indeed, it is reported that, if repetitively cultured, microorganisms can evolve, resulting in a reduced capacity to form biofilm [93]. However, isolated strains are less known and distantly related to well-described model organisms from collections, resulting in a more complex application of conventional methods and assays. Another question is how to select the most relevant microorganisms among other isolates. At the moment, no consensus exists in the field, making results very difficult to compare between different works [92]. In the study of Rzhepishevska et al. [92], 19 strains of *P. aeruginosa* originating from hospitalized patients were studied and compared to the lab reference strain PAO1 and a rmlC lipopolysaccharide PAO1 mutant. The authors observed two sets of isolates, a group with high adhesion to a polymeric anti-biofilm coating and a group with low adhesion, including PAO1. Notably, they demonstrated that the properties of clinical isolates differed from that of the lab strain. Moreover, they highlighted the importance of choosing the right model strains to provide better predictability with respect to how materials inhibit biofilm formation.

Biofilm in a natural system consists of multiple microorganisms of different species, which often results in an enhanced survival capability, including improved tolerance against antimicrobial agents and virulence infections or increased stress tolerance, biomass production, metabolic cooperation, level signalling, compared to monocultures [94–97]. Most polymeric surfaces have been tested by examining monospecies biofilm formation, and the resulting information has been translated, by a variety of approaches, to biofilms composed of multiple species. However, the results published to date have revealed that biofilm features related to multispecies consortia cannot be predicted by studies performed with monospecies [98]. The number of papers focusing on multispecies biofilms on polymeric surfaces has increased in recent years to fulfill the need to study new materials in more appropriate experimental model systems, closer to the real environment of material application. Studies with multispecies biofilm have regarded all relevant areas, including materials for medical [70,99,100], industrial [101] and marine applications [81]. The experimented microbial communities have ranged from a relatively low diversity, two to four species, to complex systems consisting of hundred taxa. Notably, the types and number of interplays within multispecies biofilms grow exponentially with the increasing number of species. Therefore, many research groups have, to date, focused on biofilms comprised of two to four species. For these studies differential imaging of single species can be obtained by marking the different taxa with different fluorescent protein genes or probes. Cossu et al. [101] evaluated a novel anti-biofilm polymer formed using poly(vinyl alcohol-*co*-ethylene) with halamine suitable for food contact surfaces by exposing the new material to high loads of *Listeria innocua* and *E. coli O157:H7*. Nowatzy et al. [70] developed a new salicylic acid-releasing polyurethane acrylate polymer for anti-biofilm urological catheter coatings purpose and tested it by using a pool of *P. aeruginosa* and *E. coli*. Kommerein et al. [102] developed a highly reproducible in vitro four-species biofilm model consisting of the highly relevant oral bacterial species *Streptococcus oralis*, *Actinomyces naeslundii*, *Veillonella dispar* and *Porphyromonas gingivalis*, with a percentage distribution closely reflected the situation in early native plaques. These systems are typically highly reproducible and fast-growing. However, they may not completely replicate communities in their native environments in terms of number and relative proportion of species, phenotypes (laboratory stock instead of wild type) or culture conditions.

In contrast, natural multispecies biofilm systems stem from isolated organisms or organisms directly taken from the environment of interest. For instance, Le Norcy et al. [81] reported the assessment of a varnish based on a biodegradable polymer, poly(ε-caprolactone-*co*-δ-valerolactone) incorporating a hemibastadin derivative, against a mixture of *Paracoccus* sp., *Pseudoalteromonas* sp. and

Bacillus sp., isolated from the Gulf of Morbihan in France. After isolation, the strains were cultivated and used in different proportions to assess the anti-biofilm performance of the new varnish. In a more complicated system, Zhang et al. [83] synthesized an anti-biofilm dental composite by combining 2-methacryloyloxyethyl phosphorylcholine with quaternary ammonium dimethylaminohexadecyl methacrylate, and evaluated the materials against an oral biofilm plaque from the saliva of 10 donors. These natural biofilm systems better mimic the species composition of the environment than do engineered model systems. However, these methods use a limited subset of isolated species, which in most of cases corresponds to the most highly abundant species within the community, giving less importance to the less abundant taxa despite their playing a key role within the community [98]. Furthermore, strains from an environment of interest can be isolated using culture-based approaches, with the risk of excluding important non-cultivable species. Another problem encountered in these systems is reproducibility, as a complex experimental design is commonly detrimental to reproducibility [103].

In light of these considerations, system selection is a trade-off between the use of a mono species system that follows a simple, easy, highly reproducible, time- and cost-effective approach, but less reflective of the real environment, and a more laborious, complex and time intensive method that closely mimics reality [98]. The ideal scenario would be to use the new material in the real environment to more easily find out the succession, organization, and role of each specific species [53]. However, in situ observations are often not feasible due to the high complexity of the system. The relevant system for testing new anti-biofilm surfaces might be one that mimics the real environment in a simplified design without losing the relevant interplays and dependencies of natural biofilm.

4. In Vitro Methods to Culture Biofilm on Anti-Biofilm Polymeric Surfaces

Biofilm culturing techniques should be chosen according to the study goals, simulating the environment and according to the availability of resources and skills (Figure 2). No less important is the fact that different devices present advantages and disadvantages, which must be considered before using them.

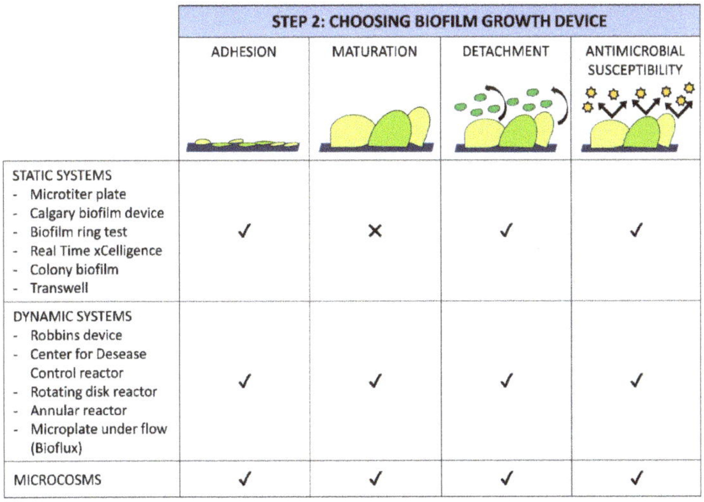

	STEP 2: CHOOSING BIOFILM GROWTH DEVICE			
	ADHESION	MATURATION	DETACHMENT	ANTIMICROBIAL SUSCEPTIBILITY
STATIC SYSTEMS - Microtiter plate - Calgary biofilm device - Biofilm ring test - Real Time xCelligence - Colony biofilm - Transwell	✓	✗	✓	✓
DYNAMIC SYSTEMS - Robbins device - Center for Desease Control reactor - Rotating disk reactor - Annular reactor - Microplate under flow (Bioflux)	✓	✓	✓	✓
MICROCOSMS	✓	✓	✓	✓

Figure 2. Scheme representing the second step in the experimental procedure for testing new anti-biofilm materials. The choice of the biofilm growth device includes the use of static, dynamic or microcosms systems, according to the step of biofilm formation to be analysed.

Technical information of the most popular laboratory devices is discussed below, and their strengths and limitations are shown in Table 1.

Table 1. Technical information of the most popular laboratory devices used to study anti-biofilm polymeric surfaces.

Apparatus	Flow Dynamic	Interface	Biofilm Analysis	Advantage	Limitations	Standard Methods
Microtiter plate	Static	Solid–liquid	- Adhesion - Detachment - Susceptibility to antimicrobial	- Easy to use - Cheap - Reproducible - Simple equipment - High-throughput screening - Multiple materials tested simultaneously - Multiple conditions tested simultaneously - Well-designed to investigate early stage of biofilm formation - Comparable experiments among different laboratories	- Not suitable to study late stage of biofilm formation - Sensitive to cell sedimentation - Poor reproducibility of real environment - Close system - Washing step can remove not loosely attached cells - Designed to study biofilms only at solid–liquid interface	None
Calgary biofilm device	Static	Solid–liquid	- Adhesion - Detachment - Susceptibility to antimicrobial	- Easy to use - Cheap - Simple equipment - Reproducible - High-throughput screening - Multiple materials tested simultaneously - Multiple conditions tested simultaneously - Well-designed to investigate early stage of biofilm formation - Reduced interference of cell sedimentation - Comparable experiments among different laboratories	- Not suitable to study late stage of biofilm formation - Poor reproducibility of real environment - Close system - Washing step can remove not loosely attached cells - Designed to study biofilms only at solid–liquid interface - Difficulty to collect individual pegs for cell enumeration	ASTM E2799-17 Standard test method for testing disinfectant efficacy against *Pseudomonas aeruginosa* biofilm using the MBEC assay [104]
Biofilm ring test	Static	Solid–liquid	- Adhesion - Detachment - Susceptibility to antimicrobial	- Easy to use - Reproducible - Rapid - High-throughput screening - Automatic analysis - Very low standard deviation - No need for staining or washing steps - Multiple conditions tested simultaneously - Comparable experiments among different laboratories - Well-designed to investigate early stage of biofilm formation	- Not suitable to study late stage of biofilm formation - Poor reproducibility of real environment - Close system - Expensive - Sensitive to cell sedimentation - Only suitable for thick biofilms - Requires specific magnetic device and scanner - Need of specified software and biofilm index to provide the results - Not suitable for multi-species biofilm - Designed to study biofilms only at solid–liquid interface - the material must display magnetic properties - Not suitable to compare multiple materials simultaneously	None

Table 1. *Cont.*

Apparatus	Flow Dynamic	Interface	Biofilm Analysis	Advantage	Limitations	Standard Methods
Real Time xCelligence	Static	Solid–liquid	- Adhesion - Detachment - Susceptibility to antimicrobial	- Easy to use - Reproducible - High-throughput screening - Non-invasive - automatic analysis - Very low standard deviation - No need for staining or washing steps - Multiple conditions tested simultaneously - Comparable experiments among different laboratories - Well-designed to investigate early stage of biofilm formation	- Not suitable to study late stage of biofilm formation - Poor reproducibility of real environment - Close system - Expensive - Sensitive to cell sedimentation - Requires specific equipment - Not suitable for multi-species biofilm - Designed to study biofilms only at solid–liquid interface - Not suitable to compare multiple materials simultaneously - Materials must have electrical properties	None
Colony biofilm	Static	Solid–air	- Adhesion - Susceptibility to antimicrobial	- Easy to use - Cheap - Simple equipment - Reproducible - Large biomass in a short period	- Planktonic cells may interfere with the biofilm assays - Biofilm detachment can not be studied - Material must be customized only in the form of semipermeable membrane-like thin film - Difficulty in manipulating surfaces when colony biomass become large - Designed to study biofilms only at solid–air interface	None
Transwell	Static	Solid–air	- Adhesion - Susceptibility to antimicrobial	- Easy to use - Cheap - Simple equipment - Reproducible - High-throughput screening - Large biomass in a short period - Possibility to collect the metabolites from biofilm culture - Independent studies in compartments with different condition	- Biofilm detachment can not be studied - Material must be customized only in the form of semipermeable membrane-like thin film - Difficulty in manipulating surfaces when colony biomass become large - Designed to study biofilms only at air–solid interface	None
Robbins Device (RD)	Dynamic (variable laminar/turbulent shear)	Solid–liquid	- Adhesion - Maturation - Detachment - Susceptibility to antimicrobial	- Multiple materials tested simultaneously (up to 12) - Suitable to study early and late stage of biofilm formation - Reproducibility of real environments - Large biomass in a short period - Can operate under differently hydrodynamic conditions (e.g., laminar/turbulent) - Autoclavable and re-useable	- Not suitable for high-throughput screening - Necessity of specialized equipment - Technically challenging - Poor experimental reproducibility - Multiple microorganisms can not be tested simultaneously - Designed to study biofilms only at solid–liquid interface - No direct observation of biofilm development - Low air–liquid exchange - Flow inside the device is difficult to be accurately adjusted - Fixed geometry of the surface (disk) - Expensive - Requires specific equipment	None

Table 1. Cont.

Apparatus	Flow Dynamic	Interface	Biofilm Analysis	Advantage	Limitations	Standard Methods
Center for Disease Control (CDC) reactor	Dynamic (high laminar/turbulent shear)	Solid–liquid	- Adhesion - Maturation - Detachment - Susceptibility to antimicrobial	- Multiple materials tested simultaneously (up to 24) - Suitable to study early and late stage of biofilm formation - Reproducibility of real environments - Large biomass in a short period - Well controlled flow within the device - All surface within the device experience the share stress - Suitable for time-course studies - Can operate under different hydrodynamic conditions (e.g., low/high and laminar/turbulent share) - Standardized biofilm method - Autoclavable and re-useable	- Not suitable for high-throughput screening - Requires specific equipment - Technically challenging - Multiple microorganisms can not be tested simultaneously - Low air-liquid exchange - Designed to study biofilms only at solid-liquid interface - No direct observation of biofilm development - Fixed geometry of the surface (disk) - Expensive - Requires a large volume of medium	- ASTM E2562-17 Standard test method for quantification of *Pseudomonas aeruginosa* biofilm grown with high shear and continuous flow using CDC biofilm reactor [105] - ASTM E2871-19 Standard test method for determining disinfectant efficacy against biofilm grown in the CDC biofilm reactor using the single tube method [106]
Rotating Disk (RD) reactor	Dynamic (intermediate laminar/turbulent shear)	Solid–liquid	- Adhesion - Maturation - Detachment - Susceptibility to antimicrobial	- Multiple materials tested simultaneously (up to 6) - Suitable to study early and late stage of biofilm formation - Reproducibility of real environments - Large biomass in a short period - Different shear can be tested simultaneously - Standardized biofilm method - Autoclavable and re-useable	- Not suitable for high-throughput screening - Requires specific equipment - Technically challenging - Multiple microorganisms can not be tested simultaneously - Low air-liquid exchange - Designed to study biofilms only at solid-liquid interface - Less suitable for time-course studies - No direct observation of biofilm development - Fixed geometry of the surface (disk) - Requires a large volume of medium - Expensive	ASTM E2196-17 Standard test method for quantification of a *Pseudomonas aeruginosa* biofilm grown with shear and continuous flow using a rotating disk reactor [107]
Annular (RA) reactor	Dynamic (variable laminar/turbulent shear)	Solid–liquid	- Adhesion - Maturation - Detachment - Susceptibility to antimicrobial	- Multiple materials tested simultaneously (up to 20) - Suitable to study early and late stage of biofilm formation - Reproducibility of real environments - Large biomass in a short period - Suitable for time-course studies - Can operate under different hydrodynamic conditions (e.g., low/high and laminar/turbulent share) - Autoclavable and re-useable	- Not suitable for high-throughput screening - Requires specific equipment - Technically challenging - Multiple microorganisms can not be tested simultaneously - Low air-liquid exchange - Designed to study biofilms only at solid-liquid interface - No direct observation of biofilm development - Fixed geometry of the surface (rectangular) - Requires a large volume of medium - Expensive	None

Table 1. Cont.

Apparatus	Flow Dynamic	Interface	Biofilm Analysis	Advantage	Limitations	Standard Methods
Drip flow (DF) reactor	Dynamic (low laminar shear)	Solid–air	- Adhesion - Maturation - Detachment - Susceptibility to antimicrobial	- Multiple materials tested simultaneously (up to 4 or 6) - Suitable to study early and late stage of biofilm formation - Reproducibility of real environments - Large biomass in a short period - Suitable for time-course studies - Standardized biofilm method - Multiple microorganisms can be tested simultaneously - Autoclavable and re-useable - Compatible with surface of various geometry - High gas transfer	- Heterogeneity of biofilm development on the coupons - Not suitable for high-throughput screening - Requires specific equipment - Technically challenging - Designed to study biofilms only at solid–liquid interface - Direct observation of the biofilm development is not allowed - Expensive	ASTM E2647-13 Standard test method for quantification of *Pseudomonas aeruginosa* biofilm grown using drip flow biofilm reactor with low shear and continuous flow [108]
Flow chamber	Dynamic (variable laminar/turbulent shear)	Solid–liquid	- Adhesion - Maturation - Detachment - Susceptibility to antimicrobial	- Multiple materials tested simultaneously (up to 6) - Suitable to study early and late stage of biofilm formation - Reproducibility of real environments - Direct inspection of living biofilm development in a non-destructive way - Multiple microorganisms can be tested simultaneously - Autoclavable and re-useable	- Low biomass - Not suitable for high-throughput screening - Requires specific equipment - Technically challenging - Designed to study biofilms only at solid–liquid interface - Biofilm recovery during experiment is difficult - Expensive - Problem of air bubble	None
Microplate under flow (Bioflux)	Dynamic (variable laminar shear)	Solid–liquid	- Adhesion - Maturation - Detachment - Susceptibility to antimicrobial	- Easy to use - Cheap - Reproducible - Simple equipment - High-throughput screening - Multiple materials tested simultaneously (up to 96) - Multiple conditions tested simultaneously - Suitable to study early and late stage of biofilm formation - Reproducibility of real environments - Direct inspection of living biofilm development in a non-destructive way - Suitable for time-course studies - Multiple microorganisms can be tested simultaneously	- Low biomass - Designed to study biofilms only at solid–liquid interface - No biofilm recovery during experiment	None
Microcosm	Static, Dynamic (variable laminar/turbulent shear)	Solid–liquid, solid–air	- Adhesion - Maturation - Detachment - Susceptibility to antimicrobial	- Hight reproducibility of real environments - Multiple materials tested simultaneously - Suitable to study early and late stage of biofilm formation - Multiple microorganisms can be tested simultaneously - Both static and dynamic systems - Compatible with surface of various geometry	- Less reproducibility - Not suitable for high-throughput screening - Technically challenging - Biofilm recovery during experiment is difficult - Complicated interpretation of results - Not suitable for time-course studies - No direct observation of biofilm development	None

4.1. Static Methods

Static methods are particularly meaningful for examining early events in biofilm development, detecting cell attachment within a 15–60 minute time frame [109]. Such assays can be used to identify the impact of innovative surfaces in modulating the transition from a planktonic to a sessile mode of existence. Indeed, they effectively identify factors that initiate biofilm formation, like flagella, pili, adhesions, enzymes associated with cyclic-di-GMP binding and metabolism [110].

Static systems are widely used because they are simple to use, high producible, and controllable, and show limited contamination, and cost-effective properties. These easy-to-use and cost-effective assays make them amenable for large-scale high-throughput screening purposes, like genetic screens, and are useful for studying multiple strains under various growth conditions [110].

However, these closed models do not allow for the flow of media, product or waste materials into or out of the system, with the consequence that the experimental conditions change progressively because of nutrient depletion and the metabolic products build-up [32]. Thus, the biofilm growth rate is rapid at the beginning when there is an ample amount of nutrients [33]. However, in the natural environment this is uncommon [44], which means that the physiological and biological features of experimentally induced biofilm are not comparable with natural biofilm, precluding a full evaluation of the effect of new materials on biofilm development and dispersion.

4.1.1. Microtiter Well Plate

The simplest experimental system to study microbial adhesion on a surface relies on the use of microtiter well plates, growing biofilm in static conditions. The surface of microtiter plates can be modified or, alternatively, a novel material can be inserted into the wells. The general protocol of microtiter plates permits the inoculation of microtiter wells with a cell suspension over a desired time period, while allowing cells to sediment on a substratum. After a specific time period in which microbial adhesion occurs, the wells are emptied or the material previously inserted in the well is carefully removed. Surfaces are then washed to remove planktonic cells and the number of adhering viable microorganisms is assessed. The removal of the liquid phase above the substratum must be done carefully to avoid the inadvertent removal of adhering cells [109].

For instance, Lin et al. [111] directly coated the surface wells of a 96-well polystyrene microtiter plate with 1,2,3,4,6-penta-O-galloyl-β-d-glucopyranose, an active plant ingredient commonly used in Chinese medicine, to test the coating efficacy against *S. aureus* biofilm. Alternatively, Swartjes et al. [112] demonstrated that polymethylmethacrylate (PMMA), a commonly employed biomaterial, coated with DNase I significantly reduced adhesion of *S. aureus* (95%) and *P. aeruginosa* (99%), and inhibited biofilm development for up to 14 h in static conditions. Salta et al. [113] coated glass discs with a paint composed by PMMA and a natural compound derived from walnut trees, and tested the new material against marine biofilm formation in a 24-well plate.

4.1.2. Calgary Biofilm Device

In this system biofilm development is studied at the coverlid, composed of pegs that fit into the wells of a microtiter plate containing nutrients and microorganisms [114]. The advantage of this approach is that the biofilm is not the result of the cell sedimentation but the adhesion of cells to the pegs. This reduces the interference of those planktonic cells that remain at the bottom of the microtiter plate wells after the washing step [115]. In order to investigate biofilm formation on specific abiotic supports, coverlid can be customized with materials with specific anti-biofilm features or pegs coated with anti-biofilm molecules. Harrison et al. [116] used the Calgary biofilm device to demonstrate that *C. tropicalis* biofilm increased on polystyrene pegs coated with L-lysine [116]. Nowatzki et al. [70] coated the peg of the Calgary biofilm device with a polyurethane acrylate polymer partly composed by salicyl acrylate, which degrades in aqueous conditions, releasing salicylic acid.

However, Calgary device assays also require the washing off of non-adherent microorganisms and cell recovery, resulting typically between 5% and 90% of the entire community [35].

4.1.3. The Biofilm Ring Test (BRT)

The principle of this assay is based on the capacity of microorganisms to immobilize magnetic microbeads when developing a biofilm at the well surface of a microtiter plate. Once a magnetic field is applied, beads are free to move and gather in the center of the well bottom. Once a biofilm has developed, the center of the well cannot accumulate the beads as the biomass prevents it, and this outcome can be measured using a specific plate reader [117,118]. After paramagnetic microbeads are added to the microbial suspension, they are loaded into the wells of a microtiter plate. The microtiter plate is then incubated, and direct measurements can be carried out [35]. The measurement of this super-paramagnetic microbead immobilization by adherent cells at different time points can be used to evaluate the kinetics of biofilm development. Indeed, the microtiter well can be modified by anti-biofilm coatings as well as customized with a desired material, and the anti-biofilm properties of the new surface can be analyzed.

This assay requires neither washing nor staining, thus avoiding procedures that can generate some significant bias in the outcomes. Moreover, it is easy to handle, and more importantly, the results are achieved in a few hours. Additionally, it could be well-suited to study the synergism of the new material with a biocide.

Unfortunately, BRT can only measure thick biofilms that develop at the bottom of the microtiter well [34]. Furthermore, it is only useful when the new anti-biofilm materials display good magnetic properties. Additionally, the procedure does not provide, in a single experiment, direct information about biofilm production on the different anti-biofilm surfaces as the strength of the magnetic field is influenced by both the type of materials and/or the thickness of the coating [119]. Indeed, there can be differences in the magnetic field strength between the new anti-biofilm material and the relative control, leading to analytical bias in the results. To date, to the best of the authors' knowledge, no studies have investigated the performance of new anti-biofilm surfaces using BRT.

4.1.4. Real-Time xCelligence

The xCelligence system uses specially designed microtiter plates with inter-digitized gold microelectrodes to non-invasively study the status of adherent cells, using electrical impedance as the readout [120]. Indeed, biofilm growth impedes the flow of an alternating microampere electric current between the electrodes. This impedance is measured automatically at intervals defined by the user, and allowes a highly sensitive readout of cell amount, cell size/shape, and cell–surface adhesion strength [121].

Because each xCelligence well can collect thousands of data, each individual well gives a complete time course for biofilm deposition or dissipation, significantly reducing the number of wells needed and the total workload. Additionally, the manual collection of endpoint data is eliminated, and multiple drugs/conditions can be analyzed simultaneously in a single plate, greatly improving throughput. Recently, the system was used to measure microbial biofilms and to study the effect of antimicrobial treatments on biofilm growth [122].

This system is non-invasive, label-free, fast, and reproducible [123]. The microtiter well can be modified by anti-biofilm coatings, as well as customized with a desired material, and the anti-biofilm properties of the new surface can be analyzed. On the other hand, the manufacture of microtiters with specific materials and correct gold biosensor insertion in each well is technically challenging. Furthermore, like BRT, xCelligence technology is not really suitable for the comparison of microbial adhesion on different surfaces as electrical impedance is influenced by both the type of material and the thickness of the coating [124]. Moreover, the xCelligence machine is costly and requires specialized detection equipment, making its availability not always affordable by the individual researcher [34].

4.1.5. Transwell Device

This consists of a plastic transwell insert support inlaid in a well plate with cultural medium, providing semi-batch working conditions and two separate chambers [125–127]. A semipermeable membrane-like thin film of the new anti-biofilm material is placed in the support, and the cell broth in the well of the culture plate. The microbial cells are not allowed to move across the two compartments, and the anti-biofilm surface to which the cells attach themselves is the only avenue for meeting nutritional needs and removing waste. The supports are periodically relocated to fresh plates, thus providing the biofilm with a semi-constant fresh supply of nutrients. After one to three incubation days, the transwell inserts are removed and the biofilm formation on the surface support is analyzed. Transwell systems have a fine control of the experimental conditions in the two chambers, a semi-constant nutrient support and the possibility to collect the metabolites by biofilm culture in the basolateral media of the plate well compartment, without the risk of contamination by planktonic cells [128]. Transwell devices are now commonly used to form biofilm under various physiological conditions [125,126,129].

4.1.6. Colony Biofilm

This technique analyzes biofilm formation at the air–surface interface, without submerging the biofilm in liquid [130]. Biofilms are cultivated directly on the anti-biofilm material that must be customized in the form of a semipermeable membrane-like thin film (e.g., wound gauzes, polycarbonate membranes), which are placed on the surface of agar Petri plates. At regular intervals, the film materials are transferred to a fresh medium, giving the biofilm a semi-continuous supply of fresh nutrients. The thick membrane is a convenient substratum that is easily maneuverable, allowing the surface-grown biofilm handling from one medium source to another. These colony biofilms can grow in a short period of time, are easy to grow and require inexpensive laboratory materials.

However, since there is no continuous flow of medium, the microorganisms are not forced to adhere to the surface, and, since there is no wash-out, planktonic cells can interfere with the biofilm assay [125]. Additionally, the stable and spatially restricted nature of this system makes cell number counts more easily attributable to cell lysis rather than detachment [109]. Furthermore, microbial taxa that differ in surface motility will spread across the material at different rates. Other disadvantages include difficulty in handling membranes when colony biomass enlarges [130].

Colony biofilm assays allowed Tran et al. [131] to successfully examine the effectiveness of cellulose discs coated with organoselenium in inhibiting *P. aeruginosa* and *S. aureus* in biofilm-related wound infections. Epstein et al. [57] used colony biofilm to show that a slippery liquid-infused porous surfaces prevented 99.6% of *P. aeruginosa* biofilm attachment over a 7-day period, as well as *S. aureus* and (97.2%) and *E. coli* (96.0%).

4.2. Dynamic Methods

Dynamic systems resemble in vivo conditions better than static ones, due to the control of nutrient delivery and flow, simulating, for instance, the flow forces in urinary and cardiovascular catheters, industrial installations and water pipelines [132].

Dynamic methods usually begin with an adhesion step performed in a low nutrient suspension, as the presence of nutrient-rich suspensions reduces the need for planktonic cells to adhere to a substratum. In subsequent steps, the continuous pumping of nutrients into the reactor leads to stress conditions that promote biofilm growth on the potential anti-biofilm surfaces [133]. Nutrient availability is accurately controlled in such a way as to promote biofilm development without producing artifacts, e.g., complete nutrient depletion that could lead to inhibition of biofilm growth.

Dynamic systems are highly suitable to assess contact-killing materials as, after the adhesion step, the suspension of non-adhered cells is flushed out of the bioreactor, allowing only adhered cells to develop into mature biofilm. On the contrary, they are less suitable to assess antimicrobial-releasing materials as the antimicrobials released are washed out of the system.

Flow systems have the advantage of simultaneously testing different surface materials, analysing samples in a non-invasive manner and with standardized protocols [134]. Additionally, bioreactors allow the sampling of materials aseptically at different time points during biofilm development, without compromising the entire experiment. Furthermore, they are convenient for studies where a large biofilm biomass amount is desirable and for those studies involving microsensor monitoring [135]. Notably, the dry weight of biofilm grown in dynamic systems is often reported to be around 100–175 g dry weight kg^{-1} biofilm, with values comparable to the solid content of centrifuged biomass from suspended cultures [136].

While each of these methods is a useful tool for studying biofilm under controlled conditions, they all need specialized apparata, are technically challenging, and are not suitable for rapid high throughput assays. Another weakness of these systems is that only a single strain can be analysed per experiment. Moreover, biofilm models are difficult to compare due to the differences in biofilm development times, growth media, and the microbial taxa employed.

4.2.1. Robbins (RO) Reactor

This reactor consists of a plug where coupons (biofilm growth surfaces) can be mounted. The plug has two ports for fluid entry and exit. Coupons of different materials can be customized and simultaneously mounted on the device.

The Robbins (RO) reactor is not designed to allow direct observation of biofilm growth. Thus, the coupons must be dislodged for further studies. Additionally, the flow dynamics inside the device need to be accurately adjusted to make sure that the flow is constant along the plug [35]. Indeed, a trend towards higher numbers adhering to the coupons at the in-flow end of the RO reactor than at the outflow end was recorded, likely reflecting reduction of adherent bacteria in the interacting stream [137].

The original RO reactor was employed to evaluate biofilm development under different fluid velocities in a simulated drinking water facility [138]. Linton et al. [137] used a modified RO reactor to compare the adhesion of *S. epidermidis* to glass, siliconized glass, plasma-conditioned glass, titanium, stainless steel and Teflon in a medical environment. Oosterhof et al. [139] tested the fungal and bacterial biofilm responses on tracheoesophageal shunt prostheses to quaternary ammonium silane coatings. Ramage et al. [140] employed an RO reactor to grow *C. albicans* on PMMA. Ginige et al. [141] installed a modified RO reactor in a full-scale water distribution system to investigate biofouling on a high-density polyethylene surface.

4.2.2. Center for Disease Control (CDC) Reactor.

This reactor is a vessel with 8 rods hosting removable coupons for a total of 24 samples. The coupons can be tailor-made from various materials that can be examined simultaneously in a single assay. Moreover, coupons can be removed or exchanged during the experiment allowing time-course studies.

The rotation of the baffled stir bar leads the coupons to undergo a consistent high shear and, as they are placed at the same radial distance, they are subjected to the same shear stress. Nutrients are continuously pumped into and out of the reactor at the same rate [133]. These stress conditions promote biofilm formation on the polymer substrata.

Two standard methods have been accepted by the American Society for Testing and Materials, namely protocols ASTM E2562-17 [105] and ASTM E2871-13 [106], which are methods for developing biofilm and for assessing disinfectant efficacy against sessile *P. aeruginosa* cells in a Center for Disease Control (CDC) reactor. In the CDC reactor, Cai et al. [142] tested the anti-biofilm performance of a diazeniumdiolate-doped poly(lactic-co-glycolic acid)-based nitric oxide releasing film applied to indwelling biomedical devices. Li et al. [143] used the CDC reactor to mimic acidogenic meals and snacks of an oral environment in order to test new dentin-composite and hydroxyapatite disks against multi-species oral biofilm. Ganewatta et al. [38] provided a new contact-killing surface by modifying the natural resin acids (from gum rosin) into quaternary ammonium compounds and employed the CDC reactor to prove the strong anti-biofilm activity of the new material against *S. aureus* and *E. coli*. Dell'Orto and colleagues [76] obtained new medical materials by grafting *p*-aminocinnamic or *p*-aminosalicylic acids on low density polyethylene surfaces, and proved their anti-biofilm efficacy against *E. coli* biofilm in the CDC reactor.

4.2.3. Rotating or Spinning Disk (RD) Reactor

Like the CDC reactor the rotating or spinning disk (RD) reactor contains coupons, made of any material, held by a disk attached to a magnet that allows an adjustable rotational speed when the reactor is kept on top of a magnetic stirrer. The disk rotation establishes a liquid shear on the coupon surfaces [134]. Different shear stresses can be assessed at the same time by placing the coupons at different radial orbits. In contrast to the CDC reactor, which allows a quick and easy removal of coupons during the experiment, the RD reactor coupon sampling can only be done by carefully removing the entire disk from the reactor and returning the disk to the reactor for further biofilm studies.

The RD reactor was originally used to evaluate the biocidal efficacy against toilet bowl sessile cells [144]. This method was subsequently developed into the standardized biofilm method ASTM E2196-17 [107] that describes the assessment of a *P. aeruginosa* biofilm grown with shear and continuous flow. For example, Cotter et al. [145] tested the ability of *S. epidermidis* biofilm to grow on polyethylene coupons by the RD reactor. Barry et al. [146] used the RD reactor to accelerate biofilm formation on latex samples from an external male catheter.

4.2.4. Annular (AN) Reactor

The annular (AN) reactor has been used for several decades to develop biofilm in turbulent flowing environments [147]. Indeed, it is well suited to mimicking biofilm formation on a water treatment process surface. The AN reactor consists of two cylinders, one a static external cylinder made of actual pipe materials and the other a rotating internal cylinder, its speed of rotation able to be finely adjusted in order to obtain the desired shear stress. The inner cylinder supports the coupons, which are in the form of rectangular slides that can be manufactured from any machinable material [147]. Some annular reactors also have a jacket to set desired temperatures.

For example, Pintar and Slawson [148] tested the incidence of temperature on a disinfectant procedure in a drinking water distribution system, using a bench-scale approach provided by an AN reactor. Indeed, there was biofilm development on the polyvinyl chloride surfaces at all the examined temperatures, but at low temperatures the disinfectant had a less biofilm inhibitory effect. Similarly, Ndiongue et al. [149] used the AN reactor to investigate the effects of temperature and biodegradable organic matter on the free chlorine residual needed to control biofilm accumulation in plastic pipes distributing water. For 15 months Jang et al. [150] investigated the effect of four pipe materials on biofilm growth and water quality, using an AN reactor under hydraulic conditions similar to a real plumbing system. The steel and copper surfaces, suffering progressive corrosion, showed substantially increased bacterial concentrations, whereas the stainless steel and polyvinyl chloride surfaces were revealed to have biofilm growth that was mainly affected by water temperature.

4.2.5. Drip flow (DF) Reactor

This is made of four/six parallel chambers with vented lids, each one containing a glass-slide-shaped coupon or tubes manufactured with a variety of materials. The medium enters the individual chambers through a needle, the reactor being kept at an angle of 10° so that the liquid flows along the length of the coupons or tubes [151]. The drip flow (DF) reactor is used in the ASTM Method E2647-13 [108] for the development, sampling and study of *P. aeruginosa* sessile cells grown under low shear and continuous flow, mimicking the environmental conditions found in indwelling devices and the human body (e.g., lung infections, tooth biofilm, microbial colonised catheters). Sawant and colleagues [152] assessed the anti-biofilm capacity of silver nanocomposites, showing that the new materials reduced E. coli biofilm development by six orders of magnitude. Pérez-Díaz et al. [84] tested the anti-biofilm properties of chitosan gels loaded with silver nanoparticles on clinical isolate strains. The preparation of a multi-species biofilm of oxacillin resistant *S. aureus* and *P. aeruginosa*, obtained from a human chronic wound infection, was performed employing a standard DF reactor under conditions that mimic the nutrient flow in the human skin. Goodwin et al. [153] used the DF reactor to investigate biofilm development on polymer nanocomposites containing carbon nanotubes when they come into contact with microorganisms in aqueous environments post-consumer use. Zaltzman et al. [58] tested the ability of nanoparticles incorporated in commercial dental resin material to inhibit biofilm formation of the cariogenic *S. mutans* by using a DF reactor.

4.2.6. Flow Cells (FC)

Flow cells (FC) were designed to evaluate biofilm processes directly using microscopy and image analysis in a non-invasive way [154]. The biofilm is grown encapsulated in a reactor (flow) chamber provided with an inspection glass that allows the microscope lens to directly record images of the biofilm [35]. The FC is connected to nutrient and waste carboys by silicone rubber tubing, and nutrients are continuously pumped inside the cells. The employment of fluorescent probes coupled with confocal laser scanning microscopy (CLSM) makes flow chambers especially useful for in situ gene expression studies. Biofilm in FC is exposed to the passage of air bubbles that could cause the detachment of biofilm parts.

Several FC devices of different design have been developed. The coupon evaluation FC are single or dual channel flow cells provided by wells (up to 3 per channel) at the bottom to accommodate coupon samples for testing. Coupons can be customized in all materials, and a standard microscope coverslip is used as a viewing window. The trasmission FC is similar to the coupon evaluation FC except that it is provided with a unique recess able to allocate any irregularly shaped materials (suture, catheter section, porous media, etc.). In the capillary FC, biofilm is grown inside glass capillaries that can be directly put under the microscope. This FC is less suitable for the study of new surfaces as it requires that the new material be cast in glass, in a capillary shape and with high optical properties. The treatment imaging FC is a round cell provided with a unique well designed to favour the quick installation of disc coupons with biofilm pre-grown in the RO, RD and CDC reactors. It is used to provide images of pre-grown biofilm during treatment with biocides and other chemical agents (See Section 6.2.1). The small liquid volume of the cell minimizes the use of valuable chemical compounds. The flow chamber is sealed with a round microscope cover glass.

Jaramillo et al. [155] used FC to test the efficacy of a polystyrene surface coated with benzalkonium chloride against early adhesion and biofilm formation of oral and dental root canal bacteria. Francolini et al. [156] loaded usnic acid, a secondary lichen metabolite, into modified polyurethane. The polymers were then incorporated in a FC and *S. aureus* and *P. aeruginosa* biofilm development was analysed using CLSM. In this research both *S. aureus* and *P. aeruginosa* were first transformed with green fluorescent proteins to make them fluorescent. In another work, Fabbri et al. [157] used a FC device to grow marine biofilms on plastic coupons coated with six different biocidal antifouling coatings and one inert non-biocidal coating for 8 weeks.

4.2.7. Microplate under Flow (Bioflux)

The device combines small volumes and high-throughput ability of microtiter plates with the biological relevance of a laminar flow cell [158]. The system consists of microtiter well plates in which reagents flow through microfluidic channels running between the wells. Indeed, a pneumatic pump forces the fresh medium from the inlet wells to the outlet, through the microfluidic channel in which biofilm develops. The pump provides for a fluid flow of up to 96 individual biofilms, allowing fine control of adjustable continuous or intermittent fluid flow rates. Once labelled with a fluorescent probe, biofilm can be viewed with a microscope or scanned with a plate reader [159]. Indeed, time-lapse

CLSM images of biofilm formation can be performed [160]. To the best of the authors' knowledge, there is no research in the literature about its use to prove the anti-biofilm performance of new materials, the Bioflux device could be suitable to easily study new coatings. However, in order not to obstruct the Biolux channels, the method is suitable for only thin coatings.

4.3. Microcosms

Microcosms are simplified systems developed under strictly controlled conditions, used to mimic natural ecosystems with their relevant microorganisms [32]. Therefore, microcosms are the systems that closely replicate the in vivo conditions of the real environment, e.g., wound, oral and stream biofilms [90].

Both static and dynamic systems can be turned into microcosms. In comparison to the previously described methods, microcosms consider more environmental parameters and better mimic the complexity and heterogeneity of natural environments. Indeed, these systems include a high diversity of species and require internal processes to reach and maintain system stability. As the complexity of these systems increases, the interpretation of the outcomes and reproducibility become more complicated, compared to both static and dynamic approaches [154].

Abdulkareema et al. [161] coated material for dental implants with zinc oxide nanoparticles and hydroxyapatite. The authors determined the anti-biofilm activity of the new material by a microcosm system using human saliva as an inoculum and artificial saliva and peri-implant sulcular fluid as medium. Li et al. [162] studied the effect of salivary pellicle on anti-biofilm activity of novel dental adhesives by means of a dental plaque microcosm biofilm model using mixed saliva from 10 donors. Similarly, Zhang et al. [83] studied the effect of water-aging on novel anti-biofilm and protein-repellent dental polymeric composite for 180 days using saliva from 10 healthy human donors who had not brushed their teeth for 24 h and had no food intake for 2 h.

5. Quantitative Analysis of Biofilm on Anti-Biofilm Polymeric Surfaces

Once biofilm has been grown on a new surface, it is necessary to quantify its biomass to assess the material's anti-biofilm performance (Figure 3).

STEP 3: CHOOSING BIOFILM ANALYSIS	
QUANTITATIVE ANALYSIS 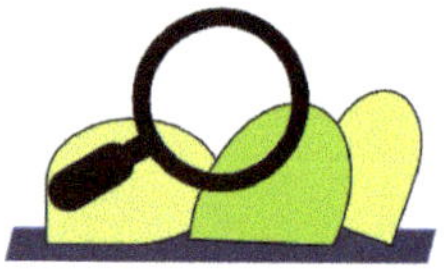	Viable cellular biomass
	Total (viable and not viable) cellular biomass
	Total biofilm (cellular + EPS components)
	EPS matrix
STRUCTURAL ASSESSMENT 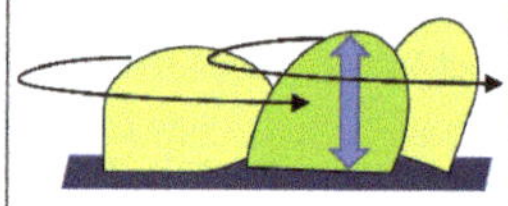	Spatial distribution of community members
	Morphology studies
	Mechanical and physical properties

Figure 3. Scheme representing the third step in the experimental procedure for testing new anti-biofilm materials. The choice of the type biofilm analysis includes quantitative and structural assessment assays.

Quantification methods include those suitable to assess only viable biomass, those able to detect both live and dead cells as well as techniques able to investigate the whole biofilm, including both cellular and EPS components. Indeed, the most appropriate method to be chosen depends on the type of materials (Table 2).

Table 2. Biofilm assays suitable for the main categories of anti-biofilm surfaces. The anti-biofilm surfaces are categorized according to Cattò et al. [36].

Topic	Method	In Situ	Ex Situ	Surface Chemistry Modification	Surface Topography Modification	Surface with Microstructure	Antimicrobial Coating	Antimicrobial-Releasing Surface	Antimicrobial-Responsive Surface	Covalent Immobilization of Antimicrobials	Metal Coating	Nanoparticles Based Materials	Anti-Biofilm Biocide-Free Surfaces
Viable cellular biomass	Plate count assay	✗	✓	✓	✓	✓	✓	✓	✓	✓	✓	✓	✓
	Biomarkers quantification (Phospholipid fatty acids, ergosterol)	✗	✓	✓	✓	✓	✓	✓	✓	✓	✓	✓	✓
	Metabolic colorimetric dyes	✓	✗	✓	✓	✓	✓	✓	✓	✓	✓	✓	✓
	ATP bioluminescence	✗	✓	✓	✓	✓	✓	✓	✓	✓	✓	✓	✓
	Isothermal microcalorimetry	✓	✗	✓	✓	✓	✓	✓	✓	✓	✓	✓	✓
	Tunable Diode Laser Absorption Spectroscopy	✓	✗	✓	✓	✓	✓	✓	✓	✓	✓	✓	✓
	Propidium monoazide-qPCR	✗	✓	✓	✓	✓	✓	✓	✓	✓	✓	✓	✓
	Chamber counting	✓	✓	✓	✓	✗	✗	✗	✗	✗	✗	✓	✓
	Dyes binding	✓	✗	✓	✓	✗	✗	✗	✗	✗	✗	✓	✓
Total (viable and not viable) cellular biomass	Biomarker quantification (total organic carbon, proteins, chlorophyll)	✗	✓	✓	✓	✗	✗	✗	✗	✗	✗	✓	✓
	Quantitative polymerase chain reaction (q-PCR)	✗	✓	✓	✓	✗	✗	✗	✗	✗	✗	✓	✓
	Flow-based cell counting	✗	✓	✓	✓	✗	✗	✗	✗	✗	✗	✓	✓
Total biofilm (cellular biomass + EPS)	Dry weight	✗	✓	✓	✓	✗	✗	✗	✗	✗	✗	✓	✓
	Optical density	✗	✓	✓	✓	✗	✗	✗	✗	✗	✗	✓	✓
	Dye-based methods	✓	✗	✓	✓	✗	✗	✗	✗	✗	✗	✓	✓
	Colour measurements	✓	✗	✓	✓	✓	✓	✓	✓	✓	✓	✓	✓
	Proteins quantification	✗	✓	✓	✓	✓	✓	✓	✓	✓	✓	✓	✓
	Polysaccharides quantification	✗	✓	✓	✓	✓	✓	✓	✓	✓	✓	✓	✓
EPS matrix	Extracellular DNA quantification	✗	✓	✓	✓	✓	✓	✓	✓	✓	✓	✓	✓
	Antibody microarrays	✗	✓	✓	✓	✓	✓	✓	✓	✓	✓	✓	✓
	Fluorescent microscopies	✓	✗	✓	✓	✓	✓	✓	✓	✓	✓	✓	✓
	Spectroscopic techniques (ATR-IR, Raman, SERS)	✓	✓	✓	✓	✓	✓	✓	✓	✓	✓	✓	✓
	Advanced techniques (HPLC, LC-UV-ESI-MS/MS, GC/MS, NMR, TXRF, ICP-MS)	✗	✓	✓	✓	✓	✓	✓	✓	✓	✓	✓	✓
Identification and spatial distribution of biofilm members	FISH and FISH-based techniques	✓	✗	✓	✓	✓	✓	✓	✓	✓	✓	✓	✓
	Immunofluorescence detection	✓	✗	✓	✓	✓	✓	✓	✓	✓	✓	✓	✓

Table 2. Cont.

Topic	Method	In Situ	Ex Situ	Surface Chemistry Modification	Surface Topography Modification	Surface with Microstructure	Antimicrobial Coating	Antimicrobial-Releasing Surface	Antimicrobial-Responsive Surface	Covalent Immobilization of Antimicrobials	Metal Coating	Nanoparticles Based Materials	Anti-Biofilm Biocide-Free Surfaces
Biofilm morphology	Confocal Laser Scanning Microscopy (CLSM, FRAP, FCS, FLIM)	✓	✗	✓	✓	✓	✓	✓	✓	✓	✓	✓	✓
	Multiphoton microscopy (MPM)	✓	✗	✓	✓	✓	✓	✓	✓	✓	✓	✓	✓
	Electronic microscopies (SEM, TEM, cryo-SEM, ESEM, FIB-SEM, ASEM)	✓	✗	✓	✓	✓	✓	✓	✓	✓	✓	✓	✓
	Raman microscopy (RM, CRM)	✓	✗	✓	✓	✓	✓	✓	✓	✓	✓	✓	✓
	Scanning transmission X-ray microscopy (STXM)	✓	✗	✓	✓	✓	✓	✓	✓	✓	✓	✓	✓
	Super-resolution microscopies (STED, GSD, RESOLFT, PALM, STORM, SIM, SSIM)	✓	✗	✓	✓	✓	✓	✓	✓	✓	✓	✓	✓
	Optical coherence tomography (OCT)	✓	✗	✓	✓	✓	✓	✓	✓	✓	✓	✓	✓
Mechanical and physical properties	Atomic force microscopy (AFM, AFM-SCFS)	✓	✗	✓	✓	✓	✓	✓	✓	✓	✓	✓	✓
	Rheometry (macro and micro-reometry, SPT, MPT)	✓	✓	✓	✓	✓	✓	✓	✓	✓	✓	✓	✓
	Quartz crystal microbalance (QCM, QCM-D)	✓	✗	✓	✓	✓	✓	✓	✓	✓	✓	✓	✓
	Surface plasma resonance (SPR)	✓	✗	✓	✓	✓	✓	✓	✓	✓	✓	✓	✓
	Fluid dynamic gauging (FDG)	✓	✗	✓	✓	✓	✓	✓	✓	✓	✓	✓	✓
	Microsensors	✓	✗	✓	✓	✓	✓	✓	✓	✓	✓	✓	✓
	Nuclear magnetic resonance (NMR, MRI, PFG-NMR)	✓	✗	✓	✓	✓	✓	✓	✓	✓	✓	✓	✓

5.1. Viable Cellular Biomass

5.1.1. Plate Count Assay

The most widely used technique to quantify a surface's viable biomass is to determine the colony forming units (CFU) on agar media, after biomass detachment from the surface [35]. The CFU technique is generally accepted as a 'gold standard'. However, the detachment procedure is a weak point as a soft procedure does not ensure the full detachment of all the sessile cells while a harsh approach, e.g., sonication, can injury cell viability and thus compromise the cell count, possibly resulting in false negative results [35]. Furthermore, many strains cannot be cultured and several cells within the biofilm, the persister cells, persevere in a non-growing, metabolically inactive state, and thus cannot be detected by the CFU approach [163]. Another important point is that CFU counting can be a valuable tool for quantifying bacterial biofilm, but it is not really suitable for the fungal biofilm that develops in filamentous structures.

5.1.2. Biomarker Quantification

Phospholipid Fatty Acids

Phospholipid fatty acids are universally distributed, and are made at a relatively constant rate among the membranes of Bacteria and fungi. Therefore, their measurement has been proposed as an accurate estimation of biomass within a biofilm [164]. Indeed, since phospholipids degrade rapidly upon cell death, they represent only the viable microbial community [165]. Indeed, the analytical identification of phospholipids can also provide early indications of the structure of the microbial community and a quantitative biomarker of microbial response to environmental stressors [166].

Many analytical methods that successfully realize the qualitative and quantitative analysis of phospholipids have been developed. Gehron and White [167] introduced a protocol based on the employment of glycerol phosphate for measuring phospholipid concentration and microbial biomass. Their procedure involves the acid hydrolysis of the phosphate from lipid glycerol, and the analysis of labile glycerol by gas chromatography coupled with mass spectrometry (GC/MS) [168]. These methods are well-established techniques for fatty acid analysis, and are the best in terms of high sensitivity and specificity, high throughput and high accuracy. In the last decade, the development of both electron and chemical ionization technologies has significantly increased the performance of MS analysis, providing rapid analysis without derivatization or additional sample handling [169].

The main drawbacks of phospholipid fatty acid determination is the microbial membrane's limited recovery rate in the extraction procedure, the amount of background lipid contamination and the sensitivity of the analytical equipment [35]. Moreover, the technique is unsuitable for microorganisms with membranes that are not composed by phospholipids, e.g., Archea [170].

Ergosterol

Ergosterol, a major component of fungal membranes, is another proper indicator for the quantification of viable fungal biomass. Based on the assumption that ergosterol is labile and undergoes rapid degradation upon cell death, many researchers employ this molecule as an indicator exclusively for living fungal biomass [171]. Ergosterol has been successfully quantified by GC/MS [172] as well as by high-performance liquid chromatography (HPLC) [171,173]. Indeed, conversion factors for microbial biomass have been obtained using representative fungal species.

5.1.3. Metabolic Assays

Colorimetric Dyes

Most common assays are based on the conversion of specific substrates to a colored product measurable with a spectrophotometer. After microbial uptake, the dyes are transformed into fluorescent compounds [174]. FDA (fluorescein-diacetate), resazurin (7-hydroxy-3H-phenoxazin-3-one-10-oxide), and tetrazolium dyes XTT (2,3-bis-(2-methoxy-4-nitro-5-sulfophenyl)-2H-tetrazolium-5-carboxanilide inner salt) and MTT (3-(4,5-dimethyl-2-thiazolyl)-2,5-diphenyl-2H-tetrazolium bromide) are examples of metabolic dyes. FDA is degraded by cellular esterases to become fluorescent yellow while resazurin, a blue dye reduced by metabolically active cells, becomes pink resorufin, also fluorescent [175]. In XTT and MTT assays, an electron transport system across the microbial plasma membrane converts the yellow tetrazolium salt to insoluble purple formazan [176].

A significant limitation of these metabolic assays is the fact that the microorganisms in biofilm do not all display the same metabolic activity, and some of them live in a dormant non-metabolic active state. Moreover, metabolic colorimetric-based assays are often calibrated against planktonic cultures, introducing significant error as the metabolic rates differ greatly between the planktonic and the biofilm states [175].

Adenosine Triphosphate (ATP) Bioluminescence

Adenosine triphosphate (ATP) reacts with luciferin when the catalyst-luciferase enzyme is present, and the effect of this oxidation reaction is the emission of light, recorded by a luminometer and quantified in relative light units [177]. The presence of ATP on the surface is a proxy of metabolic activity and consequently of microbial viability and biomass [177]. One of the major advantages of ATP detection is that it is fast and easy to carry out. However, ATP biolumiscence is an invasive assay that requires biofilm destruction. Recently, some researchers introduced a non-destructive bioluminescence assay, by producing recombinant bacteria bearing a plasmid for the endogenous production of luciferase [178]. The luminescence produced, proportional to the number of microorganisms, can be quantified via a luminometer. Other disadvantages include the inability to differentiate extracellular and intracellular ATP. Therefore, prior to any experiments, the biofilm needs to be washed with water or buffer to remove extracellular ATP. Furthermore, it is not so suitable for multi-species biofilm analysis as variation in has been observed in ATP production among diverse microbial taxa [179].

Isothermal Microcalorimetry (ICM)

Isothermal microcalorimetry (IMC) measures the heat production of biological reactions, which is directly linked to the overall metabolism [180,181]. IMC is a label-free technique that allows precise measurements in conventional, solid, and opaque media. Isothermal microcalorimeters measure less than a microwatt of heat flow possible. Consequently, IMC can detect metabolic activity from as few as 10^4 microbial cells [180]. Notably, it is suited to investigate microbiological samples in complex or heterogeneous environments as it does not necessitate optical clarity of the specimen [182]. No less important is that the samples need little preparation and after IMC measurements, the undisturbed samples can be studied by other techniques.

Tunable Diode Laser Absorption Spectroscopy (TDLAS)

Tunable diode laser absorption spectroscopy (TDLAS) allows non-invasive measurement of the microbial metabolic rate. TDLAS is used to detect change in the O_2 and CO_2 concentrations in biofilm systems, which is related to the metabolic activity of growing microorganisms [183]. Despite the TDLAS potential, there are few papers regarding its application to biofilm and its development on surfaces [181].

5.2. Total (Viable and Non-Viable) Cellular Biomass

5.2.1. Chamber Counting

At the initial developmental stage, biofilm cell counting can be carried out using microscopy and a chamber counting slide, e.g., Thoma, Burker or Petroff-Hausser chambers. Counting chambers are specialized glass microscope slides able to allocate a defined sample volume, and equipped with a 2D grid at the bottom that can be employed to evaluate the cell density of suspended biofilm [184]. This very simple procedure can be performed with unstained cells, is inexpensive and only requires an optical microscope. However, it is time consuming, requires many counts for reproducibility and is subject to manual counting bias. The biofilm has to be dislodged from the surface, homogenized and suspended in a liquid solution prior to analysis. In mature biofilm a 3D structure is formed, making counting more problematic.

5.2.2. Dye Binding

Dye binding to DNA and RNA, such as 4′,6-diamidino-2-phenylindole (DAPI) or Syto9/propidium iodide (PI), 3,3′-dihexyloxacarbocyanine iodide (DioC6)/PI, acridine orange (AO)/PI, carboxyfluorescein diacetate (CFDA)/PI, Calcein/PI, Hoechst/PI and many other combinations of dual staining, can be employed to study both live and dead microbial cells and give an insight into the total amount of microbial sessile cells [185]. Notably, these dyes do not allow discrimination between different microorganism populations in the biofilm. Fluorescence can be detected by both spectrophotometric measurements and microscopic observations [186] (Figure 4a). When relevant, the amount of dye taken up by the cells can be assayed, providing a quantitative indicator of the cellular amount within the biofilm. In most staining combinations, discrimination between viable and dead cells is based only on membrane integrity, so the effect of surfaces modified with molecules not affecting membrane integrity cannot be monitored. Moreover, the following question still remains open: how quantitative and reliable these methods are in the case of heterogeneous multi-species biofilms where variation in fluorescence emission has been observed depending on microbial strains. Stiefel et al. [187] found that staining of *S. aureus* cells with Syto9 alone resulted in equal signal intensity for both live and dead cells, whereas staining of *P. aeruginosa* cells led to 18-fold stronger signal strength for dead cells than for live ones, with an underestimation of viable cells. Indeed, the authors concluded that Gram-negative bacteria were not accessible for Syto9 staining as Gram-positive cells. Additionally, potential interference between the dyes and the surface to be tested needs to be considered, especially when the polymeric surfaces deliver specific anti-biofilm molecules. However, fluorescent staining is considered a fast and easy approach for the quantification of cellular biomass [187,188].

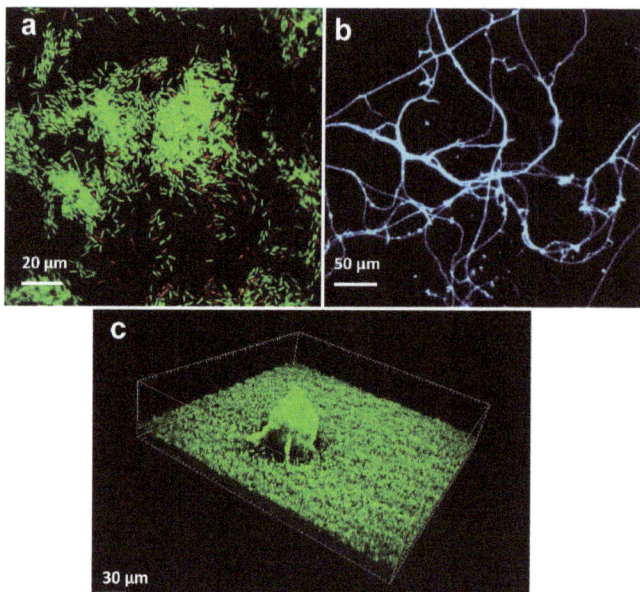

Figure 4. Epifluorescence microscope images of (**a**) *E. coli* biofilm grown on low density polyethylene surface and stained with Live/Dead BacLight; (**b**) *Aspergillus niger* biofilm grown on fluorinated coated glass surface and stained with the Fluorescent Brightener 28 dye; and (**c**) confocal laser scanning microscopy (CLSM) image of green fluorescent protein (GFP) *P. aeruginosa* biofilm grown on polycarbonate surface.

5.2.3. Biomarker Quantification

Quantification of the various components of a cell, e.g., organic carbon, proteins or other molecules, e.g., chlorophyll, have been proposed as alternative methods to indirectly quantify biofilm biomass. The number of such biomarkers is determined and then related to cellular biomass using calibration curves prepared with appropriate standards, under the assumption that their cell content is similar. However, the molecular amount often varies across species, age and culture conditions [184]. Furthermore, the biomarkers and EPS must be separated before biomolecule quantification. Therefore, it is suggested to give these results in tandem with more direct methods, such as CFU or cell counting [184].

Total organic carbon

The total organic carbon of biofilm is usually quantified by a two-step process: First, the inorganic carbon is transformed to CO_2, via heated acidification, and studied by infrared spectroscopy, then the total carbon in the sample is converted to CO_2, usually via heated oxidation, and measured. The total organic carbon is the difference between the values of total carbon and inorganic carbon [189].

Proteins

Cellular lysis releases proteins in solution, these being measured by the change in color due the dye-protein interaction via an ultraviolet–visible (UV–Vis) spectrometer at a particular wavelength. The most commonly used colorimetric assays for protein quantification include the Bradford, Lowry, and bicinchoninic acid (BCA) methods. The Bradford assay consists of adding an acidic Bradford reagent containing Coomassie Brilliant Blue G-250 dye to the lysed sample. During a brief period of incubation, the protein binds to the dye, changing the color from brown to blue. The change in absorbance at 595 nm is recorded, and converted to a total protein concentration through a standard curve [190]. The Lowry method combines the reaction of Cu+, produced by peptide bond oxidation, with the Folin phenol reagent. The result of this reaction is the reduced Folin reagent (heteropolymolybdenum Blue), an intense blue molecule of which the concentration, measured by absorbance at 750 nm, is proportional to the protein amount [191]. Like the Lowry assay, at the beginning the protein complexes with copper ions. Then, this protein-bound copper chelates BCA, resulting in a deep purple color linear with that of the amount of proteins [192]. BCA provides a more uniform response to proteins than the Bradford assay, but it is strongly affected by the amino acids tyrosine, tryptophan, and cysteine. Moreover, chemicals that react with copper (such as ammonia) can affect with the BCA assay.

Chlorophyll

Chlorophyll-*a* is one of the most employed biomarkers for quantifying microalgal and cyanobacterial biomass [193–196] compared a number of methods for cyanobacterial biomass quantification on surfaces and confirmed that chlorophyll-*a* is a good estimator of sessile biomass. Chlorophyll-*a* can be determined spectrophotometrically after extraction in DMSO following a protocol described by Fernández-Silva et al. [197]. However, this method requires an invasive manipulation of the attached cells, and a destructive sample preparation. Alternately, biofilm biomass can be achieved by measuring chlorophyll fluorescence [198]. Recently, pulse amplitude modulated (PAM) fluorometry was used by Vázquez-Nion et al. [199] to measure the in vivo fluorescence signal in a non-destructive way. By measuring the minimal fluorescence signal of dark-adapted cells and the maximal fluorescence signal after a saturating light pulse in dark-adapted cells, the maximum photochemical efficiency of photosystem II, an indicator for the general level of fitness of the photosynthetic organisms, can be quantified. Moreover, the authors developed a standard curve that allowed the correlation of the minimal fluorescence signal of dark-adapted cells with the amount of chl-*a* content as a biofilm biomass estimator.

5.2.4. Quantitative Polymerase Chain Reaction (qPCR)

Quantitative polymerase chain reaction (qPCR) has been used to study the total cellular portion of the biofilm community, evaluating the total amount of DNA from both live and dead cells [200]. Therefore, qPCR is not suitable to evaluate the anti-biofilm performance of surfaces with anti-microbial activity as it does not discern between live and dead cells. Indeed, cells might be killed but not removed from these surfaces.

This technique has limitations in that it tends to underestimate or overestimate the microbial count. Indeed, qPCR detects all the DNA in a sample, including that found in the environment [201]. To avoid the DNA quantification of not living cells, prior to DNA extraction, samples can be treated with nucleic acid intercalating dyes, such as propidium monoazide (PMA-qPCR), able to bind free extracellular DNA (eDNA) and DNA from damaged cells [202]. PMA intercalates into the DNA to which it can be covalently cross-linked when exposed to light, resulting in the suppression of PCR amplification [203].

5.2.5. Flow-Based Cell Counting

Coulter System

A more automated way to count cells involves the use of systems in which cells in liquid culture flow through narrow apertures and are measured as they pass. In the Coulter system, charged particles in an electrolyte solution alter the impedance of an electrical circuit when they pass through the aperture. Changes in voltage are correlated to particle size and, if pulsed, are counted over a period of time, providing a cell number [184]. Although simple, the technique cannot discriminate between live and dead cells. Moreover, it requires the biofilm to be homogenized and suspended in liquid solutions.

Flow Cytometry

In flow cytometry, cells, previously marked with a fluorophore, flow through a narrow opening and a laser detects them as they pass via scattering, absorbance or intrinsic and extrinsic fluorescence measurements [184]. Flow cytometry accurately assesses the cell fractions, e.g., live and dead cells. Therefore, it is well suitable to study biofilm response to antibiotics and other cytotoxic chemicals [204]. Moreover, additional information about the cells, such as dimensions, surface properties, metabolic activity and growth state, can be recorded using specific fluorescent tags [184]. The technique allows the observation of several thousands of cells in a matter of minutes, providing statistically relevant results for the analysis of sessile populations [205]. However, it is expensive and requires specific equipment and highly skilled operators. Moreover, the cell counting is often limited by cells that adhere tightly one to the other [185].

5.3. Total Biofilm (Cellular + Extracellular Polymeric Substances (EPS) Components)

5.3.1. Dry Weight

The simplest way to quantify total biofilm formation on a new anti-biofilm surface is to measure its dry weight. Measurements can be obtained by calculating the difference between the weight of surface material with biofilm and that of the same surface before biofilm formation. Dry mass is obtained by placing the biofilm in an oven at a constant temperature until water removal. Alternatively, if the biofilm surface is heat sensitive, the biofilm can be removed and suspended in a physiological buffer, precipitated with cold ethanol, and the precipitate collected for investigation [184]. Although not highly accurate, weight measurement is a very easy technique.

5.3.2. Optical Density

The reduction in intensity of a transmitted light beam, reported as optical density, is used to measure biofilm total biomass. Indeed, optical density correlates with microbial total carbon and cell mass within a fixed range of cell size and shape [206]. The biofilm is detached from the surface, dispersed in a buffer and the total biomass measured by reading the optical density at 600 nm [207]. Standard curves for cell mass vs. absorbance can be generated for any combination of reactor, microbial strain and spectrophotometer, always allowing determination of mass density by optical density.

5.3.3. Dye-Based Methods

Originally described by O'Toole and Kolter [208] to select biofilm-deficient mutants, these methods have a standard for quantifying biofilm in microtiter plates, owing to the easy use and relatively low cost. Crystal violet (CV) staining is one of the first methods used for biofilm biomass quantification [174]. Alternatively, Safranin Red and Congo Red could be used to quantify total biofilm biomass [207]. These dyes bind to negative charges and therefore target many different molecules of microorganisms and EPS [174]. Staining protocol are detailed reported by Stiefel et al. [207]. The amount of desorbed dye, measured by a spectrophotometer, is directly proportional to biofilm cell amount. Notably, the nonspecific nature of the stains does not allow species differentiation in multi-species communities. In spite it is widely used, CV has major drawbacks, including non-specific binding to anionic proteins and other negatively charged molecules, like capsules, lipopolysaccharides, and DNA/nucleic acids [34]. Additionally, this method provides no information on the actual number of living cells because both the living and dead cells, as well as the biofilm matrix, are stained [175]. Indeed, CV is quite unsuitable to evaluate the anti-biofilm efficacy of surfaces with biocidal activity. Some drawbacks of these assays also include the need for washing steps to remove the unattached cells and the unbound dye, which can lead to the detachment of some biofilm cells [35]. Finally, some studies have demonstrated that composition of cultural media dramatically alters the staining patterns, highlighting the importance of setting suitable biofilm growth conditions especially when a comparison between samples is expected [34].

5.3.4. Color Measurements

On site color measurements can be applied to quantify phototrophic biomass even before the naked eye detects the presence of biofilm [194]. The first intuitive approach to the employment of color variations for evaluating changes in biomass was reported by Young et al. [209]. However, it was Prieto et al. [210] who, for the first time, proved the correlation between modifications in the number of organisms and changes in the parameters defining color. Indeed, most works [199,211–214] performed color measurements using the CIELAB color system [215], which represents each color by means of three scalar parameters: L*, lightness or luminosity of color; a*, associated with changes in redness-greenness; and b*, associated with changes in yellowness-blueness. Each color can also be represented by three angular parameters: L*, lightness or luminosity of color, defined in both scalar and angular color sets; C^*_{ab}, chroma or saturation, related to the intensity of color; and h_{ab}, hue angle or tone of color, which refers to the dominant wavelength [214]. Sanmartín et al. [212] confirmed that CIELAB color coordinates significantly correlated with the chlorophyll-a, phycocyanin, allophycocyanin, and ATP contents. Color measurement has successfully been applied not only to quantifying biofilm growth, but also as a useful tool to assess the physiological state of phototrophic organisms on solid surfaces [216].

5.4. EPS Matrix

The amount of biomass retrieved from a substratum is an indicator of the anti-biofilm features of a new material. In fact, new materials can also act by destabilizing the biofilm matrix and its physical integrity. Therefore, EPS is a must in the assessment of the anti-biofilm performance of new materials.

In addition to water, EPS is made of extracellular polymeric substances, mainly polysaccharides, proteins, lipids and DNA. Characterization of the matrix requires the identification and quantification of each constituent. Generally, the analysis of molecules in the matrix can be investigated by ex situ and in situ methods [217].

5.4.1. Ex Situ EPS Analysis

EPS Extraction

Ex situ quantification of EPS compounds greatly depends on the extraction methods. Indeed, fractions of exopolymers, colloidal and capsular, can be extracted from each biofilm. The colloidal fraction includes compounds that are loosely bound to microorganisms, while the capsular fraction contains tightly bound carbohydrates and proteins [218].

EPS extraction is a challenge due to the different physicochemical properties. Moreover, it is necessary to detach EPS from microorganisms without destroying the cells. The physical methods include ultrasounds, blending, high speed centrifugation, steaming, heating, cation exchange resin or lyophilization, whereas the chemical ones include the use of chemical reagents such as ethanol, formaldehyde, formamide, NaOH, EDTA or glutaraldehyde [219]. Cation exchange resin is another effective technique that has been used to separate EPS from cells [220,221]. No consensus exists on the best methodology as the amount and quality of recovered compounds depends on biofilm species and EPS complexity. A combination of physical, chemical and mechanical methods is often the best solution to ensure extraction of EPS enriched fractions with few contaminates of intracellular content [196,222]. Indeed, an adequate extraction protocol often depends on the scientific goal to be addressed.

Comparing five extraction methods of EPS from alga-bacteria biofilm, Pan et al. [223] found that biofilm pre-treatment with ultrasound at low intensity doubled the extracted matrix yield without significant changes in the composition of EPS. The addition of NaOH to EDTA or formaldehyde increases yield extraction of about one order of magnitude compared to the extraction performed with only EDTA or formaldehyde. Liu et al. [224] matched estimated EPS quantities extracted by formaldehyde–NaOH with CLSM observations and found that formaldehyde–NaOH extract limited only a portion of proteins and polysaccharides. Indeed, sonication coupled with formaldehyde treatments is more efficient for extracting proteins, while EDTA is better for extracting polysaccharides and humic acid substances [224]. McSwain et al. [220] found that the use of NaOH and heat extraction produces a higher protein and polysaccharide amount from cell lysis, highlighting the importance of finding a good extraction procedure, as contamination by cell lysis and dead biomass leads incorrect conclusions.

Once extracted, the amount of extracellular components can be quantified.

Proteins

Protein quantification has principally been performed by colorimetric methods, following the same procedure reported in Section 5.2.3. For example, the Bradford assay was used successfully by Villa et al. [225] to measure the amount of proteins in the matrix of a colony biofilm growing on a polycarbonate membrane. Similarly, Cattò et al. [226] quantified the amount of proteins in the *E. coli* biofilm EPS grown on polycarbonate coupons in the CDC. Alternatively, in Jachlewski et al. [219] extracellular proteins were quantified by a modified Lowry assay.

Polysaccharides

The phenol-sulfuric acid method proposed by Masuko et al. [227] is the simplest and most rapid colorimetric method to evaluate total carbohydrates in a specimen. The method detects virtually all classes of carbohydrates, including mono-, di-, oligo-, and polysaccharides. In this method, the concentrated sulfuric acid breaks down any polysaccharides that react with phenol producing a yellow-gold color. The yellow-gold color is proportional to the amount of total polysaccharides in the sample and can be measured by absorbance at 490 nm. The amount of polysaccharides can be estimated by constructing a standard curve using xylose or glucose as a standard. The color is stable for several hours, and the accuracy of the method is within ±2% under proper conditions [228]. Moreover, it is suitable for high-throughput screening in microtiter well plates.

The major disadvantage of the method is that it does not provide really exact quantitative values as different sugars cause unequal responses [229]. Furthermore, it does not distinguish the different monomeric, oligomeric, or polymeric carbohydrates in the samples. Therefore, a suitable cultivation medium is fundamental to obtain reliable outcomes [229]. Indeed, complex media containing carbohydrate compounds should be avoided or eliminated so as to avoid false values. Additionally, the use of hot temperature and concentrated sulfuric acid and phenol necessitates special precautions with regard to personal safety and laboratory equipment. Consequently, in the last decade, variants of the method have been proposed by removing the carcinogenic phenol reagent or by reducing the reaction time and removing the heat incubation step. A detailed overview and description of different colorimetric modifications to quantify total polysaccharides is discussed extensively in Rühmann et al. [229].

The screening of specific carbohydrates or fractions has also been proposed to study EPS [230–232]. One possibility is to screen uronic acids by the hydroxydiphenyl assay [233] using alginate as standard. In the presence of m-hydroxydiphenyl, uronic acids give a color reaction that is specific for mannuronic-, glucuronic-, and galacturonic-acids. As mannuronic-, glucuronic-, and galacturonic-acids show different responses, the uronic acid quantification is reliable only when a known uronic acid is present in the biofilm [229]. Furthermore, high concentrations of neutral sugars or proteins could cause erratic results [234].

Extracellular DNA

Different approaches have been used to extract extracellular DNA (eDNA) from a matrix; these include the use of ionic exchange, chelating agents, anionic surfactants, a strong alkaline solution and enzymes [235]. In any case it is quite difficult to extract eDNA from the biofilm matrices without contamination from the genomic DNA released after cell death. Moreover, eDNA binds with other biopolymers such as polysaccharides, proteins and metabolites, making its extraction from the complex matrix even more difficult [236].

Once extracted, the easiest approach to quantify eDNA is by reading eDNA absorbance at 260 nm, and assessing its purity by calculating the ratio between the absorbance at 260 nm and 280 nm [237]. Alternatively, nucleic acids can be stained with Syto9 or DAPI and the intensity of fluorescence intensity measured [238].

Antibody Microarrays

Antibody microarrays provide a fast and reliable analysis of up to hundreds of biomarkers simultaneously. In the fluorescent sandwich microarray immunoassay, selected antibodies (primary antibodies) recognize and bind to specific EPS proteins and polysaccharides with high specificity. Detection of this binding is accomplished by directly linking a variety of fluorophores to the primary antibody or introducing them through a secondary antibody that recognizes the primary antibody. Fluorescence intensity is measured and the experimental values can be transformed into a binary matrix and visualized as a heat map. Furthermore, clustering analysis permits the association of similar immunoprofiles or patterns with samples from apparently very different environments, showing that they share similar universal biomarkers. While this assay can only detect predefined antigens without providing precise characterization, it still works as a rapid fingerprinting technique for comparing different samples [218]. In recent work, Blanco et al. [218] used 80 diverse antibodies labeled with the fluorophore Alexa-647 to provide a protein and glycosidic immunoprofile of the capsular EPS fractions extracted from 20 biofilms taken from five extreme environments. Antibodies were set up to detect specific bioanalytes from Bacteria, Archaea and Eukarya, and specific proteins related to iron storage, transporters or metal reductases.

Spectroscopic Techniques

Biofilm matrix can be analyzed by vibrational spectroscopic techniques like attenuated total reflection/ Fourier transform infrared spectrometry (ATR-IR) [217,239,240] and Raman spectroscopy [241,242].

Indeed, ATR-IR has been used to determine the chemical composition of biofilm by an analysis of the absorbance of infrared light by specific chemical groups. ATR-IR enables studies of the biofilm matrix, eliminating artefacts that can arise during the processes required to isolate specific matrix components. Raman spectroscopy measures photons scatterring from the molecule, which depend on the types of bonds in the molecule. Raman spectroscopy provides fingerprint information about the analyte of interest. As the Raman spectrum of each molecule is unique, the spectrum can be used to identify specific molecules within the biofilm. Diffraction-limited spatial resolution of Raman spectroscopy is around 1 μm, enabling detailed analysis of a complex mixture of various molecules such as proteins, carbohydrates, lipids, and nucleic acids [241]. Sample preparation is easy and there is no need for staining procedures. However, the acquisition of spectra from biomolecules can take a longer time and require higher laser power, leading to damage of the sample. In modified Raman spectroscopy-based techniques such as surface-enhanced Raman scattering (SERS), the sensitivity is significantly increased, the detection threshold is lowered and it is possible to detect EPS components that are not detectable by Raman microscopy [243].

Advanced Techniques

More sophisticated approaches allow the single components of EPS, or the entire composition, to be studied. Included are chromatographic techniques such as gel permeation chromatography [244] and HPLC [245]. The combination of liquid chromatography with UV and electrospray ionization ion trap detection (LC–UV-ESI-MS/MS) performs very well in the qualification and quantification of various sugars. Indeed, this method allowed the simultaneous analysis of hexoses, pentoses, deoxy, and amino-sugars, uronic acids as well as different sugar modifications in one single run [246]. GC/MS gave a detailed overview of the entire EPS composition [245,247] as well as of single components [239].

Matrix-assisted laser desorption/ionization (MALDI)-MS has been successfully used to detect and identify polysaccharides, proteins and lipids in complex biofilms [248,249]. Nuclear magnetic resonance (NMR) gave information about the extracellular polysaccharide composition, including the sequence of repeated units or linkages between the heteropolysaccharides [250]. Blanco et al. [218] measured the total concentrations of nine recoverable metals (Zn, Cu, Fe, Co, Ni, As, Cd, Cr and Pb) using X-ray fluorescence reflection (TXRF) and inductively coupled plasma-mass spectrometry (ICP-MS).

All these techniques have greatly advanced the state of art of biofilm matrix knowledge. However, they require complex and expensive equipment, long times to define experimental conditions, and a high level of expertise not commonly found in any laboratory. In addition, complex preparation steps of the samples are sometimes needed.

5.4.2. In Situ EPS Analysis

Microscopic Techniques

Fluorescence microscopy is the pioneering technique used to analyze in situ EPS biofilm. Indeed, CLSM is a powerful tool to assess the EPS on material surfaces (see Section 6.2.1 for details) [251]. Proteins, polysaccharides and DNA can be stained by specific dyes and visualized by the microscope. A semi-quantitative analysis of acquired pictures provides information about the general architecture and the EPS distribution, generating reconstructed 3D images of biofilm grown on a new anti-biofilm surface. Indeed, it is possible to approximate the amount, concentrations and coverage of the various components by correlating the fluorescent intensity of the biofilm components to standard solutions. Examples of protein dyes include the SYPRO Ruby, the 3-(4-carboxybenzoyl)quinoline-2-carboxaldehyde (CBQCA), or the NanoOrange [207]. Polysaccharides can be stained by the Calcofluor White that binds to β-linked polysaccharides such as cellulose and chitin [252] (Figure 4b). Alternatively, ConA-FITC binds α-D-mannopyranosyl and α-D-glucopyranosyl residues in amylopectin and dextran [207]. Fluorescein isothiocyanate (FITC) should label proteins by the reaction of the isothiocyanate group with primary and secondary amine groups [253]. Alternatively, EPS compounds can be visualized with specific antibody labelled with fluorescent probes [254]. Fluorescence microscopy offers high-quality images but limited chemical information.

Spectroscopic Techniques

Spectroscopic techniques can be used in situ to characterize biofilm matrix. The crystal of the ATR-IR can be modified using a specific coating and the real time growth of biofilm on the surface can be monitored. For example, Sportelli et al. [255] deposited a thin film of silver nanoparticle Teflon-like composite on the infrared inactive region of the waveguide of the ATR crystal. The authors used ART-IR techniques to follow, in real-time, the inhibition of sessile *P. fluorescens* cells induced by the bioactive silver ions released from the nano-antimicrobial coating. Notably, ATR-IR is a powerful tool to assess the activity of materials with antimicrobial properties, as well as being suitable to study living bacteria. Furthermore, recent developments in instrumentation have allowed Raman spectrometry to define the matrix chemistry in a given location on a specimen with high spatial resolution (down to a few micrometers). For instance, Feng et al. [256] in situ characterized *P. aeruginosa* biofilm cultivated on a chip substrate made of polydimethylsiloxane on a microfluidic platform.

6. Structural Assessment of Biofilm on Anti-Biofilm Polymeric Surfaces

6.1. Identification and Spatial Distribution of Biofilm Community Members

6.1.1. Fluorescence In Situ Hybridization (FISH)

FISH can be used to investigate the spatial organization of mixed microbial communities, especially in environmental samples, providing also semi-quantitative data of the taxa composition. This can give an insight into how microorganisms interact with each other and the key players occurring in biofilm. Standard FISH uses labeled nucleotide probes for the in situ identification of microorganisms by hybridization to the ribosomal RNA of fixed cells, which can subsequently be visualized and quantified by the microscope. Online databases containing probes developed for FISH are currently available [257]. Using probes with different fluorescent properties it is possible to distinguish and identify microorganisms of different taxa in a mixed biofilm, and assess their spatial organization by microscopy [258]. However, the method shows limitations related to cell permeability, hybridization affinity and target site accessibility, leading to sometimes poor signal-to-noise ratios and lack of target site specificity and sensitivity [259]. Indeed, cells with low rRNA copy numbers, slow growing, or starving, e.g., those in biofilms, often lie below the detection limits or are lost in high background fluorescence [258].

Peptide nucleic acid probes (PNA-FISH) present a quicker and stronger binding to DNA/RNA [259] than standard FISH. The hydrophobic nature of the PNA molecule allows easy cell penetration, and, theoretically, better diffusion through the biofilm matrix. Alternatively, in locked nucleic acids (LNA-FISH), a synthetic RNA analog with the ribose ring locked to a C3' endo-conformation is used as higher affinity, specificity, thermal stability and resistance to degradation in comparison to traditional probes [260].

Improvements have also been introduced to enhance the probe fluorescent signals. In the catalyzed reporter deposition-FISH (CARD-FISH) the fluorescence signal is amplified from 26 to 41 times via the immobilization of multiple radicalized fluorescent tyramides by the enzyme horseradish peroxidase conjugated to the oligonucleotide probes, making the visualization of hard-to-detect cells feasible [261]. However, CARD-FISH is rather expensive, time-consuming and requires a harsh sample preparation protocol, with an enzymatic pretreatment and numerous washing steps that compromise biofilm integrity [262]. In other approaches, probes are double (double labeling of oligonucleotide probes FISH, DOPE-FISH) or multilabeled (Multilabeled FISH, MIL-FISH), so that the fluorescent signal is amplified several times [258,263]. Probes can be also combined in order to increase the number of target microorganisms. In the combinatorial labeling and spectral imaging FISH (CLASI-FISH) microorganisms of interest are labeled with a repertoire of monolabeled oligonucleotide probes carrying fluorochromes of closely overlapping spectra [264]. The combination of emitted wavelengths is recorded by spectral imaging with CLSM. CLASI-FISH allows the simultaneous identification of tens to potentially hundreds of microbial taxa in a single microscope image [265].

FISH combined with microautoradiography (FISH-MAR) has been used to make suggestions about metabolic phenotypes of microorganisms [266]. Indeed, biofilm is grown with radio-isotope labeled substrates and FISH reveals radioactivity in cells that have taken up the particular substrate, and the MAR image is then overlaid with the FISH image, providing a specific substrate uptake profile of the individual bacterial cells in the microbial community [267]. However, some chemical elements, e.g., nitrogen or oxygen, do not have a radioactive isotope with a suitable half-life time for use as a labeled tracer for FISH-MAR experiments, and thus cannot be monitored. Similarly, the combination of FISH with the Nano-scale Secondary Ion Mass Spectrometry (FISH-NanoSIMS) allows the simultaneous exploration of the microbial distribution, and quantifies the utilization of C and N isotopes, allowing the detection of the metabolic activity of identified microorganisms at the single-cell level [268].

Alternatively, confocal Raman microscopy (CRM) coupled with FISH (FISH-Raman) can provide information about FISH-identifiable microbes and the non-biological components within the biofilm, e.g., embedded mineral particles and variant chemical composition of the matrix. Unfortunately, to be compatible with Raman spectroscopic techniques, probes must be labeled with quantum dots or radionuclides, with serious trade-offs regarding cost efficiency and experimental safety [269].

The combination of flow cytometry and FISH (Flow-FISH) has also been proposed for high-throughput, rapid and accurate quantification of biofilm cells with simultaneous phylogenetic specificity being provided by the oligonucleotide FISH probes [270].

6.1.2. Immunofluorescence Detection

Immunofluorescence is a very sensitive technique that exploits antibody binding to specific microorganisms in a mixed population, this binding being visualized by the fluorescence emitted by a marker molecule bound to the antibody. The location of the microbial cells can be viewed using a fluorescence microscope [271]. Indeed, antibody-based methods have been demonstrated to be very promising for high specificity and affinity detection in food and clinical samples [272,273]. The technique is also useful to visualize microorganisms bearing specific proteins accessible to antibodies [274]. For example, Vejborg et al. [275] studied the chain formation in *E. coli* K-12 biofilm on vinyl plastic surface, using an immunochemistry procedure to mark the antigen 43, a self-associating autotransporter protein that had already been implicated in auto-aggregation and biofilm development. The authors observed that Ag43 was concentrated at or near the cell poles, and that when the antigen was highly overexpressed a more uniform distribution of bacteria was present within the biofilm.

6.2. Biofilm Imaging for Biofilm Morphology Studies

6.2.1. Confocal Laser Scanning Microscopy (CLSM)

CLSM is the most powerful tool to assess biofilm architecture on material surfaces, and as it is readily available in labs and core facilities it has made a considerable contribution to biofilm research [115]. CLSM combined with fluorescent staining and high-speed computing allows the acquisition of two-dimensional cross-sections of a biofilm at different depths, resulting, upon analysis by specific software, in the representation of the 3D architecture [276]. The use of water-immersible lenses that do not require a coverslip can help avoid pressure and distortion of the biofilm structure, offering high resolution with working distances of several millimetres and allowing the visualization of fluorescently labeled single cells and an accurate examination of irregular substrata.

Coupled with the use of various probes, CLSM allows the observation of various biofilm components simultaneously. Table 3 gives an overview of the probes binding the main biofilm components. Indeed, using CLSM in a multi-channel modus it is possible to map the individual biofilm components at the same time, e.g., cellular biomass with Syto9, dead cells with PI, extracellular polysaccharides with Concanavalin A. The coupling of CLSM with FISH probes leads to more information about the identification and localization of several microbial taxa. Another option is to take advantage of the intrinsic natural auto-fluorescence property of some microorganisms, e.g., phototrophic biofilm for imaging differentiation. It is also possible to genetically modify organisms in such a way as to make them auto-fluorescent, for instance through the expression of the green fluorescent protein (GFP) or multicolor variants (Figure 4c). GFP is expressed by metabolic active cells, and can be excited using light at 396 nm, emitting green fluorescence light at 508 nm.

QQuantitative 3D digital image analysis of multichannel data sets allows the volumetric and structural quantification of each single biofilm constituent. Indeed, a number of highly advanced software packages, both commercial and free, coupled with high-speed computers, are available to analyze large data file sets [115,185,276]. Common image analysis software includes Imaris (Figure 5), ImageJ (https://imagej.nih.gov/ij/), Fiji (https://fiji.sc/), Comstat and Phlip [277–279]. A comprehensive book on digital image analysis has been edited by Miura [280].

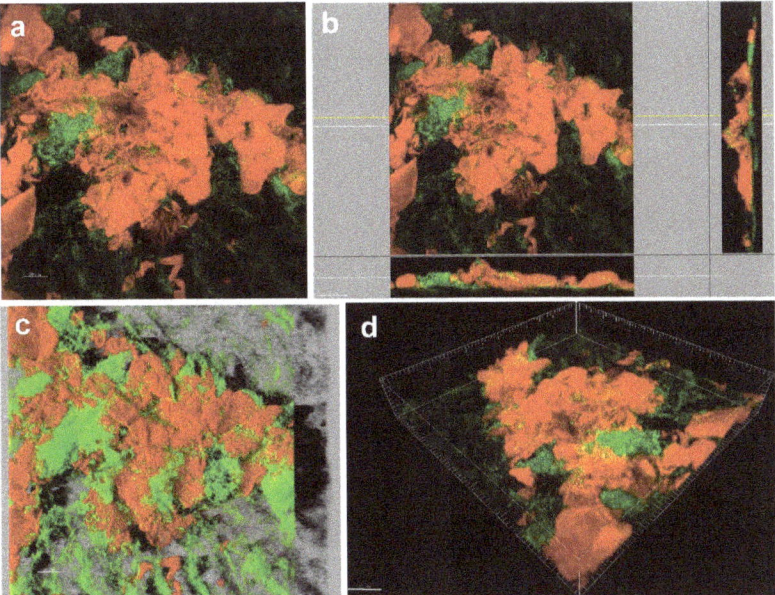

Figure 5. Comparison of different computer visualizations of a single confocal laser scanning microscopy (CLSM) image of *E. coli* biofilm grown on low density polyethylene surface. Computational analysis has been performed by Imaris software. (**a**) maximum intensity projection; (**b**) orthogonal projection; (**c**) blend projection and (**d**) 3D reconstruction. Biofilm was stained green with Syber green I (live cells) and red with Texas Red-labelled ConA (polysaccharidic matrix).

When assessing a sample, not only should the intensity of the excited fluorochrome can be measured but also its lifetime as this can reveal additional valuable information [281], e.g., the efficacy of disinfection treatment [282]. For example, the evaluation of an accurate threshold value up to which biofilm remains undisturbed on the surface under antimicrobial treatments is valuable information for their direct application in many industrial contexts where biofilm is unwanted. The technique, called time-lapse CLSM, consists in installing a disc coupon with biofilm pre-grown in a biofilm reactor in a Treatment Imaging FC (Figure 6a). Prior to being placed in the flow cell, the biofilm is stained with fluorescent dye that labels viable and dead cells (e.g., the LIVE/DEAD BacLight) or enzymatic activities (e.g., the esterase activity marker calcein acetoxymethyl ester). The imaging technique is based on evaluating the loss of fluorescence corresponding to the leakage of a fluorophore out of cells due to membrane permeabilization by the antimicrobial agent [283] (Figure 6b). In recent work, Cattò et al. [284] used time-lapse microscopy to evaluate the enhanced susceptibility of an *E. coli* biofilm pre-grown on a polyethylene surface functionalized with p-amino-cinnamic acid and p-amino-salicylic acid to ethanol. The method allows the decrease of fluorescence intensity at different locations within the biofilm to be measured, revealing that the ethanol antimicrobial action occurs very rapidly at the biofilm surface and slower where the bottom of the biofilm is in contact with the coupon substratum. Advanced CLSM-based tools including fluorescence recovery after photobleaching (FRAP), fluorescence correlation spectroscopy (FCS) and fluorescence lifetime imaging (FLIM) can also be used to assess the antibiotic diffusion-reaction within a biofilm locally. These techniques trace the diffusion of fluorescent labeled antibiotics within the biofilm, offering a spatiotemporal resolution not available with the commonly employed time-lapse CLSM imaging method [282].

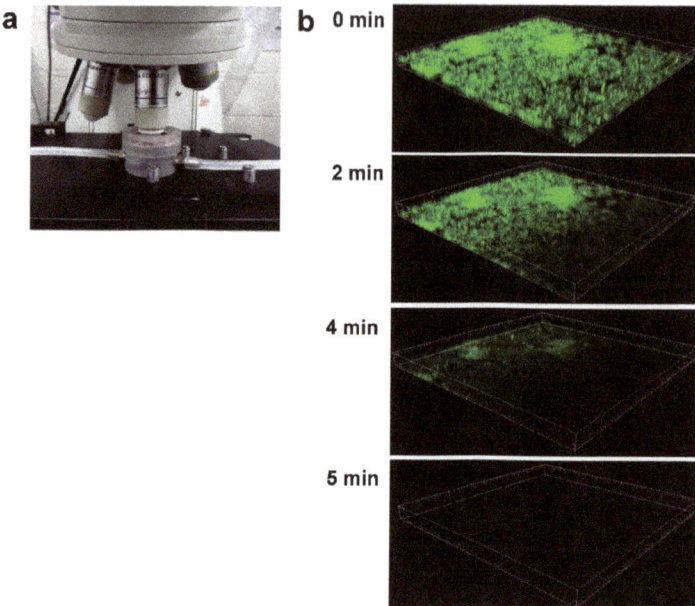

Figure 6. (a) Treatment imaging flow cell (FC) under CLSM for time lapse experiments; (b) time lapse CLSM of ethanol action performed on *E. coli* biofilm grown on low density polyethylene surfaces functionalized with *p*-aminosalicylic acid. The fluorescence loss from stained *E. coli* cells is used to monitor real-time loss in cell viability during the biocide action. Under ethanol treatment, biofilm displayed a total loss in fluorescent intensity in 5 min.

The main disadvantage of CLSM is that the depth of penetration into the sample is limited to around 20-40 μm. Indeed, as depth increases, the scattering and absorption signals of both excitation and emission light lose intensity. Thus, CLSM is not suitable for biofilm of more than 50 μm thickness.

Another limitation of CLSM is the unequal resolution in XY and Z. However, this can be avoided by increasing the objective lens numerical aperture. By employing two opposed lenses and mounting the specimen between two coverslips, equally resolved XYZ data sets can be recorded [281].

Moreover, another major disadvantage of CLSM is the scanning process, which limits temporal resolution, and the need for more excitation energy, resulting in increased photobleaching [285].

However, these drawbacks have now been partially sidestepped as CLSM has been improved tremendously in the last decade with novel optics, lasers, fluorescent proteins and probes as well as CLSM derivatives, such as multiphoton microscopy (MPM), light sheet fluorescence microscopy [286,287] and spinning-disk confocal laser systems [288,289]. For example, instead of using a light source emitting a continuous intensity, MPM uses a laser emitting high-powered (peak power >2 kW) ultrashort pulse (in the femto- or picosecond range), so that two or more photons are able to interact simultaneously with a fluorescent dye molecule at the point of focus [290]. The use of near-infrared excitation light enables MPM microscopy to minimise sample damage and increase the light penetration depth. Moreover, due to multiphoton absorption, the background signal is strongly suppressed. Furthermore, MPM overcomes drawbacks of other optical microscopy techniques such as photobleaching and phototoxicity [291].

Table 3. Examples of the most common fluorescent stains used for staining biofilm grown on polymeric surfaces with anti-biofilm properties.

Staining Pattern	Stain	Colour (Maxima Excitation/ Emission)	Cells (Viability: Live/Dead/ Both)	Matrix	Polymeric Substrate
Nucleic acids	DAPI	Blue (358/461 nm)	X (both)		- Polyurethane coated with N-vanillylnonanamide [292] - Permanox plastic coated with B-type proanthocyanidins [293] - Surfactant polymer dressing (PluroGel) [294]
	SYTO 9	Green (485/498 nm)	X (both)		- Poly(ε-caprolactone-co-δ-valerolactone) mixed with dibromohemibasta-din-1 [81] - Silycon containing (3-acrylamidopropyl) trimethylammonium chloride (AMPTMA) or quaternized polyethylenimine methacrylate [99] - Siloxane modified with non-ionic surfactants and antioxidant [295]
	SYBR green-I	Green (495/537 nm)	X (both)		- Low density polyethylene functionalyzed with p-aminocinnamic acid and p-aminosalicylic acid [284] - Low density polyethylene functionalized with α-chymotrypsin [74]
	Live/Dead Bac-Light	Green (485/498 nm) Red (585/617 nm)	X (both)		- Nanostructured silicon [55] - Black silicon with nanoprotrusion [296] - Nanoporous 1,2-polybutadiene-b-polydimethylsiloxane loaded with sodium dodecyl sulfate [297] - Nanostructured poly (methyl methacrylate) [298] - Polydimethylsiloxane with immobilized polymyxins B and E [28] - NO-releasing amine plasma polymer [299] - Low density polyethylene functionalyzed with p-aminocinnamic acid and p-aminosalicylic acid [284] - Low density polyethylene functionalized with α-chymotrypsin [74] - Poly(methyl methacrylate) with incorporated Juglone [113] - Ciprofloxacin-incorporated polyurethane polymers [300]
	Propidium Iodide	Red (585/617 nm)	X (dead)		- Nanoporous 1,2-polybutadiene-b-polydimethylsiloxane leaded with sodium dodecyl sulfate [297] - Polymer brushes based on poly(cysteine methacrylate) grafted on on the nanocellulose membranes [301]
	Acridine orange	Green (500/526 nm)	X (both)		- Urinary catheters coated with lipase-embedded polycaprolactone (PCL), coimpregnated with the antibiotic gentamicin sulfate [302]
Plasma membrane	CellMask plasma membrane orange	Red (554/567 nm)	X (both)		- Low density polyethylene functionalyzed with p-aminocinnamic acid and p-aminosalicylic acid [76]
Cell wall	Wheat Germ Agglutinin (FITC conjugated)	Green (490/525 nm)	X (both)		- Surfactant polymer dressing (PluroGel) [294]
	Calcofluor white	Blue (355/433 nm)	X (both)		- 1H,1H,2H,2H-Perfluoro-octyl-methacrylate, methyl methacrylate, Paraloid B72 acrylic resin [303]
Metabolic activity	Resazurin	Blu (575/585 nm)	X (live)		- Poly(vinyl alcohol-co-ethylene) [101]
	Calcein or fluorescein diacetate	Green (495/515 nm)	X (live)		- Poly(vinyl alcohol-co-ethylene) [101]
	SNARF-1	Green (580/640 nm)		X	- Poly(methacrylic acid) antibiotic-loaded [304]
Proteins	FITC	Green (490/525 nm)	X (both)		- Poly (ε-caprolactone)-based polyurethane coated with butanolide [53]
	SYPRO Ruby	Red (450/610 nm)		X	- Surfactant polymer dressing (PluroGel) [294] - Polymer brushes based on poly(cysteine methacrylate) grafted on on the nanocellulose membranes [301]
Polysaccharides	Concanavalin A (Texas red, Alexa Fluor 594 conjugated)	Red (Texas red: 595/613 nm; Alexa Fluor 594: 591/618 nm;)	X (both)	X	- Low density polyethylene functionalyzed with p-aminocinnamic acid and p-aminosalicylic acid [284] - Low density polyethylene functionalized with α-chymotrypsin [74] - Silica particles attached to polydimethylsiloxane [305]

6.2.2. Electron Microscopy

Conventional electron microscopy is widely used to achieve imaging of sub-nanometer resolution, providing a detailed insight into the ultrastructure of the biofilm and its environment [306,307]. Indeed, electron microscopy is often applied to visualize the initial formation of biofilm, starting with the single cells attached to an interface [308].

Several electron microscopy techniques have been used to examine the assembly of biofilm structure on solid surfaces, scanning electron microscopy (SEM) and transmission electron microscopy (TEM) being the predominant choices [309–313]. SEM and TEM have been extensively used for a qualitative observation of biofilm, but they are not generally recommended for quantitative evaluations [35,174]. A drawback of both SEM and TEM is the sample preparation, which involves fixation and dehydration, followed by coating with conductive materials such as gold or platinum. As biofilm consists mainly of water, so specimen dehydration could alter the morphology, and changes or artifacts be introduced [311–313]. Moreover, the sample is under vacuum, introducing artifacts into the biofilm structure [307].

By sidestepping the hydration and vacuum limitation, in cryo-SEM the biofilm is not dehydrated but kept frozen, thus achieving high-magnification images closer to the native state of the sample [314]. The advantage of cryo-SEM is the lack of pre- operational steps. Ultrafast freezing procedures, e.g., high-pressure freezing, are used for specimen fixation, therefore, sample preparation occurs within a maximum of one minute of time. However, compared to conventional SEM, cryo-SEM images are of poorer resolution due to the low frozen surface conductivity, compared to the dehydrated gold-sputtered surface used in conventional SEM [306]. Moreover, the heat generated by the focused electron beam causes the sample's frozen surface melts and cracks at high magnifications [314].

Environmental SEM (ESEM) allows the imaging of biological specimens in their original hydrated conditions at relatively high resolution, with a total lack of sample preparation [315]. As in the case of cryo-SEM, ESEM provides images of poorer resolution than conventional SEM, because of the lack of conductivity in the wet sample.

A more sophisticated alternative to create 3D biofilm reconstruction is the FIB–SEM. The FIB sequentially mills away 10 nm-thick sections from the surface of a resin that contains the embedded samples. Images of each slice are subsequently recorded by SEM and processed by specific software to perform the 3D volume reconstruction.

Atmospheric scanning electron microscopy (ASEM) was developed to observe biological samples at atmospheric pressure [307]. ASEM consists of an inverted SEM to observe a wet sample from below while optical microscopy simultaneously observes it from above [316]. Sugimoto et al. [307] cultured a biofilm on an electron-transparent film. The biofilm was directly imaged from below using the inverted SEM, allowing the study of biofilm formation near the substrate. The authors were able to visualize the intercellular nanostructures, including membrane vesicles, cytoplasmic proteins and a thick dendritic nanotube network between microbes, suggesting multicellular communication between microorganisms [307].

6.2.3. Super-Resolution Microscopy (Nanoscopy)

Super resolution microscopy techniques, also referred to as nanoscopy, have been developed to improve the resolving power of diffraction-limited optical and fluorescence microscopy. These tools are able to resolve structures below the limits of optical resolution (200 nm), even down to the 1 nm level [317].

Stimulated emission-depletion (STED) microscopy represents a major type of these techniques and was the first to be proposed and experimentally realized [318]. STED creates super-resolution images giving details smaller than 50 nm by the selective deactivation of fluorophores and minimizing the area of illumination at the focal point [318]. Photoactivated localization microscopy (PALM) and stochastic optical reconstruction microscopy (STORM) take advantage of a similar approach [319]. Instead, in structured illumination microscopy (SIM) and saturated structured illumination microscopy (SSIM) samples are illuminated by a pattern of light at three different angles that make visible the normally inaccessible high-resolution information. The result is a resolution increased of two times in comparison to the optical microscopies [320]. Compared to other super-resolution microscopies,

SIM is quite popular as standard fluorophores can be used, does not require special mounting and preparation techniques [321]. The technical details of these methods have been extensively reviewed by Li et al. [321] and Sydor et al. [322].

In spite of their high resolution, all these techniques have certain disadvantages that need to be considered. Super-resolution methods allow the imaging of only thick samples and only a small number of fluorochromes can be used [323]. Moreover, when super-resolution data are processed and analyzed, it is important to choose adequate controls to avoid artefacts and generating high-quality data [323].

6.2.4. Other Microscopic Techniques

CRM is a non-invasive, label-free technique to analyse in vivo biofilm formation. The sample is excited by a laser and the backscattered light signal is recorded, providing information on the chemical composition and conformation. In CRM, no fluorescent probe is necessary and, in contrast to other spectroscopic techniques, is only slightly sensitive to water, allowing the investigation of living specimens in fully hydrated conditions. The main advantage of CRM is that biofilms can be studied in their native, unaltered state, immersed in the medium. Specimen preparation is not necessary and information on the biofilm chemical nature is obtained [324]. A single Raman spectrum contains information about both organic compounds, e.g., polysaccharides, proteins, lipids, humic-like substances, and inorganic constituents like minerals. Specific Raman signals can be extracted and (semi-)quantitatively mapped [325]. CRM has been employed to map distributions of water and biomass [326], pigmented matrix and cellular content [327] and chemical components such as sugars or proteins [328]. Sandt et al. [327] used CRM to study the structure, composition and growth of fully hydrated biofilm grown on glass in a flow cell. Andrews et al. [329] demonstrated that the attachment of 11 bacterial strains on different surfaces was influenced by several extracellular compounds such as lipids, proteins, and nucleic acids, and the effects of these molecules were important to the genus level. A study reported by Wagner et al. [328] showed a change of EPS composition in heterotrophic biofilms over time, which was not detected by CLSM.

Scanning transmission X-ray microscopy (STXM) is extensively employed in mapping biofilm composition without using a probe, and also with reduced radiation damage to the sample. STXM is employed to study polymers as well as metal distribution at a microscale [330,331]. STXM can be applied to fully hydrated biological materials. This is a consequence of the ability of X-rays to penetrate water with reduced radiation damage to samples.

6.2.5. Optical Coherence Tomography (OCT)

Optical coherence tomography (OCT) measures depth-resolved reflection signals from translucent samples such as biofilms, and allows extended sample areas to be examined within millimetres [332]. Furthermore, the rapidity of measurement and the fact that there is no need for probes or fluorochromes are distinct OCT advantages over other conventional imaging techniques for structural description, including CLSM. OCT allows the acquisition of in situ and real time images, in a non-ionizing and non-invasive way [333]. Indeed, the cross-sectional images of biofilms on the micron scale of OCT offer a quantitative, high-resolution, spatially-resolved means to analyse biofilm growth, detachment, thickness, and structural heterogeneity [334]. Other advantages are the small size and mobility of an OCT device, allowing the investigation of biofilm inside the cultivation device itself [327].

Several papers have reported dynamic biofilm development on polymeric membrane surfaces under different operating conditions [334–336] as well as on medical devices [333,337] and other materials, e.g., polystyrene [338].

6.3. Mechanical and Physical Properties

Studies of the mechanical and physical behaviour of biofilms (e.g., viscosity, elasticity, adhesion, cohesion, permeability, etc.) are crucial to an understanding of biofilm physical stability, and thus of the performance of new anti-biofilm material. Indeed, materials based on matrix-degrading enzymes, or quorum-sensing inhibitors, can change a biofilm's mechanical and physical properties, making the biofilm more prone to detachment and less resistant to antimicrobial treatments. Therefore, mechanical and physical parameters can be considered quantitative biomarkers of EPS integrity. Furthermore, mechanical and physical features should also be useful to optimize cleaning strategies in an industrial setting, e.g., by determining the best flow stress to override biofilm presence, or to assess the antimicrobial penetration in the biofilm. For example, it has been hypothesized that the formation of viscoelastic extended structures by S. aureus in intravenous catheters could block the catheters, and that the breaking of these viscoelastic chains, e.g., by using matrix degrading polymeric materials, could dislodge the biofilm from the surfaces [339,340].

There are a number of varied testing methods available to study biofilm mechanical and physical parameters. Recently, Billings et al. [341] and Boudarel et al. [342] provided a good overview of such methods and guidelines by which the mechanical and physical properties of biofilms can be measured. However, the mechanical properties of biofilm remain a concern in biofilm research because there is a lack of standardized protocols for both mechanical and physical testing and associated identification methods [342]. This complicates the comparison of different materials, and thus the improvement of material engineering processes and screening. Furthermore, none of the existing methods cover the whole spectrum of biofilm behaviour as the properties describing the mechanical capacities of a biofilm are both numerous and varied [343]. Indeed, the combination of in situ experimental measurements and biofilm modelling seems a promising approach to ascertain the mechanical and physical properties of biofilms [344–347]. Unfortunately, the complexity of biofilm structure makes conventional mechanical and physical testing often unsuitable for engineered materials.

6.3.1. Atomic Force Microscopy (AFM)

Atomic force microscopy (AFM) techniques can be used to measure viscoelastic forces and those driving cell–cell and cell–substrate interactions [348]. AFM consists of a tip held in intimate contact with the surface. When the tip is scanned across the surface, it encounters surface forces and the cantilever is deflected, generating force–sample distance curves [349]. As samples can be examined in their native state, sample preparation is minimal, greatly reducing the development of artefacts [350].

The review of Lau et al. [350] reports a list of biofilm viscoelastic and adhesive studies using AFM. For example, Harapanahalli et al. [351] investigated the influence of S. aureus adhesion forces to different biomaterials, noting that the adhesion forces modulate the production of some matrix molecules. Also Feuille et al. [352] used AFM to study the forces guiding the self-association of S. aureus, focusing on a key surface protein. El-Kirat-Chatel et al. [353] measured adhesion forces between live bacteria and two copolymers based on tert-butyldimethylsilyl methacrylate dedicated to ship hulls.

These researches have provided a novel insight into the interplay of interaction forces and mechanical properties that govern the behaviour of biofilms, and their response to chemical and physical attack.

The main drawback is that AFM requires physical contact between the probe and the biofilm, which poses a challenge for biofilms grown in closed systems, e.g., in flow cells [354].

Modifications of standard AFM have been made, including AFM-based single-cell force spectroscopy (AFM-SCFS). In AFM-SCFS, the AFM tip is replaced by a single cell to measure cell–cell and cell–solid interaction forces. Taubenberger et al. [355] highlighted that AFM-SCFS is a suitable tool to quantify cell-biomaterial interactions, thus greatly contributing to the optimization of new materials for implants, scaffolding, and medical devices. For instance, Spengler et al. [356] used AFM-SCFS to investigate the adhesion strength between a single cell of S. aureus and a solid hydrophobic silane and hydrophilic silicon. The study showed a strong influence of the hydrophobic interaction on microbial adhesion, corroborating the notion that the adhesive strength of bacteria is not a matter of contact area, but rather a matter of which, and how many, molecules of the bacterial cell wall are involved in the contact with the surface.

6.3.2. Rheometry

Measurement of viscoelasticity includes both macro- and microrheology methods that quantify biofilm deformation under constant stress, in a compressive, shear or tensile mode, or measuring the stress needed to maintain constant deformation, also referred as stress relaxation [357,358]. The rheometer consists of either parallel plates or a cone and plate between which the material of interest is placed, providing data about the viscoelastic behaviour of the biofilm. In some studies the biofilms were dislodged from their original growth locations and placed in the rheometer [25,359,360], whereas in others the biofilms were grown directly on a rheometer plate [361–363], potentially altering the microarchitecture [363].

Macro-rheological studies have provided a lot of information about the viscoelastic properties of biofilms, but this is at the macro-scale level and often requires an ex situ analysis and an impractical amount of biofilm [354].

Particle-tracking microrheology uses micro-beads, embedded in the biofilm without disrupting the natural state of the biofilm system. The number of beads can be one, in single-particle tracking (SPT), or multiple, in the multi-particle tracking (MPT) technique [341]. In passive particle tracking, the beads are not manipulated by any external perturbation, but move in response to thermal or energy fluctuations. In active microrheology, external forces are used to move the probe particle through the biofilm rather than relying solely on fluctuations in thermal energy [364].

In the last decade, particle tracking micro-rheology has been combined with CLSM [341]. For example, Cao et al. [365], used SPT micro-rheology combined with CLSM to analyze biofilm behavior at different horizontal z-planes (bottom, middle, top) and to track trajectories of green fluorescent carboxylate micro-bead particles segregated in two different biofilm regions (voids and clusters). Similarly, Chew et al. [366] measured the rheological properties of *P. aeruginosa* biofilm at different stages of development, tracking, by CSLM, the natural Brownian movement of the spherical particles with marked intrinsic fluorescence within the sample. Alternatively, Galy et al. [364] used CSLM to track the motion of multiple magnetic beads embedded in growing biofilm.

6.3.3. Quartz Crystal Microbalance (QCM)

Quartz crystal microbalance (QCM) technology has been used to detect both the mass and viscoelastic changes in biofilms, in real time and in a non-destructive way. This technique is based on the measurement of changes in frequency of a system composed of a surface or thin coating adsorbed on a piezoelectric quartz sensor due to the additional of removal of small masses [367,368].

A special variation of this technique is called QCM with dissipation (QCM-D). Compared with conventional QCM, the QCM-D technique is able to simultaneously measure changes in resonant frequency and energy loss, or dissipation, of the system, allowing the detection of mass increase and structural changes of cells at the same time [369–371].

QCM and QCM-D are well suited to investigating the processes occurring at or near the anti-biofilm surface during initial cell adhesion, including the binding properties between the cell and the material [367,372–374]. Wang et al. [374] modified the QCM-D sensor surface with different glycopolymers and cationic polymers and studied the bacteria–substratum interactions on different polymer-treated sensor surfaces. The authors found that lectin-carbohydrate interactions play a significant role in *E. coli* and *P. aeruginosa* adhesion, compared to other non-specific forces, e.g., electrostatic interactions. Indeed, *P. aeruginosa* adhered to the glycopolymer surface with strong contact point stiffness in comparison to *E. coli*. In another work, Knowles et al. [375] used QCM to understand the protein interactions with a new silica nanoparticle anti-biofilm coating. This study elucidated the effect of nanoscale surface topography on fouling processes.

Both QCM and QCM-D systems are capable of detecting the kinetics of biofilm formation on materials, without differentiating between biotic and abiotic components [376]. Moreover, the miniaturization of the mass sensitive detector permits its integration into industrial plants, including the food industry, water distribution systems and clinical settings [373]. However, the interpretation of

QCM and QCM-D is often difficult, especially in the case of microbial adhesion. Indeed, many studies on microbial adhesion and biofilm formation report a decrease in resonance frequency upon microbial adhesion whereas other studies report an increase [377].

6.3.4. Surface Plasma Resonance (SPR)

Surface plasma resonance (SPR) is an emerging technique to investigate the binding kinetics and adhesion of *microorganisms* to various natural and synthetic materials. For instance, Pranzetti et al. [378] used SPR to study the initial stages of bacterial adhesion to surfaces, including non-specific contributions from electrostatic, van der Waals, and hydrophobic forces. In this study, SPR provided real-time observations of both EPS and adhesion of two marine bacteria with different hydrophobicity to model surfaces. Indeed, SPR spectral data reveal kinetics of adhesion depending on both the marine bacterial species and the backbone structures and functional groups of the substrate. Zhang et al. [379] demonstrated by SPR that nanosized TiO_2 decreased the adhesive ability of both B. *subtilis* cell and EPS, and induced biofilm detachment from different surfaces in some hours. Indeed, the decrease in adhesive strength worked against microbial aggregation. These experiments show that the differences in binding were dependent on the type of surface and microbial strains.

6.3.5. Fluid Dynamic Gauging (FDG)

Fluid dynamic gauging (FDG) has been developed to quantify the in situ and real time strength of soft deposits, immersed in a liquid environment [380]. FDG can be used to estimate the adhesive and cohesive strength of biofilm by means of flow data. For instance, Peck et al. [381] investigated E. *coli* biofilm removal by FDG during cleaning treatments under controlled hydrodynamic conditions. The authors compared three different substrates and found that mature biofilm grown on glass has a stronger surface attachment than that on stainless steel and polyethylene.

6.3.6. Microsensors

Microsensors, consisting of a needle-type sensor with a tip diameter of 10–20 microns, measure the gradient concentration of particular chemicals, e.g., the concentrations of oxygen, carbon dioxide, sulfide, pH, oxidation-reduction potential, ammonium, nitrate and nitrite. These probes are small enough to not significantly harm the biofilm upon entry, providing an in situ direct measurement of the chemical concentrations within the biofilm, in a non-invasive way [382]. Microelectrodes have the advantage of making both spatial and temporal measurements within the biofilm. Moreover, multiple microbial taxa can be profiled using different metabolic fingerprints, and the use of multiple sensors allows a better understanding of how such communities are arranged. By creating an array of microelectrodes, it is also possible to measure multiple chemical signatures simultaneously in the same location [383–385]. Microelectrodes have been widely used to analyze biofilm on a wide range of materials, including medical surfaces [386], membranes used in wastewater treatments [387,388] and other polymeric materials such as polycarbonate slides [389]. Indeed, equations for macroscale models to gain an insight into flow and transport processes within the biofilm have received much attention [390–393].

6.3.7. Magnetic Resonance Imaging (MRI) and Pulse-Field Gradient Nuclear Magnetic Resonance (PFG-NMR)

Magnetic resonance imaging (MRI) is a NMR-based technique that has been used in situ and in vivo to characterize water dynamics within biofilm, e.g., determination of flow velocity, as well as the molecular dynamics and diffusion of biomolecules in biofilm, in a non-invasive way. Notably, MRI is not impeded by biofilm thickness and is thus quite suitable for thick biofilm. Studies of mass transport processes inside biofilm on polymeric surfaces using MRI have included water diffusion measurements in biofilm on a polyether ether ketone plastic disc [394] and the transport and fate of heavy metals in biofilm on plastic surfaces [395].

Alternatively, pulse-field gradient NMR (PFG-NMR) can also be employed for the diffusion analysis of water and small molecules within the biofilm. PFG-NMR employs pulsed magnetic field gradients to obtain information about the average displacement of the spins. With PFG-NMR it is possible, in principle, to measure the self-diffusion coefficients of all NMR-detectable molecules [396].

7. Conclusions

In recent years, new techniques to study biofilm grown on polymeric surfaces have been proposed. These include microcosms able to accurately reproduce human conditions, and microfluidics that allow the precise manipulation and control of fluids in microscale channels, typically less than 100 μm, and omic-based approaches revealing physiological differences occurring in the course of sessile development in response to interactions with materials [115,397,398]. However, despite their notable contribution to the study of biofilm, these techniques are still far from being widely applied to study anti-biofilm properties. Indeed, these approaches often require specific equipment, a high level of expertise and often long experimental procedures, which make them less appropriate for screening purposes on a large and/or industrial scale. Therefore, while the development of new microbiological techniques is proceeding fast, the evolution of standards for testing the new anti-biofilm materials is proceeding rather slowly.

A key aspect toward the standardization of testing anti-biofilm materials is the sharing of specific details about the experimental technique employed and the corresponding experimental conditions. This is key aspect to replicate studies at an interlaboratory scale, favouring the spreading of methodologies that are expecting to become the standard for the field in the feature. Already there has been a lot of effort put into developing dedicated public web platforms, like that of MIABiE [399] and BiofOmics [400], for the systematic and standardized collection of guidelines, experiments and data. However, the efforts so far performed are not enough and standardization in anti-biofilm surface testing methods remains a blind spot in the biofilm material community. Indeed, standardization is still a challenging matter as biofilms are living, complex, highly heterogeneous and constantly evolving structures. Such features yield intra-sample and sample-to-sample high variability in results, which is, among others, one of the main obstacles when dealing with standardization [342]. Variability has been even reported in the results of the same test on a biofilm grown in the same conditions [342]. To complicate the scenarios, there is still a need to study the response of biofilms throughout their life-cycle in the different environment. Moreover, studies establishing the validity of laboratory biofilm models are still lacking [401].

Beside the number of issues in the field, the implementation of such standardized methods is technically demanding, and efforts to overcome limitations in their development is the direction of the future. Companies in the field urgently ask for new standardized tests to demonstrate that their new discoveries provide statistically relevant results and motivation for spreading the new products on the market. On the other hand, regulatory agencies need standard methods to assess the performance of the new materials and compare their features with the existing technology on the market.

The literature shows that inexpensive and easy assays can be performed routinely, and are more suitable to be standardized, compared to a more accurate but sophisticated assay. Indeed, although often regarded as over-simplistic, these models have contributed greatly to today's knowledge of biofilm physiology. Certainly, the direction of the future is to set up simple standardized anti-biofilm procedures that on an industrial scale can establish correlation with real outcomes, facilitating data comparison.

Given the lack of standardized procedures to evaluate the anti-biofilm properties of new polymeric materials, today the only possible approach for the scientific community is to follow common bases and good practices. These guidelines are a preliminary step in the direction of standardized protocols. At the present time, there is no single method for studies on the nature of biofilm on surfaces. Indeed, each method has its drawbacks, but it also has distinct strengths, that are important to consider when interpreting the results. Since biofilms are heterogeneous in their organization and structure, the suggestion is to use complementary approaches to confirm the anti-biofilm activity of a selected material.

Author Contributions: All authors conceived the review; C.C. Writing—Original Draft Preparation, F.C. Supervision, Writing—Review and Editing.

Funding: This research received no external funding.

Conflicts of Interest: The authors declare no conflict of interest.

References

1. Namazi, H. Polymers in our daily life. *Bioimpacts* **2017**, *7*, 73–74. [CrossRef]
2. Teo, A.J.T.; Mishra, A.; Park, I.; Kim, Y.J.; Park, W.T.; Yoon, Y.J. Polymeric biomaterials for medical implants and devices. *ACS Biomater. Sci. Eng.* **2016**, *2*, 454–472. [CrossRef]
3. Siracusa, V. Food packaging permeability behaviour: A report. *Int. J. Polym. Sci.* **2012**, *2012*, 302029. [CrossRef]
4. Agrillo, B.; Balestrieri, M.; Gogliettino, M.; Palmieri, G.; Moretta, R.; Proroga, Y.T.; Rea, I.; Cornacchia, A.; Capuano, F.; Smaldone, G.; et al. Functionalized polymeric materials with bio-derived antimicrobial peptides for "active" packaging. *Int. J. Mol. Sci.* **2019**, *20*, 601. [CrossRef] [PubMed]
5. Chen, G.F.R.; Zhao, X.Y.; Sun, Y.; He, C.B.; Tan, M.C.; Tan, D.T.H. Low loss nanostructured polymers for chip-scale waveguide amplifiers. *Sci. Rep.* **2017**, *7*, 3366. [CrossRef] [PubMed]
6. Cappitelli, F.; Zanardini, E.; Sorlini, C. The biodeterioration of synthetic resins used in conservation. *Macromol. Biosci.* **2004**, *4*, 399–406. [CrossRef]
7. Giacomucci, L.; Toja, F.; Sanmartin, P.; Toniolo, L.; Prieto, B.; Villa, F.; Cappitelli, F. Degradation of nitrocellulose-based paint by *Desulfovibrio desulfuricans* ATCC 13541. *Biodegradation* **2012**, *23*, 705–716. [CrossRef] [PubMed]
8. Haque, S.K.M.; Ardila-Rey, J.A.; Umar, Y.; Rahman, H.; Mas'ud, A.A.; Muhammad-Sukki, F.; Albarracin, R. Polymeric materials for conversion of electromagnetic waves from the sun to electric power. *Polymers* **2018**, *10*, 307. [CrossRef] [PubMed]
9. Koniuszewska, A.G.; Kaczmar, J.W. Application of polymer based composite materials in transportation. *Prog. Rubber Plast. Recycl. Technol.* **2016**, *32*, 1–24. [CrossRef]
10. Prabhu, T.N.; Prashantha, K.A. Review on present status and future challenges of starch based polymer films and their composites in food packaging applications. *Polym. Compos.* **2018**, *39*, 2499–2522. [CrossRef]
11. Costerton, J.W. Introduction to biofilm. *Int. J. Antimicrob. Agents* **1999**, *11*, 217–221. [CrossRef]
12. Plyuta, V.A.; Lipasova, V.A.; Kuznetsov, A.E.; Khmel, I.A. Effect of salicylic, indole-3-acetic, gibberellic, and abscisic acids on biofilm formation by *Agrobacterium tumefaciens* c58 and *Pseudomonas aeruginosa* PAO1. *Appl. Biochem. Microbiol.* **2013**, *49*, 706–710. [CrossRef]
13. Riga, E.K.; Vohringer, M.; Widyaya, V.T.; Lienkamp, K. Polymer-based surfaces designed to reduce biofilm formation: From antimicrobial polymers to strategies for long-term applications. *Macromol. Rapid Commun.* **2017**, *38*. [CrossRef] [PubMed]
14. Vigneron, A.; Alsop, E.B.; Chambers, B.; Lomans, B.P.; Head, I.M.; Tsesmetzis, N. Complementary microorganisms in highly corrosive biofilms from an offshore oil production facility. *Appl. Environ. Microbiol.* **2016**, *82*, 2545–2554. [CrossRef] [PubMed]
15. Cappitelli, F.; Polo, A.; Villa, F. Biofilm formation in food processing environments is still poorly understood and controlled. *Food Eng. Rev.* **2014**, *6*, 29–42. [CrossRef]
16. Douterelo, I.; Jackson, M.; Solomon, C.; Boxall, J. Spatial and temporal analogies in microbial communities in natural drinking water biofilms. *Sci. Total Environ.* **2017**, *581*, 277–288. [CrossRef] [PubMed]
17. Galie, S.; Garcia-Gutierrez, C.; Miguelez, E.M.; Villar, C.J.; Lombo, F. Biofilms in the food industry: Health aspects and control methods. *Front. Microbiol.* **2018**, *9*, 898. [CrossRef]
18. Francolini, I.; Donelli, G.; Crisante, F.; Taresco, V.; Piozzi, A. Antimicrobial polymers for anti-biofilm medical devices: State-of-art and perspectives. *Adv. Exp. Med. Biol.* **2015**, *831*, 93–117. [CrossRef]
19. Sadekuzzaman, M.; Yang, S.; Mizan, M.F.R.; Ha, S.D. Current and recent advanced strategies for combating biofilms. *Compr. Rev. Food Sci. Food Saf.* **2015**, *14*, 491–509. [CrossRef]

20. Anderson, D.J.; Podgorny, K.; Berrios-Torres, S.I.; Bratzler, D.W.; Dellinger, E.P.; Greene, L.; Nyquist, A.C.; Saiman, L.; Yokoe, D.S.; Maragakis, L.L.; et al. Strategies to prevent surgical site infections in acute care hospitals: 2014 update. *Infect. Control Hosp. Epidemiol.* **2014**, *35*, 605–627. [CrossRef]

21. Badia, J.M.; Casey, A.L.; Petrosillo, N.; Hudson, P.M.; Mitchell, S.A.; Crosby, C. Impact of surgical site infection on healthcare costs and patient outcomes: A systematic review in six European countries. *J. Hosp. Infect.* **2017**, *96*, 1–15. [CrossRef]

22. Lo, J.; Lange, D.; Chew, B.H. Ureteral stents and foley catheters-associated urinary tract infections: The role of coatings and materials in infection prevention. *Antibiotics (Basel)* **2014**, *3*, 87–97. [CrossRef]

23. Johnson, J.R.; Kuskowski, M.A.; Wilt, T.J. Systematic review: Antimicrobial urinary catheters to prevent catheter-associated urinary tract infection in hospitalized patients. *Ann. Intern. Med.* **2006**, *144*, 116–126. [CrossRef]

24. Stewart, P.S. Antimicrobial tolerance in biofilms. *Microbiol. Spectr.* **2015**, *3*. [CrossRef]

25. Bas, S.; Kramer, M.; Stopar, D. Biofilm surface density determines biocide effectiveness. *Front. Microbiol.* **2017**, *8*, 2443. [CrossRef]

26. Hoiby, N.; Bjarnsholt, T.; Givskov, M.; Molin, S.; Ciofu, O. Antibiotic resistance of bacterial biofilms. *Int. J. Antimicrob. Agents* **2010**, *35*, 322–332. [CrossRef]

27. Nisnevitch, M. Antibiotic resistance and antibiotic alternatives: Looking towards the future. *Sci. Prog.* **2016**, *99*, 92–96. [CrossRef]

28. Alves, D.; Pereira, M.O. Bio-inspired coating strategies for the immobilization of polymyxins to generate contact-killing surfaces. *Macromol. Biosci.* **2016**, *16*, 1450–1460. [CrossRef]

29. Sjollema, J.; Zaat, S.A.J.; Fontaine, V.; Ramstedt, M.; Luginbuehl, R.; Thevissen, K.; Li, J.Y.; van der Mei, H.C.; Busscher, H.J. In vitro methods for the evaluation of antimicrobial surface designs. *Acta Biomater.* **2018**, *70*, 12–24. [CrossRef]

30. Phillips, K.S.; Patwardhan, D.; Jayan, G. Biofilms, medical devices, and antibiofilm technology: Key messages from a recent public workshop. *Am. J. Infect. Control* **2015**, *43*, 2–3. [CrossRef]

31. Miquel, S.; Lagrafeuille, R.; Souweine, B.; Forestier, C. Anti-biofilm activity as a health issue. *Front. Microbiol.* **2016**, *7*, 592. [CrossRef] [PubMed]

32. Roy, R.; Tiwari, M.; Donelli, G.; Tiwari, V. Strategies for combating bacterial biofilms: A focus on anti-biofilm agents and their mechanisms of action. *Virulence* **2018**, *9*, 522–554. [CrossRef] [PubMed]

33. Yu, O.Y.; Zhao, I.S.; Mei, M.L.; Lo, E.C.; Chu, C.H. Dental biofilm and laboratory microbial culture models for cariology research. *Dent. J. (Basel)* **2017**, *5*, 21. [CrossRef]

34. Haney, E.F.; Trimble, M.J.; Cheng, J.T.; Valle, Q.; Hancock, R.E.W. Critical assessment of methods to quantify biofilm growth and evaluate antibiofilm activity of host defence peptides. *Biomolecules* **2018**, *8*, 29. [CrossRef] [PubMed]

35. Azeredo, J.; Azevedo, N.F.; Briandet, R.; Cerca, N.; Coenye, T.; Costa, A.R.; Desvaux, M.; Di Bonaventura, G.; Hébraud, M.; Jaglic, Z.; et al. Critical review on biofilm methods. *Crit. Rev. Microbiol.* **2017**, *43*, 313–351. [CrossRef] [PubMed]

36. Cattò, C.; Villa, F.; Cappitelli, F. Recent progress in bio-inspired biofilm-resistant polymeric surfaces. *Crit. Rev. Microbiol.* **2018**, *44*, 633–652. [CrossRef] [PubMed]

37. Lichter, J.A.; Van Vliet, K.J.; Rubner, M.F. Design of antibacterial surfaces and interfaces: Polyelectrolyte multilayers as a multifunctional platform. *Macromolecules* **2009**, *42*, 8573–8586. [CrossRef]

38. Ganewatta, M.S.; Miller, K.P.; Singleton, S.P.; Mehrpouya-Bahrami, P.; Chen, Y.P.; Yan, Y.; Nagarkatti, M.; Nagarkatti, P.; Decho, A.W.; Tang, C. Antibacterial and biofilm-disrupting coatings from resin acid-derived materials. *Biomacromolecules* **2015**, *16*, 3336–3344. [CrossRef]

39. Antoci, V.; Adams, C.S.; Parvizi, J.; Davidson, H.M.; Composto, R.J.; Freeman, T.A.; Wickstrom, E.; Ducheyne, P.; Jungkind, D.; Shapiro, I.M.; et al. The inhibition of *Staphylococcus epidermidis* biofilm formation by vancomycin-modified titanium alloy and implications for the treatment of periprosthetic infection. *Biomaterials* **2008**, *29*, 4684–4690. [CrossRef]

40. Francolini, I.; Donelli, G. Prevention and control of biofilm-based medical-device-related infections. *FEMS Immunol. Med. Microbiol.* **2010**, *59*, 227–238. [CrossRef]

41. Swartjes, J.; Sharma, P.K.; van Kooten, T.G.; van der Mei, H.C.; Mahmoudi, M.; Busscher, H.J.; Rochford, E.T.J. Current developments in antimicrobial surface coatings for biomedical applications. *Curr. Med. Chem.* **2015**, *22*, 2116–2129. [CrossRef] [PubMed]

42. Ashbaugh, A.G.; Jiang, X.S.; Zheng, J.; Tsai, A.S.; Kim, W.S.; Thompson, J.M.; Miller, R.J.; Shahbazian, J.H.; Wang, Y.; Dillen, C.A.; et al. Polymeric nanofiber coating with tunable combinatorial antibiotic delivery prevents biofilm-associated infection in vivo. *Proc. Natl. Acad. Sci. USA* **2016**, *113*, E6919–E6928. [CrossRef] [PubMed]
43. Barde, M.; Davis, M.; Rangari, S.; Mendis, H.C.; De La Fuente, L.; Auad, M.L. Development of antimicrobial-loaded polyurethane films for drug-eluting catheters. *J. Appl. Polym. Sci.* **2018**, *135*, 46467. [CrossRef]
44. Coenye, T.; Nelis, H.J. In vitro and in vivo model systems to study microbial biofilm formation. *J. Microbiol. Methods* **2010**, *83*, 89–105. [CrossRef] [PubMed]
45. Gao, P.; Nie, X.; Zou, M.J.; Shi, Y.J.; Cheng, G. Recent advances in materials for extended-release antibiotic delivery system. *J. Antibiot.* **2011**, *64*, 625–634. [CrossRef] [PubMed]
46. Chen, M.; Yu, Q.S.; Sun, H.M. Novel strategies for the prevention and treatment of biofilm related infections. *Int. J. Mol. Sci.* **2013**, *14*, 18488–18501. [CrossRef] [PubMed]
47. Zanini, S.; Polissi, A.; Maccagni, E.A.; Dell'Orto, E.C.; Liberatore, C.; Riccardi, C. Development of antibacterial quaternary ammonium silane coatings on polyurethane catheters. *J. Colloid Interface Sci.* **2015**, *451*, 78–84. [CrossRef] [PubMed]
48. Ergene, C.; Palermo, E.F. Cationic poly (benzyl ether) s as self-Immolative antimicrobial polymers. *Biomacromolecules* **2017**, *18*, 3400–3409. [CrossRef] [PubMed]
49. Li, X.; Wu, B.; Chen, H.; Nan, K.H.; Jin, Y.Y.; Sun, L.; Wang, B.L. Recent developments in smart antibacterial surfaces to inhibit biofilm formation and bacterial infections. *J. Mater. Chem. B* **2018**, *6*, 4274–4292. [CrossRef]
50. Gbejuade, H.O.; Lovering, A.M.; Webb, J.C. The role of microbial biofilms in prosthetic joint infections. *Acta Orthop.* **2015**, *86*, 147–158. [CrossRef]
51. Romano, C.L.; Scarponi, S.; Gallazzi, E.; Romano, D.; Drago, L. Antibacterial coating of implants in orthopaedics and trauma: A classification proposal in an evolving panorama. *J. Orthop. Surg. Res.* **2015**, *10*, 157. [CrossRef] [PubMed]
52. Adlhart, C.; Verran, J.; Azevedo, N.F.; Olmez, H.; Keinanen-Toivola, M.M.; Gouveia, I.; Melo, L.F.; Crijns, F. Surface modifications for antimicrobial effects in the healthcare setting: A critical overview. *J. Hosp. Infect.* **2018**, *99*, 239–249. [CrossRef] [PubMed]
53. Ding, W.; Ma, C.F.; Zhang, W.P.; Chiang, H.Y.; Tam, C.; Xu, Y.; Zhang, G.Z.; Qian, P.Y. Anti-biofilm effect of a butenolide/polymer coating and metatranscriptomic analyses. *Biofouling* **2018**, *34*, 111–122. [CrossRef] [PubMed]
54. Francolini, I.; Silvestro, I.; Di Lisio, V.; Martinelli, A.; Piozzi, A. Synthesis, characterization, and bacterial fouling-resistance properties of polyethylene glycol-grafted polyurethane elastomers. *Int. J. Mol. Sci.* **2019**, *20*, 1001. [CrossRef] [PubMed]
55. Hsu, L.C.; Fang, J.; Borca-Tasciuc, D.A.; Worobo, R.W.; Moraru, C.I. Effect of micro- and nanoscale topography on the adhesion of bacterial cells to solid surfaces. *Appl. Environ. Microbiol.* **2013**, *79*, 2703–2712. [CrossRef] [PubMed]
56. Fernandez, I.C.S.; van der Mei, H.C.; Lochhead, M.J.; Grainger, D.W.; Busscher, H.J. The inhibition of the adhesion of clinically isolated bacterial strains on multi-component cross-linked poly(ethylene glycol)-based polymer coatings. *Biomaterials* **2007**, *28*, 4105–4112. [CrossRef] [PubMed]
57. Epstein, A.K.; Wong, T.S.; Belisle, R.A.; Boggs, E.M.; Aizenberg, J. Liquid-infused structured surfaces with exceptional anti-biofouling performance. *Proc. Natl. Acad. Sci. USA* **2012**, *109*, 13182–13187. [CrossRef]
58. Zaltsman, N.; Ionescu, A.C.; Weiss, E.I.; Brambilla, E.; Beyth, S.; Beyth, N. Surface-modified nanoparticles as anti-biofilm filler for dental polymers. *PLoS ONE* **2017**, *12*, e0189397. [CrossRef]
59. Cao, W.W.; Zhang, Y.; Wang, X.; Li, Q.; Xiao, Y.H.; Li, P.L.; Wang, L.N.; Ye, Z.W.; Xing, X.D. Novel resin-based dental material with anti-biofilm activity and improved mechanical property by incorporating hydrophilic cationic copolymer functionalized nanodiamond. *J. Mater. Sci. Mater. Med.* **2018**, *29*, 162. [CrossRef]
60. Knowles, B.R.; Wagner, P.; Maclaughlin, S.; Higgins, M.J.; Molino, P.J. Silica nanoparticles functionalized with zwitterionic sulfobetaine siloxane for application as a versatile antifouling coating system. *ACS Appl. Mater. Interfaces* **2017**, *9*, 18584–18594. [CrossRef]
61. Gkana, E.N.; Doulgeraki, A.I.; Chorianopoulos, N.G.; Nychas, G.J.E. Anti-adhesion and anti-biofilm potential of organosilane nanoparticles against foodborne pathogens. *Front. Microbiol.* **2017**, *8*, 1295. [CrossRef] [PubMed]

62. Sufian, M.M.; Khattak, J.Z.K.; Yousaf, S.; Rana, M.S. Safety issues associated with the use of nanoparticles in human body. *Photodiagnosis Photodyn. Ther.* **2017**, *19*, 67–72. [CrossRef] [PubMed]
63. Reed, R.B.; Zaikova, T.; Barber, A.; Simonich, M.; Lankone, R.; Marco, M.; Hristovski, K.; Herckes, P.; Passantino, L.; Fairbrother, D.H.; et al. Potential environmental impacts and antimicrobial efficacy of silver and nanosilver-containing textiles. *Environ. Sci. Technol.* **2016**, *50*, 4018–4026. [CrossRef] [PubMed]
64. Resnik, D.B. How should engineered nanomaterials be regulated for public and environmental health? *AMA J. Ethics* **2019**, *21*, 363–369. [CrossRef]
65. Villa, F.; Cappitelli, F. Plant-derived bioactive compounds at sub-lethal concentrations: Towards smart biocide-free antibiofilm strategies. *Phytochem. Rev.* **2013**, *12*, 245–254. [CrossRef]
66. Rémy, B.; Mion, S.; Plener, L.; Elias, M.; Chabrière, E.; Daudé, D. Interference in bacterial quorum sensing: A biopharmaceutical perspective. *Front. Pharmacol.* **2018**, *9*, 203. [CrossRef] [PubMed]
67. Kaplan, J.B. Biofilm dispersal: Mechanisms, clinical implications, and potential therapeutic uses. *J. Dent. Res.* **2010**, *89*, 205–218. [CrossRef] [PubMed]
68. Kostakioti, M.; Hadjifrangiskou, M.; Hultgren, S.J. Bacterial biofilms: Development, dispersal, and therapeutic strategies in the dawn of the postantibiotic era. *Cold Spring Harb. Perspect. Med.* **2013**, *3*, a010306. [CrossRef] [PubMed]
69. Chifiriuc, C.; Grumezescu, V.; Grumezescu, A.M.; Saviuc, C.; Lazǎr, V.; Andronescu, E. Hybrid magnetite nanoparticles/*Rosmarinus officinalis* essential oil nanobiosystem with antibiofilm activity. *Nanoscale Res. Lett.* **2012**, *7*, 209. [CrossRef] [PubMed]
70. Nowatzki, P.J.; Koepsel, R.R.; Stoodley, P.; Min, K.; Harper, A.; Murata, H.; Donfack, J.; Hortelano, E.R.; Ehrlich, G.D.; Russell, A.J. Salicylic acid-releasing polyurethane acrylate polymers as anti-biofilm urological catheter coatings. *Acta Biomater.* **2012**, *8*, 1869–1880. [CrossRef]
71. Marcano, A.; Ba, O.; Thebault, P.; Crétois, R.; Marais, S.; Duncan, A.C. Elucidation of innovative antibiofilm materials. *Colloids Surf. B* **2015**, *136*, 56–63. [CrossRef] [PubMed]
72. Villa, F.; Secundo, F.; Polo, A.; Cappitelli, F. Immobilized hydrolytic enzymes exhibit antibiofilm activity against *Escherichia coli* at sub-lethal concentrations. *Curr. Microbiol.* **2015**, *71*, 106–114. [CrossRef] [PubMed]
73. Spadoni-Andreani, E.; Villa, F.; Cappitelli, F.; Krasowska, A.; Biniarz, P.; Lukaszewicz, M.; Secundo, F. Coating polypropylene surfaces with protease weakens the adhesion and increases the dispersion of *Candida albicans* cells. *Biotechnol. Lett.* **2017**, *39*, 423–428. [CrossRef] [PubMed]
74. Cattò, C.; Secundo, F.; James, G.; Villa, F.; Cappitelli, F. α-Chymotrypsin immobilized on a low-density polyethylene surface successfully weakens *Escherichia coli* biofilm formation. *Int. J. Mol. Sci.* **2018**, *19*, 4003. [CrossRef] [PubMed]
75. Kim, Y.G.; Lee, J.H.; Gwon, G.; Kim, S.I.; Park, J.G.; Lee, J. Essential oils and eugenols inhibit biofilm formation and the virulence of *Escherichia coli* O157:H7. *Sci. Rep.* **2016**, *6*, 36377. [CrossRef] [PubMed]
76. Dell'orto, S.; Catto, C.; Villa, F.; Forlani, F.; Vassallo, E.; Morra, M.; Cappitelli, F.; Villa, S.; Gelain, A. Low density polyethylene functionalized with antibiofilm compounds inhibits *Escherichia coli* cell adhesion. *J. Biomed. Mater. Res. A* **2017**, *105*, 3251–3261. [CrossRef] [PubMed]
77. Sajeevan, S.E.; Chatterjee, M.; Paul, V.; Baranwal, G.; Kumar, V.A.; Bose, C.; Banerji, A.; Nair, B.G.; Prasanth, B.P.; Biswas, R. Impregnation of catheters with anacardic acid from cashew nut shell prevents *Staphylococcus aureus* biofilm development. *J. Appl. Microbiol.* **2018**, *125*, 1286–1295. [CrossRef]
78. Pu, Y.; Liu, A.B.; Zheng, Y.Q.; Ye, B. In vitro damage of *Candida albicans* biofilms by chitosan. *Exp. Ther. Med.* **2014**, *8*, 929–934. [CrossRef]
79. Bregnocchi, A.; Zanni, E.; Uccelletti, D.; Marra, F.; Cavallini, D.; De Angelis, F.; De Bellis, G.; Bossu, M.; Ierardo, G.; Polimeni, A.; et al. Graphene-based dental adhesive with anti-biofilm activity. *J. Nanobiotechnol.* **2017**, *15*, 89. [CrossRef]
80. Namivandi-Zangeneh, R.; Sadrearhami, Z.; Bagheri, A.; Sauvage-Nguyen, M.; Ho, K.K.K.; Kumar, N.; Wong, E.H.H.; Boyer, C. Nitric oxide-loaded antimicrobial polymer for the synergistic eradication of bacterial biofilm. *ACS Macro Lett.* **2018**, *7*, 592–597. [CrossRef]
81. Le Norcy, T.; Niemann, H.; Proksch, P.; Linossier, I.; Vallee-Rehel, K.; Hellio, C.; Fay, F. Anti-biofilm effect of biodegradable coatings based on hemibastadin derivative in marine environment. *Int. J. Mol. Sci.* **2017**, *18*, E1520. [CrossRef]

82. Liu, H.Y.; Shukla, S.; Vera-Gonzalez, N.; Tharmalingam, N.; Mylonakis, E.; Fuchs, B.B.; Shukla, A. Auranofin releasing antibacterial and antibiofilm polyurethane intravascular catheter coatings. *Front. Cell. Infect. Microbiol.* **2019**, *9*, 37. [CrossRef]
83. Zhang, N.; Zhang, K.; Melo, M.A.S.; Weir, M.D.; Xu, D.J.; Bai, Y.X.; Xu, H.H.K. Effects of long-term water-aging on novel anti-biofilm and protein-repellent dental composite. *Int. J. Mol. Sci.* **2017**, *18*, 186. [CrossRef]
84. Perez-Nadales, E.; Nogueira, M.F.A.; Baldin, C.; Castanheira, S.; El Ghalid, M.; Grund, E.; Lengeler, K.; Marchegiani, E.; Mehrotra, P.V.; Moretti, M.; et al. Fungal model systems and the elucidation of pathogenicity determinants. *Fungal Genet. Biol.* **2014**, *70*, 42–67. [CrossRef]
85. Nett, J.E.; Andes, D.R. Fungal Biofilms: In vivo models for discovery of anti-biofilm drugs. *Microbiol. Spectr.* **2015**, *3*, E30. [CrossRef]
86. Villa, F.; Pitts, B.; Lauchnor, E.; Cappitelli, F.; Stewart, P.S. Development of a laboratory model of a phototroph-heterotroph mixed-species biofilm at the stone/air interface. *Front. Microbiol.* **2015**, *6*, 1251. [CrossRef]
87. Peng, C.; Vishwakarma, A.; Li, Z.R.; Miyoshi, T.; Barton, H.A.; Joy, A. Modification of a conventional polyurethane composition provides significant anti-biofilm activity against *Escherichia coli*. *Polym. Chem.* **2018**, *9*, 3195–3198. [CrossRef]
88. Karathia, H.; Vilaprinyo, E.; Sorribas, A.; Alves, R. *Saccharomyces cerevisiae* as a Model Organism: A Comparative Study. *PLoS ONE* **2011**, *6*, e16015. [CrossRef]
89. Russell, J.J.; Theriot, J.A.; Sood, P.; Marshall, W.F.; Landweber, L.F.; Fritz-Laylin, L.; Polka, J.K.; Oliferenko, S.; Gerbich, T.; Gladfelter, A.; et al. Non-model model organisms. *BMC Biol.* **2017**, *15*, 55. [CrossRef]
90. Lebeaux, D.; Chauhan, A.; Rendueles, O.; Beloin, C. From in vitro to in vivo models of bacterial biofilm-related infections. *Pathogens* **2013**, *2*, 288–356. [CrossRef]
91. Roder, H.L.; Sorensen, S.J.; Burmolle, M. Studying Bacterial multispecies biofilms: Where to start? *Trends Microbiol.* **2016**, *24*, 503–513. [CrossRef]
92. Rzhepishevska, O.; Limanska, N.; Galkin, M.; Lacoma, A.; Lundquist, M.; Sokol, D.; Hakobyan, S.; Sjostedt, A.; Prat, C.; Ramstedt, M. Characterization of clinically relevant model bacterial strains of *Pseudomonas aeruginosa* for anti-biofilm testing of materials. *Acta Biomater.* **2018**, *76*, 99–107. [CrossRef]
93. Eydallin, G.; Ryall, B.; Maharjan, R.; Ferenci, T. The nature of laboratory domestication changes in freshly isolated *Escherichia coli* strains. *Environ. Microbiol.* **2014**, *16*, 813–828. [CrossRef]
94. Elias, S.; Banin, E. Multi-species biofilms: Living with friendly neighbors. *FEMS Microbiol. Rev.* **2012**, *36*, 990–1004. [CrossRef]
95. Liu, W.Z.; Roder, H.L.; Madsen, J.S.; Bjarnsholt, T.; Sorensen, S.J.; Burmolle, M. Interspecific bacterial interactions are reflected in multispecies biofilm spatial organization. *Front. Microbiol.* **2016**, *7*, 1366. [CrossRef]
96. Tay, W.H.; Chong, K.K.L.; Kline, K.A. Polymicrobial-host interactions during infection. *J. Mol. Biol.* **2016**, *428*, 3355–3371. [CrossRef]
97. Parijs, I.; Steenackers, H.P. Competitive inter-species interactions underlie the increased antimicrobial tolerance in multispecies brewery biofilms. *ISME J.* **2018**, *12*, 2061–2075. [CrossRef]
98. Tan, C.H.; Lee, K.W.K.; Burmolle, M.; Kjelleberg, S.; Rice, S.A. All together now: Experimental multispecies biofilm model systems. *Environ. Microbiol.* **2017**, *19*, 42–53. [CrossRef]
99. Zhou, C.; Wu, Y.; Thappeta, K.R.V.; Subramanian, J.T.L.; Pranantyo, D.; Kang, E.T.; Duan, H.W.; Kline, K.; Chan-Park, M.B. In vivo anti-biofilm and anti-bacterial non-leachable coating thermally polymerized on cylindrical catheter. *ACS Appl. Mater. Interfaces* **2017**, *9*, 36269–36280. [CrossRef]
100. Albuquerque, M.T.P.; Nagata, J.; Bottino, M.C. Antimicrobial efficacy of triple antibiotic-eluting polymer nanofibers against multispecies biofilm. *Acta Biomater.* **2017**, *43*, S51–S56. [CrossRef]
101. Cossu, A.; Si, Y.; Sun, G.; Nitin, N. Antibiofilm effect of poly(vinyl alcohol-co-ethylene) halamine film against *Listeria innocua* and *Escherichia coli* O157:H7. *Appl. Environ. Microbiol.* **2017**, *83*, e00975-17. [CrossRef]
102. Kommerein, N.; Stumpp, S.N.; Musken, M.; Ehlert, N.; Winkel, A.; Haussler, S.; Behrens, P.; Buettner, F.F.R.; Stiesch, M. An oral multispecies biofilm model for high content screening applications. *PLoS ONE* **2017**, *12*, e0173973. [CrossRef]
103. Roeselers, G.; Zippel, B.; Staal, M.; van Loosdrecht, M.; Muyzer, G. On the reproducibility of microcosm experiments-different community composition in parallel phototrophic biofilm microcosms. *FEMS Microbiol. Ecol.* **2006**, *58*, 169–178. [CrossRef]

104. American Society for Testing and Materials. *ASTM E2799-17. Standard Test Method for Testing Disinfectant Efficacy Against Pseudomonas Aeruginosa Biofilm Using the MBEC Assay*; ASTM International: West Conshohocken, PA, USA, 2017.
105. American Society for Testing and Materials. *ASTM E2562-17. Standard Test Method for Quantification of Pseudomonas Aeruginosa Biofilm Grown with High Shear and Continuous Flow Using CDC Biofilm Reactor*; ASTM International: West Conshohocken, PA, USA, 2017.
106. American Society for Testing and Materials. *ASTM E2871-19. Standard Test Method for Determining Disinfectant Efficacy Against Biofilm Grown in the CDC Biofilm Reactor Using the Single Tube Method*; ASTM International: West Conshohocken, PA, USA, 2019.
107. American Society for Testing and Materials. *ASTM E2196-17. Standard Test Method for Quantification of Pseudomonas Aeruginosa Biofilm Grown with Medium Shear and Continuous Flow Using Rotating Disk Reactor*; ASTM International: West Conshohocken, PA, USA, 2017.
108. American Society for Testing and Materials. *ASTM E2647-13. Standard Test Method for Quantification of Pseudomonas Aeruginosa Biofilm Grown Using Drip Flow Biofilm Reactor with Low Shear and Continuous Flow*; ASTM International: West Conshohocken, PA, USA, 2013.
109. Merritt, J.H.; Kadouri, D.E.; O'Toole, G.A. Growing and analyzing static biofilms. *Curr. Protoc. Microbiol.* **2005**, *1*, 1B.1.1–1B.1.17. [CrossRef]
110. O'Toole, G.A. Microtiter dish biofilm formation assay. *J. Vis. Exp.* **2011**, *47*, 2437. [CrossRef]
111. Lin, M.H.; Chang, F.R.; Hua, M.Y.; Wu, Y.C.; Liu, S.T. Inhibitory effects of 1,2,3,4,6-penta-O-galloyl-beta-D-glucopyranose on biofilm formation by *Staphylococcus aureus*. *Antimicrob. Agents Chemother.* **2011**, *55*, 1021–1027. [CrossRef]
112. Swartjes, J.; Das, T.; Sharifi, S.; Subbiahdoss, G.; Sharma, P.K.; Krom, B.P.; Busscher, H.J.; van der Mei, H.C. A Functional DNase I coating to prevent adhesion of bacteria and the formation of biofilm. *Adv. Funct. Mater.* **2013**, *23*, 2843–2849. [CrossRef]
113. Salta, M.; Dennington, S.P.; Wharton, J.A. Biofilm inhibition by novel natural product- and biocide-containing coatings using high-throughput screening. *Int. J. Mol. Sci.* **2018**, *19*, 1434. [CrossRef]
114. Ceri, H.; Olson, M.E.; Stremick, C.; Read, R.R.; Morck, D.; Buret, A. The Calgary biofilm device: New technology for rapid determination of antibiotic susceptibilities of bacterial biofilms. *J. Clin. Microbiol. Infect.* **1999**, *37*, 1771–1776.
115. Franklin, M.J.; Chang, C.; Akiyama, T.; Bothner, B. New Technologies for studying biofilms. *Microbiol. Spectr.* **2015**, *3*. [CrossRef]
116. Harrison, J.J.; Ceri, H.; Yerly, J.; Stremick, C.A.; Hu, Y.P.; Martinuzzi, R.; Turner, R.J. The use of microscopy and three-dimensional visualization to evaluate the structure of microbial biofilms cultivated in the Calgary Biofilm Device. *Biol. Proced. Online* **2006**, *8*, 194–215. [CrossRef] [PubMed]
117. Olivares, E.; Badel-Berchoux, S.; Provot, C.; Jaulhac, B.; Prevost, G.; Bernardi, T.; Jehl, F. The biofilm ring test: A rapid method for routine analysis of *Pseudomonas aeruginosa* biofilm formation kinetics. *J. Clin. Microbiol.* **2016**, *54*, 657–661. [CrossRef] [PubMed]
118. Magana, M.; Sereti, C.; Ioannidis, A.; Mitchell, C.A.; Ball, A.R.; Magiorkinis, E.; Chatzipanagiotou, S.; Hamblin, M.R.; Hadjifrangiskou, M.; Tegos, G.P. Options and limitations in clinical investigation of bacterial biofilms. *Clin. Microbiol. Rev.* **2018**, *31*, e00084-16. [CrossRef] [PubMed]
119. Stadelmaier, H.H. Magnetic properties of materials. *Mater Sci. Eng. A Struct. Mater.* **2000**, *287*, 138–145. [CrossRef]
120. Junka, A.F.; Janczura, A.; Smutnicka, D.; Maczynska, B.; Secewicz, A.; Nowicka, J.; Bartoszewicz, M.; Gosciniak, G. Use of the real time xCelligence system for purposes of medical microbiology. *Pol. J. Microbiol.* **2012**, *61*, 191–197. [PubMed]
121. Gutierrez, D.; Hidalgo-Cantabrana, C.; Rodriguez, A.; Garcia, P.; Ruas-Madiedo, P. Monitoring in real time the formation and removal of biofilms from clinical related pathogens using an impedance-based technology. *PLoS ONE* **2016**, *11*, e0163966. [CrossRef] [PubMed]
122. Ferrer, M.D.; Rodriguez, J.C.; Alvarez, L.; Artacho, A.; Royo, G.; Mira, A. Effect of antibiotics on biofilm inhibition and induction measured by real-time cell analysis. *J. Appl. Microbiol.* **2017**, *122*, 640–650. [CrossRef] [PubMed]

123. Gutierrez, D.; Fernandez, L.; Martinez, B.; Ruas-Madiedo, P.; Garcia, P.; Rodriguez, A. Real-Time assessment of *Staphylococcus aureus* biofilm disruption by phage-derived proteins. *Front. Microbiol.* **2017**, *8*, 1632. [CrossRef]
124. Aggas, J.R.; Harrell, W.; Lutkenhaus, J.; Guiseppi-Elie, A. Metal-polymer interface influences apparent electrical properties of nano-structured polyaniline films. *Nanoscale* **2018**, *10*, 672–682. [CrossRef]
125. Wu, C.C.; Lin, C.T.; Wu, C.Y.; Peng, W.S.; Lee, M.J.; Tsai, Y.C. Inhibitory effect of *Lactobacillus salivarius* on *Streptococcus mutans* biofilm formation. *Mol. Oral Microbiol.* **2015**, *30*, 16–26. [CrossRef]
126. Wang, Z.L.; Xiang, Q.Q.; Yang, T.; Li, L.Q.; Yang, J.L.; Li, H.G.; He, Y.; Zhang, Y.H.; Lu, Q.; Yu, J.L. Autoinducer-2 of *Streptococcus mitis* as a target molecule to inhibit pathogenic multi-species biofilm formation in vitro and in an endotracheal intubation rat model. *Front. Microbiol.* **2016**, *7*, 88. [CrossRef] [PubMed]
127. Powell, L.C.; Pritchard, M.F.; Ferguson, E.L.; Powell, K.A.; Patel, S.U.; Rye, P.D.; Sakellakou, S.M.; Buurma, N.J.; Brilliant, C.D.; Copping, J.M.; et al. Targeted disruption of the extracellular polymeric network of *Pseudomonas aeruginosa* biofilms by alginate oligosaccharides. *Npj Biofilms Microbiomes* **2018**, *4*, 13. [CrossRef] [PubMed]
128. Kim, B.Y.; Thyiam, G.; Kang, J.E.; Lee, S.H.; Park, S.H.; Kim, J.S.; Abraham, M. Development of an *Escherichia coli* biofilm model on transwell. *Korean J. Clin. Lab. Sci.* **2012**, *44*, 112–117. [CrossRef]
129. Standar, K.; Kreikemeyer, B.; Redanz, S.; Munter, W.L.; Laue, M.; Podbielski, A. Setup of an in vitro test system for basic studies on biofilm behavior of mixed-species cultures with dental and periodontal pathogens. *Plos ONE* **2010**, *5*, e13135. [CrossRef] [PubMed]
130. Peterson, S.B.; Irie, Y.; Borlee, B.R.; Murakami, K.; Harrison, J.J.; Colvin, K.M.; Parsek, M.R. Different Methods for culturing biofilms in vitro. In *Biofilm Infections*; Bjarnsholt, T., Jensen, P., Moser, C., Høiby, N., Eds.; Springer: New York, NY, USA, 2011; pp. 251–266, ISBN 978-1-4419-6084-9.
131. Tran, P.L.; Hammond, A.A.; Mosley, T.; Cortez, J.; Gray, T.; Colmer-Hamood, J.A.; Shashtri, M.; Spallholz, J.E.; Hamood, A.N.; Reid, T.W. Organoselenium coating on cellulose inhibits the formation of biofilms by *Pseudomonas aeruginosa* and *Staphylococcus aureus*. *Appl. Environ. Microbiol.* **2009**, *75*, 3586–3592. [CrossRef] [PubMed]
132. Bakker, D.P.; van der Mats, A.; Verkerke, G.J.; Busscher, H.J.; van der Mei, H.C. Comparison of velocity profiles for different flow chamber designs used in studies of microbial adhesion to surfaces. *Appl. Environ. Microbiol.* **2003**, *69*, 6280–6287. [CrossRef]
133. Goeres, D.M.; Loetterle, L.R.; Hamilton, M.A.; Murga, R.; Kirby, D.W.; Donlan, R.M. Statistical assessment of a laboratory method for growing biofilms. *Microbiology* **2005**, *151*, 757–762. [CrossRef]
134. Gomes, I.B.; Meireles, A.; Goncalves, A.L.; Goeres, D.M.; Sjollema, J.; Simoes, L.C.; Simoes, M. Standardized reactors for the study of medical biofilms: A review of the principles and latest modifications. *Crit. Rev. Biotechnol.* **2018**, *38*, 657–670. [CrossRef]
135. Schwartz, K.; Stephenson, R.; Hernandez, M.; Jambang, N.; Boles, B.R. The use of drip flow and rotating disk reactors for *Staphylococcus aureus* biofilm analysis. *J. Vis. Exp.* **2010**, *46*, 2470. [CrossRef]
136. Sebestyen, P.; Blanken, W.; Bacsa, I.; Toth, G.; Martin, A.; Bhaiji, T.; Dergez, A.; Kesseru, P.; Koos, A.; Kiss, I. Upscale of a laboratory rotating disk biofilm reactor and evaluation of its performance over a half-year operation period in outdoor conditions. *Algal Res.* **2016**, *18*, 266–272. [CrossRef]
137. Linton, C.J.; Sherriff, A.; Millar, M.R. Use of a modified Robbins device to directly compare the adhesion of *Staphylococcus epidermidis* RP62A to surfaces. *J. Appl. Microbiol.* **1999**, *86*, 194–202. [CrossRef] [PubMed]
138. McCoy, W.F.; Bryers, J.D.; Robbins, J.; Costerton, J.W. Observations of fouling biofilm formation. *Can. J. Microbiol.* **1981**, *27*, 910–917. [CrossRef] [PubMed]
139. Oosterhof, J.J.H.; Buijssen, K.; Busscher, H.J.; van der Laan, B.; van der Mei, H.C. Effects of quaternary ammonium silane coatings on mixed fungal and bacterial biofilms on tracheoesophageal shunt prostheses. *Appl. Environ. Microbiol.* **2006**, *72*, 3673–3677. [CrossRef] [PubMed]
140. Ramage, G.; Wickes, B.L.; Lopez-Ribot, J.L. A seed and feed model for the formation of Candida albicans biofilms under flow conditions using an improved modified Robbins device. *Rev. Iberoam. Micol.* **2008**, *25*, 37–40. [CrossRef]
141. Ginige, M.P.; Garbin, S.; Wylie, J.; Krishna, K.C.B. Effectiveness of devices to monitor biofouling and metals deposition on plumbing materials exposed to a full-scale drinking water distribution system. *PLoS ONE* **2017**, *12*, e0169140. [CrossRef] [PubMed]
142. Cai, W.Y.; Wu, J.F.; Xi, C.W.; Meyerhoff, M.E. Diazeniumdiolate-doped poly(lactic-co-glycolic acid)-based nitric oxide releasing films as antibiofilm coatings. *Biomaterials* **2012**, *33*, 7933–7944. [CrossRef] [PubMed]

143. Li, Y.; Carrera, C.; Chen, R.; Li, J.; Lenton, P.; Rudney, J.D.; Jones, R.S.; Aparicio, C.; Fok, A. Degradation in the dentin-composite interface subjected to multi-species biofilm challenges. *Acta Biomater.* **2014**, *10*, 375–383. [CrossRef]
144. Pitts, B.; Willse, A.; McFeters, G.A.; Hamilton, M.A.; Zelver, N.; Stewart, P.S. A repeatable laboratory method for testing the efficacy of biocides against toilet bowl biofilms. *J. Appl. Microbiol.* **2001**, *91*, 110–117. [CrossRef]
145. Cotter, J.J.; O'Gara, J.P.; Stewart, P.S.; Pitts, B.; Casey, E. Characterization of a modified rotating disk reactor for the cultivation of *Staphylococcus epidermidis* biofilm. *J. Appl. Microbiol.* **2010**, *109*, 2105–2117. [CrossRef]
146. Barry, D.M.; McGrath, P.B. Rotation disk process to assess the influence of metals and voltage on the growth of biofilm. *Materials* **2016**, *9*, 568. [CrossRef]
147. Gomes, I.B.; Simoes, M.; Simoes, L.C. An overview on the reactors to study drinking water biofilms. *Water Res.* **2014**, *62*, 63–87. [CrossRef] [PubMed]
148. Pintar, K.D.M.; Slawson, R.M. Effect of temperature and disinfection strategies on ammonia-oxidizing bacteria in a bench-scale drinking water distribution system. *Water Res.* **2003**, *37*, 1805–1817. [CrossRef]
149. Ndiongue, S.; Huck, P.M.; Slawson, R.M. Effects of temperature and biodegradable organic matter on control of biofilms by free chlorine in a model drinking water distribution system. *Water Res.* **2005**, *39*, 953–964. [CrossRef] [PubMed]
150. Jang, H.J.; Choi, Y.J.; Ka, J.O. Effects of diverse water pipe materials on bacterial communities and water quality in the annular reactor. *J. Microbiol. Biotechnol.* **2011**, *21*, 115–123. [CrossRef] [PubMed]
151. Goeres, D.M.; Hamilton, M.A.; Beck, N.A.; Buckingham-Meyer, K.; Hilyard, J.D.; Loetterle, L.R.; Lorenz, L.A.; Walker, D.K.; Stewart, P.S. A method for growing a biofilm under low shear at the air-liquid interface using the drip flow biofilm reactor. *Nat. Protoc.* **2009**, *4*, 783–788. [CrossRef]
152. Sawant, S.N.; Selvaraj, V.; Prabhawathi, V.; Doble, M. Antibiofilm properties of silver and gold incorporated PU, PCLm, PC and PMMA nanocomposites under two shear conditions. *PLoS ONE* **2013**, *8*, e63311. [CrossRef] [PubMed]
153. Goodwin, D.G.; Xia, Z.; Gordon, T.B.; Gao, C.; Bouwer, E.J.; Fairbrother, D.H. Biofilm development on carbon nanotube/polymer nanocomposites. *Environ. Sci. Nano* **2016**, *3*, 545–558. [CrossRef]
154. Salli, K.M.; Ouwehand, A.C. The use of in vitro model systems to study dental biofilms associated with caries: A short review. *J. Oral Microbiol.* **2015**, *7*, 26149. [CrossRef]
155. Jaramillo, D.E.; Arriola, A.; Safavi, K.; de Paz, L.E.C. Decreased bacterial adherence and biofilm growth on surfaces coated with a solution of benzalkonium chloride. *J. Endod.* **2012**, *38*, 821–825. [CrossRef]
156. Francolini, I.; Norris, P.; Piozzi, A.; Donelli, G.; Stoodley, P. Usnic acid, a natural antimicrobial agent able to inhibit bacterial biofilm formation on polymer surfaces. *Antimicrob. Agents Chemother.* **2004**, *48*, 4360–4365. [CrossRef]
157. Fabbri, S.; Dennington, S.P.; Price, C.; Stoodley, P.; Longyear, J. A marine biofilm flow cell for in situ screening marine fouling control coatings using optical coherence tomography. *Ocean. Eng.* **2018**, *170*, 321–328. [CrossRef]
158. Tremblay, Y.D.N.; Vogeleer, P.; Jacques, M.; Harel, J. High-throughput microfluidic method to study biofilm formation and host-pathogen interactions in pathogenic *Escherichia coli*. *Appl. Environ. Microbiol.* **2015**, *81*, 2827–2840. [CrossRef]
159. Benoit, M.R.; Conant, C.G.; Ionescu-Zanetti, C.; Schwartz, M.; Matin, A. New device for high-throughput viability screening of flow biofilms. *Appl. Environ. Microbiol.* **2010**, *76*, 4136–4142. [CrossRef]
160. Moormeier, D.E.; Endres, J.L.; Mann, E.E.; Sadykov, M.R.; Horswill, A.R.; Rice, K.C.; Fey, P.D.; Bayles, K.W. Use of microfluidic technology to analyze gene expression during *Staphylococcus aureus* biofilm formation reveals distinct physiological niches. *Appl. Environ. Microbiol.* **2013**, *79*, 3413–3424. [CrossRef]
161. Abdulkareem, E.H.; Memarzadeh, K.; Allaker, R.P.; Huang, J.; Pratten, J.; Spratt, D. Anti-biofilm activity of zinc oxide and hydroxyapatite nanoparticles as dental implant coating materials. *J. Dent.* **2015**, *43*, 1462–1469. [CrossRef]
162. Li, F.; Weir, M.D.; Fouad, A.F.; Xu, H.H.K. Effect of salivary pellicle on antibacterial activity of novel antibacterial dental adhesives using a dental plaque microcosm biofilm model. *Dent. Mater.* **2014**, *30*, 182–191. [CrossRef]
163. Wood, T.K.; Knabel, S.J.; Kwan, B.W. Bacterial persister cell formation and dormancy. *Appl. Environ. Microbiol.* **2013**, *79*, 7116–7121. [CrossRef]

164. Hooijmans, C.M.; Abdin, T.A.; Alaerts, G.J. Quantification of viable biomass in biofilm reactors by extractable lipid phosphate. *Appl. Microbiol. Biotechnol.* **1995**, *43*, 781–785. [CrossRef]
165. Quideau, S.A.; McIntosh, A.C.S.; Norris, C.E.; Lloret, E.; Swallow, M.J.B.; Hannam, K. Extraction and analysis of microbial phospholipid fatty acids in soils. *J. Vis. Exp.* **2016**, *114*, 54360. [CrossRef]
166. Willers, C.; van Rensburg, P.J.J.; Claassens, S. Phospholipid fatty acid profiling of microbial communities-a review of interpretations and recent applications. *J. Appl. Microbiol.* **2015**, *119*, 1207–1218. [CrossRef]
167. Gehron, M.J.; White, D.C. Sensitive assay of phospholipid glycerol in environmental sample. *J. Microbiol. Met.* **1983**, *1*, 23–32. [CrossRef]
168. Oursel, D.; Loutelier-Bourhis, C.; Orange, N.; Chevalier, S.; Norris, V.; Lange, C.M. Identification and relative quantification of fatty acids in *Escherichia coli* membranes by gas chromatography/mass spectrometry. *Rapid Commun. Mass Spectrom.* **2007**, *21*, 3229–3233. [CrossRef]
169. Li, L.; Han, J.J.; Wang, Z.P.; Liu, J.A.; Wei, J.C.; Xiong, S.X.; Zhao, Z.W. Mass spectrometry methodology in lipid analysis. *Int. J. Mol. Sci.* **2014**, *15*, 10492–10507. [CrossRef]
170. Jain, S.; Caforio, A.; Driessen, A.J.M. Biosynthesis of archaeal membrane ether lipids. *Front. Microbiol.* **2014**, *5*, 641. [CrossRef]
171. Gors, S.; Schumann, R.; Haubner, N.; Karsten, U. Fungal and algal biomass in biofilms on artificial surfaces quantified by ergosterol and chlorophyll a as biomarkers. *Int. Biodeterior. Biodegrad.* **2007**, *60*, 50–59. [CrossRef]
172. Hippelein, M.; Rugamer, M. Ergosterol as an indicator of mould growth on building materials. *Int. J. Hyg. Environ. Health* **2004**, *207*, 379–385. [CrossRef]
173. Ng, H.E.; Raj, S.S.A.; Wong, S.H.; Tey, D.; Tan, H.M. Estimation of fungal growth using the ergosterol assay: A rapid tool in assessing the microbiological status of grains and feeds. *Lett. Appl. Microbiol.* **2008**, *46*, 113–118. [CrossRef]
174. Pantanella, F.; Valenti, P.; Natalizi, T.; Passeri, D.; Berlutti, F. Analytical techniques to study microbial biofilm on abiotic surfaces: Pros and cons of the main techniques currently in use. *Ann. Ig.* **2013**, *25*, 31–42. [CrossRef]
175. Welch, K.; Cai, Y.; Strømme, M. A method for quantitative determination of biofilm viability. *J. Funct. Biomater.* **2012**, *3*, 418–431. [CrossRef]
176. Trafny, E.A.; Lewandowski, R.; Zawistowska-Marciniak, I.; Stepinska, M. Use of MTT assay for determination of the biofilm formation capacity of microorganisms in metalworking fluids. *World J. Microbiol. Biotechnol.* **2013**, *29*, 1635–1643. [CrossRef] [PubMed]
177. Nante, N.; Ceriale, E.; Messina, G.; Lenzi, D.; Manzi, P. Effectiveness of ATP bioluminescence to assess hospital cleaning: A review. *J. Prev. Med. Hyg.* **2017**, *58*, E177–E183. [PubMed]
178. AlLuhaybi, K.A.R.; Alghaith, G.Y.; Moneib, N.A.; Yassien, M.A.M. Generation of recombinant bioluminescent *Escherichia coli* for quantitative determination of bacterial adhesion. *Pak. J. Pharm. Sci.* **2015**, *28*, 1301–1306. [PubMed]
179. Ivanova, E.P.; Alexeeva, Y.V.; Pham, D.K.; Wright, J.P.; Nicolau, D.V. ATP level variations in heterotrophic bacteria during attachment on hydrophilic and hydrophobic surfaces. *Int. Microbiol.* **2006**, *9*, 37–46. [PubMed]
180. Braissant, O.; Wirz, D.; Gopfert, B.; Daniels, A.U. Use of isothermal microcalorimetry to monitor microbial activities. *FEMS Microbiol. Lett.* **2010**, *303*, 1–8. [CrossRef] [PubMed]
181. Solokhina, A.; Bruckner, D.; Bonkat, G.; Braissant, O. Metabolic activity of mature biofilms of *Mycobacterium tuberculosis* and other non-tuberculous mycobacteria. *Sci. Rep.* **2017**, *7*, 9225. [CrossRef]
182. Said, J.; Walker, M.; Parsons, D.; Stapleton, P.; Beezer, A.E.; Gaisford, S. Development of a flow system for studying biofilm formation on medical devices with microcalorimetry. *Methods* **2015**, *76*, 35–40. [CrossRef] [PubMed]
183. Brueckner, D.; Roesti, D.; Zuber, U.G.; Schmidt, R.; Kraehenbuehl, S.; Bonkat, G.; Braissant, O. Comparison of tunable diode laser absorption spectroscopy and isothermal micro-calorimetry for non-invasive detection of microbial growth in media fills. *Sci. Rep.* **2016**, *6*, 27894. [CrossRef]
184. Wilson, C.; Lukowicz, R.; Merchant, S.; Valquier-Flynn, H.; Caballero, J.; Sandoval, J.; Okuom, M.; Huber, C.; Brooks, T.D.; Wilson, E.; et al. Quantitative and qualitative assessment methods for biofilm growth: A mini-review. *Res. Rev. J. Eng. Technol.* **2017**, *6*.

185. Bogachev, M.I.; Volkov, V.Y.; Markelov, O.A.; Trizna, E.Y.; Baydamshina, D.R.; Melnikov, V.; Murtazina, R.R.; Zelenikhin, P.V.; Sharafutdinov, I.S.; Kayumov, A.R. Fast and simple tool for the quantification of biofilm-embedded cells sub-populations from fluorescent microscopic images. *PLoS ONE* **2018**, *13*, e0193267. [CrossRef]
186. Shi, L.; Gunther, S.; Hubschmann, T.; Wick, L.Y.; Harms, H.; Muller, S. Limits of propidium iodide as a cell viability indicator for environmental bacteria. *Cytom. A* **2007**, *71A*, 592–598. [CrossRef]
187. Netuschil, L.; Auschill, T.M.; Sculean, A.; Arweiler, N.B. Confusion over live/dead stainings for the detection of vital microorganisms in oral biofilms—Which stain is suitable? *BMC Oral Health* **2014**, *14*, 2. [CrossRef] [PubMed]
188. Stiefel, P.; Schmidt-Emrich, S.; Maniura-Weber, K.; Ren, Q. Critical aspects of using bacterial cell viability assays with the fluorophores SYTO9 and propidium iodide. *BMC Microbiol.* **2015**, *15*, 36. [CrossRef] [PubMed]
189. Dobor, J.; Varga, M.; Zaray, G. Biofilm controlled sorption of selected acidic drugs on river sediments characterized by different organic carbon content. *Chemosphere* **2012**, *87*, 105–110. [CrossRef] [PubMed]
190. Bradford, M.M. A rapid and sensitive method for the quantitation of microgram quantities of protein utilizing the principle of protein-dye binding. *Anal. Biochem.* **1976**, *72*, 248–254. [CrossRef]
191. Lowry, O.H.; Rosebrough, N.J.; Farr, A.L.; Randall, R.J. Protein measurement with the folin phenol reagent. *J. Biol. Chem.* **1951**, *193*, 265–275.
192. Smith, P.K.; Krohn, R.I.; Hermanson, G.T.; Mallia, A.K.; Gartner, F.H.; Provenzano, M.D.; Fujimoto, E.K.; Goeke, N.M.; Olson, B.J.; Klenk, D.C. Measurement of protein using bicinchoninic acid. *Anal. Biochem.* **1985**, *150*, 76–85. [CrossRef]
193. Jesus, B.; Perkins, R.G.; Mendes, C.R.; Brotas, V.; Paterson, D.M. Chlorophyll fluorescence as a proxy for microphytobenthic biomass: Alternatives to the current methodology. *Mar. Biol.* **2006**, *150*, 17–28. [CrossRef]
194. Sanmartin, P.; Aira, N.; Devesa-Rey, R.; Silva, B.; Prieto, B. Relationship between color and pigment production in two stone biofilm-forming cyanobacteria (*Nostoc* sp PCC 9104 and *Nostoc* sp PCC 9025). *Biofouling* **2010**, *26*, 499–509. [CrossRef]
195. Sendersky, E.; Simkovsky, R.; Golden, S.S.; Schwarz, R. Quantification of chlorophyll as a proxy for biofilm formation in the cyanobacterium *Synechococcus Elongatus*. *Bio-Protoc.* **2017**, *7*, 14. [CrossRef]
196. Chamizo, S.; Adessi, A.; Mugnai, G.; Simiani, A.; De Philippis, R. Soil Type and Cyanobacteria species influence the macromolecular and chemical characteristics of the polysaccharidic matrix in induced biocrusts. *Microb. Ecol.* **2018**, *78*, 482–493. [CrossRef]
197. Fernandez-Silva, I.; Sanmartin, P.; Silva, B.; Moldes, A.; Prieto, B. Quantification of phototrophic biomass on rocks: Optimization of chlorophyll-a extraction by response surface methodology. *J. Ind. Microbiol. Biotechnol.* **2011**, *38*, 179–188. [CrossRef]
198. Vazquez-Nion, D.; Silva, B.; Prieto, B. Bioreceptivity index for granitic rocks used as construction material. *Sci. Total Environ.* **2018**, *633*, 112–121. [CrossRef]
199. Vazquez-Nion, D.; Silva, B.; Prieto, B. Influence of the properties of granitic rocks on their bioreceptivity to subaerial phototrophic biofilms. *Sci. Total Environ.* **2018**, *610*, 44–54. [CrossRef]
200. Dalwai, F.; Spratt, D.A.; Pratten, J. Use of quantitative PCR and culture methods to characterize ecological flux in bacterial biofilms. *J. Clin. Microbiol.* **2007**, *45*, 3072–3076. [CrossRef]
201. Alvarez, G.; Gonzalez, M.; Isabal, S.; Blanc, V.; Leon, R. Method to quantify live and dead cells in multi-species oral biofilm by real-time PCR with propidium monoazide. *Amb. Express* **2013**, *3*, 1. [CrossRef]
202. Taylor, M.J.; Bentham, R.H.; Ross, K.E. Limitations of using propidium monoazide with qpcr to discriminate between live and dead *Legionella* in biofilm samples. *Microbiol. Insights* **2014**, *7*, 15–24. [CrossRef]
203. Soto-Munoz, L.; Teixido, N.; Usall, J.; Vinas, I.; Crespo-Sempere, A.; Torres, R. Development of PMA real-time PCR method to quantify viable cells of Pantoea agglomerans CPA-2, an antagonist to control the major postharvest diseases on oranges. *Int. J. Food Microbiol.* **2014**, *180*, 49–55. [CrossRef]
204. Ambriz-Aviña, V.; Contreras-Garduño, J.A.; Pedraza-Reyes, M. Applications of flow cytometry to characterize bacterial physiological responses. *Biomed. Res. Int.* **2014**, *2014*, 461941. [CrossRef]
205. Kerstens, M.; Boulet, G.; Van Kerckhoven, M.; Clais, S.; Lanckacker, E.; Delputte, P.; Maes, L.; Cos, P. A flow cytometric approach to quantify biofilms. *Folia Microbiol.* **2015**, *60*, 335–342. [CrossRef]
206. Bakke, R.; Kommedal, R.; Kalvenes, S. Quantification of biofilm accumulation by an optical approach. *J. Microbiol. Methods* **2001**, *44*, 13–26. [CrossRef]

207. Stiefel, P.; Rosenberg, U.; Schneider, J.; Mauerhofer, S.; Maniura-Weber, K.; Ren, Q. Is biofilm removal properly assessed? Comparison of different quantification methods in a 96-well plate system. *Appl. Microbiol. Biotechnol.* **2016**, *100*, 4135–4145. [CrossRef]
208. O'Toole, G.A.; Kolter, R. Initiation of biofilm formation in *Pseudomonas fluorescens* WCS365 proceeds via multiple, convergent signalling pathways: A genetic analysis. *Mol. Microbiol.* **1998**, *28*, 449–461. [CrossRef]
209. Young, M.E.; Wakefield, R.; Urquhart, D.C.M.; Nicholson, K.; Tonge, K. Assesment in a field setting of the efficacy of various biocides on sandstone. In *Int. Coll Methods of Evaluating Products for the Conservation of Porous Building Materials in Monuments*; ICCROM: Rome, Italy, 1995; pp. 93–99, ISBN 92-9077-131-3.
210. Prieto, B.; Rivas, T.; Silva, B. Rapid quantification of phototrophic microorganisms and their physiological state through their colour. *Biofouling* **2002**, *18*, 229–236. [CrossRef]
211. Vazquez-Nion, D.; Sanmartin, P.; Silva, B.; Prieto, B. Reliability of color measurements for monitoring pigment content in a biofilm-forming cyanobacterium. *Int. Biodeterior. Biodegrad.* **2013**, *84*, 220–226. [CrossRef]
212. Sanmartin, P.; Villa, F.; Polo, A.; Silva, B.; Prieto, B.; Cappitelli, F. Rapid evaluation of three biocide treatments against the cyanobacterium *Nostoc* sp PCC 9104 by color changes. *Ann. Microbiol.* **2015**, *65*, 1153–1158. [CrossRef]
213. Sanmartin, P.; Vazquez-Nion, D.; Arines, J.; Cabo-Dominguez, L.; Prieto, B. Controlling growth and colour of phototrophs by using simple and inexpensive coloured lighting: A preliminary study in the Light4Heritage project towards future strategies for outdoor illumination. *Int. Biodeterior. Biodegrad.* **2017**, *122*, 107–115. [CrossRef]
214. Prieto, B.; Vazquez-Nion, D.; Silva, B.; Sanmartin, P. Shaping colour changes in a biofilm-forming cyanobacterium by modifying the culture conditions. *Algal Res.* **2018**, *33*, 173–181. [CrossRef]
215. Fairchild, M.D. International Commission on Illumination. In *CIE 015:2018 Colorimetry*, 4th ed.; CIE Central Bureau: Vienna, Austria, 2018; p. 111, ISBN 978-3-902842-13-8.
216. Sanmartin, P.; Villa, F.; Silva, B.; Cappitelli, F.; Prieto, B. Color measurements as a reliable method for estimating chlorophyll degradation to phaeopigments. *Biodegradation* **2011**, *22*, 763–771. [CrossRef]
217. Di Martino, P. Extracellular polymeric substances, a key element in understanding biofilm phenotype. *Aims Microbiol.* **2018**, *4*, 274–288. [CrossRef]
218. Blanco, Y.; Rivas, L.A.; González-Toril, E.; Ruiz-Bermejo, M.; Moreno-Paz, M.; Parro, V.; Palacín, A.; Aguilera, Á.; Puente-Sánchez, F. Environmental parameters, and not phylogeny, determine the composition of extracellular polymeric substances in microbial mats from extreme environments. *Sci. Total Environ.* **2019**, *650*, 384–393. [CrossRef]
219. Jachlewski, S.; Jachlewski, W.D.; Linne, U.; Bräsen, C.; Wingender, J.; Siebers, B. Isolation of extracellular polymeric substances from biofilms of the thermoacidophilic archaeon *Sulfolobus acidocaldarius*. *Front. Bioeng. Biotechnol.* **2015**, *3*, 123. [CrossRef]
220. McSwain, B.S.; Irvine, R.L.; Hausner, M.; Wilderer, P.A. Composition and distribution of extracellular polymeric substances in aerobic flocs and granular sludge. *Appl. Environ. Microbiol.* **2005**, *71*, 1051–1057. [CrossRef]
221. Cho, J.; Hermanowicz, S.W.; Hur, J. Effects of experimental conditions on extraction yield of extracellular polymeric substances by cation exchange resin. *Sci. World J.* **2012**, *2012*, 751965. [CrossRef]
222. Rossi, F.; Mugnai, G.; De Philippis, R. Complex role of the polymeric matrix in biological soil crusts. *Plant Soil* **2018**, *429*, 19–34. [CrossRef]
223. Pan, X.L.; Liu, J.; Zhang, D.Y.; Chen, X.; Li, L.H.; Song, W.J.; Yang, J.Y. A comparison of five extraction methods for extracellular polymeric substances (EPS) from biofilm by using three-dimensional excitation-emission matrix (3DEEM) fluorescence spectroscopy. *Water Sa* **2010**, *36*, 111–116. [CrossRef]
224. Liu, H.; Fang, H.H.P. Extraction of extracellular polymeric substances (EPS) of sludges. *J. Biotechnol.* **2002**, *95*, 249–256. [CrossRef]
225. Villa, F.; Remelli, W.; Forlani, F.; Gambino, M.; Landini, P.; Cappitelli, F. Effects of chronic sub-lethal oxidative stress on biofilm formation by *Azotobacter vinelandii*. *Biofouling* **2012**, *28*, 823–833. [CrossRef]
226. Cattò, C.; Grazioso, G.; Dell'Orto, S.; Gelain, A.; Villa, S.; Marzano, V.; Vitali, A.; Villa, F.; Cappitelli, F.; Forlani, F. The response of *Escherichia coli* biofilm to salicylic acid. *Biofouling* **2017**, *33*, 235–251. [CrossRef]
227. Masuko, T.; Minami, A.; Iwasaki, N.; Majima, T.; Nishimura, S.I.; Lee, Y.C. Carbohydrate analysis by a phenol-sulfuric acid method in microplate format. *Anal. Biochem.* **2005**, *339*, 69–72. [CrossRef]

228. Nielsen, S.S. Total carbohydrate by phenol-sulfuric acid method. In *Food Analysis Laboratory Manual*; Springer: Boston, MA, USA, 2010; ISBN 978-1-4419-1462-0.
229. Ruhmann, B.; Schmid, J.; Sieber, V. Methods to identify the unexplored diversity of microbial exopolysaccharides. *Front. Microbiol.* **2015**, *6*, 565. [CrossRef]
230. Mojica, K.; Elsey, D.; Cooney, M.J. Quantitative analysis of biofilm EPS uronic acid content. *J. Microbiol. Methods* **2007**, *71*, 61–65. [CrossRef]
231. Khodse, V.B.; Bhosle, N.B. Differences in carbohydrate profiles in batch culture grown planktonic and biofilm cells of *Amphora rostrata* Wm. Sm. *Biofouling* **2010**, *26*, 527–537. [CrossRef]
232. Tielen, P.; Rosenau, F.; Wilhelm, S.; Jaeger, K.E.; Flemming, H.C.; Wingender, J. Extracellular enzymes affect biofilm formation of mucoid *Pseudomonas Aeruginosa*. *Microbiology* **2010**, *156*, 2239–2252. [CrossRef]
233. Blumenkr, N.; Asboehan, G. New method for quantitative-determination of uronic acids. *Anal. Biochem.* **1973**, *54*, 484–489. [CrossRef]
234. van den Hoogen, B.M.; van Weeren, P.R.; Lopes-Cardozo, M.; van Golde, L.M.G.; Barneveld, A.; van de Lest, C.H.A. A microtiter plate assay for the determination of uronic acids. *Anal. Biochem.* **1998**, *257*, 107–111. [CrossRef]
235. Wu, J.F.; Xi, C.W. Evaluation of different methods for extracting extracellular DNA from the biofilm matrix. *Appl. Environ. Microbiol.* **2009**, *75*, 5390–5395. [CrossRef]
236. Das, T.; Sehar, S.; Manefield, M. The roles of extracellular DNA in the structural integrity of extracellular polymeric substance and bacterial biofilm development. *Environ. Microbiol. Rep.* **2013**, *5*, 778–786. [CrossRef]
237. Steinberger, R.E.; Holden, P.A. Extracellular DNA in single- and multiple-species unsaturated biofilms. *Appl. Environ. Microbiol.* **2005**, *71*, 5404–5410. [CrossRef]
238. Tang, L.; Schramm, A.; Neu, T.R.; Revsbech, N.P.; Meyer, R.L. Extracellular DNA in adhesion and biofilm formation of four environmental isolates: A quantitative study. *FEMS Microbiol. Ecol.* **2013**, *86*, 394–403. [CrossRef]
239. Jiao, Y.Q.; Cody, G.D.; Harding, A.K.; Wilmes, P.; Schrenk, M.; Wheeler, K.E.; Banfield, J.F.; Thelen, M.P. Characterization of extracellular polymeric substances from acidophilic microbial biofilms. *Appl. Environ. Microbiol.* **2010**, *76*, 2916–2922. [CrossRef]
240. Nan, L.; Yang, K.; Ren, G.G. Anti-biofilm formation of a novel stainless steel against *Staphylococcus aureus*. *Mat. Sci. Eng. C* **2015**, *51*, 356–361. [CrossRef]
241. Kelestemur, S.; Avci, E.; Culha, M. Raman and surface-enhanced raman scattering for biofilm characterization. *Chemosensors* **2018**, *6*, 5. [CrossRef]
242. Ramirez-Mora, T.; Davila-Perez, C.; Torres-Mendez, F.; Valle-Bourrouet, G. Raman spectroscopic characterization of endodontic biofilm matrices. *J. Spectrosc.* **2019**, *2019*, 1307397. [CrossRef]
243. Chao, Y.Q.; Zhang, T. Surface-enhanced Raman scattering (SERS) revealing chemical variation during biofilm formation: From initial attachment to mature biofilm. *Anal. Bioanal. Chem.* **2012**, *404*, 1465–1475. [CrossRef]
244. Xu, H.C.; He, P.J.; Wang, G.Z.; Shao, L.M. Three-dimensional excitation emission matrix fluorescence spectroscopy and gel-permeating chromatography to characterize extracellular polymeric substances in aerobic granulation. *Water Sci. Technol.* **2010**, *61*, 2931–2942. [CrossRef]
245. Bales, P.M.; Renke, E.M.; May, S.L.; Shen, Y.; Nelson, D.C. Purification and characterization of biofilm-associated eps exopolysaccharides from ESKAPE organisms and other pathogens. *PLoS ONE* **2013**, *8*, e67950. [CrossRef]
246. Ruhmann, B.; Schmid, J.; Sieber, V. Fast carbohydrate analysis via liquid chromatography coupled with ultra violet and electrospray ionization ion trap detection in 96-well format. *J. Chromatogr. A* **2014**, *1350*, 44–50. [CrossRef]
247. Ramirez-Mora, T.; Retana-Lobo, C.; Valle-Bourrouet, G. Biochemical characterization of extracellular polymeric substances from endodontic biofilms. *PLoS ONE* **2018**, *13*, e0204081. [CrossRef]
248. Hasan, N.; Gopal, J.; Wu, H.F. Rapid, sensitive and direct analysis of exopolysaccharides from biofilm on aluminum surfaces exposed to sea water using MALDI-TOF MS. *J. Mass Spectrom.* **2011**, *46*, 1160–1167. [CrossRef]
249. Gonzalez-Gil, G.; Thomas, L.; Emwas, A.H.; Lens, P.N.; Saikaly, P.E. NMR and MALDI-TOF MS based characterization of exopolysaccharides in anaerobic microbial aggregates from full-scale reactors. *Sci. Rep.* **2015**, *5*, 14316. [CrossRef]

250. Yildiz, F.; Fong, J.; Sadovskaya, I.; Grard, T.; Vinogradov, E. Structural characterization of the extracellular polysaccharide from *Vibrio cholerae* O1 El-Tor. *PLoS ONE* **2014**, *9*, e86751. [CrossRef]
251. Neu, T.R.; Lawrence, J.R. Advanced techniques for in situ analysis of the biofilm matrix (structure, composition, dynamics) by means of laser scanning microscopy. *Methods Mol. Biol.* **2014**, *1147*, 43–64. [CrossRef]
252. Cowan, S.E.; Gilbert, E.; Liepmann, D.; Keasling, J.D. Commensal interactions in a dual-species biofilm exposed to mixed organic compounds. *Appl. Environ. Microbiol.* **2000**, *66*, 4481–4485. [CrossRef]
253. Chen, M.Y.; Lee, D.J.; Tay, J.H.; Show, K.Y. Staining of extracellular polymeric substances and cells in bioaggregates. *Appl. Microbiol. Biotechnol.* **2007**, *75*, 467–474. [CrossRef]
254. Berk, V.; Fong, J.C.N.; Dempsey, G.T.; Develioglu, O.N.; Zhuang, X.W.; Liphardt, J.; Yildiz, F.H.; Chu, S. Molecular architecture and assembly principles of *Vibrio cholerae* biofilms. *Science* **2012**, *337*, 236–239. [CrossRef]
255. Sportelli, M.C.; Tutuncu, E.; Picca, R.A.; Valentini, M.; Valentini, A.; Kranz, C.; Mizaikoff, B.; Barth, H.; Cioffi, N. Inhibiting, *P. Fluorescens* biofilms with fluoropolymer-embedded silver nanoparticles: An in-situ spectroscopic study. *Sci. Rep.* **2017**, *7*, 11870. [CrossRef]
256. Feng, J.; de la Fuente-Núñez, C.; Trimble, M.J.; Xu, J.; Hancock, R.E.; Lu, X. An in situ Raman spectroscopy-based microfluidic "lab-on-a-chip" platform for non-destructive and continuous characterization of Pseudomonas aeruginosa biofilms. *Chem. Commun.* **2015**, *51*, 8966–8969. [CrossRef]
257. Greuter, D.; Loy, A.; Horne, M.; Ratteil, T. probeBase-an online resource for rRNA-targeted oligonucleotide probes and primers: New features 2016. *Nucleic Acids Res.* **2016**, *44*, D586–D589. [CrossRef]
258. Schimak, M.P.; Kleiner, M.; Wetzel, S.; Liebeke, M.; Dubilier, N.; Fuchs, B.M. MiL-FISH: Multilabeled oligonucleotides for fluorescence in situ hybridization improve visualization of bacterial cells. *Appl. Environ. Microbiol.* **2016**, *82*, 62–70. [CrossRef]
259. Almeida, C.; Azevedo, N.F.; Santos, S.; Keevil, C.W.; Vieira, M.J. Discriminating multi-species populations in biofilms with peptide nucleic acid fluorescence in situ hybridization (PNA FISH). *PLoS ONE* **2011**, *6*, e14786. [CrossRef]
260. Azevedo, A.S.; Almeida, C.; Pereira, B.; Madureira, P.; Wengel, J.; Azevedo, N.F. Detection and discrimination of biofilm populations using locked nucleic acid/2'-O-methyl-RNA fluorescence in situ hybridization (LNA/2' OMe-FISH). *Biochem. Eng. J.* **2015**, *104*, 64–73. [CrossRef]
261. Kubota, K. CARD-FISH for environmental microorganisms: Technical advancement and future applications. *Microbes Environ.* **2013**, *28*, 3–12. [CrossRef]
262. Escudero, C.; Vera, M.; Oggerin, M.; Amils, R. Active microbial biofilms in deep poor porous continental subsurface rocks. *Sci. Rep.* **2018**, *8*, 1538. [CrossRef]
263. Stoecker, K.; Dorninger, C.; Daims, H.; Wagner, M. Double labeling of oligonucleotide probes for fluorescence in situ hybridization (DOPE-FISH) improves signal intensity and increases rRNA accessibility. *Appl. Environ. Microbiol.* **2010**, *76*, 922–926. [CrossRef]
264. Valm, A.M.; Oldenbourg, R.; Borisy, G.G. Multiplexed spectral imaging of 120 different fluorescent labels. *PLoS ONE* **2016**, *11*, e0158495. [CrossRef]
265. Valm, A.M.; Welch, J.L.M.; Borisy, G.G. CLASI-FISH: Principles of combinatorial labeling and spectral imaging. *Syst. Appl. Microbiol.* **2012**, *35*, 496–502. [CrossRef]
266. Congestri, R. FISH methods in phycology: Phototrophic biofilm and phytoplankton applications. *Plant Biosyst.* **2008**, *142*, 337–342. [CrossRef]
267. Musat, N.; Foster, R.; Vagner, T.; Adam, B.; Kuypers, M.M.M. Detecting metabolic activities in single cells, with emphasis on nanoSIMS. *FEMS Microbiol. Rev.* **2012**, *36*, 486–511. [CrossRef]
268. Li, T.; Wu, T.D.; Mazeas, L.; Toffin, L.; Guerquin-Kern, J.L.; Leblon, G.; Bouchez, T. Simultaneous analysis of microbial identity and function using NanoSIMS. *Environ. Microbiol.* **2008**, *10*, 580–588. [CrossRef]
269. Kniggendorf, A.K.; Nogueira, R.; Kelb, C.; Schadzek, P.; Meinhardt-Wollweber, M.; Ngezahayo, A.; Roth, B. Confocal Raman microscopy and fluorescent in situ hybridization-a complementary approach for biofilm analysis. *Chemosphere* **2016**, *161*, 112–118. [CrossRef]
270. Manti, A.; Boi, P.; Amalfitano, S.; Puddu, A.; Papa, S. Experimental improvements in combining CARD-FISH and flow cytometry for bacterial cell quantification. *J. Microbiol. Methods* **2011**, *87*, 309–315. [CrossRef]
271. Janse, J.D.; Kokoskova, B. Indirect immunofluorescence microscopy for the detection and identification of plant pathogenic bacteria (in particular for *Ralstonia solanacearum*). *Methods Mol. Biol.* **2009**, *508*, 89–99.

272. Bruneval, P.; Choucair, J.; Paraf, F.; Casalta, J.P.; Raoult, D.; Scherchen, F.; Mainardi, J.L. Detection of fastidious bacteria in cardiac valves in cases of blood culture negative endocarditis. *J. Clin. Pathol.* **2001**, *54*, 238–240. [CrossRef]
273. Lin, M.; Todoric, D.; Mallory, M.; Luo, B.S.; Trottier, E.; Dan, H.H. Monoclonal antibodies binding to the cell surface of *Listeria monocytogenes* serotype 4b. *J. Med. Microbiol.* **2006**, *55*, 291–299. [CrossRef]
274. Foulston, L.; Elsholz, A.K.W.; DeFrancesco, A.S.; Losick, R. The extracellular matrix of *Staphylococcus aureus* biofilms comprises cytoplasmic proteins that associate with the cell surface in response to decreasing pH. *MBio* **2014**, *5*, e01667-14. [CrossRef]
275. Vejborg, R.M.; Klemm, P. Cellular chain formation in *Escherichia coli* biofilms. *Microbiology* **2009**, *155*, 1407–1417. [CrossRef]
276. Luo, T.L.; Eisenberg, M.C.; Hayashi, M.A.L.; Gonzalez-Cabezas, C.; Foxman, B.; Marrs, C.F.; Rickard, A.H. A Sensitive thresholding method for confocal laser scanning microscope image stacks of microbial biofilms. *Sci. Rep.* **2018**, *8*, 13013. [CrossRef]
277. Heydorn, A.; Nielsen, A.T.; Hentzer, M.; Sternberg, C.; Givskov, M.; Ersboll, B.K.; Molin, S. Quantification of biofilm structures by the novel computer program COMSTAT. *Microbiology* **2000**, *146*, 2395–2407. [CrossRef]
278. Mueller, L.N.; de Brouwer, J.F.; Almeida, J.S.; Stal, L.J.; Xavier, J.B. Analysis of a marine phototrophic biofilm by confocal laser scanning microscopy using the new image quantification software PHLIP. *BMC Ecol.* **2006**, *6*, 1. [CrossRef]
279. Sommerfeld Ross, S.S.; Tu, M.H.; Falsetta, M.L.; Ketterer, M.R.; Kiedrowski, M.R.; Horswill, A.R.; Apicella, M.A.; Reinhardt, J.M.; Fiegel, J. Quantification of confocal images of biofilms grown on irregular surfaces. *J. Microbiol. Methods* **2014**, *100*, 111–120. [CrossRef]
280. Miura, K. *Bioimage Data Analysis*, 1st ed.; Wiley-VCH Verlag GmbH & Co KGaA: Weinheim, Germany, 2016; ISBN 978-3-527-80092-6.
281. Neu, T.R.; Manz, B.; Volke, F.; Dynes, J.J.; Hitchcock, A.P.; Lawrence, J.R. Advanced imaging techniques for assessment of structure, composition and function in biofilm systems. *FEMS Microbiol. Ecol.* **2010**, *72*, 1–21. [CrossRef]
282. Oubekka, S.D.; Briandet, R.; Fontaine-Aupart, M.P.; Steenkeste, K. Correlative time-resolved fluorescence microscopy to assess antibiotic diffusion-reaction in biofilms. *Antimicrob. Agents Chemother.* **2012**, *56*, 3349–3358. [CrossRef]
283. Davison, W.M.; Pitts, B.; Stewart, P.S. Spatial and temporal patterns of biocide action against *Staphylococcus epidermidis* biofilms. *Antimicrob. Agents Chemother.* **2010**, *54*, 2920–2927. [CrossRef]
284. Cattò, C.; James, G.; Villa, F.; Villa, S.; Cappitelli, F. Zosteric acid and salicylic acid bound to a low density polyethylene surface successfully control bacterial biofilm formation. *Biofouling* **2018**, *34*, 440–452. [CrossRef]
285. Schneider, J.P.; Basler, M. Shedding light on biology of bacterial cells. *Philos. Trans. R. Soc. Lond. B Biol. Sci.* **2016**, *371*, 20150499. [CrossRef]
286. Power, R.M.; Huisken, J. A guide to light-sheet fluorescence microscopy for multiscale imaging. *Nat. Methods* **2017**, *14*, 360–373. [CrossRef]
287. Parthasarathy, R. Monitoring microbial communities using light sheet fluorescence microscopy. *Curr. Opin. Microbiol.* **2018**, *43*, 31–37. [CrossRef]
288. Janissen, R.; Murillo, D.M.; Niza, B.; Sahoo, P.K.; Nobrega, M.M.; Cesar, C.L.; Temperini, M.L.A.; Carvalho, H.F.; de Souza, A.A.; Cotta, M.A. Spatiotemporal distribution of different extracellular polymeric substances and filamentation mediate Xylella fastidiosa adhesion and biofilm formation. *Sci. Rep.* **2015**, *5*, 9856. [CrossRef]
289. Yan, J.; Sharo, A.G.; Stone, H.A.; Wingreen, N.S.; Bassler, B.L. *Vibrio cholerae* biofilm growth program and architecture revealed by single-cell live imaging. *Proc. Natl. Acad. Sci. USA* **2016**, *113*, E5337–E5343. [CrossRef]
290. Bryers, J.D. Two-photon excitation microscopy for analyses of biofilm processes. *Methods Enzymol.* **2001**, *337*, 259–269. [CrossRef]
291. Thomsen, H.; Graf, F.E.; Farewell, A.; Ericson, M.B. Exploring photoinactivation of microbial biofilms using laser scanning microscopy and confined 2-photon excitation. *J. Biophotonics* **2018**, *11*, e201800018. [CrossRef]
292. Villa, F.; Giacomucci, L.; Polo, A.; Principi, P.; Toniolo, L.; Levi, M.; Turri, S.; Cappitelli, F. N-vanillylnonanamide tested as a non-toxic antifoulant, applied to surfaces in a polyurethane coating. *Biotechnol. Lett.* **2009**, *31*, 1407–1413. [CrossRef]

293. Trentin, D.S.; Silva, D.B.; Frasson, A.P.; Rzhepishevska, O.; da Silva, M.V.; Pulcini, E.E.L.; James, G.; Soares, G.V.; Tasca, T.; Ramstedt, M.; et al. Natural Green coating inhibits adhesion of clinically important bacteria. *Sci. Rep.* **2015**, *5*, 8287. [CrossRef]
294. Das Ghatak, P.; Mathew-Steiner, S.S.; Pandey, P.; Roy, S.; Sen, C.K. A surfactant polymer dressing potentiates antimicrobial efficacy in biofilm disruption. *Sci. Rep.* **2018**, *8*, 873. [CrossRef]
295. Akuzov, D.; Franca, L.; Grunwald, I.; Vladkova, T. Sharply reduced biofilm formation from cobetia marina and in black sea water on modified siloxane coatings. *Coatings* **2018**, *8*, 136. [CrossRef]
296. Ivanova, E.P.; Hasan, J.; Webb, H.K.; Gervinskas, G.; Juodkazis, S.; Truong, V.K.; Wu, A.H.F.; Lamb, R.N.; Baulin, V.A.; Watson, G.S.; et al. Bactericidal activity of black silicon. *Nat. Commun.* **2013**, *4*, 2838. [CrossRef]
297. Li, L.; Molin, S.; Yang, L.; Ndoni, S. Sodium dodecyl sulfate (SDS)-loaded nanoporous polymer as anti-biofilm surface coating material. *Int. J. Mol. Sci.* **2013**, *14*, 3050–3064. [CrossRef]
298. Dickson, M.N.; Liang, E.I.; Rodriguez, L.A.; Vollereaux, N.; Yee, A.F. Nanopatterned polymer surfaces with bactericidal properties. *Biointerphases* **2015**, *10*, 021010. [CrossRef]
299. Ho, K.K.K.; Ozcelik, B.; Willcox, M.D.P.; Thissen, H.; Kumar, N. Facile solvent-free fabrication of nitric oxide (NO)-releasing coatings for prevention of biofilm formation. *Chem. Commun.* **2017**, *53*, 6488–6491. [CrossRef]
300. Xu, Y.C.; Wang, J.Z.; Hao, Z.Y.; Wang, S.; Liang, C.Z. Biodegradable ciprofloxacin-incorporated waterborne polyurethane polymers prevent bacterial biofilm formation in vitro. *Exp. Ther. Med.* **2019**, *17*, 1831–1836. [CrossRef]
301. Valencia, L.; Kumar, S.; Jalvo, B.; Mautner, A.; Salazar-Alvarez, G.; Mathew, A.P. Fully bio-based zwitterionic membranes with superior antifouling and antibacterial properties prepared via surface-initiated free-radical polymerization of poly(cysteine methacrylate). *J. Mater. Chem. A* **2018**, *6*, 16277–16712. [CrossRef]
302. Dave, R.N.; Joshi, H.M.; Venugopalan, V.P. Novel biocatalytic polymer-based antimicrobial coatings as potential ureteral biomaterial: Preparation and in vitro performance evaluation. *Antimicrob. Agents Chemother.* **2011**, *55*, 845–853. [CrossRef]
303. Sabatini, V.; Cattò, C.; Cappelletti, G.; Cappitelli, F.; Antenucci, S.; Farina, H.; Ortenzi, M.A.; Camazzola, S.; Di Silvestro, G. Protective features, durability and biodegration study of acrylic and methacrylic fluorinated polymer coatings for marble protection. *Prog. Org. Coat.* **2018**, *114*, 47–57. [CrossRef]
304. Albright, V.; Zhuk, I.; Wang, Y.H.; Selin, V.; van de Belt-Gritter, B.; Busscher, H.J.; van der Mei, H.C.; Sukhishvili, S.A. Self-defensive antibiotic-loaded layer-by-layer coatings: Imaging of localized bacterial acidification and pH-triggering of antibiotic release. *Acta Biomater.* **2017**, *61*, 66–74. [CrossRef]
305. Lagree, K.; Mon, H.H.; Mitchell, A.P.; Ducker, W.A. Impact of surface topography on biofilm formation by *Candida albicans*. *PLoS ONE* **2018**, *13*, e0197925. [CrossRef]
306. Alhede, M.; Qvortrup, K.; Liebrechts, R.; Hoiby, N.; Givskov, M.; Bjarnsholt, T. Combination of microscopic techniques reveals a comprehensive visual impression of biofilm structure and composition. *FEMS Immunol. Med. Microbiol.* **2012**, *65*, 335–342. [CrossRef]
307. Sugimoto, S.; Okuda, K.; Miyakawa, R.; Sato, M.; Arita-Morioka, K.; Chiba, A.; Yamanaka, K.; Ogura, T.; Mizunoe, Y.; Sato, C. Imaging of bacterial multicellular behaviour in biofilms in liquid by atmospheric scanning electron microscopy. *Sci. Rep.* **2016**, *6*, 25889. [CrossRef]
308. Bridier, A.; Meylheuc, T.; Briandet, R. Realistic representation of Bacillus subtilis biofilms architecture using combined microscopy (CLSM, ESEM and FESEM). *Micron* **2013**, *48*, 65–69. [CrossRef]
309. Asahi, Y.; Miura, J.; Tsuda, T.; Kuwabata, S.; Tsunashima, K.; Noiri, Y.; Sakata, T.; Ebisu, S.; Hayashi, M. Simple observation of *Streptococcus mutans* biofilm by scanning electron microscopy using ionic liquids. *AMB Express* **2015**, *5*, 6. [CrossRef]
310. Gonzalez-Ramirez, A.I.; Ramirez-Granillo, A.; Medina-Canales, M.G.; Rodriguez-Tovar, A.V.; Martinez-Rivera, M.A. Analysis and description of the stages of Aspergillus fumigatus biofilm formation using scanning electron microscopy. *BMC Microbiol.* **2016**, *16*, 243. [CrossRef]
311. Gomes, L.C.; Mergulhao, F.J. SEM analysis of surface impact on biofilm antibiotic treatment. *Scanning* **2017**, *2017*, 2960194. [CrossRef]
312. Mohmmed, S.A.; Vianna, M.E.; Penny, M.R.; Hilton, S.T.; Mordan, N.; Knowles, J.C. Confocal laser scanning, scanning electron, and transmission electron microscopy investigation of *Enterococcus faecalis* biofilm degradation using passive and active sodium hypochlorite irrigation within a simulated root canal model. *Microbiologyopen* **2017**, *6*, e00455. [CrossRef]

313. McCutcheon, J.; Southam, G. Advanced biofilm staining techniques for TEM and SEM in geomicrobiology: Implications for visualizing EPS architecture, mineral nucleation, and microfossil generation. *Chem. Geol.* **2018**, *498*, 115–127. [CrossRef]
314. Hrubanova, K.; Nebesarova, J.; Ruzicka, F.; Krzyzanek, V. The innovation of cryo-SEM freeze-fracturing methodology demonstrated on high pressure frozen biofilm. *Micron* **2018**, *110*, 28–35. [CrossRef]
315. Liu, M.H.; Wu, X.X.; Li, J.K.; Liu, L.; Zhang, R.G.; Shao, D.Y.; Du, X.D. The specific anti-biofilm effect of gallic acid on *Staphylococcus aureus* by regulating the expression of the ica operon. *Food Control* **2017**, *73*, 613–618. [CrossRef]
316. Nishiyama, H.; Koizumi, M.; Ogawa, K.; Kitamura, S.; Konyuba, Y.; Watanabe, Y.; Ohbayashi, N.; Fukuda, M.; Suga, M.; Sato, C. Atmospheric scanning electron microscope system with an open sample chamber: Configuration and applications. *Ultramicroscopy* **2014**, *147*, 86–97. [CrossRef]
317. Sahl, S.J.; Hell, S.W.; Jakobs, S. Fluorescence nanoscopy in cell biology. *Nat. Rev. Mol. Cell. Biol.* **2017**, *18*, 685–701. [CrossRef]
318. Blom, H.; Widengren, J. Stimulated emission depletion microscopy. *Chem. Rev.* **2017**, *117*, 7377–7427. [CrossRef]
319. Coltharp, C.; Xiao, J. Superresolution microscopy for microbiology. *Cell Microbiol.* **2012**, *14*, 1808–1818. [CrossRef]
320. Xiao, J.; Dufrêne, Y.F. Optical and force nanoscopy in microbiology. *Nat. Microbiol.* **2016**, *1*, 16186. [CrossRef]
321. Li, C.K.; Kuang, C.F.; Liu, X. Prospects for fluorescence nanoscopy. *ACS Nano* **2018**, *12*, 4081–4085. [CrossRef]
322. Sydor, A.M.; Czymmek, K.J.; Puchner, E.M.; Mennella, V. Super-resolution microscopy: From single molecules to supramolecular assemblies. *Trends Cell. Biol.* **2015**, *25*, 730–748. [CrossRef]
323. Ball, G.; Demmerle, J.; Kaufmann, R.; Davis, I.; Dobbie, I.M.; Schermelleh, L. SIMcheck: A toolbox for successful super-resolution structured illumination microscopy. *Sci. Rep.* **2015**, *5*, 15915. [CrossRef]
324. Virdis, B.; Harnisch, F.; Batstone, D.J.; Rabaey, K.; Donose, B.C. Non-invasive characterization of electrochemically active microbial biofilms using confocal Raman microscopy. *Energy Environ. Sci.* **2012**, *5*, 7017–7024. [CrossRef]
325. Wagner, M.; Horn, H. Optical coherence tomography in biofilm research: A comprehensive review. *Biotechnol. Bioeng.* **2017**, *114*, 1386–1402. [CrossRef]
326. Sandt, C.; Smith-Palmer, T.; Comeau, J.; Pink, D. Quantification of water and biomass in small colony variant PAO1 biofilms by confocal Raman microspectroscopy. *Appl. Microbiol. Biotechnol.* **2009**, *83*, 1171–1182. [CrossRef]
327. Sandt, C.; Smith-Palmer, T.; Pink, J.; Brennan, L.; Pink, D. Confocal Raman microspectroscopy as a tool for studying the chemical heterogeneities of biofilms in situ. *J. Appl. Microbiol.* **2007**, *103*, 1808–1820. [CrossRef]
328. Wagner, M.; Ivleva, N.P.; Haisch, C.; Niessner, R.; Horn, H. Combined use of confocal laser scanning microscopy (CLSM) and Raman microscopy (RM): Investigations on EPS-Matrix. *Water Res.* **2009**, *43*, 63–76. [CrossRef]
329. Andrews, J.S.; Rolfe, S.A.; Huang, W.E.; Scholes, J.D.; Banwart, S.A. Biofilm formation in environmental bacteria is influenced by different macromolecules depending on genus and species. *Environ. Microbiol.* **2010**, *12*, 2496–2507. [CrossRef]
330. Lawrence, J.R.; Swerhone, G.D.W.; Dynes, J.J.; Hitchcock, A.P.; Korber, D.R. Complex organic corona formation on carbon nanotubes reduces microbial toxicity by suppressing reactive oxygen species production. *Environ. Sci. Nano* **2016**, *3*, 181–189. [CrossRef]
331. Yang, S.I.; George, G.N.; Lawrence, J.R.; Kaminskyj, S.G.W.; Dynes, J.J.; Lai, B.; Pickering, I.J. Multispecies biofilms transform selenium oxyanions into elemental selenium particles: Studies using combined synchrotron x-ray fluorescence imaging and scanning transmission x-ray microscopy. *Environ. Sci. Technol.* **2016**, *50*, 10343–10350. [CrossRef]
332. Blauert, F.; Horn, H.; Wagner, M. Time-resolved biofilm deformation measurements using optical coherence tomography. *Biotechnol. Bioeng.* **2015**, *112*, 1893–1905. [CrossRef]
333. Heidari, A.E.; Moghaddam, S.; Truong, K.K.; Chou, L.; Genberg, C.; Brenner, M.; Chena, Z.P. Visualizing biofilm formation in endotracheal tubes using endoscopic three-dimensional optical coherence tomography. *J. Biomed. Opt.* **2016**, *21*, 126010. [CrossRef]
334. Farid, M.U.; Guo, J.X.; An, A.K. Bacterial inactivation and in situ monitoring of biofilm development on graphene oxide membrane using optical coherence tomography. *J. Memb. Sci.* **2018**, *564*, 22–34. [CrossRef]

335. Dreszer, C.; Wexler, A.D.; Drusova, S.; Overdijk, T.; Zwijnenburg, A.; Flemming, H.C.; Kruithof, J.C.; Vrouwenvelder, J.S. In-situ biofilm characterization in membrane systems using optical coherence tomography: Formation, structure, detachment and impact of flux change. *Water Res.* **2014**, *67*, 243–254. [CrossRef]
336. Fortunato, L.; Jeong, S.; Leiknes, T. Time-resolved monitoring of biofouling development on a flat sheet membrane using optical coherence tomography. *Sci. Rep.* **2017**, *7*, 15. [CrossRef]
337. Ogrodzki, P.; Cheung, C.S.; Saad, M.; Dahmani, K.; Coxill, R.; Liang, H.D.; Forsythe, S.J. Rapid in situ imaging and whole genome sequencing of biofilm in neonatal feeding tubes: A clinical proof of concept. *Sci. Rep.* **2017**, *7*, 15948. [CrossRef]
338. de Andrade, M.C.L.; de Oliveira, M.A.S.; dos Santos, F.D.G.; Vilela, P.D.X.; da Silva, M.N.; Macedo, D.P.C.; Neto, R.G.D.; Neves, H.J.P.; Brandao, I.D.L.; Chaves, G.M.; et al. A new approach by optical coherence tomography for elucidating biofilm formation by emergent Candida species. *PLoS ONE* **2017**, *12*, e0188020. [CrossRef]
339. Rupp, C.J.; Fux, C.A.; Stoodley, P. Viscoelasticity of *Staphylococcus aureus* biofilms in response to fluid shear allows resistance to detachment and facilitates rolling migration. *Appl. Environ. Microbiol.* **2005**, *71*, 2175–2178. [CrossRef]
340. Kim, M.K.; Drescher, K.; Pak, O.S.; Bassler, B.L.; Stone, H.A. Filaments in curved streamlines: Rapid formation of *Staphylococcus aureus* biofilm streamers. *New J. Phys.* **2014**, *16*, 065024. [CrossRef]
341. Billings, N.; Birjiniuk, A.; Samad, T.S.; Doyle, P.S.; Ribbeck, K. Material properties of biofilms—A review of methods for understanding permeability and mechanics. *Rep. Progr. Phys.* **2015**, *78*, 036601. [CrossRef]
342. Boudarel, H.; Mathias, J.D.; Blaysat, B.; Grediac, M. Towards standardized mechanical characterization of microbial biofilms: Analysis and critical review. *NPJ Biofilms Microbiomes* **2018**, *4*, 17. [CrossRef]
343. Bol, M.; Ehret, A.E.; Albero, A.B.; Hellriegel, J.; Krull, R. Recent advances in mechanical characterisation of biofilm and their significance for material modelling. *Crit. Rev. Biotechnol.* **2013**, *33*, 145–171. [CrossRef]
344. Martin, K.J.; Bolster, D.; Derlon, N.; Morgenroth, E.; Nerenberg, R. Effect of fouling layer spatial distribution on permeate flux: A theoretical and experimental study. *J. Membr. Sci.* **2014**, *471*, 130–137. [CrossRef]
345. Li, C.Y.; Wagner, M.; Lackner, S.; Horn, H. Assessing the influence of biofilm surface roughness on mass transfer by combining optical coherence tomography and two-dimensional modeling. *Biotechnol. Bioeng.* **2016**, *113*, 989–1000. [CrossRef]
346. Jafari, M.; Desmond, P.; van Loosdrecht, M.C.M.; Derlon, N.; Morgenroth, E.; Picioreanu, C. Effect of biofilm structural deformation on hydraulic resistance during ultrafiltration: A numerical and experimental study. *Water Res.* **2018**, *145*, 375–387. [CrossRef]
347. Picioreanu, C.; Blauert, F.; Horn, H.; Wagner, M. Determination of mechanical properties of biofilms by modelling the deformation measured using optical coherence tomography. *Water Res.* **2018**, *145*, 588–598. [CrossRef]
348. Dufrene, Y.F. Sticky microbes: Forces in microbial cell adhesion. *Trends Microbiol.* **2015**, *23*, 376–382. [CrossRef]
349. James, S.A.; Powell, L.C.; Wright, C.J. Atomic force microscopy of biofilms-imaging, interactions, and mechanics. In *Microbial Biofilms—Importance and Applications*; Dhanasekaran, D., Thajuddin, N., Eds.; IntechOpen limited: London, UK, 2016; pp. 95–118. [CrossRef]
350. Lau, P.C.; Dutcher, J.R.; Beveridge, T.J.; Lam, J.S. Absolute quantitation of bacterial biofilm adhesion and viscoelasticity by microbead force spectroscopy. *Biophys. J.* **2009**, *96*, 2935–2948. [CrossRef]
351. Harapanahalli, A.K.; Chen, Y.; Li, J.; Busscher, H.J.; van der Mei, H.C. Influence of adhesion force on icaA and cidA Gene expression and production of matrix components in *Staphylococcus aureus* biofilms. *Appl. Environ. Microbiol.* **2015**, *81*, 3369–3378. [CrossRef]
352. Feuillie, C.; Formosa-Dague, C.; Hays, L.M.; Vervaeck, O.; Derclaye, S.; Brennan, M.P.; Foster, T.J.; Geoghegan, J.A.; Dufrêne, Y.F. Molecular interactions and inhibition of the staphylococcal biofilm-forming protein SdrC. *Proc. Natl. Acad. Sci. USA* **2017**, *114*, 3738–3743. [CrossRef]
353. El-Kirat-Chatel, S.; Puymege, A.; Duong, T.H.; Van Overtvelt, P.; Bressy, C.; Belec, L.; Dufrêne, Y.F.; Molmeret, M. Phenotypic heterogeneity in attachment of marine bacteria toward antifouling copolymers unraveled by AFM. *Front. Microbiol.* **2017**, *8*, 1399. [CrossRef]
354. Kundukad, B.; Seviour, T.; Liang, Y.; Rice, S.A.; Kjelleberg, S.; Doyle, P.S. Mechanical properties of the superficial biofilm layer determine the architecture of biofilms. *Soft Matter* **2016**, *12*, 5718–5726. [CrossRef]

355. Taubenberger, A.V.; Hutmacher, D.W.; Muller, D.J. Single-cell force spectroscopy, an emerging tool to quantify cell adhesion to biomaterials. *Tissue Eng. Part B Rev.* **2014**, *20*, 40–55. [CrossRef]
356. Spengler, C.; Thewes, N.; Jung, P.; Bischoff, M.; Jacobs, K. Determination of the nano-scaled contact area of staphylococcal cells. *Nanoscale* **2017**, *9*, 10084–10093. [CrossRef]
357. Klapper, I.; Rupp, C.J.; Cargo, R.; Purvedorj, B.; Stoodley, P. Viscoelastic fluid description of bacterial biofilm material properties. *Biotechnol. Bioeng.* **2002**, *80*, 289–296. [CrossRef]
358. Peterson, B.W.; He, Y.; Ren, Y.; Zerdoum, A.; Libera, M.R.; Sharma, P.K.; van Winkelhoff, A.J.; Neut, D.; Stoodley, P.; van der Mei, H.C.; et al. Viscoelasticity of biofilms and their recalcitrance to mechanical and chemical challenges. *FEMS Microbiol. Rev.* **2015**, *39*, 234–245. [CrossRef]
359. Stojkovic, B.; Sretenovic, S.; Dogsa, I.; Poberaj, I.; Stopar, D. Viscoelastic properties of levan-DNA mixtures important in microbial biofilm formation as determined by micro-and macrorheology. *Biophys. J.* **2015**, *108*, 758–765. [CrossRef]
360. Kesel, S.; Grumbein, S.; Gumperlein, I.; Tallawi, M.; Marel, A.K.; Lieleg, O.; Opitz, M. Direct comparison of physical properties of *Bacillus subtilis* NCIB 3610 and B-1 Biofilms. *Appl. Environ. Microbiol.* **2016**, *82*, 2424–2432. [CrossRef]
361. Di Stefano, A.; D'Aurizio, E.; Trubiani, O.; Grande, R.; Di Campli, E.; Di Giulio, M.; Di Bartolomeo, S.; Sozio, P.; Iannitelli, A.; Nostro, A.; et al. Viscoelastic properties of *Staphylococcus aureus* and *Staphylococcus epidermidis* mono-microbial biofilms. *Microb. Biotechnol.* **2009**, *2*, 634–641. [CrossRef]
362. Pavlovsky, L.; Younger, J.G.; Solomon, M.J. In situ rheology of *Staphylococcus epidermidis* bacterial biofilms. *Soft Matter* **2013**, *9*, 122–131. [CrossRef]
363. Grumbein, S.; Werb, M.; Opitz, M.; Lieleg, O. Elongational rheology of bacterial biofilms in situ. *J. Rheol.* **2016**, *60*, 1085–1094. [CrossRef]
364. Galy, O.; Latour-Lambert, P.; Zrelli, K.; Ghigo, J.M.; Beloin, C.; Henry, N. Mapping of bacterial biofilm local mechanics by magnetic microparticle actuation. *Biophys. J.* **2012**, *103*, 1400–1408. [CrossRef]
365. Cao, H.Y.; Habimana, O.; Safari, A.; Heffernan, R.; Dai, Y.H.; Casey, E. Revealing region-specific biofilm viscoelastic properties by means of a micro-rheological approach. *NPJ Biofilms Microbiomes* **2016**, *2*, 5. [CrossRef]
366. Chew, S.C.; Kundukad, B.; Seviour, T.; van der Maarel, J.R.C.; Yang, L.; Rice, S.A.; Doyle, P.; Kjelleberg, S. Dynamic remodeling of microbial biofilms by functionally distinct exopolysaccharides. *Mbio* **2014**, *5*, e01536-14. [CrossRef]
367. Olofsson, A.C.; Hermansson, M.; Elwing, H. Use of a quartz crystal microbalance to investigate the antiadhesive potential of N-acetyl-L-cysteine. *Appl. Environ. Microbiol.* **2005**, *71*, 2705–2712. [CrossRef]
368. Chen, J.Y.; Penn, L.S.; Xi, J. Quartz crystal microbalance: Sensing cell-substrate adhesion and beyond. *Biosens. Bioelectron.* **2018**, *99*, 593–602. [CrossRef]
369. Dixon, M.C. Quartz crystal microbalance with dissipation monitoring: Enabling real-time characterization of biological materials and their interactions. *J. Biomol. Tech.* **2008**, *19*, 151–158.
370. Costa, F.; Sousa, D.M.; Parreira, P.; Lamghari, M.; Gomes, P.; Martins, M.C.L. N-acetylcysteine-functionalized coating avoids bacterial adhesion and biofilm formation. *Sci. Rep.* **2017**, *7*. [CrossRef]
371. Tonda-Turo, C.; Carmagnola, I.; Ciardelli, G. Quartz crystal microbalance with dissipation monitoring: A powerful method to predict the in vivo behavior of bioengineered surfaces. *Front. Bioeng. Biotechnol.* **2018**, *6*, 17374. [CrossRef]
372. Reipa, V.; Almeida, J.; Cole, K.D. Long-term monitoring of biofilm growth and disinfection using a quartz crystal microbalance and reflectance measurements. *J. Microbiol. Methods* **2006**, *66*, 449–459. [CrossRef]
373. Sprung, C.; Wahlisch, D.; Huttl, R.; Seidel, J.; Meyer, A.; Wolf, G. Detection and monitoring of biofilm formation in water treatment systems by quartz crystal microbalance sensors. *Water Sci. Technol.* **2009**, *59*, 543–548. [CrossRef]
374. Wang, Y.N.; Narain, R.; Liu, Y. Study of bacterial adhesion on different glycopolymer surfaces by quartz crystal microbalance with dissipation. *Langmuir* **2014**, *30*, 7377–7387. [CrossRef]
375. Knowles, B.R.; Yang, D.; Wagner, P.; Maclaughlin, S.; Higgins, M.J.; Molino, P.J. Zwitterion functionalized silica nanoparticle coatings: The effect of particle size on protein, bacteria, and fungal spore adhesion. *Langmuir* **2019**, *35*, 1335–1345. [CrossRef]
376. Tam, K.; Kinsinger, N.; Ayala, P.; Qi, F.; Shi, W.; Myung, N.V. Real-time monitoring of *Streptococcus mutans* biofilm formation using a quartz crystal microbalance. *Caries Res.* **2007**, *41*, 474–483. [CrossRef]

377. Olsson, A.L.; van der Mei, H.C.; Busscher, H.J.; Sharma, P.K. Influence of cell surface appendages on the bacterium-substratum interface measured real-time using QCM-D. *Langmuir* **2009**, *25*, 1627–1632. [CrossRef]
378. Pranzetti, A.; Salaun, S.; Mieszkin, S.; Callow, M.E.; Callow, J.A.; Preece, J.A.; Mendes, P.M. Model organic surfaces to probe marine bacterial adhesion kinetics by surface plasmon resonance. *Adv. Funct. Mater.* **2012**, *22*, 3672–3681. [CrossRef]
379. Zhang, P.; Guo, J.S.; Yan, P.; Chen, Y.P.; Wang, W.; Dai, Y.Z.; Fang, F.; Wang, G.X.; Shen, Y. Dynamic dispersal of surface layer biofilm induced by nanosized tio2 based on surface plasmon resonance and waveguide. *Appl. Environ. Microbiol.* **2018**, *84*, e00047-18. [CrossRef]
380. Gordon, P.W.; Brooker, A.D.M.; Chew, Y.M.J.; Wilson, D.I.; York, D.W. A scanning fluid dynamic gauging technique for probing surface layers. *Meas. Sci. Technol.* **2010**, *21*, 085103. [CrossRef]
381. Peck, O.P.W.; Chew, Y.M.J.; Bird, M.R.; Bolhuis, A. Application of fluid dynamic gauging in the characterization and removal of biofouling deposits. *Heat Transf. Eng.* **2015**, *36*, 685–694. [CrossRef]
382. Beyenal, H.; Babauta, J. Microsensors and microscale gradients in biofilms. *Adv. Biochem. Eng. Biotechnol.* **2014**, *146*, 235–256. [CrossRef]
383. Lee, J.H.; Seo, Y.; Lim, T.S.; Bishop, P.L.; Papautsky, I. MEMS needle-type sensor array for in situ measurements of dissolved oxygen and redox potential. *Environ. Sci. Technol.* **2007**, *41*, 7857–7863. [CrossRef]
384. Moya, A.; Guimera, X.; del Campo, F.J.; Prats-Alfonso, E.; Dorado, A.D.; Baeza, M.; Villa, R.; Gabriel, D.; Gamisans, X.; Gabriel, G. Biofilm oxygen profiling using an array of microelectrodes on a micro fabricated needle. *Procedia Eng.* **2014**, *87*, 256–259. [CrossRef]
385. Masi, E.; Ciszak, M.; Santopolo, L.; Frascella, A.; Giovannetti, L.; Marchi, E.; Viti, C.; Mancuso, S. Electrical spiking in bacterial biofilms. *J. R. Soc. Interface* **2015**, *12*, 20141036. [CrossRef]
386. James, G.A.; Zhao, A.G.; Usui, M.; Underwood, R.A.; Nguyen, H.; Beyenal, H.; Pulcini, E.D.; Hunt, A.A.; Bernstein, H.C.; Fleckman, P.; et al. Microsensor and transcriptomic signatures of oxygen depletion in biofilms associated with chronic wounds. *Wound Repair Regen.* **2016**, *24*, 373–383. [CrossRef]
387. Ito, T.; Okabe, S.; Satoh, H.; Watanabe, Y. Successional development of sulfate-reducing bacterial populations and their activities in a wastewater biofilm growing under microaerophilic conditions. *Appl. Environ. Microbiol.* **2002**, *68*, 1392–1402. [CrossRef]
388. Hibiya, K.; Terada, A.; Tsuneda, S.; Hirata, A. Simultaneous nitrification and denitrification by controlling vertical and horizontal microenvironment in a membrane-aerated biofilm reactor. *J. Biotechnol.* **2003**, *100*, 23–32. [CrossRef]
389. Lee, W.H.; Wahman, D.G.; Pressman, J.G. Amperometric carbon fiber nitrite microsensor for in situ biofilm monitoring. *Sens. Actuators B Chem.* **2013**, *188*, 1263–1269. [CrossRef]
390. von der Schulenburg, D.A.G.; Pintelon, T.R.R.; Picioreanu, C.; Van Loosdrecht, M.C.M.; Johns, M.L. Three-dimensional simulations of biofilm growth in porous media. *AIChE J.* **2009**, *55*, 494–504. [CrossRef]
391. Bottero, S.; Storck, T.; Heimovaara, T.J.; van Loosdrecht, M.C.M.; Enzien, M.V.; Picioreanu, C. Biofilm development and the dynamics of preferential flow paths in porous media. *Biofouling* **2013**, *29*, 1069–1086. [CrossRef]
392. Davit, Y.; Byrne, H.; Osborne, J.; Pitt-Francis, J.; Gavaghan, D.; Quintard, M. Hydrodynamic dispersion within porous biofilms. *Phys. Rev.* **2013**, *87*, 012718. [CrossRef]
393. Qin, C.Z.; Hassanizadeh, S.M. Pore-network modeling of solute transport and biofilm growth in porous media. *Transp. Porous Med.* **2015**, *110*, 345–367. [CrossRef]
394. McLean, J.S.; Ona, O.N.; Majors, P.D. Correlated biofilm imaging, transport and metabolism measurements via combined nuclear magnetic resonance and confocal microscopy. *ISME J.* **2008**, *2*, 121–131. [CrossRef]
395. Phoenix, V.R.; Holmes, W.M. Magnetic resonance imaging of structure, diffusivity, and copper immobilization in a phototrophic biofilm. *Appl. Environ. Microbiol.* **2008**, *74*, 7454. [CrossRef]
396. Vogt, M.; Flemming, H.C.; Veeman, W.S. Diffusion in *Pseudomonas aeruginosa* biofilms: A pulsed field gradient NMR study. *J. Biotechnol.* **2000**, *77*, 137–146. [CrossRef]
397. Gabrilska, R.A.; Rumbaugh, K.P. Biofilm models of polymicrobial infection. *Future Microbiol.* **2015**, *10*, 1997–2015. [CrossRef]
398. Brann, M.; Suter, J.D.; Addleman, R.S.; Larimer, C. Monitoring bacterial biofilms with a microfluidic flow chip designed for imaging with white-light interferometry. *Biomicrofluidics* **2017**, *11*, 044113. [CrossRef]

399. Lourenco, A.; Coenye, T.; Goeres, D.M.; Donelli, G.; Azevedo, A.S.; Ceri, H.; Coelho, F.L.; Flemming, H.C.; Juhna, T.; Lopes, S.P.; et al. Minimum information about a biofilm experiment (MIABiE): Standards for reporting experiments and data on sessile microbial communities living at interfaces. *Pathog. Dis.* **2014**, *70*, 250–256. [CrossRef]
400. Lourenco, A.; Ferreira, A.; Veiga, N.; Machado, I.; Pereira, M.O.; Azevedo, N.F. BiofOmics: A Web platform for the systematic and standardized collection of high-throughput biofilm data. *PLoS ONE* **2012**, *7*, e39960. [CrossRef]
401. Coenye, T.; Goeres, D.; Van Bambeke, F.; Bjarnsholt, T. Should standardized susceptibility testing for microbial biofilms be introduced in clinical practice? *Clin. Microbiol. Infect.* **2018**, *24*, 570–572. [CrossRef]

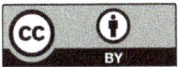

© 2019 by the authors. Licensee MDPI, Basel, Switzerland. This article is an open access article distributed under the terms and conditions of the Creative Commons Attribution (CC BY) license (http://creativecommons.org/licenses/by/4.0/).

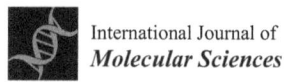

Review

Antimicrobial Polymers for Additive Manufacturing

Carmen Mabel González-Henríquez [1,2,*], **Mauricio A. Sarabia-Vallejos** [3,4] **and Juan Rodríguez Hernandez** [5,*]

[1] Departamento de Química, Facultad de Ciencias Naturales, Matemáticas y del Medio Ambiente, Universidad Tecnológica Metropolitana, Las Palmeras 3360, Santiago 7800003, Chile
[2] Programa Institucional de Fomento a la Investigación, Desarrollo e Innovación, Universidad Tecnológica Metropolitana, Ignacio Valdivieso 2409, Santiago 8940577, Chile
[3] Departamento de Ingeniería Estructural y Geotecnia, Escuela de Ingeniería, Pontificia Universidad Católica de Chile, Avenida Vicuña Mackenna 4860, Santiago 7820436, Chile; masarabi@puc.cl
[4] Instituto de Ingeniería Biológica y Médica, Pontificia Universidad Católica de Chile, Avenida Vicuña Mackenna 4860, Santiago 7820436, Chile
[5] Polymer Functionalization Group, Departamento de Química Macromolecular Aplicada, Instituto de Ciencia y Tecnología de Polímeros-Consejo Superior de Investigaciones Científicas (ICTP-CSIC), Juan de la Cierva 3, 28006 Madrid, Spain
* Correspondence: carmen.gonzalez@utem.cl (C.M.G.-H.); jrodriguez@ictp.csic.es (J.R.H.); Tel.: +56-2-27877188 (C.M.G.H.); + 34-912587505 (J.R.H.)

Received: 15 February 2019; Accepted: 5 March 2019; Published: 10 March 2019

Abstract: Three-dimensional (3D) printing technologies can be widely used for producing detailed geometries based on individual and particular demands. Some applications are related to the production of personalized devices, implants (orthopedic and dental), drug dosage forms (antibacterial, immunosuppressive, anti-inflammatory, etc.), or 3D implants that contain active pharmaceutical treatments, which favor cellular proliferation and tissue regeneration. This review is focused on the generation of 3D printed polymer-based objects that present antibacterial properties. Two main different alternatives of obtaining these 3D printed objects are fully described, which employ different polymer sources. The first one uses natural polymers that, in some cases, already exhibit intrinsic antibacterial capacities. The second alternative involves the use of synthetic polymers, and thus takes advantage of polymers with antimicrobial functional groups, as well as alternative strategies based on the modification of the surface of polymers or the elaboration of composite materials through adding certain antibacterial agents or incorporating different drugs into the polymeric matrix.

Keywords: additive manufacturing; antibacterial polymers; biocompatible systems; drug delivery systems; 3D printing

---

1. Introduction

According to the International Organization for Standardization/American Society for Testing and Materials (ISO/ASTM) standards (from a report of Technical Committee F42), additive manufacturing (AM) is defined as "the process of joining materials to make parts from 3D model data, usually, layer by layer" [1]. In the last years, several advances have been performed in AM technologies by the scientific community, thus generating an abrupt and quick evolution in the development of these methods. As mentioned by Campbell and Ivanova [2], AM is today widely considered a disruptive technology that offers a new paradigm for engineering design and manufacturing that could have significant economic, geopolitical, environmental, intellectual property, and security implications.

The use of additive manufacturing (AM) methods, which are commonly known as three-dimensional (3D) printing, has allowed the fabrication of an endless variety of devices with a wide myriad of potential applications in several fields, and particularly in the bioengineering area [3,4]. 3D printing methodologies permitted us, for instance, to manufacture or fabricate structures with architectures closely similar to biological tissues, such as bones, cartilages, or heart valves. With AM technology, complex geometrical cues with high accuracy can be straightforwardly achieved. Moreover, the increasing demands and applications of tissue engineering, antimicrobial/anti-biofouling devices, and regenerative medicine, researchers are seeking new manufacturing technologies that could solve the supply shortage of tissues or organs and the immunological requirements of implanted devices [5]. The fields of biomedicine, food fabrication, packaging, paintings, and naval [6], among others, have not been the exception. For example, there are several examples of polymeric-based biomedical devices, including artificial hips and knee implants or systems such as stents, heart valves, or even vascular grafts, which are commonly used both to improve the quality of life and, in some cases, increase life expectancy.

In spite of this, a still remaining fundamental problem in the employment of polymeric materials for biomedical purposes is related to material contamination by a wide variety of microorganisms. This issue is nowadays a critical limitation for the use of polymeric materials in this application field. Particularly, in the biomedical area, this topic is important because it is highly possible that bacteria could be present in the media, affecting the integrity of the medical devices and healthcare products [7].

Another common problem associated with contamination by microorganisms, which needs to be solved in a short time, is the biofilm formation over 3D printed structures [8]. Understanding the relationship between the extracellular matrix and the 3D topography of the material could be fundamental for describing the mechanisms of matrix formation, mechanosensing, matrix remodeling, and the modulation of cell–cell or cell–matrix interactions during biofilm formation [9], which would allow one more step toward the solution for avoiding biofilm formation.

In this context, this short review will attempt to briefly describe the most relevant and recent advances in the elaboration of antimicrobial 3D printed devices and objects. We will first briefly describe the principles of additive manufacturing and the basics of antimicrobial polymers. The following sections will be devoted to the description of illustrative examples of the different strategies that have been reported for the fabrication of antimicrobial objects using natural occurring polymers, but also using synthetic polymer blends with antimicrobial agents.

2. Principles of Additive Manufacturing

As described in Figure 1, AM starts with the design of a three-dimensional (3D) model (Step 1), which is then transferred to the printing machine (steps 2 to 3). Then, the model is digitalized and sliced into several layers. Set-up parameters are introduced (Step 4), including the energy source (temperature, laser intensity, etc.) or z-resolution (provided by the layer thickness). Once the experimental conditions are selected, the AM system prints the layers in a build, adding each new layer on top of the prior one (Step 5). The final steps involve post-processing to remove the supporting material (steps 6 to 7), and finally, its use for the application for which it was designed (Step 8).

There are several types of AM methodologies; the most common types are the ones based on material extrusion, such as fused deposition modeling (FDM) or bio-plotting [10], which are particularly interesting for this review, because it enables manufacturing parts with several types of biocompatible or biodegradable polymers, and in some cases, with living cells or bacteria [11]. Other common technologies are the stereolithography (SLA), technologies based on partially-melting powder such as selective laser sintering (SLS), and full-melting powder such as selective laser melting (SLM) or binder jetting.

Additive manufacturing offers important advantages over other currently employed technologies for prototyping [12]. AM permits the fabrication of fully customized geometrically complex products in an economic manner for limited production. Some reports established that AM is cost-effective in comparison, for instance, with plastic injection molding for targeted production runs ranging from 50 to 5000 units. Other authors estimated that AM is competitive with plastic injection molding for the targeted fabrications below 1000 items [13]. The basis of the low production cost is related to not needing molds or costly tools, there being no requirements for milling or sanding processes, and the full automatization of the process.

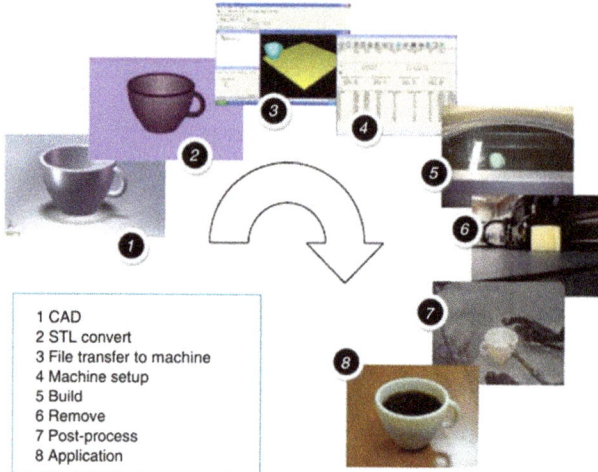

Figure 1. Steps involved in the fabrication of a cup by additive manufacturing (AM). Reproduced with permission from Ref. [1].

Another crucial advantage is related to the design of the AM printed parts. Designs can be easily created and modified according to any required change, and can be shared so that manufacturing can be easily carried out in many different places simultaneously. In fact, AM allows for the quick fabrication of prototypes with different versions for lab testing without the need for costly retooling. Moreover, replacement parts can be produced by third-party providers utilizing the original designs provided by the manufacturer. As a result, an inventory is not required that can suppose additional costs if finished goods remain unsold.

Finally, it is worth mentioning that AM offers important improvements in terms of environmental implications, because it results in an efficient use of the materials and permits an environment-friendly design.

As shown in Figure 2, which was extracted from Mawale et al. [14], a clear evolution from rapid prototyping to series production can be observed in the latest years. The future of AM should be focused, according to Mawale et al., on the efficiency of AM processes to decrease the final fabrication time and price.

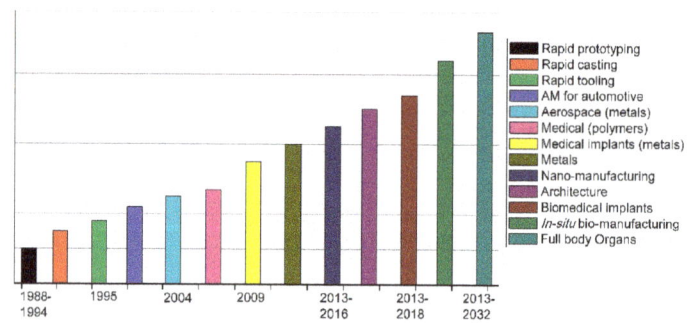

Figure 2. AM timeline for different applications. Reproduced with permission from Ref. [14].

In terms of applications, the future still requires further investigations in areas of biomedical devices, in situ biomanufacturing, or in the fabrication of full body organs. AM technologies have been steadily growing during the last 20 years, and today, AM parts accomplish the requirements of many different industrial areas, particularly in biomedical applications including implants/prosthetics, dental, and surgical devices/aids [12,15]. Some of these devices use ceramics or bioceramics as a base for 3D printing [16], but in this review, we will be focused on the usage of polymeric materials (or some polymeric composites) for fabricating antimicrobial devices and objects.

A crucial disadvantage for bio-related applications that needs to be solved quickly for some of the materials that are used in AM methodologies is their natural cytotoxicity. Zhu et al. showed that several SLA resins are highly toxic, impeding the developing of zebrafish embryos [17]. The authors have postulated that chip-based devices manufactured using SLA processes leached toxic chemicals to the culture media, causing significant toxicity, as evidenced by the highly sensitive zebrafish embryo toxicity biotest [17]. Other groups focused their studies on the potential chemical hazard profiles and limitations associated with the fabrication of biocompatible devices using SLA, FDM, and multi-jet modeling (MJM) processes [18]. Here, three distinctive biotests were selected for testing the potential chemical hazard risks associated with 3D printed polymer leachates. These results show that the majority of SLA and MJM polymers exhibit toxic effects, which is a problem for biological applications. Table 1 contains a summary of the toxicity data available for some of the composites that are used in SLA printing.

Table 1. Summary of toxicity data available for the photoinitiators, photopolymers, and auxiliary compounds used in stereolithography (SLA). Reproduced with permission from Ref. [19].

Compounds	Available	Toxicological Information
Photoinitiators		
Phosphine oxide compounds [1]	FORMlabs (Dental and E-Shell series)	Fertility-impairing effect [20], acute and chronic toxic for aquatic organisms [21], toxic effect on mouse NIH 3T3 cells [22]. Not readily biodegradable by Organization for Economic Cooperation and Development (OECD) criteria [21,23,24].
Benzophenone compounds [2]	UV-cured inks	Causes liver hypertrophy and kidney adenoma in rats [25,26].
Triarylsulfonium salt (Cationic) [3]	3D Systems	EC_{50} (24 h) Daphnia magna—4.4 mg/L [27]. EC_{50} (48 h) Daphnia magna—0.68 mg/L [27].
Photopolymers		
Acrylate monomers, Acrylate and Urethane acrylate oligomers	FORMlabs Autodesk Envisiontec 3D Systems	Toxic or harmful to various species of fish, algae, and water microorganisms [23]. Potential mutagens and a reproductive and developmental toxicant [28,29].
Methyl methacrylate monomers [3] and oligomers	FORMlabs (Envisiontec Dental resin)	Assessment of repeated dose toxicity indicates the potential to affect the liver and kidneys, as indicated in animal studies [30]. Potential mutagen, and a reproductive and developmental toxicant, aquatic toxicant, and genotoxic in mammalian cell culture [31–33].
Bisphenol A-diglycidyl dimethacrylate (Bis-GMA)	Dental resins	EC_{50} mouse fibroblast—9.35 µM [34].
Auxiliary compounds		
Butylated hydroxytoluene	Dental resins	Toxic or harmful to various species of fish, algae, and water microorganisms [35].
Sebacate compounds [4]	FORMlabs (Dental Envisiontec)	Toxic to aquatic life with long-lasting effects [23], not readily biodegradable (OECD 301B) [23,36].
Hydroquinone	Dental resins	Evidence of mutagenicity in mammal studies, toxic to aquatic life; absorption, in sufficient concentrations, leads to cyanosis [37].

[1] Including diphenyl(2,4,6-trimethylbenzoyl) phosphine oxide (TPO) and bis acyl phosphine oxide (BAPO). [2] Including benzophenone-3 (BP-3) and benzophenone-4 (BP-4) [38]. [3] Degrades to methacrylic acid: LD_{50} Oral rat—1320 mg/kg, LC_{50} (96 h) Oncorhynchus mykiss—85 mg/L [39]. [4] Bis(2,2,6,6-tetramethyl-4-piperidyl) sebacate, Pentamethyl-piperidyl sebacate.

3. Innovative AM Technologies

To carry out a deep discussion about the antimicrobial polymers used in AM methodologies, it is important to first mention some of the most common types and innovative AM technologies. The

ASTM technical committee F42 define the criteria that has been employed for classifying the AM technologies into seven different categories: (a) material extrusion, (b) powder bed fusion, (c) vat photopolymerization, (d) material jetting, (e) binder jetting, (f) sheet lamination, and (g) directed energy deposition [40,41]. While it is true that today there exists a wide variety of materials that are used in AM including thermoplastics, photopolymers, ceramics, and metallic powders, we will center our attention on those techniques that exclusively employ polymeric materials and composites, and particularly those that use antimicrobial polymers for biomedical or biotechnological applications. Among these methods, material extrusion, powder bed fusion, and vat photopolymerization are the most common techniques to create 3D printed devices, and consequently, they have been extensively employed in conjunction with polymeric antimicrobial composites.

There are also some innovative technologies that are based on one or more of the previously mentioned technologies. A novel methodology is for example that reported by Chang et al. [42], who developed a technique for 3D printing that was coined electrohydrodynamic printing (EHD), which is based on the application of a controlled electric current through a syringe that follows a predetermined path layer-by-layer to form a 3D printing part. Another interesting example is the reported by Malinauskas et al. [43] from the year 2017, which developed an ultrafast laser lithography methodology by using a femtosecond laser to create micro-optical devices (lenses) with optical clearness and high resilence. Additionally, they proved a controlled pyrolysis procedure as a method to shrink the printed parts in order to achieve smaller dimensions without compromising the resolution of the printed part. Malinauskas et al. achieved a 40% volumetric shrinkage by removing the organic constituents of their printed parts via pyrolysis.

Similarly, the group of Jeon et al. [44] developed a method coined high-resolution 3D interference printing, which is based on the optical interference phenomenon with restricted near-field diffraction generated by conformal binary gratings. The advantage of this methodology is that it involves only one single ultrashort exposure step. The design of the conformal grating allows controlling the geometry of the printed parts, permitting obtaining high-resolution printing devices in a short amount of time. Another similar methodology that allows obtaining high-resolution devices of multiple materials in a single exposure step is that coined by the group of Hawker et al. [45] as Solution Mask Liquid Lithography (SMaLL). In this case, photochromic molecules are used to control the polymerization kinetics through coherent bleaching fronts, providing large curing depths and rapid build rates without the need for moving parts. The coupling of these photoswitches with some resin mixtures allows the simultaneous and selective curing of multiple networks, providing access to 3D printed parts with chemically and mechanically distinct domains.

The group of Watanabe et al. [46] reported an innovative method for 3D printing based on a plasma ion beam. They used a high-current plasma focused ion beam (FIB) to generate customized microelectromechanical systems (MEMS). This methodology allows creating capacitive MEMS vibration sensors, which were compared to their counterparts fabricated with conventional lithography methods. The difference in measured resonance frequency was small (less than 4%), but the fabrication times were reduced by more than 80% using this methodology.

There are some innovative printing method that are not directly linked with the topic of this review (antimicrobial 3D printing), but deserve to be mentioned due to their originality and novel applications; one of these is the so-called 3D ice printing [47] developed by the group of Zhang et al., which uses this technique to print microcapsule chip arrays over different substrates for target detection. This printing method allows storing the microcapsule arrays in ice form before use, guaranteeing their long-term stability. Other methods, such as that reported by Shear et al. [48], enable 3D printing bacterial communities that are encapsulated in polypeptide matrices of particular and complex shapes and forms. In this article, the authors described a strategy that enabled printing multiple bacteria populations that could be organized within essentially any 3D geometry, including adjacent, nested, and free-floating colonies. The printing method works with a laser-based lithographic technique that permits the formation of microscopic containers around selected bacteria suspended in gelatin via focal cross-linking of the after-mentioned polypeptide molecules.

4. Antibacterial Polymers: Few Elementary Aspects

Pioneer studies on antimicrobial molecules have been mainly focused on the use of low molecular weight substances. However, Boman [49] et al. discovered that a particular family of peptides, i.e., antimicrobial peptides (AMPs), were excellent candidates to remove gram-positive and gram-negative bacteria, as well as also fungi. Since these initial reports AMPs have been extensively investigated, and a large amount of peptides have been reported, classified, and gathered in an antimicrobial peptide database (APD) [50]. The investigations that were carried out at that time concluded that a major part of the AMPs presented a common characteristic, i.e., they were formed by a combination of amino acids with polar and non-polar side chains, thus leading to amphiphilic structures. The polar units are typically formed by amino acids such as lysine or glutamic acid, and the non-polar parts are formed by the incorporation of amino acids such as tryptophan. This amphiphilic characteristic has been demonstrated to play a key role in the interaction of the AMPs with the bacterial membrane, and was employed as a starting point to develop antimicrobial polymers mimicking this polar/non-polar characteristic. [51] As a result, a variety of synthetic polymers with variable chemical structures and functional groups have been employed for the preparation of antimicrobial macromolecules, in some cases with effective antimicrobial activity. [52–57] In this section, we aim to briefly summarize the most relevant characteristics of the antimicrobial polymers reported, taking into account their structure and functionality.

4.1. Polymer Requirements: Polymeric Structures and Other Relevant Characteristics

Matsuzaki [58] proposed a list of four major features that an antimicrobial polymer should have in order to exhibit efficient antimicrobial activity. These features are based on the analysis of the structure of the bacterial membrane and the mechanisms involved in the disruption of this membrane. The four major characteristics are:

(a) able to establish enough contact with the microorganisms,
(b) the polymer should have enough cationic groups so that the adhesion to the microorganism cell can occur,
(c) the polymer should also be designed with hydrophobic moieties that are responsible for the attachment and integration inside the cellular membrane.
(d) the polymer must selectively kill the microbes in the presence of other cells such as mammalian cells.

These initial four major characteristics were complemented with another proposed by Kenawy et al. [7], taking into account the antibacterial mechanism and the synthetic aspects involved in the fabrication of the polymer. Then, these authors proposed that a model antimicrobial polymer should also:

(1) be synthesized using easy and cost-effective strategies
(2) be stable for the applications that can in some cases require long-term usage and storage at a certain temperature
(3) the polymer should remain insoluble in aqueous solution
(4) not decompose or release toxic products, and should not be toxic or irritating to users
(5) ideally be regenerated, maintaining its activity, and finally,
(6) be able to target different pathogenic microorganisms in a relatively short period of time.

4.2. Types of Antimicrobial Groups Integrated in Polymers

From a synthetic point of view, several aspects can be tailored for the synthesis of antimicrobial polymers. Herein, we will briefly discuss these aspects, which are divided in two main groups. On the one hand, the functional groups that were inserted in the polymer structure play a key role in the interaction with the microorganism membrane. On the other hand, those polymer characteristics are related with the structure of the polymer, including the molecular weight and distribution of the functional groups.

For instance, it is today widely admitted that bacterial cell membranes (both gram positive and gram negative) are formed by phospholipids and teichoic acids with a negative net surface charge, among other materials. Therefore, polymers bearing positively charged functional groups are in principle able to interact better with the bacterial cell wall in comparison to neutral or negatively charged functional groups.

4.2.1. Positively Charged Functional Groups

Without any doubt, quaternary ammonium/phosphonium groups are the most extensively employed functional groups for the preparation of cationic polymers and have been reported to act as efficient antimicrobial agents.

Pioneer works using ammonium chlorides were reported in the early 1980s by Ikeda et al. [59,60], which described the preparation of polyvinylbenzyl ammonium chloride. In their studies, Ikeda et al. evidenced high antimicrobial activity, and associated this activity with the possibility of interaction between the polymer and the cell membrane [61]. In addition to the above-depicted quaternary amine functional groups, other functional groups that are able to be protonated, depending on the environmental pH, have been equally reported. In this context, primary, secondary, and tertiary amino groups have been also explored. An illustrative example was reported by Gelman et al. [62]. This group synthesized a wide range of polymers based on polystyrene comprising tertiary amine groups. After the protonation of the tertiary amino groups, the authors observed an activity similar to that exhibited for quaternary amine functional groups. Dimethylamino ethyl methacrylate (DMAEMA) is a monomer with tertiary amino side functional groups that can be protonated when in contact with humidity or in aqueous media. This monomer was employed by Vigliotta et al. [63] to prepare a wide range of polymers based on DMAEMA that resulted in materials with excellent antimicrobial activity.

While the above-depicted functional groups are reported to have excellent antimicrobial activity, they present a major drawback: the toxicity against mammalian cells. In order to reduce this undesirable side effect, several groups have worked on the use of alternative cationic groups. In this context, phosphonium groups were demonstrated to be less toxic to mammalian cells, which together with an improved thermal stability, have been proposed as candidates for the incorporation in the elaboration of antimicrobial polymers [64,65]. Dehelean et al. [66], Ao et al. [67], and Zhao et al. [68] employed this type of functionality for the preparation of different antimicrobial polymers. For instance, Ao et al. [67] employed quaternary phosphonium groups to modify epoxy natural rubber, and evidenced an improved antibacterial activity of these materials in comparison to the non-modified ones. Also, Zhao et al. [68] employed quaternary phosphonium groups, but for the fabrication of terpolymers also bearing polyacrylamide. Interestingly, the authors evidenced an excellent activity in particular for adenovirus (ADV). Furthermore, the authors showed that the antibacterial activity is directly related to the amount of quaternary phosphonium within the polymer.

4.2.2. Other Antimicrobial Functional Groups

In addition to the cationic quaternary ammonium and phosphonium groups, *N*-halamine groups [69,70], sulfonium [71], zwitterionic polymers [72], and nitric oxide-containing polymers [73] are a few examples of the groups with excellent antimicrobial activity.

For instance, N-halamines are interesting candidates that have been extensively studied during the last decade, and have been reported as having a large activity against a wide variety of microorganisms while also being safe for the environment and humans. N-halamines can be regenerated, and can be produced at low cost. [69] According to Hui et al. [74], N-halamines have been incorporated in polymers by using different alternatives that include the polymerization approach (homopolymerization and heteropolymerization), the electrogeneration of biocidal coatings, or by grafting or coating on different substrates (typically by using epoxides, hydroxyl groups, and alkoxy silanes as anchoring groups).

Another example is the case of zwitterionic polymers. These groups present simultaneously negative and positively charged groups that result in a net neutral charge. Illustrative studies on the use of these functional groups were reported by Lowe et al. [72,73]. Jiang et al. [75] investigated a large number of these polymers, and they found some of them to present excellent antimicrobial activities in particular toward *E. Coli.* and *S. Aureus.* In a recent minireview, Jiang et al. summarized the capabilities of zwitterionic polymers as antimicrobial and simultaneously non-fouling groups [75]. They reported the recent advances of the different chemical structures of zwitterionic polymers and divided the groups into functional types depending on the microbiological application, i.e., non-fouling, non-fouling and surface bactericidal, and non-fouling and bulk antimicrobial (Figure 3). A particularly interesting example is the development of polymers that are able to kill, release, and be regenerated to restore the antimicrobial activity. In effect, for many purposes, such as reusable medical devices, the recovery of the bactericidal activity is needed. In many applications, such as most reusable surgical devices, renewable bactericidal surfaces are often needed. For this purpose, Cao et al. designed zwitterionic polymers that have the ability to undergo a reversible lactonization reaction that served to create reversible cycles between bactericidal and non-fouling states (Figure 4) [76,77].

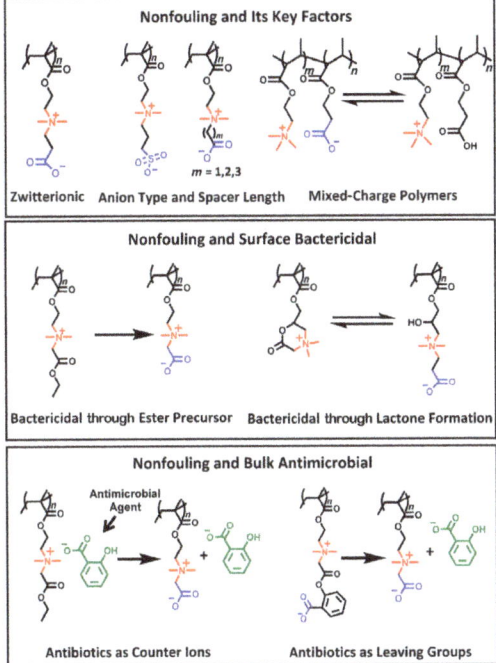

Figure 3. Chemical structures and microbiological applications of several zwitterionic polymers and their derivatives. Reproduced with permission from Ref. [75].

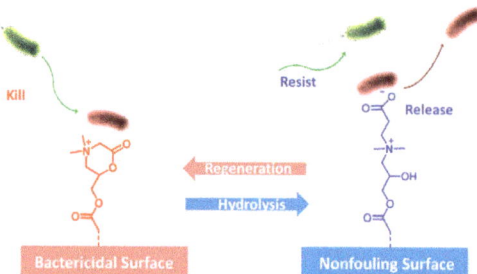

Figure 4. Illustrative scheme of the reversible lactonization that enables the system to kill bacteria (cationic state) and the release of inactivated bacterial cells occurring upon ring-opening and formation of the zwitterionic state. Reproduced with permission from Ref. [75].

4.3. Macromolecular Characteristics and their Role in the Antibacterial Activity

In addition to the chemical functional groups, several other parameters related to the polymer design play an important role. It is outside of the scope of this review to provide a detailed description of all the aspects involved; instead, we will just focus on briefly describing the most relevant characteristics, which include the hydrophilic/hydrophobic balance, the molecular weight, or the polymer topology (block/random copolymers or branched/linear polymers).

Without any doubt, one of the most critical aspects is the amphiphilicity of the polymer, i.e., the hydrophobic/hydrophilic balance. The amphiphilic character affects both the antimicrobial activity as well as the selectivity toward mammalian cells. An ideal amphiphilic polymer is formed by hydrophilic moieties, which are typically positively charged groups, and hydrophobic moieties (usually alkyl chains) forming the main polymer chain [78]. The design of this polymeric structure is based on two main ideas. First of all, it provides electrostatic interactions between the negatively charged cell membrane and the cationic groups in the polymers. Second, the hydrophobic segments within the polymer chain will be able to establish interactions with the lipid domains within the cell membrane.

As a result of this configuration, the negatively charged cell membrane will interact with the positively charge moieties and the hydrophobic main chain will be in contact with the lipid domains of the membrane [79]. However, an appropriate balance has appeared to be crucial. For instance, it has been reported that large hydrophilic moieties bind better to the cell membrane. While this is true for the hydrophilic segment, it has been proved that too large hydrophobic segments result in an increase of the cytotoxicity for all cell types [80].

Also, the molecular weight of the polymer plays a key role in both the antimicrobial activity as well as the hemolytic activity; however, it is worth mentioning that, in this case, the results that are reported largely depend on the type of cells employed and the type of polymer. In principle, the interaction between the polymer and the cell wall depend on the positive charges within the polymer structure; it is expected that higher molecular weight polymers provide better antimicrobial activities in comparison to small-sized polymers or oligomers. Nevertheless, high molecular weight polymers present important limitations such as their solubility or eventual aggregation in biological medium, but more importantly, increasing hemolytic activity (directly related to the polymer size).

Finally, also, the polymer topology significantly affects the antimicrobial activity of the polymer. Since the arrangement of polar and non-polar groups within the macromolecular structure affects the antimicrobial activity, the behavior of block copolymers and random copolymers can be significantly different. In general, random copolymers present rather good antimicrobial activities, but lack the required selectivity [81], although some studies have used alternative monomers that can be activated in acid conditions but have little hemolytic activity at neutral pH [81], or used long hydrophilic and cationic polymers [82]. In the case of amphiphilic block copolymers, they present the unique capability of forming different types of nano-objects in solution by self-assembly. The morphologies that they can form depend on the hydrophilic to hydrophobic volume ratio, but also on the molecular weight, as well as other experimental conditions such as the temperature or solvent employed. While it is true that there are not many examples in the literature, some reports indicated that the block copolymers are much less hemolytic compared to the highly hemolytic random copolymers. In an interesting manuscript, Oda et al. [83] compared the antimicrobial activity and the hemolytic activity of copolymers based on isobutyl vinyl ether (IBVE) and phthalimide-protected amine vinyl ether (PIVE) with similar chain lengths and monomer compositions. The block copolymers displayed selective activity against E. coli over red blood cells (RBCs), while the random copolymers did not and were hemolytic.

5. Antimicrobial Polymers, Blends, and Composites in Additive Manufacturing

Antimicrobial 3D printed parts have been intensively investigated in recent years due to the wide range of applications, including bone tissue engineering regeneration [84,85] to treat bone fractures [86], the fabrication of biomedical devices that are able to prevent biofilm formation [8], the fabrication of wound dressings [87], or the fabrication of scaffolds, just to mention few of them [88].

Independently of the application, in order to provide antimicrobial or antibacterial activity to a 3D printed part, different alternative strategies can be employed, which include among others the use of antimicrobial polymeric materials, the incorporation and release of antimicrobial agents, or introducing an antibacterial functionality through the surface modification of the part [89]. As will be depicted, both natural and synthetic polymers have been employed to fabricate antimicrobial 3D pritned parts. Moreover, not only polymeric but also composite materials, i.e., raw materials that present antibacterial characteristics or polymeric composites that are mixed with bactericide compounds to create antibacterial materials, have been reported.

In the following sections, we will describe the fabrication of different antimicrobial 3D printed parts depending on the nature of the polymer employed (natural or synthetic). In Sections 5 and 6, we attempt to differentiate among the alternative approaches that have been depicted to fabricate the parts such as the incorporation of antimicrobial monomers, antimicrobial agents (non-polymeric/monomeric), and surface modification. The following Section 7 will be focused on the description of those systems based on polymer composites with antimicrobial properties.

6. Naturally Occurring Antimicrobial Polymers

The use of naturally occurring polymers for AM applications has been increasing in recent years. In this context, without any doubt, cellulose—and most recently nanocellulose—is the most extensively employed natural type of polymer due to its intrinsic antimicrobial properties. The rationale behind this selection relies on cellulose being one of the primary reinforcement structures of most of the biological organisms, and indeed, it is one of the most abundant polymers on Earth [90]. Cellulose is also mechanically robust, inexpensive, biorenewable, biodegradable, chemically versatile, and also has antimicrobial properties [91]. All of these characteristics make this polymer considerably attractive for use in AM technologies, and for biomedical applications in particular. For instance, Pattinson and Hart [92] reported a method for printing a cellulose-based material via the extrusion of cellulose acetate (CA). The CA feedstock was prepared by dissolving it in acetone; then, the extrusion was performed via a gantry-style 3D printer with a capillary nozzle connected to a liquid dispenser. Once the material was extruded from the tip, the acetone evaporated, thus leaving a CA printed layer-by-layer device. In their work, Pattinson and Hart, changed the printing parameters such as liquid pressure/flow, print velocity, and distance from tip to the print bed, and solution viscosity. Figure 5a shows a schematic description of the CA printing process. Figure 5b shows a close-up of the printing process.

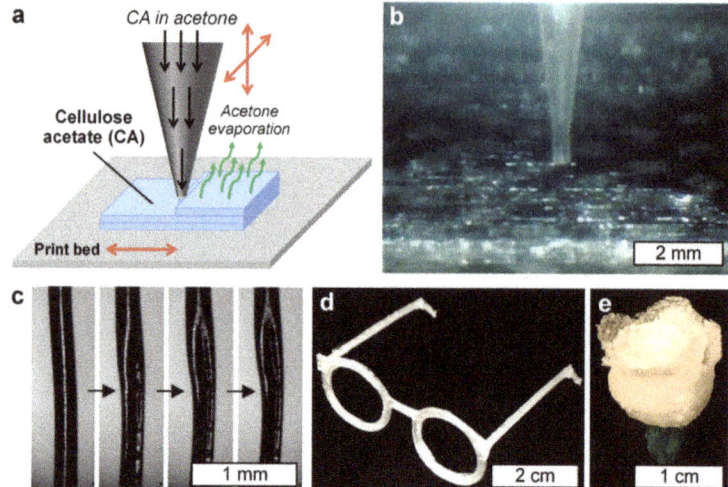

Figure 5. (a) Schematic description of the three-dimensional (3D) printing process using cellulose acetate (CA) dissolved in acetone. (b) Photograph of a close-up of printing tip during the manufacturing process. (c) Micrographs that show the acetone evaporating process. 3D printed parts, (d) eyeglass frames, and (e) a rose. Reproduced with permission from Ref. [92].

Uniaxial tests of CA printed parts were carried out to test the mechanical properties of the resulting parts. For that purpose, dogbone samples, which were printed at different printing directions (parallel and perpendicular) and with variable material treatments (for instance, with NaOH), were mechanically tested. The results demonstrated a favorable mechanical performance compared with other common thermoplastic AM materials (Acrylonitrile Butadiene Styrene (ABS), poly(lactic acid) (PLA), and nylon). The NaOH treatment effectively transforms the CA into cellulose via a deacetylation process, as evidenced by Fourier transform infrared (FTIR). It is important to remark that the mechanical behavior of the CA probes is not considerably altered. Finally, the antimicrobial effectivity of the printed parts was tested using *E. coli*. To compare the results, small amounts of known antimicrobial agent dyes (toluidine blue and rose bengal) were added to Petri dishes with the CA printed material and exposed to a fluorescent lamp; additionally, polyethylene substrates were used as a control. Different set-ups were tested, which were namely as follows. D+L+: Bacteria exposed to cellulose acetate with dye and light. D+L−: Bacteria exposed to cellulose acetate with dye, but left in the dark. D−L+: Bacteria exposed to cellulose acetate without dye, but with light. D−L−: Bacteria exposed to cellulose acetate with no dye and left in the dark. PL+: Bacteria exposed to polyethylene and light. PL−: Bacteria exposed to polyethylene and left in the dark. Figure 6 shows some of the results obtained from viable bacteria count. This data demonstrates that the dyed CA printed parts enabled a large reduction in the bacterial count by simple exposure to fluorescent light.

Recently, Gatenholm et al. [93] reported an innovative 3D printing method based on nanocellulose hydrogels aiming to provide an alternative treatment to serious auricular defects. A matrix phase of alginate mixed with nanofibrillated cellulose particles was cross-linked by using a CaCl$_2$ solution (Figure 7b). Human nasal chondrocytes (hNC) were mixed with the ink to obtain the bioink used for print (20 × 10^6 cells/mL), and then were printed into auricular constructs with open porosity (Figure 7c). Cell viability was examined at different stages of the bioprinting process: before embedding the hNCs, before embedding and cross-linking, and after embedding, bioprinting, and cross-linking. The mean cell viability after the embedding and cross-linking processes was found to be significantly lower than the samples before embedding the hNCs (Figure 7a). Furthermore, no significant difference between after embedding and after bioprinting was founded, indicating that the printing process had no significant influence on cell vitality. Based on these results, it was concluded that this bioink is promising for auricular cartilage tissue engineering and many other biomedical applications.

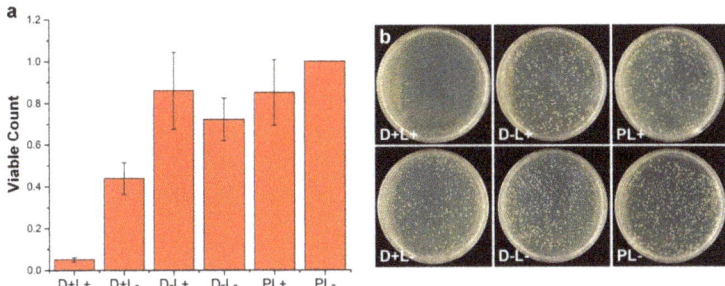

Figure 6. (**a**) Evaluation of the antimicrobial performance of the 3D printed CA parts, in which the viable bacteria count was normalized with the PL- results; and (**b**) Images of the bacteria cultured Petri dishes exposed to different conditions. Adapted with permission from Ref. [92].

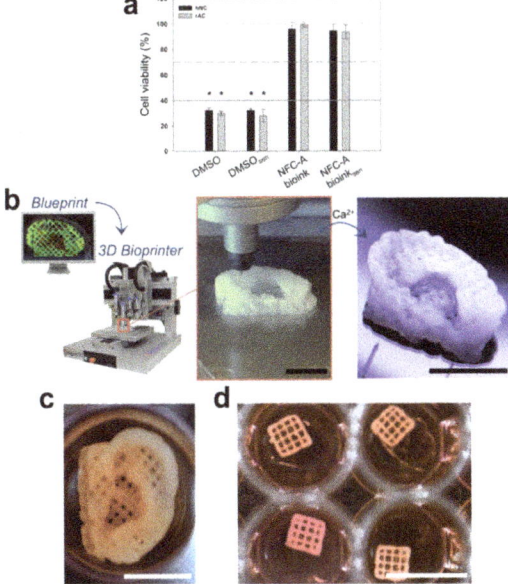

Figure 7. (**a**) In vitro cytotoxicity test of Nanofibrillated cellulose (NFC) bioink. Human nasal chondrocytes (hNC) and rabbit auricular chondrocytes (rAC) were used as indicator cells to determine the cytotoxic effects potentially caused by bioink components, cross-linking, or the bioprinting process. (**b**) 3D bioprinting process of chondrocyte-laden NFC-A auricular construct with open porosity. (**c**) 3D bioprinted auricular and (**d**) lattice-structured constructs, laden with hNCs, after 28 days of culture. Reproduced with permission from Ref. [93].

7. Synthetic Polymers with Bactericidal Properties

7.1. Antimicrobial Functional Monomers as Components in SLA Resins

Monomers with antimicrobial properties have been proposed for the elaboration of photosensitive resins to be employed in stereolithography (SLA). An interesting example was reported by the group of Herrmann and Ren et al. [94], which developed a 3D printable polymeric resin based on monomers containing antimicrobial positively charged quaternary ammonium groups. Diurethanedimethacrylate/glycerol dimethacrylate (UDMA/GDMA) linear chains were photocured via light-induced polymerization. The antimicrobial dental parts were printed using a stereolithography set-up (Figure 8a). Interestingly, the printed parts kill bacteria on contact when positively charged quaternary ammonium groups are incorporated into the photocurable UDMA/GDMA resins. A post-functionalization process permits gradually quaternizing the samples as well as modifying the methacrylate monomers with different alkyl chain lengths (QA_C_n). According to their results, the modification with an alkyl chain with a length of $n = 12$ presents the best antimicrobial performances (QA_C_{12}). The contact killing efficacy was tested on Petri dishes by using *S. mutans* as a gram-positive model. A parallel, long-term antimicrobial effect was also measured after six days of culturing. The results demonstrated that the quaternization of the material considerably improved the killing rate of the printed parts. Finally, the printed parts were also mechanically tested (Figure 8b), showing performances quite similar to those of the other common 3D printed materials.

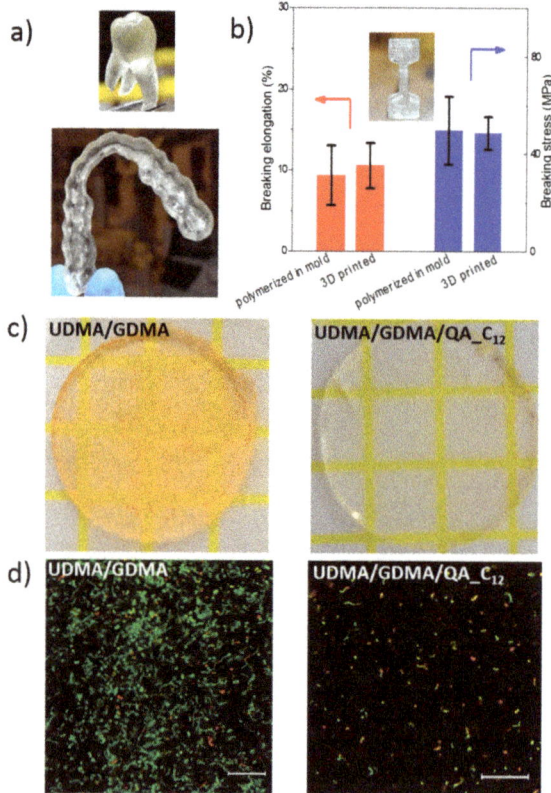

Figure 8. (a) 3D printed dental parts using diurethanedimethacrylate/glycerol dimethacrylate (UDMA/GDMA) composites. (b) Uniaxial tensile tests of 14 mol% UDMA/GDMA with the modified methacrylate monomers with an alkyl chain length of $n = 12$ (QA_C_{12}). (c) Comparison of the contact-killing efficacy of 3D printed UDMA/GDMA and UDMA/GDMA/QA_C_{12} and (d) comparison of the long-term contact-killing efficacy of 3D printed UDMA/GDMA and UDMA/GDMA/QA_C_{12} six days after live/dead staining. Reproduced with permission from Ref. [94].

Similarly, the group of Yang and Wang et al. [5] performed some modifications to a commercial 3D printing resin called MiiCraft, which comprises acrylate-based pre-polymers, cross-linking agents, and a phosphine oxide-based compound as a photoinitiator (Figure 9a). Then, by using a stereolithography method, 3D printed parts were fabricated. In order to change the surface properties of the material, polymer brushes were grown on the printed structure via the surface-initiated atomic transfer data polymerization (SI-ATRP) grafting method. In this study, a thin layer of 3-sulfopropyl methacrylate potassium salt (SPMA) was grown on the printed polymer structure to bring antimicrobial properties to the printed part. Finally, bacterial adhesion and inhibition tests were carried out for the grafted samples. Both gram-negative (*E. coli*) and gram-positive (*B. subtilis*) bacteria were used as model microorganisms (Figure 9b). The results demonstrate that the functionalized surface can not only reduce the adhesion of the bacteria, but also inhibit the growth on the surface. The technique developed by Yang and Wang et al. has significantly expanded the capability of 3D printing technology for biomedical applications.

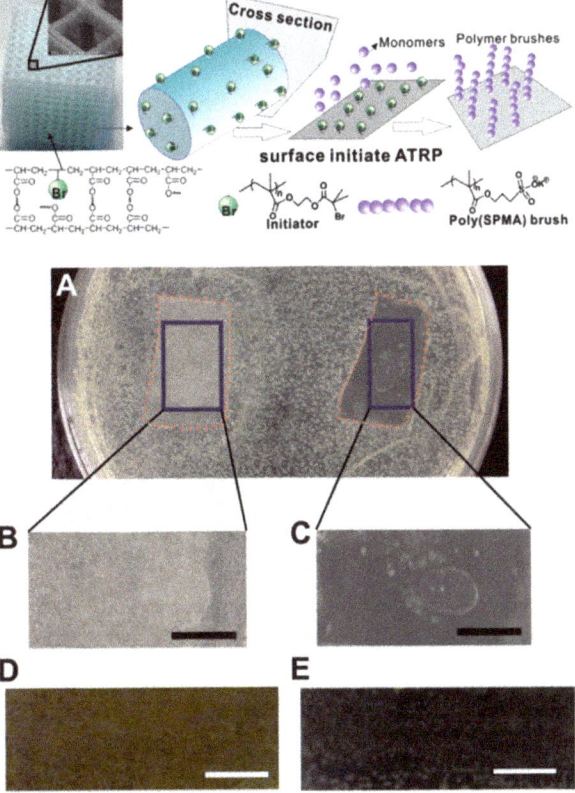

Figure 9. **Above** Schematic representation of the synthesis and grafting process of the 3D printed parts. **Below** (**a**) Photographs of the inhibition tests performed after 24 hours of bacteria growth, (**b**) the control sample and (**c**) 3-sulfopropyl methacrylate potassium salt (SPMA)-treated sample. Similar results after 48 hours for the (**d**) control and (**e**) SPMA-treated sample. Reproduced with permission from Ref. [5].

Another example was recently reported by Garcia et al. [95]. The group reported the preparation of both 3D printed pH-responsive and antimicrobial hydrogels with micrometric resolution using stereolithography. In particular, the authors prepared hydrogels using a resin formed by polyethylene glycol dimethacrylate (PEGDMA), with variable chain lengths (ranging from two up to 14 units) polyethylene glycol monomethacrylate, and acrylic acid (AA) as a linear monomer. Additionally, a photoabsorber (Sudan I) was employed in order to control the UV penetration depth. This allowed the authors to improve the printing model accuracy and simultaneously increase the z-axis resolution (Figure 7). Depending on the ratio between the components, a wide variety of smart hydrogels with variable swelling-responsive capacities were obtained. The groups reported that the hydrogel prepared by additive manufacturing was able to swell and shrink depending on the environmental pH. This effect is the consequence of the protonation and deprotonation of the carboxylic acid groups. Thus, the swelling observed is dependent on the amount of acrylic acid incorporated in the hydrogel formulation. Finally, as depicted in Figure 10, the hydrogels that were reported presented excellent antimicrobial properties for all of the compositions that were explored when exposed to S. aureus (bacteria employed as a model in this study).

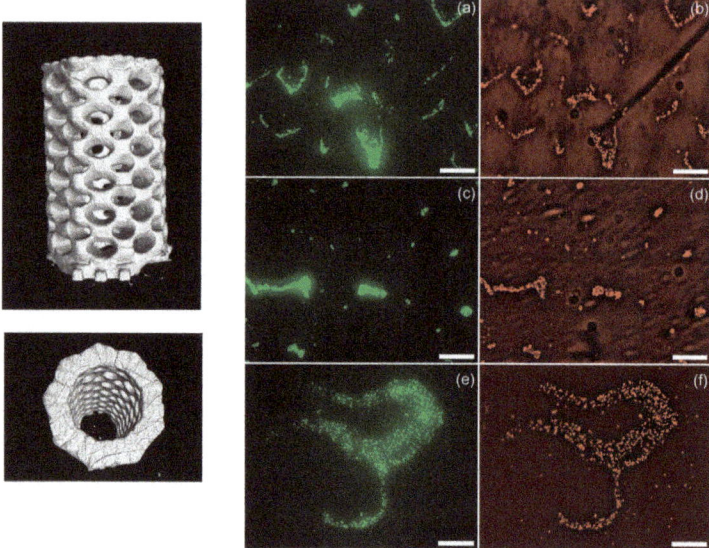

Figure 10. Left: Lateral and top 3D views of the micro-computed topography (μ-CT) images of the fabricated parts. **Right:** Bacterial viability on the different hydrogels with a variable amount of acrylic acid (AA). (**a,b**) 25 wt% AA, (**c,d**) 20 wt% AA, and (**e,f**) 10 wt% AA. Green fluorescence corresponds to the emission of all the bacteria, while the red one is related to the emission of propidium iodide (dead bacteria). Reproduced with permission from Ref. [95].

7.2. Antimicrobial Polymers for FDM

Antimicrobial thermoplastics or the elaboration of blends of thermoplastics with antimicrobial agents is a direct approach to prepare antimicrobial filaments that can be employed in FDM. For instance, Water et al. [96] characterized the physicochemical properties of the printed materials using thermoplastics charged with antimicrobial agents. More precisely, they used a custom-developed PLA feedstock material containing nitrofurantoin (NF) as an antimicrobial drug (10%, 20% or 30%) with and without the addition of 5% hydroxyapatite (HA) in polylactide strands. This mixture was used as a feedstock for the 3D printing process (Figure 11a). Figure 11b shows SEM images of the extrude and 3D materials where the surface morphology is highly dependent on the composition, which is to say, a sample with higher drug loading (30%) had an apparent rougher surface than those with lower drug content based on visual observations. The results indicated that the loading and release of NF from the printed PLA matrices showed an increased accumulated release after increasing the drug loading. Additionally, the materials showed resistance to bacterial adhesion and biofilm formation over a period of seven days. This research demonstrates the potential of custom-made, drug-loaded feedstock materials for the 3D printing of pharmaceutical products for controlled release. Similar studies that were carried out by Sandler et al. reported the possibility of incorporating NF in the PLA matrix in 5:95 (w/w) NF:PLA; this new material favored an 85% decrease of the biofilm formation on the 3D printed geometries over the 18-h time interval [8].

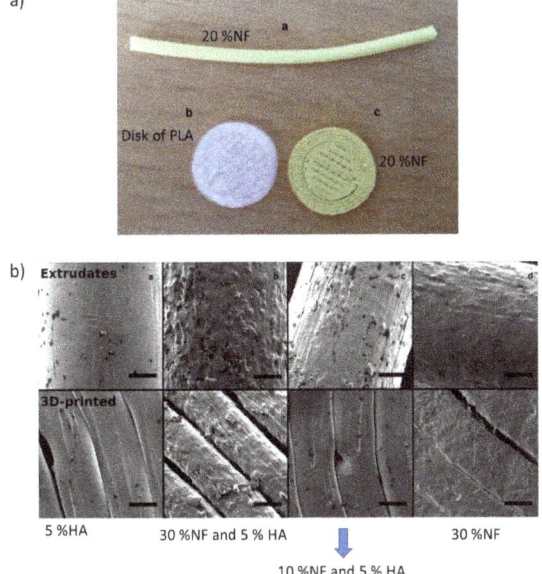

Figure 11. (a) Extrudated and 3D-printed and (b) SEM images of extruded and 3D-printed geometries. Reproduced with permission from Ref. [96].

In a recent study, Mills et al. [97] reported the cytocompatibility, mechanical, and antimicrobial properties of 3D printed poly(methyl methacrylate) (PMMA) and poly(lactic acid) (PLA) beads loaded with a calculated amount of a drug in powdered form, i.e., gentamicin sulfate (GS). In this study, they showed that all the antibiotics that were studied were successfully doped into PMMA and in PLA, and antibiotic-doped 3D printed beads, disks, and filaments were easily printed by FDM. The growth inhibition capacity of the antibiotic-loaded PMMA 3D printed constructs was also demonstrated. The 1 wt% and 2.5 wt% gentamicin-doped PLA filaments and PMMA filaments were tested on bacterial plates (Figure 5). As depicted in Figure 12, those filaments without GS did not show any inhibition, whereas both PLA and PMMA presented an inhibition zone of around 23 mm.

Another interesting example is that reported by the group of Wang et al. [42], who fabricated patches using AM technologies from polycaprolactone (PCL) and polyvinyl pyrrolidone (PVP). The parts also were charged with antibiotic drugs (tetracycline hydrochloride, TE-HCL) during the printing procedure. An interesting printing technique was used to fabricate the patches, the so-called electrohydrodynamic (EHD) technique, which is based on the application of an electric current through a nozzle that moves over a particular path to form a 3D printing part layer-by-layer (Figure 11a). This technique is very similar to electrospinning or the electrospray technique, but uses much lower voltages and currents to create the fibers. FTIR demonstrated successful TE-HCL encapsulation in the printed material. Patches prepared using PVP and TE-HCL displayed enhanced hydrophobicity compared to the rest. Also, uniaxial tensile mechanical tests were performed on the different materials; the printed parts exhibited changes in their mechanical properties arising from printing parameters such as fibrous strut orientation, variable inter-strut pore size, and film width. The release of antibiotics from PCL-PVP dosage forms was shown over five days, and was slower compared to pure PCL or PVP; also, the printed patch void size influenced antibiotic release behavior (Figure 13b–d).

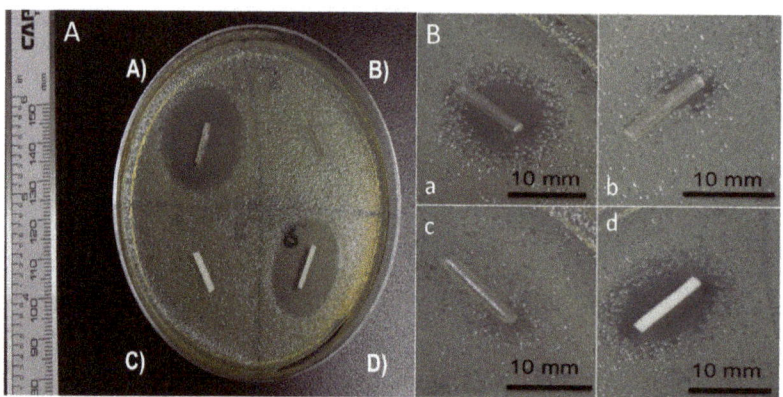

Figure 12. A. Gentamicin sulfate (GS)-doped poly(lactic acid) (PLA) and poly(methyl methacrylate) (PMMA) filaments. (**A**) 2.5 wt% gentamicin PLA filament; (**B**) Control PLA filament; (**C**) Control PMMA filament; (**D**) 2.5 wt% gentamicin PMMA filament. **B.** (**a**–**c**) 1 wt% gentamicin PLA filament; (**d**) 1 wt% gentamicin PMMA filament. Reproduced with permission from Ref. [97].

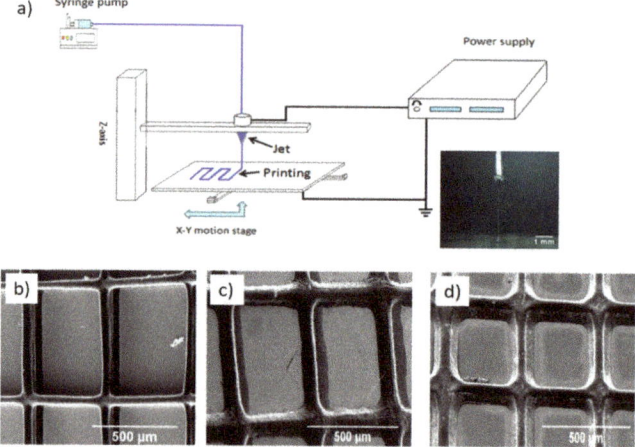

Figure 13. (**a**) Schematic description of the electrohydrodynamic (EHD) technique. SEM images of drug-loaded polycaprolactone (PCL)/polyvinyl pyrrolidone (PVP) patches at selected time intervals for the in vitro release study. (**b**) At 30 min; (**c**) At 60 min; and (**d**) At 90 min. Reproduced with permission from Ref. [42].

7.3. Surface Modification (Patterning and Functionalization) of 3D Printed Parts

An additional alternative to fabricating 3D printed parts with antimicrobial properties involves the surface modification of the part with antimicrobial agents.

In this context, an illustrative strategy of this approach was recently reported by Vargas-Alfredo et al. [98] who reported a strategy that combines the use of high-impact polystyrene (HIPS) to fabricate 3D parts with surface functionalization methodologies to provide antimicrobial 3D objects. The scaffolds were first fabricated by FDM using commercially available HIPS filaments. Then, the object surface was modified, generating 3D parts with a particular strategy that permits simultaneously controlling the surface chemistry and the topography. In particular, the authors used the breath figures

(BFs) approach. The BF strategy involves the scaffold immersion in a polymeric solution during a short (seconds) period of time. The immersion time was reported to be directly related to the pore size, and also help improve the bonding of the 3D printed layers. The results of the research showed evidence that the combination of BF and wet surface treatment is an interesting approach to control the surface microtopography (pore size) and surface functionality (a type of functional group and distribution) of 3D printed objects [98].

The 3D printed parts were fabricated via FDM using commercial polystyrene filament. The 3D porous structure was obtained via solvent evaporation from a polymeric solution: high molecular weight polystyrene (0 to 30 mg/mL) dissolved in chloroform, and water droplet condensation at the solvent/air interface occurring in a moist atmosphere. This procedure was carried out in a closed chamber with a saturated relative humidity at room temperature at different reaction time (one to five seconds). The results demonstrated that decreasing the polymeric solution produced a surface with smaller pores, which is an effect that is related to the viscosity of the reaction mixture. Additionally, a larger evaporation time finally produced pores with larger than average pore sizes. Subsequently, the surface chemical modification was carried out by immersion of the parts in the reactive chlorosulfonic acid solution at 20 °C at different reaction times (0 to 10 min).

More interestingly, by using polymer solutions comprising blends of PS and PS-b-PAA (PS$_{23}$-b-PAA$_{18}$) and a quaternized PS-b-poly(dimethylaminoethyl methacrylate) (PS$_{42}$-b-PDMAEMA$_{17}$), it was possible to simultaneously chemically modify the surface of the scaffold and therefore enable the incorporation of antimicrobial functional groups (Figure 14). Finally, the biological response of the surface-modified scaffolds against bacteria was investigated. The porous surfaces prepared using quaternized PDMAEMA as well as those prepared with PAA as the main component confer antimicrobial activity to the 3D printed parts, permitting killing *S. aureus* bacteria on contact. It should be mentioned that these functional supports are currently evaluated for the fabrication of functional devices such as biocompatible/antifouling tubes, screws for reparative surgery, or scaffolds in which the interactions' cell support can be improved by finely tuning the surface properties (chemistry and structure) [99].

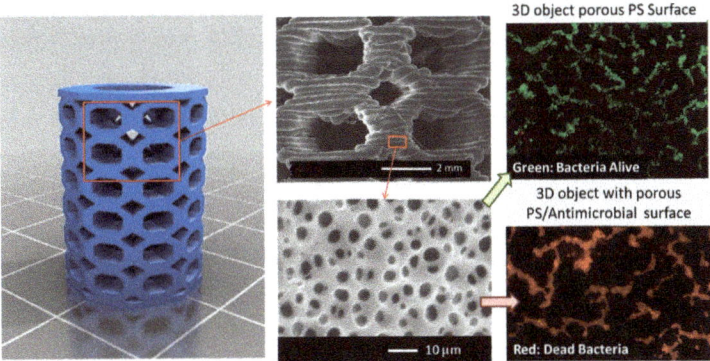

Figure 14. Left: 3D CAD model of scaffold selected for the fabrication by fused deposition modeling (FDM). **Middle:** SEM images of the scaffold surface revealing the layered structure obtained via FDM but also the formation of micropores. **Right:** Effect of the chemical composition on the antimicrobial properties of the 3D printed part. Above, without the antimicrobial functional group, and below, with the antimicrobial functional group. Reproduced with permission from Ref. [99].

8. 3D Printed Polymeric Composites with Antibacterial Capacities

Finally, polymer composites have been explored also for the preparation of antimicrobial 3D printed parts. These composites have been fabricated using graphene [100] metals such as zinc, copper, or silver [87,101,102], and TiO$_2$ [103] among others.

A good example of this strategy was described by Advincula et al. [100], which blended a thermoplastic polyurethane (TPU), poly(lactic acid) (PLA), and graphene oxide (GO), which is a material that is known to be an excellent antimicrobial agent that could also enhance the mechanical properties of the final printed part. In this article, FDM methodology was used to print complex structures. To generate the FDM filament, TPU was dissolved in dimethylformamide (DMF), as well as GO nanocomposite; in parallel, PLA was dissolved in dichloromethane (DCM). Then, the three solutions were mixed under stirring overnight; then, the polymer–composite material was precipitated in alcohol and dried at 40 °C under vacuum. Finally, the resultant precipitate was melted in an extruder to form the FDM filament. According to the proportions of TPU and PLA, the material could have elastic characteristics, which were tested via mechanical tensile and compression experiments. The addition of GO has significantly enhanced the mechanical properties of the polymer matrix by 167% in a compression modulus, and 75.5% in a tensile modulus. Filaments with different GO loadings were tested as antimicrobial and biocompatible materials via live/dead studies. Figure 15 shows a scheme of FDM filament fabrication and some results from cell culture live/dead tests. The fluorescence images in Figure 15 demonstrate that none of the samples showed dead cells, which indicates a high level of material biocompatibility, thus demonstrating that the addition of GO has no obvious toxicity to cell growth, and a small amount of GO is beneficial for cell proliferation.

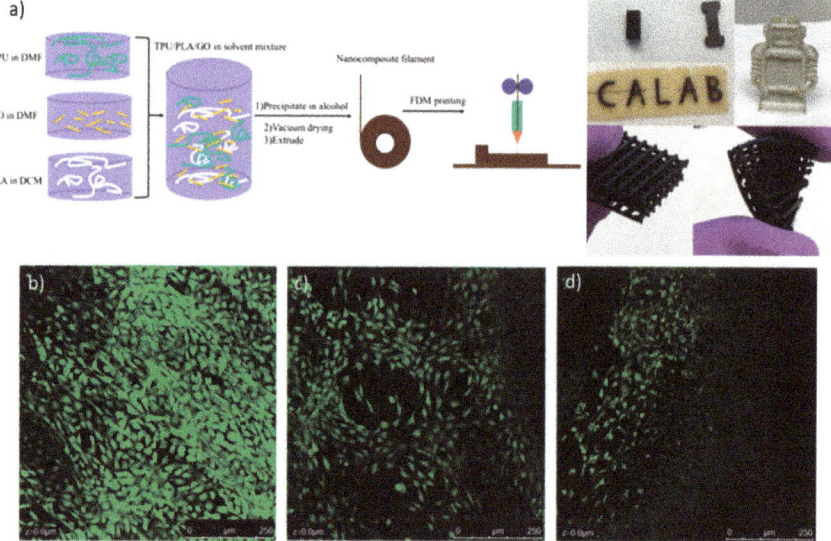

Figure 15. (**a**) Schematic description of FDM filament formation. Also, images of thermoplastic polyurethane (TPU)/poly(lactic acid) (PLA)/graphene oxide (GO) printed parts are shown. Green fluorescence images of cellular live/dead tests of the samples with different GO loads: (**b**) 0.5 wt%; (**c**) 2 wt%; and (**d**) 5 wt%. Reproduced with permission from Ref. [100].

Muwaffak et al. [87] studied the use of antimicrobial metals such as zinc, copper, and silver incorporated into an FDA (Food and Drug Administration)-approved polymer (polycaprolactone, or PCL) to produce filaments for 3D printing (Figure 16a). 3D scanning was used to construct 3D models of a nose and ear to provide the opportunity to customize the shape and size of a wound dressing to an individual patient (Figure 16b). Experimentally, this research was based on the formation of a filament composed by different metal concentrations, whose release was studied by inductively coupled plasma atomic emission spectroscopy. Surface morphology and a cross-section of the filament were obtained by SEM analysis. Additionally, the possible bond of the metals with the PCL matrix was studied via

FTIR spectra. The antibacterial efficacy of wound dressing was tested against *S. aureus*. To perform this type of study, a circular dressing was created using Tinkercard, which is a browser-based 3D design and modeling tool. According to these results, the silver and copper wound dressing had the most potent bactericidal properties.

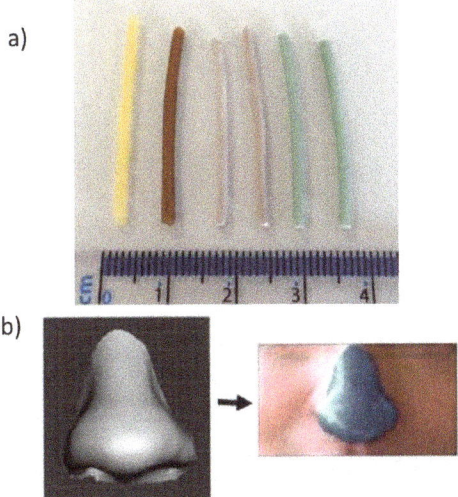

Figure 16. (**a**) Metal-loaded filaments and (**b**) 3D scan of a nose to create a designed wound dressing. Reproduced with permission from Ref. [87].

Similarly, Cristache et al. [103] obtained a poly(methylmethacrylate) (PMMA)–TiO$_2$ nanocomposite material with improved antibacterial characteristics, which was suitable for manufacturing 3D printed dental prosthesis. Different percentages of TiO$_2$ nanoparticles (0.2, 0.4, 0.6, 1 and 2.5 weight %) were added gradually into PMMA solution. In parallel, the nanoparticles were synthesized through a sol–gel procedure from titanium tetrabutoxide, in the presence of dimedone, which was acting as a chelating agent, and dimethylacetamide. Structural and morphological analyses were carried out by FTIR, SEM, and Energy-Dispersive X-ray Spectroscopy (EDX), respectively. Finally, antimicrobial efficacy against bacterial cultures from *Candida species* (*C. Scotti*) was tested. The results proved that TiO$_2$ nanoparticles modified the polymeric structure and their properties, especially the 0.4 % TiO$_2$. This concentration was used to fabricate a prototype of a complete denture using the SLA printing method (Figure 17).

Similarly, Tiimob et al. [101] studied the effect of different proportions of eggshell/silver (ES-Ag) on the microstructure, thermal, tensile, and antimicrobial properties of 70/30 poly(butylene-*co*-adipate-terephthalate)/polylactic acid (PBAT/PLA). Additionally, the release kinetics of Ag nanoparticles (NPs) from the films was also studied. The thin films were prepared using hot melt extrusion and 3D printing for mechanical and antimicrobial testing. In vitro assessment of the antimicrobial activity of these films conducted on *L. monocytogenes* and *S. Enteritidis* bacteria at two different concentrations revealed that the blend composite film possessed bacteriostatic effects, which were due to the immobilized ES-Ag nanomaterials in the blend matrix. However, these were not released into distilled water or chicken breast after 72 h and 168 h of exposure, respectively.

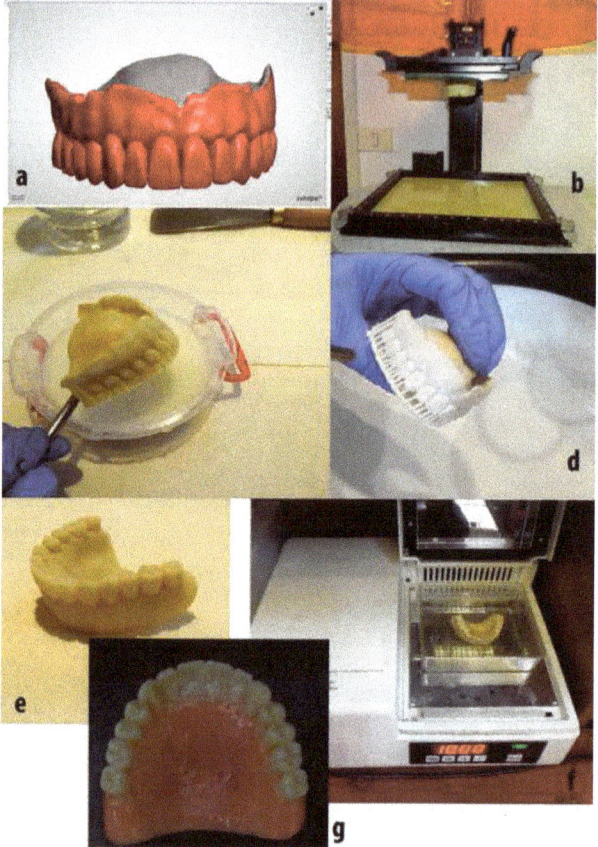

Figure 17. The protocol used to fabricate a complete denture, using the SLA printing technique. (**a**) Design in software. (**b**) Final construction in the 3D printer platform. (**c**) Denture cleaning with isopropanol. (**d**) Denture drying and supports removal. (**e**) Prototype denture polished. (**f**) Final post-curing procedure. (**g**) Esthetic adjustment. Reproduced with permission from Ref. [103].

Zuñiga [102] developed 3D printed prosthesis using antibacterial filaments, verifying their properties to kill certain bacteria. The author indicated that this information is relevant for the implementation of 3D printed prostheses as post-operative or transitional prostheses. Figure 18a shows a patient with a traumatic index finger at the proximal phalange. In Figure 18b,c, the patient was fitted with a 3D printed antibacterial finger prosthesis, and subsequently performed the Box and Block Test of manual gross dexterity (Figure 18d). *S. aureus* and *E. coli* were chosen to test the antibacterial capacity of the material, because these bacteria strains are the main causes of a variety of home-acquired and hospital-acquired infections. The prosthesis was performed using PLACTIVE™ (1% antibacterial nanoparticles additive, Copper 3D, Santiago-Chile), which is a high-quality polylactic acid polymer. The main result of this research was to prove that the antibacterial 3D oriented filament can be effectively used for prostheses, and that their antibacterial properties after extrusion were not affected.

The current investigation found that polylactic acid with 1% copper nanoparticles additives had up to 99.99% effectivity against *S. aureus* and *E. coli* after a 24-h incubation period.

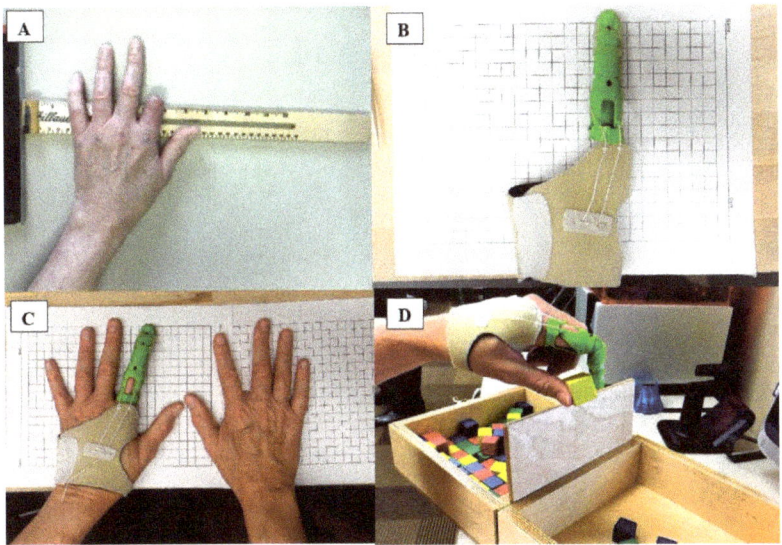

Figure 18. (**A**) Research participant with an index finger amputation. (**B**) 3D printer finder prothesis using PLACTIVE™ antibacterial 3D filament. (**C**) Patient using the antibacterial 3D finger prosthesis; and (**D**) Patient performing the Box and Block Test. Reproduced with permission from Ref. [102].

9. Conclusions

In this review, we attempted to provide a general overview about the state of the art in the preparation of antimicrobial objects fabricated by additive manufacturing. We described first the main principles of the currently employed AM technologies, as well as the evolution of these technologies, including the large impact that this technology has had in society. After this brief description, we discussed the main antimicrobial polymers, including the functional groups providing antimicrobial response as well as the macromolecular parameters involved in the antimicrobial response. We discussed the alternatives that have been reported to fabricate 3D antimicrobial parts, depending on the source of the polymers employed (natural or synthetic), as well as the strategy employed to introduce them in 3D printed parts (which were covalently linked if they acted as monomers in a photopolymerization, as additives, or simply by surface functionalization). Finally, the elaboration of composites that involve a polymeric matrix and charges including graphene or metals/metal oxide have been also reviewed.

3D printing technologies have enabled the preparation of personalized geometries with a wide variety of potential applications ranging from wound dressings, prosthesis, dental pieces, or complete denture. All of these biomedical applications without any doubt may benefit from the incorporation of antimicrobial polymers and additives that reduce the risk of infection by microorganisms.

Author Contributions: C.M.G.-H., M.A.S.V., and J.R.H. All of the authors wrote the article and provided critical feedback.

Funding: This research was funded by FONDECYT NO 1170209 and Project MAT2016-78437-R, FONDOS FEDER.

Acknowledgments: M.A.S.V. acknowledges the financial support given by CONICYT through the doctoral program Scholarship Grant.

Conflicts of Interest: The authors declare no conflict of interest.

References

1. Gibson, I.; Rosen, D.; Stucker, B. *Introduction and Basic Principles in Additive Manufacturing Technologies*; Springer New York: New York, NY, USA, 2015; pp. 1–18, ISBN 978-1-4939-2112-6.
2. Campbell, T.A.; Ivanova, O.S. Additive Manufacturing as a Disruptive Technology: Implications of Three-Dimensional Printing. *Technol. Innov.* **2013**, *15*, 67–79. [CrossRef]
3. Villar, G.; Graham, A.D.; Bayley, H. A Tissue-Like Printed Material. *Science* **2013**, *340*, 48–52. [CrossRef] [PubMed]
4. Duarte Campos, D.F.; Blaeser, A.; Weber, M.; Jäkel, J.; Neuss, S.; Jahnen-Dechent, W.; Fischer, H. Three-dimensional printing of stem cell-laden hydrogels submerged in a hydrophobic high-density fluid. *Biofabrication* **2013**, *5*, 015003. [CrossRef] [PubMed]
5. Guo, Q.; Cai, X.; Wang, X.; Yang, J. "Paintable" 3D printed structures via a post-ATRP process with antimicrobial function for biomedical applications. *J. Mater. Chem. B* **2013**, *1*, 6644–6649. [CrossRef]
6. Sun, J.; Zhou, W.; Huang, D.; Fuh, J.Y.H.; Hong, G.S. An Overview of 3D Printing Technologies for Food Fabrication. *Food Bioprocess Technol.* **2015**, *8*, 1605–1615. [CrossRef]
7. Kenawy, E.-R.; Worley, S.D.; Broughton, R. The Chemistry and Applications of Antimicrobial Polymers: A State-of-the-Art Review. *Biomacromolecules* **2007**, *8*, 1359–1384. [CrossRef] [PubMed]
8. Sandler, N.; Salmela, I.; Fallarero, A.; Rosling, A.; Khajeheian, M.; Kolakovic, R.; Genina, N.; Nyman, J.; Vuorela, P. Towards fabrication of 3D printed medical devices to prevent biofilm formation. *Int. J. Pharm.* **2014**, *459*, 62–64. [CrossRef] [PubMed]
9. Koo, H.; Yamada, K.M. Dynamic cell-matrix interactions modulate microbial biofilm and tissue 3D microenvironments. *Curr. Opin. Cell Biol.* **2016**, *42*, 102–112. [CrossRef] [PubMed]
10. Jung, J.W.; Lee, J.S.; Cho, D.W. Computer-Aided multiple-head 3D printing system for printing of heterogeneous organ/tissue constructs. *Sci. Rep.* **2016**, *6*, 21685. [CrossRef] [PubMed]
11. Melocchi, A.; Parietti, F.; Maroni, A.; Foppoli, A.; Gazzaniga, A.; Zema, L. Hot-melt extruded filaments based on pharmaceutical grade polymers for 3D printing by fused deposition modeling. *Int. J. Pharm.* **2016**, *509*, 255–263. [CrossRef] [PubMed]
12. Berman, B. 3-D printing: The new industrial revolution. *Bus. Horiz.* **2012**, *55*, 155–162. [CrossRef]
13. Sedacca, B. Hand built by lasers [additive layer manufacturing]. *Eng. Technol.* **2011**, *6*, 58–60. [CrossRef]
14. Mawale, M.B.; Kuthe, A.M.; Dahake, S.W. Additive layered manufacturing: State-of-the-art applications in product innovation. *Concur. Eng.* **2016**, *24*, 94–102. [CrossRef]
15. Gausemeier, J.; Echterhoff, N.; Wall, M. *Thinking ahead the Future of Additive Manufacturing—Analysis of Promising Industries*; Direct Manufacturing Research Center, University of Paderborn: Paderborn, Germany, 2012; pp. 1–103.
16. Inzana, J.A.; Trombetta, R.P.; Schwarz, E.M.; Kates, S.L.; Awad, H.A. 3D printed bioceramics for dual antibiotic delivery to treat implant-associated bone infection. *Eur. Cells Mater.* **2015**, *30*, 232–247. [CrossRef]
17. Zhu, F.; Skommer, J.; Macdonald, N.P.; Friedrich, T.; Kaslin, J.; Wlodkowic, D. Three-dimensional printed millifluidic devices for zebrafish embryo tests. *Biomicrofluidics* **2015**, *9*, 046502. [CrossRef] [PubMed]
18. Zhu, F.; Skommer, J.; Friedrich, T.; Kaslin, J.; Wlodkowic, D. *3D Printed Polymers Toxicity Profiling: A Caution for Biodevice Applications*; Eggleton, B.J., Palomba, S., Eds.; International Society for Optics and Photonics: San Diego, CA, USA, 2015; p. 96680Z.
19. Carve, M.; Wlodkowic, D. 3D-Printed Chips: Compatibility of Additive Manufacturing Photopolymeric Substrata with Biological Applications. *Micromachines* **2018**, *9*, 91. [CrossRef] [PubMed]
20. Formlabs. *SAFETY DATA SHEET: Clear Photoreactive Resin for Formlabs 3D Printers*; Formlabs: Somerville, MA, USA, 2016.
21. Sigma-Aldrich. *SAFETY DATA SHEET: Diphenyl(2,4,6-trimethylbenzoyl)phosphine Oxide*, version 5.4; Sigma-Aldrich: St. Louis, MO, USA, 2016.
22. Bail, R.; Patel, A.; Yang, H.; Rogers, C.M.; Rose, F.R.A.J.; Segal, J.I.; Ratchev, S.M. The Effect of a Type I Photoinitiator on Cure Kinetics and Cell Toxicity in Projection-Microstereolithography. *Procedia CIRP* **2013**, *5*, 222–225. [CrossRef]
23. Formlabs. *SAFETY DATA SHEET: Dental LT Clear (Photoreactive Resin for Form 2)*; Formlabs: Somerville, MA, USA, 2017.
24. Vertex Dental. *SAFETY DATA SHEET: NextDent Ortho IBT*; Vertex Dental: Zeist, The Netherlands, 2015.

25. Anadón, A.; Bell, D.; Binderup, M.-L.; Bursch, W.; Castle, L.; Crebelli, R.; Engel, K.-H.; Gontard, N.; Haertlé, T.; Husøy, T.; et al. Toxicological evaluation of benzophenone. *EFSA J.* **2009**, *7*, 1–30.
26. Sigma-Aldrich. *SAFETY DATA SHEET: Benzophenone*, version 3.12; Sigma-Aldrich: St. Louis, MO, USA, 2017.
27. 3D Systems Inc. *SAFETY SATA SHEETt: VisiJet SL Clear, ID: 24672-S12-04-A*; 3D Systems Inc.: Rock Hill, SC, USA, 2016.
28. DeltaMed. *SAFETY DATA SHEET: E-Shell 600 Clear*; DeltaMed: Friedberg, Germany, 2016.
29. Autodesk-Inc. *SAFETY DATA SHEET: Autodesk Resin: PR57-K-v.2 Black*; Autodesk-Inc.: San Rafael, CA, USA, 2016.
30. Dormer, W.; Gomes, R.; Meek, M. *Concise International Chemical Assessment Document: Methyl Methacrylate*; World Health Organization: Geneva, Switzerland, 1998.
31. BASF CORPORATION. *SAFETY DATA SHEET: Methyl Acrylate*, version: 3; BASF CORPORATION: Ludwigshafen, Germany, 2016.
32. Sigma-Aldrich. *SAFETY DATA SHEET: Methyl Methacrylate*; Version 5.4; Sigma-Aldrich: St. Louis, MO, USA, 2015.
33. Sigma-Aldrich. *SAFETY DATA SHEET: Methyl Acrylate*; Version 3.9; Sigma-Aldrich: St. Louis, MO, USA, 2015.
34. Schamazls, G.; Arenholt-Bindslev, D. *Biocompatibility of Dental Materials*; Springer: Berlin/Heidelberg, Germany, 2009; ISBN 978-3-540-77781-6.
35. Sigma-Aldrich. *SAFETY DATA SHEET: Butylated Hydroxytoluene*, version 5.2; Sigma-Aldrich: St. Louis, MO, USA, 2014.
36. Sigma-Aldrich. *SAFETY DATA SHEET: 1-Bis(2,2,6,6-tetramethyl-4-piperidyl) Sebacate*, version 4.4; Sigma-Aldrich: St. Louis, MO, USA, 2015.
37. Sigma-Aldrich. *SAFETY DATA SHEET: Hydroquinone*, version 4.2; Sigma-Aldrich: St. Louis, MO, USA, 2017.
38. Du, Y.; Wang, W.-Q.; Pei, Z.-T.; Ahmad, F.; Xu, R.-R.; Zhang, Y.-M.; Sun, L.-W. Acute Toxicity and Ecological Risk Assessment of Benzophenone-3 (BP-3) and Benzophenone-4 (BP-4) in Ultraviolet (UV)-Filters. *Int. J. Environ. Res. Public Health* **2017**, *14*, 1414. [CrossRef] [PubMed]
39. Sigma-Aldrich. *SAFETY DATA SHEET: Methacrylic Acid*, version 4.7; Sigma-Aldrich: St. Louis, MO, USA, 2014.
40. Manabe, K.; Nishizawa, S.; Shiratori, S. Porous Surface Structure Fabricated by Breath Figures that Suppresses Pseudomonas aeruginosa Biofilm Formation. *ACS Appl. Mater. Interfaces* **2013**, *5*, 11900–11905. [CrossRef] [PubMed]
41. Bourell, D.L. Perspectives on Additive Manufacturing. *Annu. Rev. Mater. Res.* **2016**, *46*, 1–18. [CrossRef]
42. Wang, J.-C.; Zheng, H.; Chang, M.-W.; Ahmad, Z.; Li, J.-S. Preparation of active 3D film patches via aligned fiber electrohydrodynamic (EHD) printing. *Sci. Rep.* **2017**, *7*, 43924. [CrossRef] [PubMed]
43. Jonušauskas, L.; Gailevičius, D.; Mikoliunaite, L.; Sakalauskas, D.; Šakirzanovas, S.; Juodkazis, S.; Malinauskas, M. Optically clear and resilient free-form µ-optics 3D-printed via ultrafast laser lithography. *Materials* **2017**, *10*, 12. [CrossRef] [PubMed]
44. Park, J.; Kim, K.-I.; Kim, K.; Kim, D.-C.; Cho, D.; Lee, J.H.; Jeon, S. Rapid, High-Resolution 3D Interference Printing of Multilevel Ultralong Nanochannel Arrays for High-Throughput Nanofluidic Transport. *Adv. Mater.* **2015**, *27*, 8000–8006. [CrossRef] [PubMed]
45. Dolinski, N.D.; Page, Z.A.; Callaway, E.B.; Eisenreich, F.; Garcia, R.V.; Chavez, R.; Bothman, D.P.; Hecht, S.; Zok, F.W.; Hawker, C.J. Solution Mask Liquid Lithography (SMaLL) for One-Step, Multimaterial 3D Printing. *Adv. Mater.* **2018**, *30*, 1800364. [CrossRef] [PubMed]
46. Watanabe, K.; Kinoshita, M.; Mine, T.; Morishita, M.; Fujisaki, K.; Matsui, R.; Sagawa, M.; Machida, S.; Oba, H.; Sugiyama, Y.; et al. Plasma ion-beam 3D printing: A novel method for rapid fabrication of customized MEMS sensors. In Proceedings of the 2018 IEEE Micro Electro Mechanical Systems (MEMS), Belfast, UK, 21–25 January 2018; pp. 459–462.
47. Zhang, H.Z.; Zhang, F.T.; Zhang, X.H.; Huang, D.; Zhou, Y.L.; Li, Z.H.; Zhang, X.X. Portable, Easy-to-Operate, and Antifouling Microcapsule Array Chips Fabricated by 3D Ice Printing for Visual Target Detection. *Anal. Chem.* **2015**, *87*, 6397–6402. [CrossRef] [PubMed]
48. Connell, J.L.; Ritschdorff, E.T.; Whiteley, M.; Shear, J.B. 3D printing of microscopic bacterial communities. *Proc. Natl. Acad. Sci. USA* **2013**, *110*, 18380–18385. [CrossRef] [PubMed]

49. Steiner, H.; Hultmark, D.; Engström, Å.; Nature, H.B. Sequence and specificity of two antibacterial proteins involved in insect immunity. *Nature* **1981**, *292*, 246. [CrossRef] [PubMed]
50. Wang, Z.; Wang, G. APD: The antimicrobial peptide database. *Nucleic Acids Res.* **2004**, *32* (Suppl. 1), D590–D592. [CrossRef]
51. Palermo, E.F.; Kuroda, K. Structural determinants of antimicrobial activity in polymers which mimic host defense peptides. *Appl. Microbiol. Biotechnol.* **2010**, *87*, 1605–1615. [CrossRef] [PubMed]
52. Thoma, L.M.; Boles, B.R.; Kuroda, K. Cationic Methacrylate Polymers as Topical Antimicrobial Agents against *Staphylococcus aureus* Nasal Colonization. *Biomacromolecules* **2014**, *15*, 2933–2943. [CrossRef] [PubMed]
53. King, A.; Chakrabarty, S.; Zhang, W.; Zeng, X.; Ohman, D.E.; Wood, L.F.; Abraham, S.; Rao, R.; Wynne, K.J. High Antimicrobial Effectiveness with Low Hemolytic and Cytotoxic Activity for PEG/Quaternary Copolyoxetanes. *Biomacromolecules* **2014**, *15*, 456–467. [CrossRef] [PubMed]
54. Liu, R.; Chen, X.; Chakraborty, S.; Lemke, J.J.; Hayouka, Z.; Chow, C.; Welch, R.A.; Weisblum, B.; Masters, K.S.; Gellman, S.H. Tuning the Biological Activity Profile of Antibacterial Polymers via Subunit Substitution Pattern. *J. Am. Chem. Soc.* **2014**, *136*, 4410–4418. [CrossRef] [PubMed]
55. Liu, R.; Chen, X.; Falk, S.P.; Mowery, B.P.; Karlsson, A.J.; Weisblum, B.; Palecek, S.P.; Masters, K.S.; Gellman, S.H. Structure–Activity Relationships among Antifungal Nylon-3 Polymers: Identification of Materials Active against Drug-Resistant Strains of *Candida albicans*. *J. Am. Chem. Soc.* **2014**, *136*, 4333–4342. [CrossRef] [PubMed]
56. Stratton, T.R.; Applegate, B.M.; Youngblood, J.P. Effect of Steric Hindrance on the Properties of Antibacterial and Biocompatible Copolymers. *Biomacromolecules* **2011**, *12*, 50–56. [CrossRef] [PubMed]
57. Thaker, H.D.; Cankaya, A.; Scott, R.W.; Tew, G.N. Role of Amphiphilicity in the Design of Synthetic Mimics of Antimicrobial Peptides with Gram-Negative Activity. *ACS Med. Chem. Lett.* **2013**, *4*, 481–485. [CrossRef] [PubMed]
58. Matsuzaki, K. Control of cell selectivity of antimicrobial peptides. *Biochim. Biophys. Acta BBA Biomembr.* **2009**, *1788*, 1687–1692. [CrossRef] [PubMed]
59. Ikeda, T.; Tazuke, S. Biologically active polycations: Antimicrobial activities of Poly[trialkyl(vinylbenzyl)ammonium chloride]-type polycations. *Die Makromol. Chem. Rapid Commun.* **1983**, *4*, 459–461. [CrossRef]
60. Ikeda, T.; Tazuke, S. Synthesis and antimicrobial activity of poly (trialkylvinylbenzylammonium ch1oride) s. *Synthesis* **1984**, *876*, 869–876.
61. Timofeeva, L.; Kleshcheva, N. Antimicrobial polymers: Mechanism of action, factors of activity, and applications. *Appl. Microbiol. Biotechnol.* **2011**, *89*, 475–492. [CrossRef] [PubMed]
62. Gelman, M.A.; Weisblum, B.; Lynn, D.M.; Gellman, S.H. Biocidal activity of polystyrenes that are cationic by virtue of protonation. *Org. lett.* **2004**, *6*, 557–560. [CrossRef] [PubMed]
63. Vigliotta, G.; Mella, M.; Rega, D.; Izzo, L. Modulating Antimicrobial Activity by Synthesis: Dendritic Copolymers Based on Nonquaternized 2-(Dimethylamino)ethyl Methacrylate by Cu-Mediated ATRP. *Biomacromolecules* **2012**, *13*, 833–841. [CrossRef] [PubMed]
64. Ornelas-Megiatto, C.; Wich, P.R.; Fréchet, J.M.J. Polyphosphonium Polymers for siRNA Delivery: An Efficient and Nontoxic Alternative to Polyammonium Carriers. *J. Am. Chem. Soc.* **2012**, *134*, 1902–1905. [CrossRef] [PubMed]
65. Hemp, S.T.; Smith, A.E.; Bryson, J.M.; Allen, M.H.; Long, T.E. Phosphonium-Containing Diblock Copolymers for Enhanced Colloidal Stability and Efficient Nucleic Acid Delivery. *Biomacromolecules* **2012**, *13*, 2439–2445. [CrossRef] [PubMed]
66. Popa, A.; Davidescu, C.M.; Trif, R.; Ilia, G.; Iliescu, S.; Dehelean, G. Study of quaternary "onium"salts grafted on polymers: Antibacterial activity of quaternary phosphonium salts grafted on "gel-type"styrene–divinylbenzene copolymers. *React. Funct. Polym.* **2003**, *55*, 151–158. [CrossRef]
67. Li, C.; Liu, Y.; Zeng, Q.Y.; Ao, N.J. Preparation and antimicrobial activity of quaternary phosphonium modified epoxidized natural rubber. *Mater. Lett.* **2013**, *93*, 145–148. [CrossRef]
68. Xue, Y.; Pan, Y.; Xiao, H.; Zhao, Y. Novel quaternary phosphonium-type cationic polyacrylamide and elucidation of dual-functional antibacterial/antiviral activity. *RSC Adv.* **2014**, *4*, 46887–46895. [CrossRef]
69. Sun, Y.; Sun, G. Novel Refreshable *N*-Halamine Polymeric Biocides: N-Chlorination of Aromatic Polyamides. *Ind. Eng. Chem. Res.* **2004**, *43*, 5015–5020. [CrossRef]

70. Sun, Y.; Chen, T.-Y.; Worley, S.D.; Sun, G. Novel refreshable N-halamine polymeric biocides containing imidazolidin-4-one derivatives. *J. Polym. Sci. Part A Polym. Chem.* **2001**, *39*, 3073–3084. [CrossRef]
71. Hirayama, M. The antimicrobial activity, hydrophobicity and toxicity of sulfonium compounds, and their relationship. *Biocontrol Sci.* **2011**, *16*, 23–31. [CrossRef] [PubMed]
72. Ward, M.; Sanchez, M.; Elasri, M.O.; Lowe, A.B. Antimicrobial activity of statistical polymethacrylic sulfopropylbetaines against gram-positive and gram-negative bacteria. *J. Appl. Polym. Sci.* **2006**, *101*, 1036–1041. [CrossRef]
73. Lowe, A.; Deng, W.; Smith, D.W.; Balkus, K.J. Acrylonitrile-Based Nitric Oxide Releasing Melt-Spun Fibers for Enhanced Wound Healing. *Macromolecules* **2012**, *45*, 5894–5900. [CrossRef]
74. Hui, F.; Debiemme-Chouvy, C. Antimicrobial N-Halamine Polymers and Coatings: A Review of Their Synthesis, Characterization, and Applications. *Biomacromolecules* **2013**, *14*, 585–601. [CrossRef] [PubMed]
75. Mi, L.; Jiang, S. Integrated Antimicrobial and Nonfouling Zwitterionic Polymers. *Angew. Chem. Int. Ed.* **2014**, *53*, 1746–1754. [CrossRef] [PubMed]
76. Cao, Z.; Brault, N.; Xue, H.; Keefe, A.; Jiang, S. Manipulating Sticky and Non-Sticky Properties in a Single Material. *Angew. Chem.* **2011**, *123*, 6226–6228. [CrossRef]
77. Cao, Z.; Mi, L.; Mendiola, J.; Ella-Menye, J.-R.; Zhang, L.; Xue, H.; Jiang, S. Reversibly Switching the Function of a Surface between Attacking and Defending against Bacteria. *Angew. Chem. Int. Ed.* **2012**, *51*, 2602–2605. [CrossRef] [PubMed]
78. Engler, A.C.; Wiradharma, N.; Ong, Z.Y.; Coady, D.J.; Hedrick, J.L.; Yang, Y.Y. Emerging trends in macromolecular antimicrobials to fight multi-drug-resistant infections. *Nano Today* **2012**, *7*, 201–222. [CrossRef]
79. Cheng, C.-Y.; Wang, J.-Y.; Kausik, R.; Lee, K.Y.C.; Han, S. Nature of Interactions between PEO-PPO-PEO Triblock Copolymers and Lipid Membranes: (II) Role of Hydration Dynamics Revealed by Dynamic Nuclear Polarization. *Biomacromolecules* **2012**, *13*, 2624–2633. [CrossRef] [PubMed]
80. Palermo, E.F.; Sovadinova, I.; Kuroda, K. Structural Determinants of Antimicrobial Activity and Biocompatibility in Membrane-Disrupting Methacrylamide Random Copolymers. *Biomacromolecules* **2009**, *10*, 3098–3107. [CrossRef] [PubMed]
81. Jiang, Y.; Yang, X.; Zhu, R.; Hu, K.; Lan, W.-W.; Wu, F.; Yang, L. Acid-Activated Antimicrobial Random Copolymers: A Mechanism-Guided Design of Antimicrobial Peptide Mimics. *Macromolecules* **2013**, *46*, 3959–3964. [CrossRef]
82. Yang, X.; Hu, K.; Hu, G.; Shi, D.; Jiang, Y.; Hui, L.; Zhu, R.; Xie, Y.; Yang, L. Long Hydrophilic-and-Cationic Polymers: A Different Pathway toward Preferential Activity against Bacterial over Mammalian Membranes. *Biomacromolecules* **2014**, *15*, 3267–3277. [CrossRef] [PubMed]
83. Oda, Y.; Kanaoka, S.; Sato, T.; Aoshima, S.; Kuroda, K. Block versus Random Amphiphilic Copolymers as Antibacterial Agents. *Biomacromolecules* **2011**, *12*, 3581–3591. [CrossRef] [PubMed]
84. Correia, T.R.; Figueira, D.R.; de Sá, K.D.; Miguel, S.P.; Fradique, R.G.; Mendonça, A.G.; Correia, I.J. 3D printed scaffolds with bactericidal activity aimed for bone tissue regeneration. *Int. J. Biol. Macromol.* **2016**, *93*, 1432–1445. [CrossRef] [PubMed]
85. Tardajos, M.G.; Cama, G.; Dash, M.; Misseeuw, L.; Gheysens, T.; Gorzelanny, C.; Coenye, T.; Dubruel, P. Chitosan functionalized poly-ε-caprolactone electrospun fibers and 3D printed scaffolds as antibacterial materials for tissue engineering applications. *Carbohydr. Polym.* **2018**, *191*, 127–135. [CrossRef] [PubMed]
86. Chou, Y.-C.; Lee, D.; Chang, T.-M.; Hsu, Y.-H.; Yu, Y.-H.; Chan, E.-C.; Liu, S.-J. Combination of a biodegradable three-dimensional (3D)—Printed cage for mechanical support and nanofibrous membranes for sustainable release of antimicrobial agents for treating the femoral metaphyseal comminuted fracture. *J. Mech. Behav. Biomed. Mater.* **2017**, *72*, 209–218. [CrossRef] [PubMed]
87. Muwaffak, Z.; Goyanes, A.; Clark, V.; Basit, A.W.; Hilton, S.T.; Gaisford, S. Patient-specific 3D scanned and 3D printed antimicrobial polycaprolactone wound dressings. *Int. J. Pharm.* **2017**, *527*, 161–170. [CrossRef] [PubMed]
88. Cheng, Y.L.; Chen, F. Preparation and characterization of photocured poly (ε-caprolactone) diacrylate/poly (ethylene glycol) diacrylate/chitosan for photopolymerization-type 3D printing. *Mater. Sci. Eng. C* **2017**, *81*, 66–73. [CrossRef] [PubMed]

89. Kargupta, R.; Bok, S.; Darr, C.M.; Crist, B.D.; Gangopadhyay, K.; Gangopadhyay, S.; Sengupta, S. Coatings and surface modifications imparting antimicrobial activity to orthopedic implants. *Wiley Interdiscip. Rev. Nanomed. Nanobiotechnol.* **2014**, *6*, 475–495. [CrossRef] [PubMed]
90. Klemm, D.; Cranston, E.D.; Fischer, D.; Gama, M.; Kedzior, S.A.; Kralisch, D.; Kramer, F.; Kondo, T.; Lindström, T.; Nietzsche, S.; et al. Nanocellulose as a natural source for groundbreaking applications in materials science: Today's state. *Mater. Today* **2018**, *21*, 720–748. [CrossRef]
91. Sultan, S.; Siqueira, G.; Zimmermann, T.; Mathew, A.P. 3D printing of nano-cellulosic biomaterials for medical applications. *Curr. Opin. Biomed. Eng.* **2017**, *2*, 29–34. [CrossRef]
92. Pattinson, S.W.; Hart, A.J. Additive Manufacturing of Cellulosic Materials with Robust Mechanics and Antimicrobial Functionality. *Adv. Mater. Technol.* **2017**, *2*, 1600084. [CrossRef]
93. Martínez Ávila, H.; Schwarz, S.; Rotter, N.; Gatenholm, P. 3D bioprinting of human chondrocyte-laden nanocellulose hydrogels for patient-specific auricular cartilage regeneration. *Bioprinting* **2016**, *1–2*, 22–35. [CrossRef]
94. Yue, J.; Zhao, P.; Gerasimov, J.Y.; Van De Lagemaat, M.; Grotenhuis, A.; Rustema-Abbing, M.; Van Der Mei, H.C.; Busscher, H.J.; Herrmann, A.; Ren, Y. 3D-Printable Antimicrobial Composite Resins. *Adv. Funct. Mater.* **2015**, *25*, 6756–6767. [CrossRef]
95. Garcia, C.; Gallardo, A.; López, D.; Azzahti, A.; Lopez-Martinez, E.; Cortajarena, A.L.; Gonzalez-Henriquez, C.M.; Sarabia-Vallejos, M.A.; Rodríguez-Hernández, J. Smart pH-responsive antimicrobial hydrogel scaffolds prepared by additive manufacturing. *ACS Appl. Bio Mater* **2018**, *1*, 1337–1347. [CrossRef]
96. Water, J.J.; Bohr, A.; Boetker, J.; Aho, J.; Sandler, N.; Nielsen, H.M.; Rantanen, J. Three-dimensional printing of drug-eluting implants: Preparation of an antimicrobial polylactide feedstock material. *J. Pharm. Sci.* **2015**, *104*, 1099–1107. [CrossRef] [PubMed]
97. Mills, D.K.; Jammalamadaka, U.; Tappa, K.; Weisman, J. Studies on the cytocompatibility, mechanical and antimicrobial properties of 3D printed poly(methyl methacrylate) beads. *Bioact. Mater.* **2018**, *3*, 157–166. [CrossRef] [PubMed]
98. Vargas-Alfredo, N.; Dorronsoro, A.; Cortajarena, A.L.; Rodríguez-Hernández, J. Antimicrobial 3D Porous Scaffolds Prepared by Additive Manufacturing and Breath Figures. *ACS Appl. Mater. Interfaces* **2017**, *9*, 37454–37462. [CrossRef] [PubMed]
99. Vargas-Alfredo, N.; Reinecke, H.; Gallardo, A.; del Campo, A.; Rodríguez-Hernández, J. Fabrication of 3D printed objects with controlled surface chemistry and topography. *Eur. Polym. J.* **2018**, *98*, 21–27. [CrossRef]
100. Chen, Q.; Mangadlao, J.D.; Wallat, J.; De Leon, A.; Pokorski, J.K.; Advincula, R.C. 3D printing biocompatible polyurethane/poly(lactic acid)/graphene oxide nanocomposites: Anisotropic properties. *ACS Appl. Mater. Interfaces* **2017**, *9*, 4015–4023. [CrossRef] [PubMed]
101. Tiimob, B.J.; Mwinyelle, G.; Abdela, W.; Samuel, T.; Jeelani, S.; Rangari, V.K. Nanoengineered Eggshell-Silver Tailored Copolyester Polymer Blend Film with Antimicrobial Properties. *J. Agric. Food Chem.* **2017**, *65*, 1967–1976. [CrossRef] [PubMed]
102. Zuniga, J. 3D Printed Antibacterial Prostheses. *Appl. Sci.* **2018**, *8*, 1651. [CrossRef]
103. Totu, E.E.; Nechifor, A.C.; Nechifor, G.; Aboul-Enein, H.Y.; Cristache, C.M. Poly(methyl methacrylate) with TiO2 nanoparticles inclusion for stereolitographic complete denture manufacturing—The fututre in dental care for elderly edentulous patients? *J. Dent.* **2017**, *59*, 68–77. [CrossRef] [PubMed]

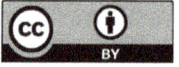

© 2019 by the authors. Licensee MDPI, Basel, Switzerland. This article is an open access article distributed under the terms and conditions of the Creative Commons Attribution (CC BY) license (http://creativecommons.org/licenses/by/4.0/).

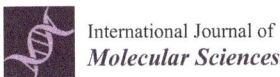

Review

Antimicrobial Polymers: The Potential Replacement of Existing Antibiotics?

Nor Fadhilah Kamaruzzaman [1,*], Li Peng Tan [1], Ruhil Hayati Hamdan [1], Siew Shean Choong [1], Weng Kin Wong [2], Amanda Jane Gibson [3], Alexandru Chivu [4] and Maria de Fatima Pina [5]

1. Faculty of Veterinary Medicine, Locked bag 36, Universiti Malaysia Kelantan, Pengkalan Chepa 16100, Kelantan, Malaysia; li.peng@umk.edu.my (L.P.T.); ruhil@umk.ed.my (R.H.H.); shean.cs@umk.edu.my (S.S.C.)
2. School of Health Sciences, Universiti Sains Malaysia, Kubang Kerian 16150, Kelantan, Malaysia; wengkinwong@usm.my
3. Royal Veterinary College, Pathobiology and Population Sciences, Hawkshead Lane, North Mymms, Hatfield AL9 7TA, UK; ajgibson@rvc.ac.uk
4. UCL Centre for Nanotechnology and Regenerative Medicine, Division of Surgery & Interventional Science, University College London, London NW3 2PF, UK; a.chivu.14@ucl.ac.uk
5. Medicines and Healthcare Regulatory Products Agency, 10 South Colonnade, Canary Wharf, London E14 4PU, UK; mfatimagpina@gmail.com
* Correspondence: norfadhilah@umk.edu.my

Received: 21 January 2019; Accepted: 11 April 2019; Published: 4 June 2019

Abstract: Antimicrobial resistance is now considered a major global challenge; compromising medical advancements and our ability to treat infectious disease. Increased antimicrobial resistance has resulted in increased morbidity and mortality due to infectious diseases worldwide. The lack of discovery of novel compounds from natural products or new classes of antimicrobials, encouraged us to recycle discontinued antimicrobials that were previously removed from routine use due to their toxicity, e.g., colistin. Since the discovery of new classes of compounds is extremely expensive and has very little success, one strategy to overcome this issue could be the application of synthetic compounds that possess antimicrobial activities. Polymers with innate antimicrobial properties or that have the ability to be conjugated with other antimicrobial compounds create the possibility for replacement of antimicrobials either for the direct application as medicine or implanted on medical devices to control infection. Here, we provide the latest update on research related to antimicrobial polymers in the context of ESKAPE (*Enterococcus faecium*, *Staphylococcus aureus*, *Klebsiella pneumoniae*, *Acinetobacter baumannii*, *Pseudomonas aeruginosa*, and *Enterobacter* spp.) pathogens. We summarise polymer subgroups: compounds containing natural peptides, halogens, phosphor and sulfo derivatives and phenol and benzoic derivatives, organometalic polymers, metal nanoparticles incorporated into polymeric carriers, dendrimers and polymer-based guanidine. We intend to enhance understanding in the field and promote further work on the development of polymer based antimicrobial compounds.

Keywords: antimicrobial resistance; antimicrobial polymers; ESKAPE pathogens

---

1. Introduction

Antimicrobial resistance (AMR) is currently widespread across 22 countries with an estimated 500,000 people infected worldwide [1]. A report by O'Neill and colleagues has estimated 10 million deaths in 2050 will be due to AMR (Figure 1) [2]. Such data informed and shaped the Global Action Plan on Antimicrobial Resistance and has encouraged governments and public health agencies to increase efforts in AMR surveillance and research. To date, 52 countries (25 high-income, 20 middle-income and 7 low-income countries) have provided information about their national surveillance systems and data on levels of AMR [2].

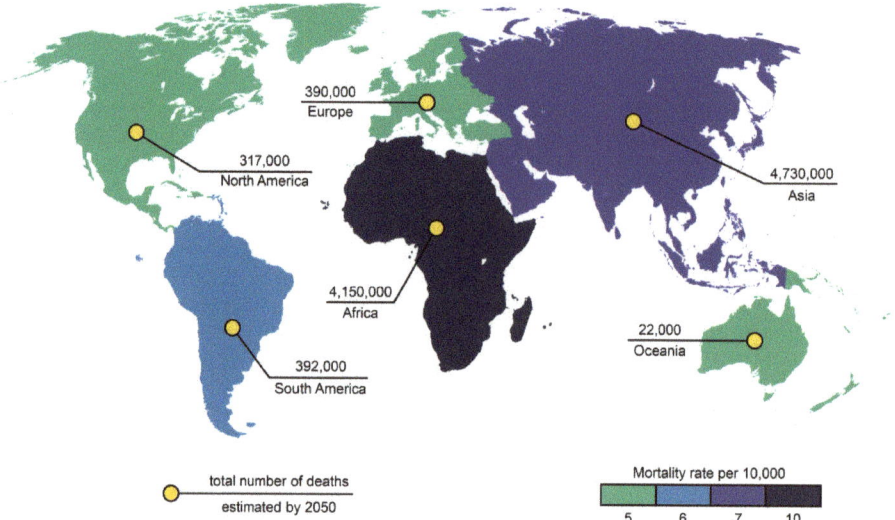

Figure 1. The estimated number of deaths at every continent in 2050 attributed to antimicrobial resistance (AMR). Image adapted from [2].

This surveillance and data are important in monitoring and clarifying the epidemiology of AMR, in order to allow priorities to be set and to develop public health policy and strategies targeting this global concern. In this first section of the review, we provide the current epidemiology of multidrug-resistant organisms (MDROs) globally, focusing mainly on ESKAPE pathogens (*Enterococcus faecium, Staphylococcus aureus, Klebsiella pneumoniae, Acinetobacter baumannii, Pseudomonas aeruginosa*, and *Enterobacter* spp.). These ESKAPE pathogens are capable of "escaping" from common antibacterial treatments and have been listed as World Health Organization (WHO) priority pathogens with critical and high priority [3]. Although extensive studies on the prevalence of antimicrobial resistance pathogens were conducted, these studies were largely limited to certain countries and we believe that these data are not able to showcase the overall picture of antimicrobial resistance around the globe. Hence, we sought to evaluate the current global prevalence of ESKAPE pathogens by reviewing published work performed between the years 2013–2018 (Table 1).

Table 1. The global prevalence of AMR among ESKAPE (*Enterococcus faecium*, *Staphylococcus aureus*, *Klebsiella pneumoniae*, *Acinetobacter baumannii*, *Pseudomonas aeruginosa*, and *Enterobacter* spp.) pathogens.

Pathogens / Country	Enterococcus faecium	Staphylococcus aureus	Klebsiella pneumoniae	Acinetobacter baumannii	Pseudomonas aeruginosa	Enterobacter spp.	References
Thailand	-	-	ER	ER	-	-	[4]
South India	-	-	ER	-	S	-	[5]
India	ER	ER	ER	ER	ER	ER	[6]
India (Veterinary Cases)	ER	ER	ER	ER	ER	ER	[7]
Iran	ER	HR	R	ER	ER	HR	[14]
Asia-Pacific	-	-	S	ER	S	S	[8]
Southern Italy	S	R	R	ER	R	-	[9]
Romania	HR	R	HR	HR	HR	-	[10]
Romania	H	ER	ER	ER	S	-	[11]
South Africa	R	S	ER	H	S	-	[12]
Brazil	ER	ER	HR	HR	ER	ER	[13]
Latin-America	-	-	R	ER	S	S	[8]

- (N/A) = data on the AMR prevalence are not available in the study, S (Susceptible) = 50% of the organism does not show resistance against any antibacterial agent; R (Resistant) = 50% of the organism must show resistance against an antibacterial agent from 1 of the antibiotic groups; HR (Highly Resistant) = 50% of the organism must show resistance against antibacterial agents from at least 2 of the antibiotic groups; ER (Extremely Resistant) = 50% of the organism must show resistance against antibacterial agents from at least 3 of the antibiotic groups. Antibiotic groups: Aminoglycosides, Carnapenems, Cephalosporins, Glycopeptides, Lincosamides, Lipopeptide, Macrolides, Monobactams, Nitrofurans, Penicillin, Fluoroquinolones, Sulfonamides, Tetracycline.

The claim on the global prevalence status of AMR among ESKAPE pathogens is rather challenging as standardisation of resistance testing across antibiotic groups being employed by the available studies is lacking. In order to give a simple visualization on the current global prevalence of antimicrobial resistance among ESKAPE pathogens, we compiled a meta-analysis of works conducted in different geographical locations and classified them into 4 major classes namely, susceptible, resistant; highly resistant and extremely resistant by having 50% of the organism show resistance against none, one or more of the 13 antibiotic groups stated.

According to the summarized work in Table 1, *A. baumannii* is reported as extremely resistant i.e., 50% resistant to at least 3 drug classes for all selected countries. It is considered one of the most challenging ESKAPE pathogens due to its particular antimicrobial resistance characteristics, having developed resistance to almost all known antimicrobials [14]. The increasing trend of multidrug resistant (MDR) pathogens has diminished the options of effective therapeutic drugs for bacterial infection. The return to the previously abandoned antimicrobial, colistin, considered to be the 'last resort' treatment is also challenging as emerging resistant clinical isolates to colistin has been reported globally [15,16].

Limiting overuse and misuse of antimicrobials were proposed as the solution to limit and even reduce the MDR pathogens. However, the theory of reduction in resistance in the absence of a given antimicrobial is no longer a novel approach [17]. Although theoretically attractive, the reversibility of resistance has proven difficult in practice as the success rate is highly dependent on many other factors such as the fitness cost of the resistance mechanism, the epidemic potential of the bacteria/strain, and the transmission route of the species [18]. Efforts to develop new antimicrobials concurrently have diminished due to a combination of market forces and the inability to match the fast-paced growth of antimicrobial resistance in superbugs [19].

Decisively, although antimicrobial resistance does not seem obviously reversible, efforts must still be focused on imposing measures that might postpone the increase in antimicrobial resistance. The overall use of antimicrobials must be reduced. The prudent use of antimicrobials should always be promoted. Alternative and preventive measures (such as vaccination) that can ultimately replace the use of antimicrobials should always be explored ahead of administration of antimicrobials.

2. ESKAPE (*Enterococcus faecium, Staphylococcus aureus, Klebsiella pneumoniae, Acinetobacter baumannii, Pseudomonas aeruginosa,* and *Enterobacter* spp.) pathogens

The acronym ESKAPE paradoxically denotes the ability of the panel of constituent bacteria, namely *Enterococcus faecium, Staphylococcus aureus, Klebsiella pneumoniae, Acinetobacter baumannii, Pseudomonas aeruginosa,* and *Enterobacter* spp., to escape the antimicrobial activities of most commonly used products in clinical treatment. The AMR capabilities of this bacterial group have been reported to severely exacerbate the condition of hospitalised patients with noncommunicable diseases, such as diabetes, cancer, cardiovascular diseases, and chronic respiratory diseases; breakage of skin barrier such as wounds; and diseases that lead to immunosuppression [4]. Exposure of these patients to ESKAPE pathogens could occur during hospitalisation through contact with medical equipment (commonly related to central line bloodstream infections, ventilator pneumonia, and urinary catheterisation), other infected patients, and healthcare staff. WHO has recently published a list of bacteria that urgently require new antibiotics and ESKAPE bacteria were identified among Priority 1 and 2 lists; as these are multidrug resistant microorganisms that pose serious threats in healthcare facilities [20].

2.1. Enterococcus faecium

Enterococci are gram-positive, facultative anaerobic organisms that form part of the normal intestinal flora. Among the 17 species of Enterococci, *Enterococcus faecium* and *E. faecalis* were most frequently reported to be pathogenic in humans. The pathogenic strains of these organisms cause a variety of infections, involving the endocardium, urinary tract, prostate, intra-abdominal organs, skin (particularly if present within a wound) [5]. If bacteria enter the normally sterile bloodstream through parenteral injections, catheterisation, surgery and open wounds, this can result in metastatic or systemic infections that eventually result in sepsis and septic shock. Research has shown that various virulence factors are present on the capsule, cell wall, membrane and within the cytoplasm of *Enterococcus faecium* that contributed to AMR and pathogenicity of the organism through formation of a protective and persistent biofilm, ß-lactamase production, and proteins directed against recruited inflammatory cells [6,7]. Reports submitted to the National Healthcare Safety Network (NHSN) at the Centres for Disease Control and Prevention (CDC) indicated that the *Enterococcus* group is the second most common pathogen across all hospital-acquired infections types (HAI) types. While *Enterococcus faecium* was ranked among the top ten organisms across all types of HAI, including central line-associated bloodstream infection (CLABSI), catheter-associated urinary tract infection (CAUTI), and surgical site infections (SSIs) [21].

2.2. Staphylococcus aureus

Staphylococcus aureus is a Gram-positive coccus that is frequently isolated from the skin, respiratory tract, and female lower reproductive tract as it forms part of the normal flora on the human body [8,9]. *S. aureus* infection has shown increased resistance towards penicillin, which led to the introduction of methicillin for the treatment of *S. aureus* showing resistance to penicillin in 1960 [10]. However, *S. aureus* developed resistance towards methicillin, thus giving rise to methicillin-resistant *S. aureus* (MRSA) clones [11]. MRSA is the second most common cause of HAI in the USA according to a report from the CDC [12]. The ability of the organism to form biofilms on tissues such as the skin and inert indwelling device surfaces such as intravenous catheters and surgical implants, further exposes susceptible individuals as the most common route of MRSA transmission is through direct contact [13]. Additionally, *S. aureus* can invade host cells and evade the antimicrobial effects of administered therapies [20,22]. Successful treatment of MRSA infection is restricted by worldwide antibiotic resistance towards first-line therapies such as vancomycin and teicoplanin [13]. Together, these characteristics allow this microorganism to remain an important pathogen and alternative therapeutic measures are critically needed.

2.3. Pseudomonas aeruginosa

P. aeruginosa is a Gram-negative, rod-shaped, facultative anaerobe that is ubiquitous in the environment and forms part of the normal gut flora. *P. aeruginosa* is capable of forming biofilms on medical device surfaces, thus patients dependent on breathing machines or fitted with an invasive device such as a catheter are at risk of severe and life-threatening illness [23–25]. Reported illnesses include endocardial valve infection through endocardial tubes, ventilator-associated pneumonia (VAP) and CAUTI. Additionally, *P. aeruginosa* has also been reported to be able to grow in intravenous fluid and could enter the bloodstream and cause sepsis [26–28]. The emergence of extremely drug-resistant (XDR) *P. aeruginosa* towards multiple antibiotics, e.g., cephalosporins and carbapenems, increases the problem of treatment globally and clinicians need to resort to the last available medication, colistin, a polymyxin antibiotic which was avoided for the past thirty years as it has been implicated in both neuro- and nephrotoxicity [29–32].

2.4. Klebsiella pneumoniae

K. pneumoniae is a non-fastidious, Gram-negative bacillus and commonly encapsulated. Although *K. pneumoniae* is among the population of normal flora found in the mouth, skin, and intestine, it has been reported to cause infections in the lungs, urinary tract, and bloodstreams of patients from hospitals, nursing homes and other healthcare facilities [30]. This bacterium is a remarkably resilient pathogen, instead of actively suppressing many components of the immune system, it successfully evades the body's defence mechanisms and survives in the most harsh environments. This organism can survive and grow within the intravenous fluid and form biofilm on medical devices such as the urinary catheter, leading to detrimental septicaemia in patients [33]. Furthermore, the bacteria have developed resistance towards almost all available antibiotics: fluoroquinolones, third-generation cephalosporins and aminoglycosides [34]. The emergence of the carbapenem-resistant *K. pnemoniae* strains circulating across the globe has forced the administration of colistin, an old antibiotic and considered the last available. Nevertheless, resistance towards colistin was recently reported, rendering treatment of multidrug resistant *K. pneumoniae* even more difficult [35].

2.5. Acinetobacter baumnannii

Acinetobacter baumnannii is a Gram-negative coccobacillus, of unknown natural habitat, that causes nosocomial infections in immunocompromised patients, including bacteraemia, pneumonia, meningitis, urinary tract infection, and wound infection [36]. The *Acinetobacter* species have a great capacity of extensive antimicrobial resistance resulting from its relatively impermeable outer membrane, the presence of efflux pumps, and lack of protein channels. Additionally, the bacteria produce various enzymes, such as beta-lactamases, to render multiple antibiotics ineffective; persistent adherence to surface through biofilm formation; as well as insertion of resistance genes from other bacterial species through genomic mutation [37]. Over the past three decades, *A. baumnannii* has been reported to be resistant to most known antibiotics, even in some cases towards colistin, the last resort of antibiotics in human medicine albeit with adverse side effects [38–40]. A combination of antibiotic treatment using colistin methansulfonate (CMS), a carbapenem, and ampicillin-sulbactam was reported to have the highest rate of success for colistin-resistant *A. baumnannii* [40]. The source of infection could originate from numerous sites and medical equipment within the healthcare facilities, including the door handle, curtains, keyboard, etc. However, the most detrimental effects involve patients infected through treatment involving the use of ventilator and venipuncture catheterisation where the mortality rates can reach 35% [41,42].

2.6. Enterobacter spp.

Enterobacter is a genus of Gram-negative bacilli from the family Enterobacteriaceae. These bacteria are facultative anaerobes that do not form spores but may be encapsulated. Two of the most clinically relevant species are *Enterobacter aerogenes*, and *Enterobacter cloacae* [43]. The worldwide emergence of colistin resistance genes (mcr-1, -2, -3, -4, -5, -6, -7, and the latest -8) in Enterobacteriaceae bacteria has detrimentally threatened global health as this polymyxin compound is considered the last resort of treatment [44]. According to the report provided by Weiner et al., *Enterobacter* spp. are among the top 10 pathogens detected in CAUTI, CLABSI, SSI and VAP, accounting for 17,235 HAI incidence recorded at NHSN [45]. In the same report, Enterobacter spp. were found to be resistant to extended-spectrum cephalosporin (ESC4, i.e., cefepime, cefotaxime, ceftazidime, ceftriaxone); carbapenems (imipenem, meropenem, doripenem); and multidrug-resistance (MDR1) at 12.8 to 38.2%, 1.9 to 6.6%, and 2.9 to 10.2% respectively [21]. On another note, unchecked antimicrobial misuse in the livestock industry may exacerbate colistin resistance in the general population as the medication has been added in feed as a growth promoter, or for treatment and prevention of infectious diseases in many countries.

3. The Progress in Antimicrobial Development

The development of a new antimicrobial is a lengthy and expensive process. The big pharmaceutical companies were once the major drivers in antimicrobial discoveries, are now no longer stand at the forefront of the arena [46]. Beginning in the late 1990s, due to lack of success, low financial returns and emergence of antimicrobial resistance, these companies began to withdraw antimicrobial discovery and development from their portfolio, with the final company Novartis followed suit in July 2018 [47]. Therefore, the task for novel discovery of antimicrobials is now left to university laboratories and small and medium-sized companies [46]. Only recently, German Ministry of Education and Research has showed interest to provide funds to Global Antibiotic Research and Development Partnership (GARDP) to accelerate discovery, development and delivery of affordable antibiotics to treat Gram-negative infections [48]. Understanding that the discovery of a novel compounds is a lengthy and expensive process, utilising the current knowledge and compounds would be one approach to ensure the continuous development of antimicrobials.

4. Antimicrobial Polymers Are the New Generation of Antimicrobials

Continuous research and understanding in the field of chemistry has opened up the possibility to design and synthesise a compound that has antibacterial activities. A new kind of antimicrobial must not only be effective against bacteria, but it must also resist the possible development of bacterial resistance. Antimicrobial polymers (AMP) are materials that have the ability to inhibit or kill the bacteria. AMP can either display the antibacterial activities through its own inherent chemical structure; e.g., quaternary nitrogen groups, halamines and poly lysine or it can serve as a backbone to improve the potency of existing antibiotics [49]. AMPs were designed based on the chemical templates provided by the antimicrobial peptides, a class of peptides of the innate immune system which protects the body from invading pathogens (Figure 2) [50]. Antimicrobial peptides (APs) are relatively small in size (10–50 amino acids), amphiphilic with cationic charge. With these physical characteristics, APs accumulate on the cell membranes and form pores on the structure, thus killing the bacteria [51]. With multimodal mechanisms of action, APs can resist acquired resistance by the bacteria. For a detailed understanding of the mechanism of action of APs, readers are invited to refer to the following article [52]. The structural and chemical diversity allow for polymer chemists to design, manipulate and construct a variety of polymers with cationic and amphiphilic structures that can function as antimicrobials. In this review, we have selected a few antimicrobial polymers that have been designed and tested against multidrug-resistant pathogens.

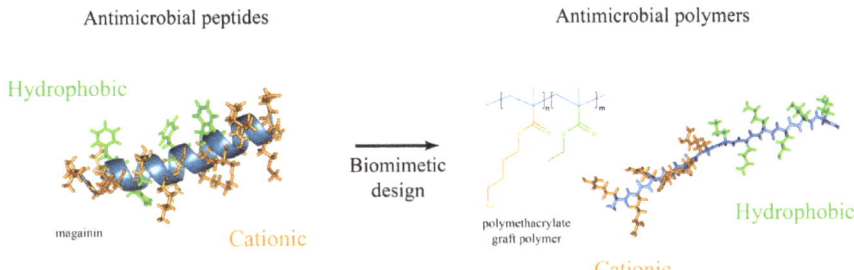

Figure 2. The structural similarities between antimicrobial polymers and antimicrobial peptides. Image was adapted with permission from [53].

4.1. Amphiphilic Antibacterial Polymers

Advancement in natural/synthetic antimicrobial polymers exploratory has also expanded researchers' interests in other amphiphilic polymers structures that conferred with antimicrobial activity [53]. Polymer structures and physicochemical properties such as molecular weight, polymer architecture, ratio of amphiphilic and its molecular arrangement are the potential determinants of materials' antimicrobial potency and selectivity [54]. An ideal amphiphilic antibacterial polymer harboring a cationic arm, low molecular weight and low-level lipophilicity would likely to incur adequate antibacterial activity against Gram-positive bacteria and has minimum hemolysis activity toward human red blood cells i.e., <4% hemolysis at a given minimum inhibitory concentration (MIC) [55]. Nonetheless, Locock et al., 2014 suggested that the combinational effect offered by the specific pendant functional groups may alter the potency, selectivity and mechanisms of synthetic AMP polymers. Some empirical data showed that optimization of the degree of hydrophobicity and cationic charge is crucial for a amphiphilic polymers to attain the best antibacterial activity and minimum red blood cells haemolysis [56]. For instance, AMP-mimicking polyurethanes with a lower ratio of hydrophobic region and higher cationic strength conferred the polymers with higher bactericidal activity and lower haemolysis rate [57]. In the comparison of cationic amine- and guanidine-copolymers, the latter of low to moderate molecular weight and hydrophobicity showed higher antimicrobial activity against *S. epidermis* and lower toxicity toward red blood cells [55]. On the other hand, auto-degradation or biodegradation of polymers is an essential consideration in choosing the right antimicrobial materials [54,58]. Degradable properties of antimicrobial material avoid or minimize undesired complication caused by prolonged retention of the materials in human body or towards the environment. Controlled degradation rate of the polymers by tuning of monomer composition and amine functionality could enhance precise control of the lifespan of antimicrobial activity [47,59]. Table 2 presents a variety of amphiphilic polymers synthesized by a random synthesis approach was tested against ESKAPE pathogens.

Table 2. Amphiphilic antimicrobial polymers activities against ESKAPE pathogens.

Polymers	Class	Description	Susceptibility						Haemolytic Activity	References
			E	S	K	A	P	E		
4-aminobutylene side chain coupled with hydrophobic ethylmethacrylate in a roughly 70/30 ratio	Amphiphilic Methacrylate Copolymers	Cationic amphiphilic random copolymers with ethyl methacrylate (EMA) comonomer were prepared with a range of comonomer fractions, and the library of copolymers was screened for antimicrobial and hemolytic activities.	BC	BS	-	BS	BS	BS	Low	[60]
PDMAEMA-g-rosin	Cationic polymers	Quaternary ammonium-containing poly(N,N-dimethylaminoethyl methacrylate) with natural rosin as the pendant group.	BS	BS	-	-	-	-	NA	[61]
Methacrylate Copolymer (E429)	Methacrylate Copolymer	Amphiphilic random copolymers with modulated cationic side chain spacer arms structure which include 2-aminoethylene, 4-aminobutylene, and 6-aminohexylene groups.	BS	BS	-	BS	BS	BS	NA	[62]
PAPMA	Amphiphilic Methacrylamide Copolymers	A series of copolymers containing lysine mimicking aminopropyl methacrylamide (APMA) and arginine mimicking guanadinopropyl methacrylamide (GPMA).	BS	BS	-	-	BS	-	NA	[63]

Table 2. *Cont.*

Polymers	Class	Description	Susceptibility						Haemolytic Activity	References
			E	S	K	A	P	E		
Cationic polyester-based copolymer	Self-Degradable Antibacterial Polymers	Auto-degradable antimicrobial copolymers bearing cationic side chains and main-chain ester linkages synthesized using the simultaneous chain- and step-growth radical polymerization of t-butyl acrylate and 3-butenyl 2-chloropropionate, followed by the transformation of t-butyl groups into primary ammonium salts.	BS	-		-	-	-	Low-Moderate	[58]
AMP-mimicking polyurethanes	Peptidomimetic Polyurethanes	Peptidomimetic polyurethanes with pendant functional groups that mimic lysine and valine amino acid residues	BC	-		-	-	-	Low	[57]
Block Amphiphilic Copolymers	Amphiphilic copolymers of Poly(Vinyl Ether)s	A series of amphiphilic block copolymers of poly(vinyl ether) derivatives prepared by base-assisting living cationic polymerization.	BS	-		-	-	-	Low	[64]
Random Amphiphilic Copolymers	Amphiphilic copolymers of Poly(Vinyl Ether)s	A series of amphiphilic random copolymers of poly(vinyl ether) derivatives prepared by base-assisting living cationic polymerization.	BS	-		-	-	-	High	[64]

Note: ESKAPE—*Enterococcus faecium*, *Staphylococcus aureus*, *Klebsiella pneumoniae*, *Acinetobacter baumannii*, *Pseudomonas aeruginosa* and *Enterobacter* spp.; antibacterial effect: BC—Bactericidal, BS—Bacteriostatic. Colour code for toxicity: White—data not available, Yellow—low haemolytic activity, Red—high haemolytic activity.

4.2. Polymers Containing Natural Peptides

APs are produced by living hosts as part of innate immune responses. These protective biologics are relatively rich at various sites such as epithelial layers, phagocytic cells and body fluids such as tears and sweat [65,66]. For instance, the major epidermal APs are reported to include cathelicidins and defensins, which exhibit broad spectrum antimicrobial activities against bacterial, fungal and viral infections [67]. The mechanism of action is non-receptor dependent; and commonly activated by the alteration of bacterial membrane structure or enveloped-components, although the interruption of internal cellular function has gained increasing evidence as illustrated in Figure 3 [68,69]. In addition, APs confer a higher affinity towards negatively charge bacterial cell membranes compared to mammalian cell membranes increasing their selectivity [70,71]. However, the clinical implementation of APs are at the early stages of translation due to the following reasons: (a) susceptibility to degradation by host proteases (b) potential toxicity to the host due to high concentration needed for antimicrobial activity and (c) short half-life due to protein binding [72]. Thus, these limitations encourage the development of synthetic AMP mimics as an alternative approach.

Current studies on synthetic antimicrobial peptides focus on the compound's susceptibility to pathogens and its toxicity effect towards the host. The susceptibility towards the pathogen is determined by the minimum inhibitory concentration of the compound that leads to either 50% (MIC_{50}) or 90% (MIC_{90}) bacterial growth, wherein the presence of activity was determined if the MIC_{50} or MIC_{90} was less than 100 µg/mL. Compound toxicity towards the host is determined by erythrocytosis activity. The degree of haemolytic activity of erythrocytes at MIC_{50} or the compound concentration leading to 50% red blood cell lysis determines the degree of the toxicity [70].

Selected studies of synthetic antimicrobial peptides and its mimics on ESKAPE pathogens are highlighted in Table 3. The model ESKAPE species were *S. aureus* and *P. aeruginosa*, as the selected Gram-positive and Gram-negative organisms, respectively. The studies showed bactericidal and/or bacteriostatic outcomes. Out of many reported compounds, only selected AMPs such as Brilacidin (also known as PMX-30063), an arylamide-peptide, has been tested in Phase II clinical trials. According to the fact sheet, a good prognosis in topical treatment of MRSA-infected wound and minimal side effects were reported [73]. Another AMP mimic, LTX 109, a membrane disrupting compound targeting Gram-positive and Gram-negative bacteria is currently under phase II clinical trials for the treatment of impetigo [73]. These two AMPs were indicated for topical used only, owing to the uncertainty from the aforementioned AMP limitations.

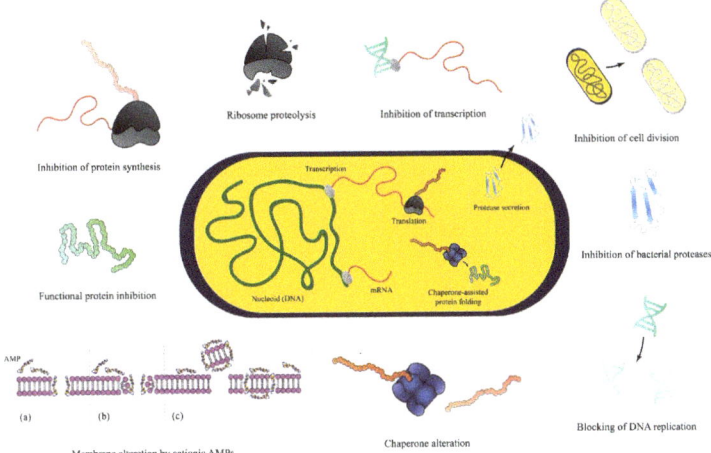

Figure 3. The proposed mechanism of bacterial killing activities by antimicrobial peptides. Image was adapted with permission from [69].

Table 3. Synthetic antimicrobial polymers mimicking peptides activities against ESKAPE pathogens.

Polymers	Class	Description	Susceptibility						Haemolytic Activity	References
			E	S	K	A	P	E		
Idolidicin variants	Peptide	A 13-residue cationic antimicrobial peptide (sequence carboxy-terminal amidated ILPWKPWPWWPWRR-NH$_2$)		BC					High	[66,73]
Gratisin analogues	Peptide	cyclo(-Val^1-Orn^2-Leu^3-D-Phe^4-Pro^5-D-Tyr^6-)$_2$		BS			BS		Low	[69]
LL-37	Peptide	A cathelin-associated antimicrobial peptide		BS			BS		None	[74]
α/β-Peptides	Peptide	Helix-forming α/β-peptides, i.e., oligomers containing a 1:1 pattern of α- and β- amino acid residues in the backbone	BS	BS					None	[75]
cecropin/melittin	Peptide	Hybrid peptide produced by recombinant DNA technology in S. aureus					BC		NA	[76]
Maleic anhydride copolymers	Peptide mimics	Peptides Mimicking Copolymers of Maleic Anhydride and 4-Methyl-1-pentene		None			None		High	[77]
Brilacidin	Peptide mimics	also known as PMX-30063, a defensin-mimetic and a membrane-targeting arylamide oligomer		BC					NA	[71]
cecropin/melittin	Synthetic peptide	Recombinant hybrid peptide					BC		NA	[76]
LL-37LTX 109	Peptide mimics	a synthetic antimicrobial peptidomimetic containing a modified tryptophan derivate as lipophilic bulk, displayed a combination of high antibacterial activity against MRSA and Staphylococcus spp. biofilm		BC			BS		Low	[78]
poly(m-phenylene ethynylene)s	Peptide mimics	Nonhemolytic abiogenic polymers	BS	BS	BS	BS	BS	BS	Low	[79]
Pandinin 2	Peptide Variants	A scorpion venom AMP contains a central proline residue		BC					High	[80]
Pyridinium Functionalized Polynorbornenes	Synthetic peptide	Amphiphilic polyoxanorbornene with different quaternary alkyl pyridinium side-chains		BS					NA	[81]
Amino-Functionalized Poly(norbornene)	Synthetic peptide	Homopolymers of the amine bearing monomers and random copolymers of amine- and alkyl-substituted monomers of high average molar mass was produced by ring-opening metathesis polymerization.		BS			BS		None	[82]

Note: ESKAPE:—Enterococcus faecium, Staphylococcus aureus, Klebsiella pneumoniae, Acinetobacter baumannii, Pseudomonas aeruginosa and Enterobacter spp.; antibacterial effect: BC—Bactericidal; BS—Bacteriostatic. Colour code for toxicity: White—data not available, Green—No haemolytic activity detected, Yellow—low haemolytic activity, Red—High haemolytic activity.

4.3. Halogen-Containing Polymers

Halogen (fluorine, chlorine, bromine, iodine) containing polymers with antimicrobial properties are attractive materials based on unique properties afforded by the associated halogen (Figure 4). Halogen-containing antimicrobials are well described. Several antimicrobials produced by *Streptomyces* spp. contain chlorine; chloramphenicol, chlortetracycline and vancomycin. Fluoroquinolones, effective against Gram-positive and Gram-negative organisms, are a class of antimicrobials where fluorine is incorporated within the quinolone structure [83].

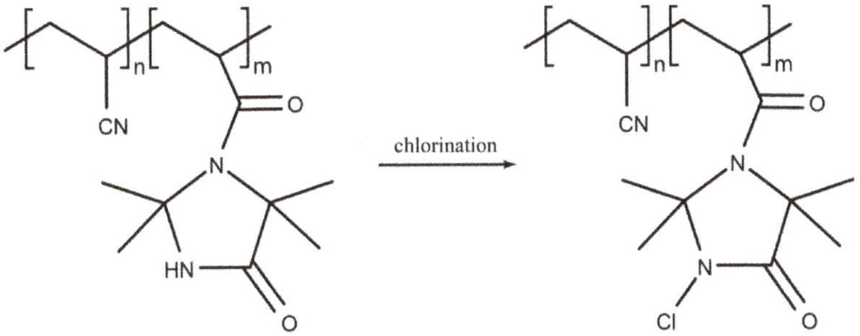

Figure 4. Chlorine-containing polymer.

Polymers containing fluorine offer antimicrobial activity due to their hydrophobic nature. A review by Munoz-Bonilla et al. highlights the use of such polymers, including the creation of a polymeric fluorine containing surfactant known as Quaterfluo® [67]. The surfactant subunit alone showed robust antimicrobial activity against *P. aeruginosa, S. aureus, C. albicans* and *A. niger* [74]. When formed as a polymer, the activity against *S. aureus* increased with the length of the active perfluorakyl chains [74]. Recently, cationic fluorinated polymer emulsions have been used to create antibacterial fabrics where the presence of fluorine greatly enhanced both the antibacterial and anti-adhesion properties of the material when tested against *E. coli* and *S. aureus* [75].

Fluorinated polymers containing antimicrobials such as ciprofloxacin, a second-generation fluoroquinolone, have been investigated to improve solubility and bioavailability. Mesallati and colleagues prepared amorphous solid dispersions (ASDs) of ciprofloxacin with acidic polymers such as Eudragit L100, Carbopol and hydroxy propyl methyl cellulose acetate succinate (HPMCAS) [76]. When incorporated in the polymer matrix, the solubility of ciprofloxacin was improved both in water and in simulated intestinal fluid. When tested against *E. coli, S. aureus, P. aeruginosa* and *K. pneumoniae*, formulations with HPMCAS drastically improved MIC and MBC concentrations as compared to monomeric ciprofloxacin [76]. Conjugation of ciprofloxacin with polymers have also been used to create biomedical nanomaterials for use in wound dressings [77]. Ciprofloxacin-PLA (poly L-lactic acid) conjugated polymers increased the solubility of ciprofloxacin for use in the fabrication of biodegradable non-woven nanofibers by electrospinning. ciprofloxacin released from the PLA non-woven nanofibers was effective at inhibiting the growth of *E. coli* and *S. aureus* indicating the utility of ciprofloxacin conjugated polymers as an antimicrobial biomedical material [77].

An effective antimicrobial group of polymers contain N-halamines, in which at least one nitrogen-halogen covalent bond is formed by the chlorination of imide, amide and amine groups. A new N-halamine, hydantoin acrylamide (HA), copolymerised with siloxane (SL) to create PHASL, was used to coat cotton fabric which was shown to be effective against *E. coli* O157: H7 and *S. aureus* within 5 min once activated by chlorination [78]. More recently the halogenated 2,2,5,5-tetramethyl-1,3-imidazolidinone (TMIO) by chlorination to form 1-chloro-2,2,5,5-tetramethyl-4-imidazolidinone (MC) was found to be effective in reducing bacterial colony-forming units (CFU) of both *S. aureus* and *P. aeruginosa* when coated on wound dressings. Bactericidal activity was observed in 15 min for *S. aureus* (6-log reduction) and within 30 min for

P. aeruginosa (7-log reduction) [79]. In this form, MC was also found to be stable when stored in the dark for 6 months, highlighting an additional utility of *N*-halamine-coated medical materials designed for wound dressings.

4.4. Polymers Containing Phosphor and Sulfo Derivatives

Polyphosphonium and polysulfonium are phospo- and sulfo- containing polymers, respectively (Figure 5). They share their mode of action with polymers comprising quaternary ammonium in causing damage to the bacterial cell wall. Phosphonium containing polycationic agents are typically considered to be more microbicidal than quaternary ammonium salt polymers with their antimicrobial potency positively related to the number of phosphonium units within the polymer [67]. Until recently, polyphosphoniums studies have been restricted to alkyl and aryl derivatives with the polymers exhibiting both hydrophobic and hydrophilic domains—a feature considered to be required for antimicrobial activity. Cuthbert and colleagues unexpectedly discovered that control polymers lacking hydrophobic alkyl chains exhibit high antimicrobial activity against *E. coli* and *S. aureus* while at the same time low lytic action on erythrocytes [80]. These findings were uncovered when investigating the ability of 'baited' phosphonium polymers to exert increased microbicidal effects, taking advantage of bacterial affinity to mannose sugars [80]. This work challenges the assumed requirement for balanced hydrophilic and lipophilic components within biocidal polymers and warrants further investigation into this promising class of antimicrobial polymers.

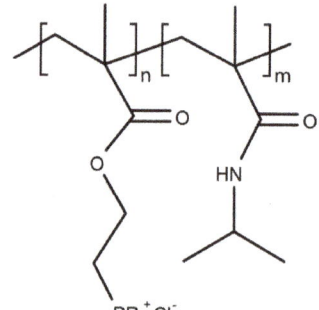

Figure 5. Polymer-containing phosphor-derivatives.

4.5. Phenol and Benzoic Derivative Polymers

Polymers containing the organic and aromatic compounds such as phenol and benzoic acid have intrinsic antimicrobial properties (Figure 6). Phenol is a strong antimicrobial agent able to disrupt the cellular membrane, while benzoic acid has broad spectrum inhibitory activity and is used as an environmentally safe antimicrobial. Vinyl polymers containing phenol or benzoic acid pendant groups were synthesised by Park and colleagues and tested for activity against *S. aureus* and *P. aeruginosa* [81]. While the polymers exhibited lower antimicrobial activity than the monomer when tested by halo diffusion, they have been used as coating materials. Nevertheless, phenol pendant vinyl polymers were marginally more effective against *S. aureus* than *P. aeruginosa* while the converse was observed for benzoic acid pendant vinyl polymers [81]. In contrast, aminated polyacrylonitrile (PAN) polymers where benzaldehyde derivatives were immobilized via their amine-terminal, were found to exhibit increased antimicrobial activity with additional bioactive groups [82]. Inhibition zone diameters significantly increased with the number of bioactive groups in each prepared polymer for several microbes, including *E. coli*, *P aeruginosa*, *S. aureus* and *A. niger* [81].

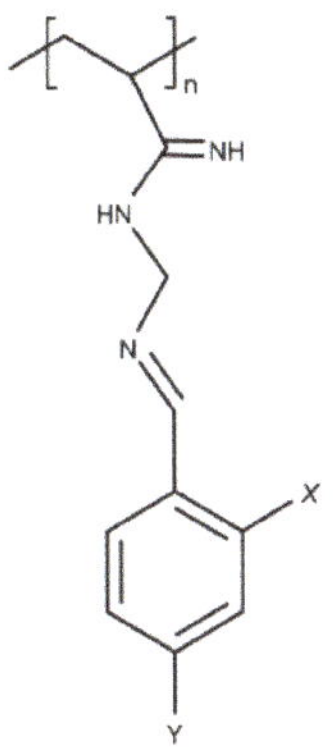

Figure 6. Polyacrynitrilbenzaldehyde.

4.6. Organometallic Polymers

Organometallic polymers contain metals bonded to at least one organic molecule carbon by pi-bonds, by coordination bonds or by sigma-/pi-bonds to other elements. Antimicrobial formulations of organometallic polymers are extensive and are reviewed in depth in [67]. Silver-containing polymers are prevalent, having potent antimicrobial activity in solid form across a wide range of organisms including key ESKAPE organisms; *E. coli*, *S. aureus*, *P. aeruginosa* and *A. niger*. The same polymers in aqueous solutions, however, showed reduced efficacy in Gram-positive bacteria and yeasts [67]. Recently, Awad and colleagues took a novel approach by creating Eco-friendly silver-polystyrene nanocomposite using touline extracted orange peel to reduce silver nitrate to silver nanoparticles (AgNP) before creating a polymer with polystyrene. Antibacterial activity was observed by disk diffusion against *E. coli*, *K. pneumoniae* and *S. aureus* for both AgNP and AgNP/polystyrene polymers, although reduced for the latter in comparison [83]. Creating AgNP via this simple method, requires further investigation in the quest for novel, environmentally sound biomaterials. In general, those polymeric resins containing Cu(II), in comparison to other metal ions, show enhanced antimicrobial activity against a range of microorganisms which has been attributed to the stability of the Cu(II) ion [67].

4.7. Metal Nanoparticles Included in Polymeric Carriers

4.7.1. Polymeric Systems Containing Silver Nanoparticles

Silver nanoparticles (AgNPs) alone have a well-established use in the treatment of bacterial infections. AgNPs show an efficient antimicrobial property due to their extremely large surface area, which provides better contact with microorganisms [84]. Wen-Ru et al. have studied the antibacterial activity and acting mechanism of AgNPs on *E. coli* [85,86]. The authors investigated the growth, permeability, and morphology of the bacterial cell wall following the treatment with AgNPs. Their results showed that, based on transmission electron microscopy (TEM) imaging, the bacteria membrane vesicles were dissolved and dispersed, and the membrane components became disorganized and scattered from their original ordered and close arrangement [87]. These observations suggested that AgNPs may damage the structure of the bacterial cell membrane and depress the activity of some membranous enzymes. Studies have also shown that AgNPs are able to interact with sulfur-containing proteins present in the bacterial membrane, in the same way as they can interact with phosphorus groups present in the cell DNA [88]. AgNPs seem to preferably attack the respiratory chain, and cell division.

The use of AgNPs in biomedical applications has been extended by the incorporation of AgNPs into polymeric systems forming multilayer films, polymeric nanotubes and nanofibres, and polymeric gels. The development of organic–inorganic hybrid nanomaterials has allowed the combination of the tunable properties of soft nanomaterials with the unique optical and electronic properties of metal nanoparticles. Due to their tunable surface, morphology and porosity, soft organic materials such as polymers that are derived from various synthetic or natural compounds can easily incorporate metal nanoparticles of different shapes and sizes. A large number of polymers have been investigated for this purpose. AgNPs can be synthesized in situ using the polymer matrix as a reaction medium, or alternatively, the AgNPs are prepared ex situ and then incorporated into the polymeric matrix [89–91].

Numerous studies have been carried out using different polymer systems [91–94]. Sanchez-Valdes et al. have prepared multilayer films of polyethylene and AgNPs and evaluated their antimicrobial activity towards *Pseudomonas oleovorans* and *Aspergillus niger* [95]. The authors showed that the release of the Ag^+ ions, and therefore the efficacy of this system, was dependent on the size of the AgNPs. Other authors have focused their attention on the modification of the nanocomposite surface, at the nanometer level, by combining the effects of oxygen plasma treatment and silver nanoparticles on the poly(lactic-co-glycolic acid) (PLGA) polymer matrix [96]. In this study, PLGA nanocomposite films were produced by solvent casting with 1 wt% and 7 wt% of AgNPs. The PLGA (used as a control) and PLGA/Ag nanocomposite surfaces were then treated with oxygen plasma. Antibacterial tests were performed using *E. coli* and *S. aureus*. The plasma-treated PLGA/Ag^+ system showed the best bactericidal effect in comparison to untreated PLGA/Ag^+ or oxygen plasma-treated PLGA matrix for both strains [96].

A different approach to prepare antibacterial coatings has been described by Taheri et al. where AgNPs were encapsulated into a phospholipid bilayer and their surface immobilised to a functional plasma polymer for application on medical devices such as catheters and wound dressings. The antibacterial efficacy of the coatings was evaluated against *S. aureus*, *S.epidermidis* and *P. aeruginosa*. The innate immune response was studied in culture of primary bone marrow-derived macrophages (BMDM) and the potential cytotoxicity was assessed in culture of primary human fibroblasts. The authors also observed a reduced expression of pro-inflammatory cytokines from BMDM which suggested a reduced inflammatory response. The prepared coatings were able to reduce the growth of *S.aureus* and *P. aeruginosa* by 70% and 80%, respectively, while colonization by *S. epidermidis* was almost completely inhibited.

Studies have also moved towards the inclusion of additional materials to the AgNPs-polymer containing systems. An example is the incorporation of growth factors (bone morphology protein-2, BMP-2) and AgNPs into hydroxyapatite (HA) coatings on metallic implant surfaces for enhancing osteo-inductivity and antibacterial properties. In this complex system, BMP-2 and AgNPs containing HA coating were prepared on titanium (Ti) surfaces by electrochemical deposition (ED). In addition, chitosan (CS) was used as a stabilising agent for the generation of the AgNPs, and simultaneously reduced their toxicity. A schematic representation of this system is shown in Figure 7. Results of antibacterial tests indicated that the CS/Ag/HA coatings have high antibacterial properties against both *S. epidermidis* and *E. coli*. Additionally, bone marrow stromal cells (BMSCs) culture results indicated that the BMP/CS/Ag/HA coatings have good osteoinductivity and promote the differentiation of BMSCs. Implantation of Ti bars with BMP/CS/Ag/HA coatings into the femur of rabbits showed that BMP/CS/Ag/HA coatings favour bone formation in vivo. Other studies can be found in the literature reporting the inclusion of other biological or synthetic compounds into the AgNPs-polymers systems such as bovine serum albumin and tiopronin.

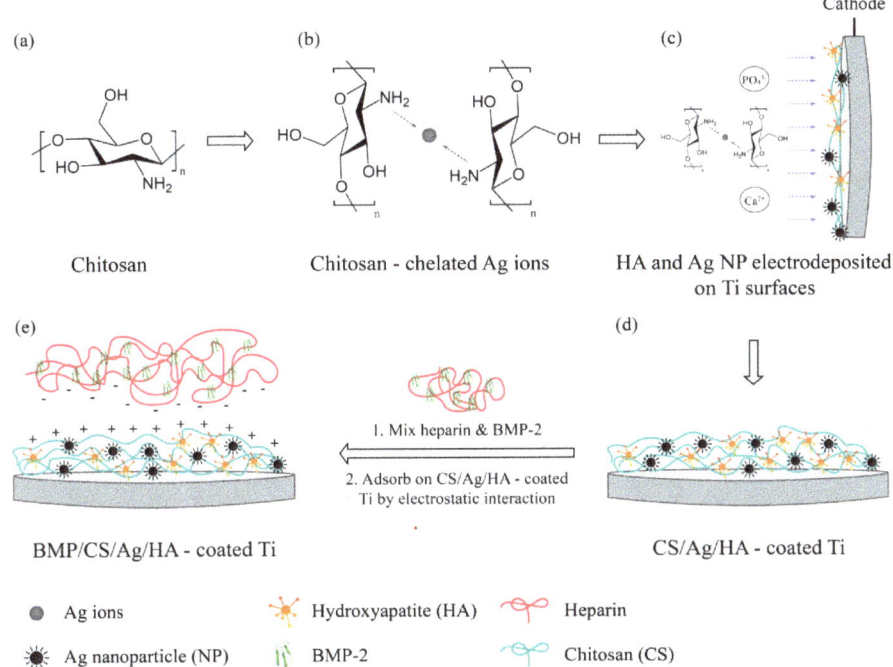

Figure 7. Schematic representation of the electrochemical deposition process and immobilization of bone morphology protein-2 (BMP-2_ on HA coatings on a Ti metal surface). Image was adapted with permission from [97].

4.7.2. Nanofiber Systems Containing Silver Nanoparticles

The development of hybrid organic–metallic systems containing AgNPs embedded in nanofibers has gained increasing interest due to the dual benefits of each individual system. Due to their high surface-to-volume ratio, polymeric nanofibers can provide a larger number of reaction sites and higher permeability. By embedding AgNPs into polymer nanofiber matrices, the composites are promising candidates for scaffolding biomaterials with antimicrobial properties [85].

Nanofibers are mostly prepared by electrospinning. Either in combination with other polymers, or on its own, biodegradable polymers such as PLGA, poly-caprolactone (PCL) and chitosan can be electrospun and further functionalised to achieve the desired antibacterial properties [86]. Other studies reported the one-step fabrication of silver nanoparticles embedded into poly(2-(tert-butylaminoethyl) methacrylate) (PTBAM) nanofibers by radical-mediated dispersion polymerization. PTBAM is a cationic polymer, which may increase the antimicrobial properties of the nanofibers loaded with AgNPs against Gram-negative *E. coli* and Gram-positive *S. aureus* [98].

A few interesting studies have used bacterial cellulose functionalized with AgNPs for wound-healing treatment [98,99]. Bacterial-derived cellulose, commonly known as bacterial cellulose (BC), is produced by the fermentation of Gram-negative bacterium *Acetobacter xylinum*, which can produce high aspect ratio nanofibers, with three-dimensional (3D) porous networks Authors showed that AgNPs sized from 5 to 12 nm, with narrow size distribution, were successfully deposited on the BC matrix. The studies showed a slow release of the AgNPs from the BC matrix, with the antibacterial effect lasting after 7 days.

4.7.3. Hydrogels Containing Silver Nanoparticles

Hydrogel-based dressings containing antimicrobial components have seen an increase in research activity in wound-care applications. Boonkaew B. et al. have prepared 2-acrylamido-2-methylpropane sulfonic acid sodium salt hydrogels containing AgNPs via ultraviolet radiation [100]. None of the hydrogels were found to be toxic to any of the tested cell lines. The measurement of cumulative release of silver indicated that 70–82% of silver was released within 72 h. The antibacterial activities against Gram-positive *S. aureus* showed a log reduction >3 after 6 h of treatment. In the case of Gram-negative *P. aeruginosa*, the results showed faster inhibition as the log reduction was >3 within 3 h. The fact that Gram-positive bacteria are less susceptible to silver ions than Gram-negative bacteria could be related to a) the fact that the cell wall of Gram-positive bacteria is thicker than that of Gram negative bacteria; b) silver may get trapped by the negative charge of the peptidoglycan cell wall.

Hydrogel based wound dressing membranes have been developed using a combination of the following polymers, polyvinylpyrrolidone (PVP), polyethylene glycol (PEG), agar and carboxymethyl cellulose (CMC) [101]. Silver ions were dispersed in the polymer matrix and its reduction with formation of a hydrogel and AgNPs was performed using gamma irradiation. In vitro and in vivo results showed increased cicatrisation with the presence of large quantity of fibroblasts being detected with little formation of collagen. Other studies explore the possibility of generating photo-activated in situ poly (ethylene glycol) diacrylate (PEGDA) and PVP hydrogel composite containing AgNPs with sustained anti-fouling/anti-bacterial activities [102]. The authors showed that the in situ method is more effective than the two-step method since a) there is minimal gel softening; b) less dispersal of nanoparticles; and c) lower concentration of metallic nanoparticles is needed, which reduces toxicity to cells. The ability of the AgNPs-hydrogel composite to control bacterial growth was evaluated by measuring bacterial growth rates in media immersed with the composite. The AgNP-PEGDA-PVP gel composite limited the bacterial growth even at the silver concentration of 0.2 mM. At a concentration of 10 mM, the system was able to inhibit bacterial growth over 5 days.

4.7.4. Inclusion of Other Metal Nanoparticles

Other metal particles are also known for their antimicrobial activity, although they are relatively less studied than silver. Gold NPs (AuNPs) have exploited their unique chemical and physical properties for transporting and unloading pharmaceutical compounds. The gold core is essentially inert and non-toxic when compared to AgNPs [103]. Furthermore, AuNPs are chemically stable and allow easy surface functionalization [104]. One of the most attractive modifications is the coating of AuNPs with biocompatible polymers such as PEG and chitosan, which by creating composites with a modulate mechanical strength can improve their features as biomedical scaffolds [105,106].

Chitosan-AuNPs nanocomposites prepared by a solvent evaporation method showed high antibacterial activity and simultaneously low cytotoxicity. It has been shown that the molecular weight (Mw) and deacetylation degree of chitosan influences the size of the AuNPs formed. The resulting nanocomposites demonstrated total bactericidal effect against two biofilm forming antimicrobial resistant strains (*S. aureus* and *P. aeruginosa*) [107]. Other studies showed that chitosan- AuNPs systems have concentration-dependent bactericidal ability without damaging human macrophages in an in vitro infection model, causing bacterial wall damage as the killing mechanism [108].

Hybrid PEG-AuNPs nanocomplexes can be effectively bio-conjugated with the enzymes or proteins [109,110]. More recently, a study has demonstrated that engineered hybrid PEG-AuNPs covalently conjugated with a peptide called innate defense regulator (IDR)-1018 showed both bactericidal and antibiofilm properties at micromolar concentration bacteria [111]. The surface of the AuNPs can also be modified with molecules that serve as the main structural components of β-lactam antimicrobials, such as 6-aminopenicillanic acid (6-APA) [112]. The APA-modified AuNPs were electrospun with PCL/gelatin to obtain biocompatible antibacterial wound dressings. The antibacterial activity in skin wound healing by a dorsal wound model of a rat exposed to *E. coli*, MDR *E. coli*, *P. aeruginosa* and MDR *P. aeruginosa* was investigated. The results showed that wounds treated with Au-APA electrospun nanofibers had better wound-healing ability than gauze and PCL/gelatin nanofibers even against MDR bacterial wound infection.

Copper nanoparticles (CuNPs) have been shown to have excellent antimicrobial properties. This could be due to an increased concentration of copper inside the cell which causes oxidative stress and forms hydrogen peroxide. Furthermore, excess copper causes a decrease of the membrane integrity of microorganisms, leading to the loss of vital nutritional cell elements, causing desiccation and eventually cell death [113]. Incorporation of CuNPs into medical grade polymers has also been described. CuNPs incorporated into polyurethane and silicone polymers displayed potent antibacterial activity against methicillin-resistant *S. aureus* and *E. coli* within 6 h [114].

Lu et al. added CuNPs to the mixture of anionic carboxymethyl chitosan (CMC) and alginate (Alg) polymers [115]. The authors found that the CMC/Alg/Cu scaffolds showed significantly improved capabilities of osteogenesis and killing clinical bacteria compared to CMC/Alg scaffolds fabricated by the same procedure but without adding CuNPs. Furthermore, in vivo studies demonstrated that CMC/Alg/Cu scaffolds could induce the formation of vascularized new bone tissue in 4 weeks while avoiding clinical bacterial infection even when the implantation sites were challenged with clinically relevant *S. aureus* bacteria.

4.7.5. Inclusion of Titanium Dioxide and Zinc Oxide

Titanium-based alloys as biomaterials have many advantages due to their lower modulus, intensive corrosion resistance and superior biocompatibility [116]. Furthermore, titanium dioxide (TiO_2) is a chemically stable and inert material, and when illuminated, can continuously exert antimicrobial effects by the generation of superoxide and hydroxyl radicals [117]. Similarly to what has been reported for other metal NPs, TiO_2 nanoparticles (TiO_2NPs) have also been incorporated into polymeric systems by different techniques and their antibacterial properties demonstrated against a variety of microorganisms. Chitosan, PLA and PLGA remain the most widely used polymers for this purpose.

Fonseca et al. prepared PLA composites containing TiO_2NPs, with a diameter of 10 nm and homogeneously dispersed in the polymer matrix. The PLA nanocomposites containing 8 wt% of TiO_2NPs when irradiated with light and ultraviolet-A (UVA), showed a reduction of ~94.3% and 99.9% against *E. coli* and *Aspergillus fumigatus*, respectively. Toniatto, T.V. and his co-authors also used PLA polymer but in the fiber shape. They prepared electrospun PLA fibers with high loadings of TiO_2NPs (1–5 wt%), which possessed bactericidal activity against *S. aureus*, however which showed no in vitro cytotoxicity using a L929 cell line [118]. Furthermore, studies have also evaluated the feasibility of PLGA-TiO_2NPs composite biofilms under UV light irradiation, on wound healing in vitro, human keratinocytes (HaCaTs), fibroblasts (L929s), and bovine carotid artery endothelial cells (BECs) [87]. These results showed that the biofilms for artificial dressing applications, containing 10% TiO_2NPs, were effective against *E. coli* and *S. aureus* and had a good biocompatibility on HaCaTs and L929s, however they had some cytotoxic effects on BECs.

An interesting study of porous scaffolds of collagen and chitosan-containing TiO_2NPs were evaluated as tissue engineering for wound repair. The collagen–chitosan composite scaffolds with various concentrations of TiO_2NPs were prepared by freeze-drying technique. The scaffolds showed an inhibitory effect on *S. aureus*, good permeability and it may provide a humid environment for wound repairing [119]. Chitosan has been used in other studies combined with TiO_2NPs for antibacterial applications [120]. Other binary polymer combinations containing poly(ether ether ketone) (PEEK)/poly(ether imide) (PEI) blends reinforced with bioactive TiO_2NPs were fabricated via ultrasonication followed by melt-blending [121]. The nanocomposites showed significant antibacterial properties against human pathogenic bacteria with and without UV illumination, and the effect on *S. aureus* was systematically stronger than that on *E. coli*.

Zinc oxide (ZnO) nanoparticles (ZnONPs) have been widely investigated thanks to its multifunctional properties coupled with the ease of preparing various morphologies, such as nanowires, nanorods, and nanoparticles [122]. Three-dimensional and interconnected porous granules of nanostructured hydroxyapatite (nanoHA) incorporated with different amounts of ZnONPs have been prepared by a simple polymer sponge replication method [123]. Granules loaded with 2% ZnONPs showed a strong antibacterial effect against *S. aureus* and *S. epidermidis*. In vivo studies used nanoHA porous granules with and without ZnONPs implanted into the subcutaneous tissue in rats and their inflammatory response after 3, 7 and 30 days was examined. The results showed the potential of these systems in reducing bacterial activity in vitro and in vivo, with a low cell growth inhibition in vitro and no differences in the connective tissue growth and inflammatory response in vivo. Sustained release preparations of polymers containing ZnONPs have been described by the formation of crosslinked polymer networks with ZnNPs in the form of hydrogels [124].

4.8. Dendrimers

Dendrimers are a class of molecule and the word is derived from dendron which means tree for their characteristic branch-like appearances (Figure 8). The most common dendrimers used for biological applications are based on polyamidoamines (PAMAM) and polypropylene imine (PPI), (Figure 9). Dendrimers are synthesized from the core and develop into a globular structure with the size between 2–5 nm. The core structure provides attachment of the dendrons and each section represents a generation (G1, G2, G3) (Figure 8). The higher generation the dendrimer is built of, the more branched and exposed number of end groups are available for conjugation with other molecules including small molecule antibiotics [125]. Dendrimers' chemical branches can be tailored according to the solubility and degradability to enhance biological activity of interest [126].

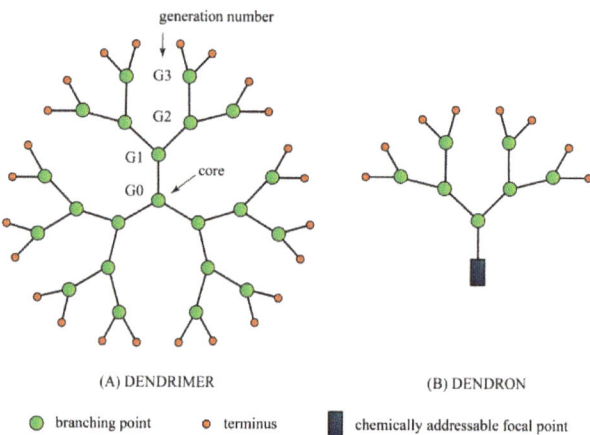

Figure 8. The physical structure of a dendrimer.

Dendrimers can demonstrate its own antibacterial activities through interaction with the bacterial lipid bilayer and causes destabilisation of the bacterial structure [127]. Mofrad et al., 2018 demonstrated the efficacy of G3-poly-amidoamine dendrimer (G3-PAD) against seven species of Gram-negative and -positive bacteria. Interestingly, the highest sensitivity was observed for *Salmonella* species with the least susceptibility were observed in *Klebsiella* species. The author suggested differences in the bacterial membrane composition contributed to the strong barriers against the entrance of dendrimers inside the bacteria [128]. Additionally, Pires et al. 2015 demonstrated effective antimicrobial activities of peptide dendrimer, G3KL against multidrug resistant *Acinetobactor baumanii* and *P. aeruginosa* [129]. These two examples are only selected research on dendrimers' antibacterial activities and readers are invited to refer more on related information as provided by [125]. Due to the multi- functional group within dendrimers, the molecules can also be conjugated with existing antibiotics to potentiate their activities. Interestingly, stimulus-controlled antibiotic released from the dendrimer can be achieved by specific triggers, for example, light, pH or temperature. Some examples of the successful functionalization of antibiotics are summarized in Table 4.

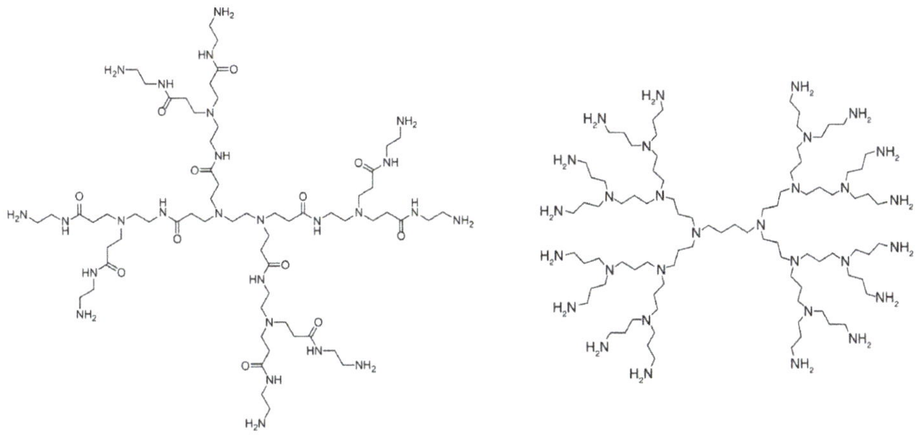

(a) Polyamidoamine dendrimer G1

(b) Polypropyleneimine dendrimer G3

Figure 9. Examples of common dendrimers for biological application.

Table 4. Examples of dendrimers conjugated with antibiotics.

Dendrimers	Antibiotics Conjugates	Pathogens Tested	Mechanism of Antibiotic Release	References
Polyamidoamines (PAMAM)	Ciprofloxacin	E. coli	Light-active release	[130]
PAMAM	Vancomycin	S. aureus	Temperature-active release	[131]
PAMAM	Vancomycin	S. aureus	NA	[132]
PAMAM	Erythromycin	S. aureus	Hydrolysis of the ester linkage	[133]
Polypropylene imine (PPI)-modified maltose	Amoxicillin	E. coli and P. aeruginosa	NA	[134]
PPI	Ceftazidime	P. aeruginosa	pH-active release	[135]
Polyesters	Fusidic acid	S. aureus	Water-active release	[136]
Carbohydrate-glycopeptide	Tobramycin	P. aeruginosa	Temperature-active release	[137]

4.9. Polymer-Based Guanidine

Guanidine-like compounds have been investigated for the past three decades and have given benefit in diverse medicinal field (Figure 10a) [138,139]. Guanidine can be found in natural terrestrial and marine environments such as microorganisms, plants and invertebrates [140]. Guanidine displays cationic properties and this allows for interaction with the anionic counterpart. The side chain diversity of guanidine allows for further development of guanidine scaffold for different therapeutic purposes [141]. Compounds containing guanidine have attracted interest and have been successfully applied as therapeutics for the central nervous system, anti-inflammatory agents, anti-thrombotic agents, anti-diabetic agents and antimicrobial agents [138]. One of the most commonly used antimicrobial polymers is polyhexamethylene biguanide (PHMB) or also known as polyhexanide (Figure 11). PHMB is synthesized by oligomirazation of guanidine salts and hexamethylenediaemine [141]. PHMB has been widely used in domestic applications, as an antiseptic in medicine, and in the food industry. PHMB applications include impregnation of wound dressings, water treatment, mouthwash and disinfection in contact lenses [142–144].

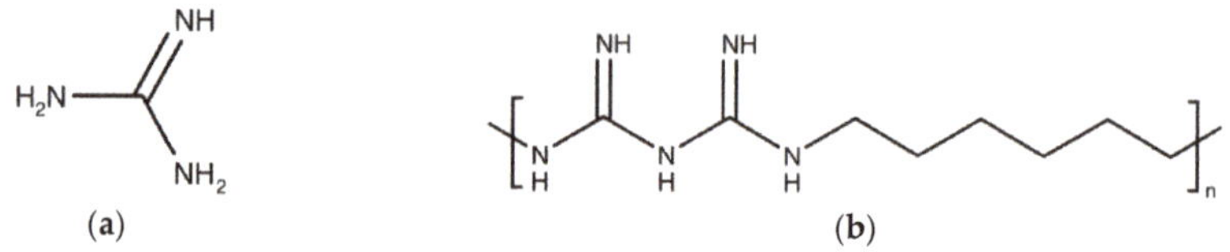

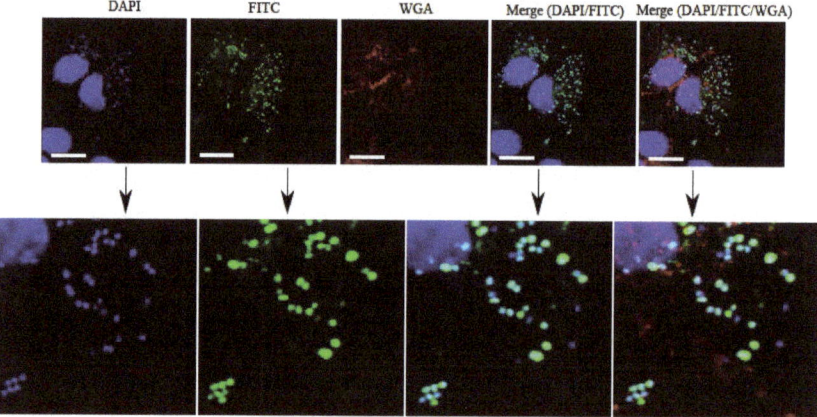

Figure 10. (a) The guanidine structure (b) The polyhexamethylene biguanide (PHMB) structure. PHMB is a cationic polymer of repeating hexamethylene biguanide groups, with n average = 10–12 (n is the number of structural unit repeats) and molecular weight (mw) 3025 g/mol.

Figure 11. Intracellular localization and bactericidal activities of PHMB against intracellular methicillin-resistant *S. aureus* (MRSA). Colocalization of fluorescence-tagged PHMB (PHMB-FITC) with intracellular *S. aureus* strain EMRSA-15 in keratinocytes. Keratinocytes were infected with EMRSA-15 followed by treatment with PHMB-FITC (green). Keratinocytes were labelled with DAPI (blue) for keratinocytes and EMRSA-15 nuclei staining and WGA (red) for keratinocyte membrane stain. Upper panels are images of infected cells and merged images. Lower panels are enlarged images that clearly show colocalization between PHMB-FITC (green) and EMRSA-15 (blue). White scale bar is 25 µm. Image is reprinted from [22].

PHMB is a potent topical antimicrobial against Gram-positive and Gram-negative bacteria, fungi, parasites and viruses [144–148]. PHMB antimicrobial activities involve the interaction of biguanide groups with the cytoplasmic membrane, lipopolysaccharide and peptidoglycan of the bacterial cell wall. This binding is believed to displace the divalent cation Ca^{2+} causing membrane destabilization and cellular leakages [145]. Simultaneously, the hexamethylene segment can interact with phospholipids on the membrane, causing a phase separation that disturbs random distribution of lipids, further destabilizing the membrane structure. Furthermore, Chindera et al. demonstrated that PHMB enters bacteria cells and this leads to chromosome condensation [148]. Therefore, PHMB may have at least two mechanisms of action, and this may help to explain why acquired antimicrobial resistance to PHMB has not yet been reported, despite being used in the clinic and domestic application for the past 40 years.

PHMB has also been reported to enter mammalian cells and kill intracellular bacteria (MRSA) and parasites (*Leishmania* spp.) at low dosage (Figure 11) [22,149]. Additionally, due to the cationic nature of the molecules, PHMB is able to form nanoparticles with other small antibiotic molecules thus potentiate its antibacterial activities [20,148,149]. PHMB is considered less toxic towards mammalian cells compared to other compounds in its class. Muller and Kramer, 2008 compared the cellular cytotoxicity of PHMB and other commonly used antiseptics in the clinic and found that PHMB has a higher biocompatibility index towards mammalian cells than other antiseptics tested [150].

5. Challenges in Bringing Antimicrobial Polymers into Clinics

Now comes the main question as to whether bench to bedside translation of these antimicrobial polymers would come into reality or remains as the research output and ends only in the publication repository. Before choosing to embark to the clinical journey, it is mandatory for the researcher to assess the in-vitro and in-vivo toxicity, biocompatibility, evaluation of the cell viability, biodistribution, immunogenicity in order to reach the go/no go decision. Mignani et al. provide an excellent guideline on the translational requirements for dendrimers and nanoparticles to move the compounds towards the investigational new drug (IND) application, which is the evaluation of the safe profile before initiating clinical trials, the first essential step to entering the clinic phase [139]. We believe the guideline is also applicable for antimicrobial polymers and readers are invited to refer to this excellent review for comprehensive information [139].

Once the researcher establish the risk/benefit ratio, it is a wise decision to understand from the early stages the potential route of application for the compound. If the compound shows good efficacy and has potential for development as oral drugs, the researcher must understand what are the suitable requirements for the oral route, and understand the Lipinsky rule of five could be a good start [151]. However, based on the history of antibiotics development and commercialisation, antibiotics generally do not obey these rules [152]. If the compound turns out to be less likely to be developed in the oral route, other routes of administration can be an alternative, for example, topical. The guideline for development of a topical product are extensively reviewed by Chang et al. 2015 [153].

6. Conclusions and Future Considerations

We are living in an era where the globe is increasingly connected with highly mobile populations, moving easily between different countries, which is a compounding factor in the global AMR challenge [154]. Indeed, in 2016 at a UN General Assembly, countries worldwide affirmed their commitment to develop national action plans based on the WHO Global Action Plan for Antibiotic Resistance (2015) [2]. In principle, the plan aims to ensure "treatment and prevention of infectious diseases with quality-assured, safe and effective medicines". A key relevant objective within the proposed WHO action plan is to strengthen knowledge through surveillance and research.

In order to provide a tangible new medicine as part of the solution for the increasing AMR problem, we propose that a network based multidisciplinary approach is vital. A continuous collaboration between chemists, microbiologists and clinicians is paramount to further develop and translate promising antimicrobial polymers for use in the clinic. One such polymer group to highlight is those containing guanidine; specifically, polyhexamethylene biguanide (PHMB) and its nanoparticle constructs, and this has been used for topical/local application. Despite PHMB being in use both for clinical and domestic purposes for over 40 years, there are no reports of resistance to date. Lack of acquired resistance is likely due to multimodal antimicrobial [145,148]. PHMB is particularly interesting for exhibiting broad spectrum activity against intracellular bacteria and parasites in nanoparticle form. Of note, PHMB demonstrates antimicrobial effects at low concentrations and has been shown to have lower toxicity than other agents of its class [20,150,155]. Future studies exploring the delivery options for PHMB, novel formulations with small molecule antibiotics, and interactions with ESKAPE isolates are required.

Clearly, going forward, the success of any existing, novel or reformulated antimicrobial of the polymer class must (i) be effective at controlling infection, (ii) exhibit low toxicity towards the host and (iii) ideally harness a multimodal arsenal of antimicrobial activity in order to provide long-term sustainability. Finally, we call on national research funding agencies to continue their commitment to the global AMR challenge. Strategic, allocated funding will play a key role in supporting the development and in vivo application of novel polymeric systems to treat resistant microbial infections that, currently, available therapeutics are failing to treat.

Author Contributions: For research articles with several authors, a short paragraph specifying their individual contributions must be provided. The following statements should be used "Conceptualization, N.F.K.; Writing-Original Draft Preparation, N.F.K., L.P.T., R.H.H., S.S.C., W.K.W., A.J.G. & M.d.F.P.; Writing-Review & Editing, N.F.K, L.P.T., W.K.W., A.J.G. & M.d.F.P. Visualization, A.C.

Funding: A.J.G. is supported by BBSRC grant BB/N004590/1.

Conflicts of Interest: The views expressed by M.d.F.P are those of the author; they do not reflect in any way the views of the agency.

References

1. WHO High Levels of Antibiotic Resistance Found Worldwide, New Data Shows. WHO, News Release. Available online: https://www.who.int/mediacentre/news/releases/2018/antibiotic-resistance-found/en/ (accessed on 29 January 2018).
2. O'Neill, J. Antimicrobial Resistance: Tackling a crisis for the health and wealth of nations. *Rev. Antimicrob. Resist.* **2014**, *1*, 1–16.
3. Boucher, H.W.; Talbot, G.H.; Bradley, J.S.; Edwards, J.E.; Gilbert, D.; Rice, L.B.; Scheld, M.; Spellberg, B.; Bartlett, J. Bad bugs, no drugs: No ESKAPE! An update from the Infectious Diseases Society of America. *Clin. Infect. Dis.* **2009**, *48*, 1–12. [CrossRef]
4. Bjarnsholt, T. The role of bacterial biofilms in chronic infections. *APMIS* **2013**, *121*, 1–58. [CrossRef] [PubMed]
5. Natarajan, S.V.; Dhanasekar, U. Trends in antibiotic resistance pattern against ESKAPE pathogens from tertiary care teaching institute – South India. *Infect. Dis. Heal.* **2016**, *21*, 142–143. [CrossRef]
6. Mohamed, J.A.; Huang, D.B. Biofilm formation by enterococci. *J. Med. Microbiol.* **2007**, *56*, 1581–1588. [CrossRef] [PubMed]
7. Gao, W.; Howden, B.P.; Stinear, T.P. Evolution of virulence in Enterococcus faecium, a hospital-adapted opportunistic pathogen. *Curr. Opin. Microbiol.* **2018**, *41*, 76–82. [CrossRef] [PubMed]
8. Al-Talib, H.; Yean, C.; Al-Jashamy, K.; Hasan, H. Methicillin-resistant Staphylococcus aureus nosocomial infection trends in Hospital Universiti Sains Malaysia during 2002–2007. *Ann. Saudi Med.* **2010**, *30*, 358–363. [CrossRef] [PubMed]
9. Harch, S.A.J.; MacMorran, E.; Tong, S.Y.C.; Holt, D.C.; Wilson, J.; Athan, E.; Hewagama, S. High burden of complicated skin and soft tissue infections in the Indigenous population of Central Australia due to dominant Panton Valentine leucocidin clones ST93-MRSA and CC121-MSSA. *BMC Infect. Dis.* **2017**, *17*, 405. [CrossRef] [PubMed]
10. Enright, M.C.; Robinson, D.A.; Randle, G.; Feil, E.J.; Grundmann, H.; Spratt, B.G. The evolutionary history of methicillin-resistant Staphylococcus aureus (MRSA). *Proc. Natl. Acad. Sci. USA* **2002**, *99*, 7687–7692. [CrossRef] [PubMed]
11. Macmorran, E.; Harch, S.; Athan, E.; Lane, S.; Tong, S.; Crawford, L.; Krishnaswamy, S.; Hewagama, S. The rise of methicillin resistant Staphylococcus aureus: Now the dominant cause of skin and soft tissue infection in Central Australia. *Epidemiol. Infect.* **2017**, *145*, 2817–2826. [CrossRef]
12. Malani, P.N. National burden of invasive methicillin-resistant Staphylococcus aureus infection. *Jama* **2014**, *311*, 1438–1439. [CrossRef] [PubMed]
13. Sisirak, M.; Zvizdic, A.; Hukic, M. Methicillin-resistant Staphylococcus aureus (MRSA) as a cause of nosocomial wound infections. *Bosn J. Basic Med. Sci.* **2010**, *10*, 32–37. [CrossRef] [PubMed]
14. Xie, R.; Zhang, X.D.; Zhao, Q.; Peng, B.; Zheng, J. Analysis of global prevalence of antibiotic resistance in Acinetobacter baumannii infections disclosed a faster increase in OECD countries. *Emerg. Microbes Infect.* **2018**, *7*. [CrossRef] [PubMed]
15. Olaitan, A.O.; Morand, S.; Rolain, J.M. Emergence of colistin-resistant bacteria in humans without colistin usage: A new worry and cause for vigilance. *Int. J. Antimicrob. Agents* **2016**, *47*, 1–3. [CrossRef] [PubMed]

16. Rossi, F.; Girardello, R.; Cury, A.P.; Di Gioia, T.S.R.; de Almeida, J.N.; Duarte, A.J.D.S. Emergence of colistin resistance in the largest university hospital complex of São Paulo, Brazil, over five years. *Brazilian J. Infect. Dis.* **2017**, *21*, 98–101. [CrossRef] [PubMed]
17. Sun, L.; Klein, E.Y.; Laxminarayan, R. Seasonality and temporal correlation between community antibiotic use and resistance in the United States. *Clin. Infect. Dis.* **2012**, *55*, 687–694. [CrossRef] [PubMed]
18. Sundqvist, M. Reversibility of antibiotic resistance. *Ups. J. Med. Sci.* **2014**, *119*, 142–148. [CrossRef] [PubMed]
19. Biotech Connection. Trends and Opportunities in Antibiotic Development for Multidrug-Resistant Bacterial Infections. 2018. Available online: https://biotechconnectionbay.org/market-reports/antibioticdevelopment/ (accessed on 1 March 2019).
20. Kamaruzzaman, N.; Pina, M.; Chivu, A.; Good, L. Polyhexamethylene biguanide and nadifloxacin self-assembled nanoparticles: Antimicrobial effects against intracellular methicillin-resistant Staphylococcus aureus. *Polymers* **2018**, *10*, 521. [CrossRef] [PubMed]
21. Weiner, L.M.; Webb, A.K.; Limbago, B.; Dudeck, M.A.; Patel, J.; Kallen, A.J.; Edwards, J.R.; Sievert, D.M. Antimicrobial-Resistant Pathogens Associated With Healthcare-Associated Infections: Summary of Data Reported to the National Healthcare Safety Network at the Centers for Disease Control and Prevention, 2011-2014. *Infect. Control. Hosp. Epidemiol.* **2016**, *37*, 1288–1301. [CrossRef]
22. Kamaruzzaman, N.F.; Firdessa, R.; Good, L. Bactericidal effects of polyhexamethylene biguanide against intraclualar Staphylococcus aureus EMRSA-15 and USA 300. *J. Antimicrob. Chemother.* **2016**, *71*, 1252–1259. [CrossRef]
23. Ruparelia, J.P.; Chatterjee, A.K.; Duttagupta, S.P.; Mukherji, S. Strain specificity in antimicrobial activity of silver and copper nanoparticles. *Acta Biomater.* **2008**, *4*, 707–716. [CrossRef] [PubMed]
24. Golan, Y. Empiric therapy for hospital-acquired, Gram-negative complicated intra-abdominal infection and complicated urinary tract infections: A systematic literature review of current and emerging treatment options. *BMC Infect. Dis.* **2015**, *15*, 313. [CrossRef] [PubMed]
25. Cornejo-Juárez, P.; Vilar-Compte, D.; Pérez-Jiménez, C.; Ñamendys-Silva, S.A.; Sandoval-Hernández, S.; Volkow-Fernández, P. The impact of hospital-acquired infections with multidrug-resistant bacteria in an oncology intensive care unit. *Int. J. Infect. Dis.* **2015**, *31*, e31–e34. [CrossRef] [PubMed]
26. Jamal, M.; Ahmad, W.; Andleeb, S.; Jalil, F.; Imran, M.; Nawaz, M.A.; Hussain, T.; Ali, M.; Rafiq, M.; Kamil, M.A. Bacterial biofilm and associated infections. *J. Chin. Med. Assoc.* **2018**, *81*, 7–11. [CrossRef] [PubMed]
27. Chaftari, A.M.; El Zakhem, A.; Jamal, M.A.; Jiang, Y.; Hachem, R.; Raad, I. The use of minocycline-rifampin coated central venous catheters for exchange of catheters in the setting of staphylococcus aureus central line associated bloodstream infections. *BMC Infect. Dis.* **2014**, *14*, 518. [CrossRef] [PubMed]
28. McGuffie, B.A.; Vallet-Gely, I.; Dove, S.L. sigma Factor and Anti-sigma Factor That Control Swarming Motility and Biofilm Formation in *Pseudomonas aeruginosa*. *J. Bacteriol.* **2015**, *198*, 755–765. [CrossRef] [PubMed]
29. Solomkin, J.S.; Mazuski, J.E.; Bradley, J.S.; Rodvold, K.A.; Goldstein, E.J.; Baron, E.J.; O'Neill, P.J.; Chow, A.W.; Dellinger, E.P.; Eachempati, S.R.; et al. Diagnosis and management of complicated intra-abdominal infection in adults and children: Guidelines by the Surgical Infection Society and the Infectious Diseases Society of America. *Surg. Infect.* **2010**, *11*, 79–109. [CrossRef] [PubMed]
30. Codjoe, F.; Donkor, E. Carbapenem Resistance: A Review. *Med. Sci.* **2017**, *6*, 1. [CrossRef] [PubMed]
31. Johansen, H.K.; Moskowitz, S.M.; Ciofu, O.; Pressler, T.; Høiby, N. Spread of colistin resistant non-mucoid *Pseudomonas aeruginosa* among chronically infected Danish cystic fibrosis patients. *J. Cyst. Fibros.* **2008**, *7*, 391–397. [CrossRef]
32. Fiaccadori, E.; Antonucci, E.; Morabito, S.; d'Avolio, A.; Maggiore, U.; Regolisti, G. Colistin Use in Patients With Reduced Kidney Function. *Am. J. Kidney Dis.* **2016**, *68*, 296–306. [CrossRef]
33. Singla, S.; Harjai, K.; Chhibber, S. Artificial Klebsiella pneumoniae biofilm model mimicking in vivo system: Altered morphological characteristics and antibiotic resistance. *J. Antibiot.* **2014**, *67*, 305–309. [CrossRef] [PubMed]
34. ECDC. *Surveillance of Antimicrobial Resistance in Europe 2016*; European Centre for Disease Prevention and Control: Stockholm, Sweden, 2017; ISBN 9789294980991.

35. Otter, J.A.; Doumith, M.; Davies, F.; Mookerjee, S.; Dyakova, E.; Gilchrist, M.; Brannigan, E.T.; Bamford, K.; Galletly, T.; Donaldson, H.; et al. Emergence and clonal spread of colistin resistance due to multiple mutational mechanisms in carbapenemase-producing *Klebsiella pneumoniae* in London. *Sci. Rep.* **2017**, *7*, 1–8. [CrossRef] [PubMed]
36. Maragakis, L.L.; Perl, T.M. Acinetobacter baumannii: Epidemiology, antimicrobial resistance, and treatment options. *Clin. Infect. Dis.* **2008**, *46*, 1254–1263. [CrossRef] [PubMed]
37. Bonomo, R.A.; Szabo, D. Mechanisms of Multidrug Resistance in *Acinetobacter* Species and *Pseudomonas aeruginosa*. *Clin. Infect. Dis.* **2006**, *44106*, 49–56. [CrossRef] [PubMed]
38. Nation, R.L.; Li, J.; Cars, O.; Couet, W.; Dudley, M.N.; Kaye, K.S.; Mouton, J.W.; Paterson, D.L.; Tam, V.H.; Theuretzbacher, U.; et al. Framework for optimisation of the clinical use of colistin and polymyxin B: The Prato polymyxin consensus. *Lancet Infect. Dis.* **2015**, *15*, 225–234. [CrossRef]
39. Potron, A.; Poirel, L.; Nordmann, P. Emerging broad-spectrum resistance in *Pseudomonas aeruginosa* and *Acinetobacter baumannii*: Mechanisms and epidemiology. *Int. J. Antimicrob Agents* **2015**, *45*, 568–585. [CrossRef]
40. Qureshi, Z.A.; Hittle, L.E.; O'Hara, J.A.; Rivera, J.I.; Syed, A.; Shields, R.K.; Pasculle, A.W.; Ernst, R.K.; Doi, Y. Colistin-resistant Acinetobacter baumannii: Beyond carbapenem resistance. *Clin. Infect. Dis.* **2015**, *60*, 1295–1303. [CrossRef]
41. Wilks, M.; Wilson, A.; Warwick, S.; Price, E.; Kennedy, D.; Ely, A.; Millar, M.R. Control of an outbreak of multidrug-resistant *Acinetobacter baumannii*-calcoaceticus colonization and infection in an intensive care unit (ICU) without closing the ICU or placing patients in isolation. *Infect. Control. Hosp. Epidemiol.* **2006**, *27*, 654–658. [CrossRef]
42. Antunes, L.C.; Visca, P.; Towner, K.J. *Acinetobacter baumannii*: Evolution of a global pathogen. *Pathog. Dis.* **2014**, *71*, 292–301. [CrossRef]
43. Davin-Regli, A.; Pagès, J.-M. Enterobacter aerogenes and Enterobacter cloacae; versatile bacterial pathogens confronting antibiotic treatment. *Front. Microbiol.* **2015**, *6*, 392. [CrossRef]
44. Wang, X.; Wang, Y.; Zhou, Y.; Li, J.; Yin, W.; Wang, S.; Zhang, S.; Shen, J.; Shen, Z.; Wang, Y. Emergence of a novel mobile colistin resistance gene, mcr-8, in NDM-producing *Klebsiella pneumoniae*. *Emerg. Microbes Infect.* **2018**, *7*, 122. [CrossRef] [PubMed]
45. Robinson, K.M.; Janes, M.S.; Pehar, M.; Monette, J.S.; Ross, M.F.; Hagen, T.M.; Murphy, M.P.; Beckman, J.S. Selective fluorescent imaging of superoxide in vivo using ethidium-based probes. *Proc. Natl. Acad. Sci. USA* **2006**, *103*, 15038–15043. [CrossRef]
46. Jackson, N.; Czaplewski, L.; Piddock, L.J.V. Discovery and development of new antibacterial drugs: Learning from experience? *J. Antimicrob. Chemother.* **2018**, *73*, 1452–1459. [CrossRef] [PubMed]
47. Delplace, V.; Nicolas, J. Degradable vinyl polymers for biomedical applications. *Nat. Chem.* **2015**, *7*, 771–784. [CrossRef]
48. Frade, S. German Government Funds GARDP's Efforts to Discover, Develop, and Deliver Affordable Antibiotics: Funding Supports Delivery of R&D Strategy That Focuses on Treating Gram-Negative Infections. Available online: https://www.gardp.org/2018/news-resources/press-releases/german-government-funds-gardp-discover-develop-deliver-affordable-antibiotics/ (accessed on 15 March 2019).
49. Jain, A.; Duvvuri, L.S.; Farah, S.; Beyth, N.; Domb, A.J.; Khan, W. Antimicrobial Polymers. *Adv. Healthc. Mater.* **2014**, *3*, 1969–1985. [CrossRef]
50. Mowery, B.P.; Lee, S.E.; Kissounko, D.A.; Epand, R.F.; Epand, R.M.; Weisblum, B.; Stahl, S.S.; Gellman, S.H. Mimicry of Antimicrobial Host-Defense Peptides by Random Copolymers. *J. Am. Chem. Soc.* **2007**, *129*, 15474–15476. [CrossRef] [PubMed]
51. Bechinger, B.; Gorr, S.U. Antimicrobial Peptides: Mechanisms of Action and Resistance. *J. Dent. Res.* **2017**, *96*, 254–260. [CrossRef]
52. Park, A.J.; Okhovat, J.P.; Kim, J. Antimicrobial peptides. *Clin. Basic Immunodermatol. Second Ed.* **2017**, *1548*, 81–95. [CrossRef]
53. Takahashi, H.; Palermo, E.F.; Yasuhara, K.; Caputo, G.A.; Kuroda, K. Molecular Design, Structures, and Activity of Antimicrobial Peptide-Mimetic Polymers. *Macromol. Biosci.* **2013**, *13*, 1285–1299. [CrossRef]
54. Foster, L.L.; Mizutani, M.; Oda, Y.; Palermo, E.F.; Kuroda, K. Polymers for Biomedicine. John Wiley & Sons: Hoboken, NJ, USA, 2017.
55. Locock, K.E.S.; Michl, T.D.; Griesser, H.J.; Haeussler, M.; Meagher, L. Structure–activity relationships of guanylated antimicrobial polymethacrylates. *Pure Appl. Chem.* **2014**, *86*, 1281–1291. [CrossRef]

56. Palermo, E.F.; Lienkamp, K.; Gillies, E.R.; Ragogna, P.J. Antibacterial Activity of Polymers: Discussions on the Nature of Amphiphilic Balance. *Angew. Chem. Int. Ed.* **2019**, *58*, 3690–3693. [CrossRef] [PubMed]
57. Mankoci, S.; Kaiser, R.L.; Sahai, N.; Barton, H.A.; Joy, A. Bactericidal Peptidomimetic Polyurethanes with Remarkable Selectivity against *Escherichia coli*. *ACS Biomater. Sci. Eng.* **2017**, *3*, 2588–2597. [CrossRef]
58. Mizutani, M.; Palermo, E.F.; Thoma, L.M.; Satoh, K.; Kamigaito, M.; Kuroda, K. Design and synthesis of self-degradable antibacterial polymers by simultaneous chain- and step-growth radical copolymerization. *Biomacromolecules* **2012**, *13*, 1554–1563. [CrossRef]
59. Holden, M.T.G.; Hauser, H.; Sanders, M.; Ngo, T.H.; Cherevach, I.; Cronin, A.; Goodhead, I.; Mungall, K.; Quail, M.; Price, C.; et al. Rapid evolution of virulence and drug resistance in the emerging zoonotic pathogen *Streptococcus suis*. *PLoS ONE* **2009**, *4*, 6072. [CrossRef] [PubMed]
60. Palermo, E.F.; Vemparala, S.; Kuroda, K. Cationic spacer arm design strategy for control of antimicrobial activity and conformation of amphiphilic methacrylate random copolymers. *Biomacromolecules* **2012**, *13*, 1632–1641. [CrossRef] [PubMed]
61. Chen, A.; Fei, J.; Deirmegian, C. Diagnosis of periprosthetic infection: Novel developments. *J. Knee Surg.* **2014**, *27*, 259–265. [CrossRef] [PubMed]
62. Kuroda, K.; Caputo, G.A. Antimicrobial polymers as synthetic mimics of host-defense peptides. *Wiley Interdiscip. Rev. Nanomed. Nanobiotechnol.* **2012**, *5*, 49–66. [CrossRef] [PubMed]
63. Exley, S.E.; Paslay, L.C.; Sahukhal, G.S.; Abel, B.A.; Brown, T.D.; McCormick, C.L.; Heinhorst, S.; Koul, V.; Choudhary, V.; Elasri, M.O.; et al. Antimicrobial Peptide Mimicking Primary Amine and Guanidine Containing Methacrylamide Copolymers Prepared by Raft Polymerization. *Biomacromolecules* **2015**, *16*, 3845–3852. [CrossRef]
64. Oda, Y.; Kanaoka, S.; Sato, T.; Aoshima, S.; Kuroda, K. Block versus random amphiphilic copolymers as antibacterial agents. *Biomacromolecules* **2011**, *12*, 3581–3591. [CrossRef]
65. Burian, M.; Schittek, B. The secrets of dermcidin action. *Int. J. Med. Microbiol.* **2015**, *305*, 283–286. [CrossRef]
66. McDermott, A.M. Antimicrobial compounds in tears. *Exp. Eye Res.* **2013**, *117*, 53–61. [CrossRef] [PubMed]
67. Muñoz-Bonilla, A.; Fernández-García, M. Polymeric materials with antimicrobial activity. *Prog. Polym. Sci.* **2012**, *37*, 281–339. [CrossRef]
68. Friedrich, C.L.; Moyles, D.; Beveridge, T.J.; Hancock, R.E.W. Antibacterial Action of Structurally Diverse Cationic Peptides on Gram-Positive Bacteria. *Antimicrob. Agents Chemother.* **2000**, *44*, 2086. [CrossRef] [PubMed]
69. Le, C.-F.; Fang, C.-M.; Sekaran, S.D. Intracellular Targeting Mechanisms by Antimicrobial Peptides. *Antimicrob. Agents Chemother.* **2017**, *61*, e02340-16. [CrossRef] [PubMed]
70. Dartois, V.; Sanchez-Quesada, J.; Cabezas, E.; Chi, E.; Dubbelde, C.; Dunn, C.; Granja, J.; Gritzen, C.; Weinberger, D.; Ghadiri, M.R. Systemic antibacterial activity of novel synthetic cyclic peptides. *Antimicrob. Agents Chemother.* **2005**, *49*, 3302–3310. [CrossRef] [PubMed]
71. Aoki, W.; Ueda, M. Characterization of Antimicrobial Peptides toward the Development of Novel Antibiotics. *Pharmaceuticals* **2013**, *6*, 1055–1081. [CrossRef]
72. Peters, B.M.; Shirtliff, M.E.; Jabra-Rizk, M.A. Antimicrobial peptides: Primeval molecules or future drugs? *PLoS Pathog.* **2010**, *6*, 4–7. [CrossRef] [PubMed]
73. Butler, M.S.; Blaskovich, M.A.T.; Cooper, M.A. Antibiotics in the clinical pipeline at the end of 2015. *J. Antibiot.* **2016**, *70*, 3. [CrossRef]
74. Caillier, L.; Taffin de Givenchy, E.; Levy, R.; Vandenberghe, Y.; Geribaldi, S.; Guittard, F. Polymerizable semi-fluorinated gemini surfactants designed for antimicrobial materials. *J. Colloid Interface Sci.* **2009**, *332*, 201–207. [CrossRef]
75. Lin, J.; Chen, X.; Chen, C.; Hu, J.; Zhou, C.; Cai, X.; Wang, W.; Zheng, C.; Zhang, P.; Cheng, J.; et al. Durably Antibacterial and Bacterially Antiadhesive Cotton Fabrics Coated by Cationic Fluorinated Polymers. *ACS Appl. Mater. Interfaces* **2018**, *10*, 6124–6136. [CrossRef]
76. Mesallati, H.; Umerska, A.; Paluch, K.J.; Tajber, L. Amorphous Polymeric Drug Salts as Ionic Solid Dispersion Forms of Ciprofloxacin. *Mol. Pharm.* **2017**, *14*, 2209–2223. [CrossRef] [PubMed]
77. Parwe, S.P.; Chaudhari, P.N.; Mohite, K.K.; Selukar, B.S.; Nande, S.S.; Garnaik, B. Synthesis of ciprofloxacin-conjugated poly (L-lactic acid) polymer for nanofiber fabrication and antibacterial evaluation. *Int. J. Nanomed.* **2014**, *9*, 1463–1477. [CrossRef]

78. Kocer, H.B.; Worley, S.D.; Broughton, R.M.; Huang, T.S. A novel N-halamine acrylamide monomer and its copolymers for antimicrobial coatings. *React. Funct. Polym.* **2011**, *71*, 561–568. [CrossRef]
79. Demir, B.; Broughton, R.M.; Qiao, M.; Huang, T.S.; Worley, S.D. N-halamine biocidal materials with superior antimicrobial efficacies for wound dressings. *Molecules* **2017**, *22*, 1582. [CrossRef] [PubMed]
80. Cuthbert, T.J.; Hisey, B.; Harrison, T.D.; Trant, J.F.; Gillies, E.R.; Ragogna, P.J. Surprising Antibacterial Activity and Selectivity of Hydrophilic Polyphosphoniums Featuring Sugar and Hydroxy Substituents. *Angew. Chem. Int. Ed.* **2018**, *57*, 12707–12710. [CrossRef] [PubMed]
81. Park, E.S.; Moon, W.S.; Song, M.J.; Kim, M.N.; Chung, K.H.; Yoon, J.S. Antimicrobial activity of phenol and benzoic acid derivatives. *Int. Biodeterior. Biodegrad.* **2001**, *47*, 209–214. [CrossRef]
82. Alamri, A.; El-Newehy, M.H.; Al-Deyab, S.S. Biocidal polymers: Synthesis and antimicrobial properties of benzaldehyde derivatives immobilized onto amine-terminated polyacrylonitrile. *Chem. Cent. J.* **2012**, *6*, 1. [CrossRef] [PubMed]
83. Awad, M.A.; Mekhamer, W.K.; Merghani, N.M.; Hendi, A.A.; Ortashi, K.M.O.; Al-Abbas, F.; Eisa, N.E. Green Synthesis, Characterization, and Antibacterial Activity of Silver/Polystyrene Nanocomposite. *J. Nanomater.* **2015**, *2015*. [CrossRef]
84. Rai, M.; Yadav, A.; Gade, A. Silver nanoparticles as a new generation of antimicrobials. *Biotechnol. Adv.* **2009**, *27*, 76–83. [CrossRef]
85. Zhang, S.; Tang, Y.; Vlahovic, B. A Review on Preparation and Applications of Silver-Containing Nanofibers. *Nanoscale Res. Lett.* **2016**, *11*, 80. [CrossRef]
86. de Faria, A.F.; Perreault, F.; Shaulsky, E.; Arias Chavez, L.H.; Elimelech, M. Antimicrobial Electrospun Biopolymer Nanofiber Mats Functionalized with Graphene Oxide–Silver Nanocomposites. *ACS Appl. Mater. Interfaces* **2015**, *7*, 12751–12759. [CrossRef]
87. Wu, J.-Y.; Li, C.-W.; Tsai, C.-H.; Chou, C.-W.; Chen, D.-R.; Wang, G.-J. Synthesis of antibacterial TiO_2/PLGA composite biofilms. *Nanomed. Nanotechnol. Biol. Med.* **2014**, *10*, e1097–e1107. [CrossRef]
88. Liu, J.; Sonshine, D.A.; Shervani, S.; Hurt, R.H. Controlled release of biologically active silver from nanosilver surfaces. *ACS Nano* **2010**, *4*, 6903–6913. [CrossRef]
89. Hussain, M.A.; Shah, A.; Jantan, I.; Shah, M.R.; Tahir, M.N.; Ahmad, R.; Bukhari, S.N.A. Hydroxypropylcellulose as a novel green reservoir for the synthesis, stabilization, and storage of silver nanoparticles. *Int. J. Nanomed.* **2015**, *10*, 2079–2088. [CrossRef]
90. Sharma, V.K.; Yngard, R.A.; Lin, Y. Silver nanoparticles: Green synthesis and their antimicrobial activities. *Adv. Colloid Interface Sci.* **2009**, *145*, 83–96. [CrossRef]
91. Divya, K.P.; Miroshnikov, M.; Dutta, D.; Vemula, P.K.; Ajayan, P.M.; John, G. In Situ Synthesis of Metal Nanoparticle Embedded Hybrid Soft Nanomaterials. *Acc. Chem. Res.* **2016**, *49*, 1671–1680. [CrossRef]
92. Francesko, A.; Cano Fossas, M.; Petkova, P.; Fernandes, M.M.; Mendoza, E.; Tzanov, T. Sonochemical synthesis and stabilization of concentrated antimicrobial silver-chitosan nanoparticle dispersions. *J. Appl. Polym. Sci.* **2017**, *134*, 45136. [CrossRef]
93. Ayala Valencia, G.; Cristina de Oliveira Vercik, L.; Ferrari, R.; Vercik, A. Synthesis and characterization of silver nanoparticles using water-soluble starch and its antibacterial activity on *Staphylococcus aureus*. *Starch Stärke* **2013**, *65*, 931–937. [CrossRef]
94. An, J.; Luo, Q.; Li, M.; Wang, D.; Li, X.; Yin, R. A facile synthesis of high antibacterial polymer nanocomposite containing uniformly dispersed silver nanoparticles. *Colloid Polym. Sci.* **2015**, *293*, 1997–2008. [CrossRef]
95. Sánchez-Valdes, S.; Ortega-Ortiz, H.; Ramos-de Valle, L.F.; Medellín-Rodríguez, F.J.; Guedea-Miranda, R. Mechanical and antimicrobial properties of multilayer films with a polyethylene/silver nanocomposite layer. *J. Appl. Polym. Sci.* **2009**, *111*, 953–962. [CrossRef]
96. Fortunati, E.; Mattioli, S.; Visai, L.; Imbriani, M.; Fierro, J.L.G.; Kenny, J.M.; Armentano, I. Combined Effects of Ag Nanoparticles and Oxygen Plasma Treatment on PLGA Morphological, Chemical, and Antibacterial Properties. *Biomacromolecules* **2013**, *14*, 626–636. [CrossRef]
97. Xie, C.-M.; Lu, X.; Wang, K.-F.; Meng, F.-Z.; Jiang, O.; Zhang, H.-P.; Zhi, W.; Fang, L.-M. Silver Nanoparticles and Growth Factors Incorporated Hydroxyapatite Coatings on Metallic Implant Surfaces for Enhancement of Osteoinductivity and Antibacterial Properties. *ACS Appl. Mater. Interfaces* **2014**, *6*, 8580–8589. [CrossRef]
98. Song, J.; Kang, H.; Lee, C.; Hwang, S.H.; Jang, J. Aqueous Synthesis of Silver Nanoparticle Embedded Cationic Polymer Nanofibers and Their Antibacterial Activity. *ACS Appl. Mater. Interfaces* **2012**, *4*, 460–465. [CrossRef]

99. Wu, C.-N.; Fuh, S.-C.; Lin, S.-P.; Lin, Y.-Y.; Chen, H.-Y.; Liu, J.-M.; Cheng, K.-C. TEMPO-Oxidized Bacterial Cellulose Pellicle with Silver Nanoparticles for Wound Dressing. *Biomacromolecules* **2018**, *19*, 544–554. [CrossRef]
100. Boonkaew, B.; Suwanpreuksa, P.; Cuttle, L.; Barber, P.M.; Supaphol, P. Hydrogels containing silver nanoparticles for burn wounds show antimicrobial activity without cytotoxicity. *J. Appl. Polym. Sci.* **2014**, *131*. [CrossRef]
101. de Lima, G.G.; de Lima, D.W.F.; de Oliveira, M.J.A.; Lugão, A.B.; Alcântara, M.T.S.; Devine, D.M.; de Sá, M.J.C. Synthesis and in Vivo Behavior of PVP/CMC/Agar Hydrogel Membranes Impregnated with Silver Nanoparticles for Wound Healing Applications. *ACS Appl. Bio Mater.* **2018**. [CrossRef]
102. Baek, K.; Liang, J.; Lim, W.T.; Zhao, H.; Kim, D.H.; Kong, H. In Situ Assembly of Antifouling/Bacterial Silver Nanoparticle-Hydrogel Composites with Controlled Particle Release and Matrix Softening. *ACS Appl. Mater. Interfaces* **2015**, *7*, 15359–15367. [CrossRef]
103. Ghosh, P.; Han, G.; De, M.; Kim, C.K.; Rotello, V.M. Gold nanoparticles in delivery applications. *Adv. Drug Deliv. Rev.* **2008**, *60*, 1307–1315. [CrossRef]
104. Zhou, Y.; Kong, Y.; Kundu, S.; Cirillo, J.D.; Liang, H. Antibacterial activities of gold and silver nanoparticles against Escherichia coli and bacillus Calmette-Guérin. *J. Nanobiotechnol.* **2012**, *10*, 19. [CrossRef]
105. Jokerst, J.V.; Lobovkina, T.; Zare, R.N.; Gambhir, S.S. Nanoparticle PEGylation for imaging and therapy. *Nanomedicine* **2011**, *6*, 715–728. [CrossRef]
106. Niidome, T.; Yamagata, M.; Okamoto, Y.; Akiyama, Y.; Takahashi, H.; Kawano, T.; Katayama, Y.; Niidome, Y. PEG-modified gold nanorods with a stealth character for in vivo applications. *J. Control. Release* **2006**, *114*, 343–347. [CrossRef]
107. Regiel-Futyra, A.; Kus-Liśkiewicz, M.; Sebastian, V.; Irusta, S.; Arruebo, M.; Stochel, G.; Kyzioł, A. Development of Noncytotoxic Chitosan–Gold Nanocomposites as Efficient Antibacterial Materials. *ACS Appl. Mater. Interfaces* **2015**, *7*, 1087–1099. [CrossRef]
108. Mendoza, G.; Regiel-Futyra, A.; Andreu, V.; Sebastián, V.; Kyzioł, A.; Stochel, G.; Arruebo, M. Bactericidal Effect of Gold–Chitosan Nanocomposites in Coculture Models of Pathogenic Bacteria and Human Macrophages. *ACS Appl. Mater. Interfaces* **2017**, *9*, 17693–17701. [CrossRef]
109. Politi, J.; Spadavecchia, J.; Fiorentino, G.; Antonucci, I.; De Stefano, L. Arsenate reductase from *Thermus thermophilus* conjugated to polyethylene glycol-stabilized gold nanospheres allow trace sensing and speciation of arsenic ions. *J. R. Soc. Interface* **2016**, *13*. [CrossRef]
110. Politi, J.; Spadavecchia, J.; Iodice, M.; de Stefano, L. Oligopeptide–heavy metal interaction monitoring by hybrid gold nanoparticle based assay. *Analyst* **2015**, *140*, 149–155. [CrossRef]
111. Palmieri, G.; Tatè, R.; Gogliettino, M.; Balestrieri, M.; Rea, I.; Terracciano, M.; Proroga, Y.T.; Capuano, F.; Anastasio, A.; De Stefano, L. Small Synthetic Peptides Bioconjugated to Hybrid Gold Nanoparticles Destroy Potentially Deadly Bacteria at Submicromolar Concentrations. *Bioconjug. Chem.* **2018**, *29*, 3877–3885. [CrossRef]
112. Yang, X.; Yang, J.; Wang, L.; Ran, B.; Jia, Y.; Zhang, L.; Yang, G.; Shao, H.; Jiang, X. Pharmaceutical Intermediate-Modified Gold Nanoparticles: Against Multidrug-Resistant Bacteria and Wound-Healing Application via an Electrospun Scaffold. *ACS Nano* **2017**, *11*, 5737–5745. [CrossRef]
113. Manzl, C.; Enrich, J.; Ebner, H.; Dallinger, R.; Krumschnabel, G. Copper-induced formation of reactive oxygen species causes cell death and disruption of calcium homeostasis in trout hepatocytes. *Toxicology* **2004**, *196*, 57–64. [CrossRef]
114. Sehmi, S.K.; Noimark, S.; Weiner, J.; Allan, E.; MacRobert, A.J.; Parkin, I.P. Potent Antibacterial Activity of Copper Embedded into Silicone and Polyurethane. *ACS Appl. Mater. Interfaces* **2015**, *7*, 22807–22813. [CrossRef]
115. Lu, Y.; Li, L.; Zhu, Y.; Wang, X.; Li, M.; Lin, Z.; Hu, X.; Zhang, Y.; Yin, Q.; Xia, H.; et al. Multifunctional Copper-Containing Carboxymethyl Chitosan/Alginate Scaffolds for Eradicating Clinical Bacterial Infection and Promoting Bone Formation. *ACS Appl. Mater. Interfaces* **2018**, *10*, 127–138. [CrossRef]
116. Liu, X.; Chu, P.K.; Ding, C. Surface modification of titanium, titanium alloys, and related materials for biomedical applications. *Mater. Sci. Eng. R Rep.* **2004**, *47*, 49–121. [CrossRef]
117. Liou, J.-W.; Chang, H.-H. Bactericidal Effects and Mechanisms of Visible Light-Responsive Titanium Dioxide Photocatalysts on Pathogenic Bacteria. *Arch. Immunol. Ther. Exp.* **2012**, *60*, 267–275. [CrossRef]

118. Toniatto, T.V.; Rodrigues, B.V.M.; Marsi, T.C.O.; Ricci, R.; Marciano, F.R.; Webster, T.J.; Lobo, A.O. Nanostructured poly (lactic acid) electrospun fiber with high loadings of TiO_2 nanoparticles: Insights into bactericidal activity and cell viability. *Mater. Sci. Eng. C* **2017**, *71*, 381–385. [CrossRef]
119. Fan, X.; Chen, K.; He, X.; Li, N.; Huang, J.; Tang, K.; Li, Y.; Wang, F. Nano-TiO_2/collagen-chitosan porous scaffold for wound repairing. *Int. J. Biol. Macromol.* **2016**, *91*, 15–22. [CrossRef]
120. Archana, D.; Singh, B.K.; Dutta, J.; Dutta, P.K. In vivo evaluation of chitosan–PVP–titanium dioxide nanocomposite as wound dressing material. *Carbohydr. Polym.* **2013**, *95*, 530–539. [CrossRef]
121. Díez-Pascual, A.M.; Díez-Vicente, A.L. Nano-TiO_2 Reinforced PEEK/PEI Blends as Biomaterials for Load-Bearing Implant Applications. *ACS Appl. Mater. Interfaces* **2015**, *7*, 5561–5573. [CrossRef]
122. Laurenti, M.; Cauda, V. ZnO Nanostructures for Tissue Engineering Applications. *Nanomaterials* **2017**, *7*, 374. [CrossRef]
123. Grenho, L.; Salgado, C.L.; Fernandes, M.H.; Monteiro, F.J.; Ferraz, M.P. Antibacterial activity and biocompatibility of three-dimensional nanostructured porous granules of hydroxyapatite and zinc oxide nanoparticles—An in vitro and in vivo study. *Nanotechnology* **2015**, *26*, 315101. [CrossRef]
124. Wahid, F.; Yin, J.-J.; Xue, D.-D.; Xue, H.; Lu, Y.-S.; Zhong, C.; Chu, L.-Q. Synthesis and characterization of antibacterial carboxymethyl Chitosan/ZnO nanocomposite hydrogels. *Int. J. Biol. Macromol.* **2016**, *88*, 273–279. [CrossRef]
125. García-Gallego, S.; Franci, G.; Falanga, A.; Gómez, R.; Folliero, V.; Galdiero, S.; De La Mata, F.J.; Galdiero, M. Function oriented molecular design: Dendrimers as novel antimicrobials. *Molecules* **2017**, *22*, 1581. [CrossRef]
126. Gupta, U.; Perumal, O. *Dendrimers and Its Biomedical Applications*, 1st ed.; Elsevier Inc.: Amsterdam, The Netherlands; ISBN 9780123969835.
127. Winnicka, K.; Wroblewska, M.; Wieczorek, P.; Sacha, P.T.; Tryniszewska, E.A. The effect of PAMAM dendrimers on the antibacterial activity of antibiotics with different water solubility. *Molecules* **2013**, *18*, 8607–8617. [CrossRef]
128. Mofrad, A.S.; Mohammadi, M.J.; Mansoorian, H.J.; Khaniabadid, Y.O.; Jebeli, M.A.; Khanjani, N.; Khoshgoftar, M.; Yari, A.R. The antibacterial effect of g3-poly-amidoamine dendrimer on gram negative and gram positive bacteria in aqueous solutions. *Desalin. Water Treat.* **2018**, *124*, 223–231. [CrossRef]
129. Siriwardena, T.N.; Stach, M.; Tinguely, R.; Kasraian, S.; Luzzaro, F.; Leib, S.L.; Darbre, T.; Reymond, J.; Endimiani, A. In Vitro Activity of the Novel Antimicrobial Peptide Dendrimer G3KL against Multidrug-Resistant *Acinetobacter baumannii* and *Pseudomonas aeruginosa*. *Antimicrob. Agents Chemother.* **2015**, *59*, 7915–7918. [CrossRef]
130. Wong, P.T.; Tang, S.; Mukherjee, J.; Tang, K.; Gam, K.; Isham, D.; Murat, C.; Sun, R.; Baker, J.R.; Choi, S.K. Light-Controlled Active Release of Photocaged Ciprofloxacin for Lipopolysaccharide-Targeted Drug Delivery using Dendrimer Conjugates Pamela. *Chem. Commun.* **2016**, *52*, 10357–10360. [CrossRef]
131. Serri, A.; Mahboubi, A.; Zarghi, A.; Moghimi, H.R. PAMAM-dendrimer Enhanced Antibacterial Effect Hydrochloride Against Gram-Negative Bacteria of Vancomycin. *J. Pharm. Sci.* **2019**, *22*, 10–21. [CrossRef]
132. Choi, S.K.; Myc, A.; Silpe, J.E.; Sumit, M.; Wong, P.T.; McCarthy, K.; Desai, A.M.; Thomas, T.P.; Kotlyar, A.; Holl, M.M.B.; et al. Dendrimer-based multivalent vancomycin nanoplatform for targeting the drug-resistant bacterial surface. *ACS Nano* **2013**, *7*, 214–228. [CrossRef]
133. Bosnjakovic, A.; Mishra, M.K.; Ren, W.; Kurtoglu, Y.E.; Shi, T.; Fan, D.; Kannan, R.M. Poly(amidoamine) dendrimer-erythromycin conjugates for drug delivery to macrophages involved in periprosthetic inflammation. *Nanomed. Nanotechnol. Biol. Med.* **2011**, *7*, 284–294. [CrossRef]
134. Wrońska, N.; Felczak, A.; Zawadzka, K.; Poszepczy Nska, M.; Rózalska, S.; Bryszewska, M.; Appelhans, D.; Lisowska, K. Poly(propylene imine) dendrimers and amoxicillin as dual-action antibacterial agents. *Molecules* **2015**, *20*, 19330–19342. [CrossRef]
135. Aghayari, M.; Salouti, M.; Kazemizadeh, A.R.; Zabihian, A.; Hamidi, M.; Shajari, N.; Moghtader, F. Enhanced antibacterial activity of ceftazidime against pseudomonas aeruginosa using poly (propyleneimine) dendrimer as a nanocarrier. *Sci. Iran. F* **2015**, *22*, 1330–1336.
136. Sikwal, D.R.; Kalhapure, R.S.; Jadhav, M.; Rambharose, S.; Mocktar, C.; Govender, T. Non-ionic self-assembling amphiphilic polyester dendrimers as new drug delivery excipients. *RSC Adv.* **2017**, *7*, 14233–14246. [CrossRef]
137. Michaud, G.; Visini, R.; Bergmann, M.; Salerno, G.; Bosco, R.; Gillon, E.; Richichi, B.; Nativi, C.; Imberty, A.; Stocker, A.; et al. Overcoming antibiotic resistance in *Pseudomonas aeruginosa* biofilms using glycopeptide dendrimers. *Chem. Sci.* **2016**, *7*, 166–182. [CrossRef]

138. Saczewski, F.; Balewski, Ł. Biological activities of guanidine compounds. *Expert Opin. Therap. Patents* **2009**, *19*, 1417–1448. [CrossRef]
139. Mignani, S.; Rodrigues, J.; Tomas, H.; Roy, R.; Shi, X.; Majoral, J. Bench-to-bedside translation of dendrimers: Reality or utopia? A concise analysis. *Adv. Drug Deliv. Rev.* **2017**, *136–137*, 73–81. [CrossRef]
140. Berlinck, R.G.S.; Burtoloso, A.C.B.; Kossuga, M.H. The chemistry and biology of organic guanidine derivatives. *Nat. Prod. Rep.* **2005**, *22*, 919–954. [CrossRef]
141. Zhang, Y.; Jiang, J.; Chen, Y. Synthesis and antimicrobial activity of polymeric guanidine and biguanidine salts. *Polymer* **1999**, *40*, 6189–6198. [CrossRef]
142. Moore, K.; Gray, D. Using PHMB antimicrobial to prevent wound infection. *Wounds* **2007**, *3*, 96.
143. Kusnetsov, J.M.; Tulkki, I.; Ahonen, H.E.; Martikainen, P.J. Efficacy of three prevention strategies against legionella in cooling water systems. *J. Appl. Microbiol.* **1997**, *82*, 763–768. [CrossRef]
144. Hiti, K. Viability of Acanthamoeba after exposure to a multipurpose disinfecting contact lens solution and two hydrogen peroxide systems. *Br. J. Ophthalmol.* **2002**, *86*, 144–146. [CrossRef]
145. Gilbert, P.; Moore, L.E. Cationic antiseptics: Diversity of action under a common epithet. *J. Appl. Microbiol.* **2005**, *99*, 703–715. [CrossRef]
146. Messick, C.R.; Pendland, S.L.; Moshirfar, M.; Fiscellac, R.G.; Losnedah, K.J.; Schriever, C.A.; Schreckenb, P.C. In-vitro activity of polyhexamethylene biguanide (PHMB) against fungal isolates associated with infective keratitits. *J. Antimicrob. Chemother.* **1999**, *44*, 291–302. [CrossRef]
147. Romanowski, E.G.; Yates, K.A.; Connor, K.E.O.; Francis, S.; Shanks, R.M.Q.; Kowalski, R.P.; Ascp, M.S.M. The Evaluation of Polyhexamethylene Biguanide (PHMB) as a Disinfectant for Adenovirus. *JAMA Opthalmol.* **2013**, *131*, 495–498. [CrossRef]
148. Chindera, K.; Mahato, M.; Kumar Sharma, A.; Horsley, H.; Kloc-Muniak, K.; Kamaruzzaman, N.F.; Kumar, S.; McFarlane, A.; Stach, J.; Bentin, T.; et al. The antimicrobial polymer PHMB enters cells and selectively condenses bacterial chromosomes. *Sci. Rep.* **2016**, *6*, 23121. [CrossRef]
149. Firdessa, R.; Good, L.; Amstalden, M.C.; Chindera, K.; Kamaruzzaman, N.F.; Schultheis, M.; Röger, B.; Hecht, N.; Oelschlaeger, T.A.; Meinel, L.; et al. Pathogen- and Host-Directed Antileishmanial Effects Mediated by Polyhexanide (PHMB). *PLoS Negl. Trop. Dis.* **2015**, *9*. [CrossRef]
150. Müller, G.; Kramer, A. Biocompatibility index of antiseptic agents by parallel assessment of antimicrobial activity and cellular cytotoxicity. *J. Antimicrob. Chemother.* **2008**, *61*, 1281–1287. [CrossRef]
151. Lewis, K. Platforms for antibiotic discovery. *Nat. Publ. Gr.* **2013**, *12*, 371–387. [CrossRef]
152. Shea, R.O.; Moser, H.E. Physicochemical Properties of Antibacterial Compounds: Implications for Drug Discovery. *J. Med. Chem.* **2008**, *51*. [CrossRef]
153. Chang, R.-K.; Raw, A.; Lionberger, R.; Yu, L.X. Generic development of topical dermatologic products: Formulation development, process development, and testing of topical dermatologic products. *AAPS J.* **2013**, *15*, 41–52. [CrossRef]
154. Nellums, L.B.; Thompson, H.; Holmes, A.; Castro-Sánchez, E.; Otter, J.A.; Norredam, M.; Friedland, J.S.; Hargreaves, S. Antimicrobial resistance among migrants in Europe: A systematic review and meta-analysis. *Lancet Infect. Dis.* **2018**, *18*, 796–811. [CrossRef]
155. Kamaruzzaman, N.F.; Chong, S.Q.Y.; Edmondson-Brown, K.M.; Ntow-Boahene, W.; Bardiau, M.; Good, L. Bactericidal and anti-biofilm effects of polyhexamethylene Biguanide in models of intracellular and biofilm of Staphylococcus aureus isolated from bovine mastitis. *Front. Microbiol.* **2017**, *8*, 1–10. [CrossRef]

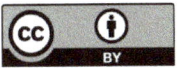

© 2019 by the authors. Licensee MDPI, Basel, Switzerland. This article is an open access article distributed under the terms and conditions of the Creative Commons Attribution (CC BY) license (http://creativecommons.org/licenses/by/4.0/).

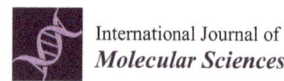

Review

Novel Bioactive and Therapeutic Dental Polymeric Materials to Inhibit Periodontal Pathogens and Biofilms

Minghan Chi [1,2,†], Manlin Qi [1,2,†], Lan A [1,2,†], Ping Wang [3], Michael D. Weir [3], Mary Anne Melo [3], Xiaolin Sun [1,2], Biao Dong [4], Chunyan Li [1,2,*], Junling Wu [5,*], Lin Wang [1,2,3,*] and Hockin H. K. Xu [3,6,7]

1. Department of Oral Implantology, School of Dentistry, Jilin University, Changchun 130021, China; minghan93@hotmail.com (M.C.); qml1992@126.com (M.Q.); hi_alan2001@163.com (L.A); sxl2673366@126.com (X.S.)
2. Jilin Provincial Key Laboratory of Sciences and Technology for Stomatology Nanoengineering, Changchun 130021, China
3. Department of Advanced Oral Sciences and Therapeutics, University of Maryland School of Dentistry, Baltimore, MD 21201, USA; dentistping@hotmail.com (P.W.); mweir@umaryland.edu (M.D.W.); mmelo@umaryland.edu (M.A.M.); hxu@umaryland.edu (H.H.K.X.)
4. State Key Laboratory on Integrated Optoelectronics, College of Electronic Science and Engineering, Jilin University, Changchun 130012, China; dongb@jlu.edu.cn
5. Shandong Provincial Key Laboratory of Oral Tissue Regeneration, Department of Prosthodontics, School of Stomatology, Shandong University, Jinan 250012, China
6. Center for Stem Cell Biology and Regenerative Medicine, University of Maryland School of Medicine, Baltimore, MD 21201, USA
7. University of Maryland Marlene and Stewart Greenebaum Cancer Center, University of Maryland School of Medicine, Baltimore, MD 21201, USA

* Correspondence: wanglin1982@jlu.edu.cn (L.W.); jlcyspring@126.com (C.L.); doctorwujunling@163.com (J.W.)
† These authors contribute equally to this work.

Received: 19 December 2018; Accepted: 9 January 2019; Published: 11 January 2019

Abstract: Periodontitis is a common infectious disease characterized by loss of tooth-supporting structures, which eventually leads to tooth loss. The heavy burden of periodontal disease and its negative consequence on the patient's quality of life indicate a strong need for developing effective therapies. According to the World Health Organization, 10–15% of the global population suffers from severe periodontitis. Advances in understanding the etiology, epidemiology and microbiology of periodontal pocket flora have called for antibacterial therapeutic strategies for periodontitis treatment. Currently, antimicrobial strategies combining with polymer science have attracted tremendous interest in the last decade. This review focuses on the state of the art of antibacterial polymer application against periodontal pathogens and biofilms. The first part focuses on the different polymeric materials serving as antibacterial agents, drug carriers and periodontal barrier membranes to inhibit periodontal pathogens. The second part reviews cutting-edge research on the synthesis and evaluation of a new generation of bioactive dental polymers for Class-V restorations with therapeutic effects. They possess antibacterial, acid-reduction, protein-repellent, and remineralization capabilities. In addition, the antibacterial photodynamic therapy with polymeric materials against periodontal pathogens and biofilms is also briefly described in the third part. These novel bioactive and therapeutic polymeric materials and treatment methods have great potential to inhibit periodontitis and protect tooth structures.

Keywords: polymers; antibacterial; drug delivery; periodontitis; periodontal biofilms

1. Introduction

Periodontitis is a dental plaque (bacteria)-induced, and host-mediated, breakdown of soft and hard tissues surrounding the teeth [1]. It is a persistent disease with no appreciable decrease in the prevalence of periodontitis in any of the world's regions between 1990 and 2010 [2]. In 1999, nearly 35% of individuals ≥30 years of age showed signs of periodontitis in the United States [3]. Severe periodontitis was reported as the sixth most prevalent chronic condition in 2010, affecting 10.8% of the population 15–99 years of age, or 743 million people [2]. Furthermore, the prevalence of periodontal disease increases with age. More than 70% of adults aged 65 or older are diagnosed with some form of periodontal disease [4].

Microbial biofilms are the aggravative factor of periodontitis [5]. The conventional treatment for periodontitis involves mechanical processing (such as supragingival scaling, subgingival scaling, and root planing) advantageously accompanied by the adjuvant administration of antibiotics, which can be applied by systemic or local administration [6]. The periodontal pocket provides a natural reservoir, which is easily accessible for the insertion of a delivery device. Therefore, intra-pocket drug delivery systems are highly desirable due to the potentially lower incidence of undesirable side effects, improved efficacy and enhanced patient compliance. Recent progress in polymer sciences have produced bioactive polymeric materials, which can be modified to meet pharmacological and biological requirements [7]. First, polymers can possess strong antibacterial properties against periodontal pathogens and could be used as an alternative to low molecular weight antimicrobial agents in periodontitis treatment due to their low cost, versatility, and processability [8–11]. Second, polymeric materials can serve as intra-pocket drug delivery devices for the treatment of periodontitis in various formulations and forms. Third, polymeric materials can be applied in fabrication of biodegradable periodontal membranes for guided tissue regeneration (GTR) [12–16]. The periodontal membrane acts as a mechanical barrier which protects the clot, and allows periodontal ligament and bone tissue to selectively repopulate the root surface during healing [12]. The main risk that contributes to unsuccessful tissue regeneration by GTR membrane treatment is the action of periodontal pathogens. Therefore, multifunctional GTR membranes were recently developed to possess not only barrier and tissue regenerative properties, but also antibacterial effects against periodontal pathogens. Several meritorious reviews on polymeric materials have described their antibacterial effects against pathogenic microorganisms [17–19], drug delivery capabilities [20–22] and periodontal regeneration for periodontitis treatment [23–25], which is not repeated here.

Tooth-colored polymeric composites and bonding agents are the primary materials for restoring tooth cavities [26–30]. This is because advances in polymer chemistry and filler particle compositions have enhanced the composite restoration properties [31–36]. As the world population ages, there is an increasing trend of root caries in senior people. Root caries can be treated with Class-V restorations. However, they often have subgingival margins which are difficult to clean and can provide pockets for periodontal bacterial growth. This in turn leads to the worsening of periodontitis and the damage of the periodontal attachment. To make matters worse, the currently available dental polymer-based Class-V composites not only have no antibacterial effect, but actually accumulate more biofilms and plaque than other materials such as metals. The present article reviews new developments in polymeric materials for periodontitis treatment, periodontal tissue regeneration and Class-V restorations, focusing on bioactive and therapeutic effects against periodontal pathogens and biofilms.

2. Polymeric Materials as Drug Carrier for Combating Periodontal Biofilm

The origin of periodontitis is closely related with a dramatic shift from a symbiotic microbial community to a dysbiotic microbial community that is mainly composed of anaerobic genera [37]. As the treatment of periodontitis mainly focuses on the elimination of the periodontal pathogens or biofilms from the tooth surface, antibiotics are commonly used to treat the disease. Therefore, intra-pocket drug delivery systems are highly desirable because they can maintain effective high levels of antibiotics in the gingival crevicular fluid for a prolonged period of time [7]. Meanwhile, they have lower risks of undesirable side effects, superior efficacy and enhanced patient compliance [7]. Due to the relatively low price, higher stability, nontoxicity, biocompatibility, nonimmunogenicity and biodegradability, a variety of polymers are investigated as drug carriers in various formulations and forms such as fibers [38–41], strips [42], films [43,44], gels [45,46], micro-particles [47–49], nanoparticles [11,50–52], and vesicular system [53,54]. Table 1 shows various polymer-based local drug delivery systems delivering a variety of antibiotics, such as metronidazole, doxycycline, tetracycline and secnidazole, for combating periodontal pathogens.

Table 1. Polymeric materials as drug delivery systems for combating periodontal pathogens.

Type	Polymer/Polymer-Based Product	Drug/Antibiotics	Periodontal Pathogens	References
Film	Chitosan	Chlirhexidine (Chx) gluconate Taurine (Amino acid)	P. gingivalis	[9]
	Cellulose acetate phthalate and Pluronic F-127 (CCAP)	Metronidazole	>P. gingivalis	[55]
	PLGA	Secnidazole (SC) Doxycycline hydrochloride (DH)	P. gingivalis F. nucleatum	[56]
Gel	Arestin®	Minocycline	>A. actinomycetemcomitans	[57]
	Polyester	Doxycycline hyclate Metronidazole	>P. gingivalis	[46]
	Badam gum Karaya gum Chitosan	Moxifloxacin	>A. actinomycetemcomitans	[58]
	Atridox®	Doxycycline hyclate	P. gingivalis F. nucleatum	[59,60]
Chip	PLGA	Chlorhexidine (CHX) CHX digluconate	P. gingivalis	[61]
Strip	Hydroxypropylcellulose	Green tea catechin	P. gingivalis Prevotella spp.	[62]
Cube	poly(glycerol sebacate) (PGS)	Berbereine chlorhexidine	P. gingivalis A. actinomycetemcomitans	[63]
Microparticles	Gelatin	Doxycycline	P. gingivalis	[64]
Nanoparticles	PLGA Polymersomes	Minicycline Metronidazole Doxycycline	P. gingivalis T. forsythia T. denticola P. gingivalis	[65,66]
	PEGylated PLGA	Minocycline	A. actinomycetemcomitans	[67]
	PLGA	H.madagascariensis leaf extract (HLE)	Prevotella species	[68]

Gels as semisolid systems could easily apply to the site of action with fast drug release rate, adhere to wide area of mucosa in the dental pockets, and maintain the concentration of antibiotics due to their bio-adhesive characteristics [69]. Polymers such as chitosan, poly (DL-lactide-co-glycolide) (PLGA) and polyacrylic acid are used for the preparation of gels. Gad et al. formulated PLGA "in situ implants" containing secnidazole and doxycycline by a non-solvent-induced phase separation mechanism [56]. The antibacterial evaluation against *Porphyromonas gingivalis* (*P. gingivalis*) showed that implants with 25% PLGA showed a greater zone of inhibition than a commercial control Atridox®, which is a locally delivered antimicrobial product containing doxycycline hyclate [56].

In addition, films are widely used for intra-pocket delivery. Films could be fabricated either by solvent-casting or direct milling. The drugs are distributed throughout the polymer and released by diffusion and/or matrix dissolution or erosion [70]. Importantly, the shape of the film can be easily adjusted according to the dimensions of the intra-pocket. Solvent-cast PLGA films were aminolyzed and modified by a Layer-by-Layer technique to obtain a nano-layered coating with poly(sodium4-styrenesulfonate) and poly(allylamine hydrochloride) as polyelectrolytes [71]. A water-soluble antibiotic, metronidazole (MET), was incorporated to successfully endow the film with excellent antibacterial properties against the keystone periodontal pathogen *P. gingivalis*, without compromising the in vitro biocompatibility.

Recently, intensive efforts are being made all over the world to improve the effectiveness of delivery systems. Due to the rapid advancement in nanotechnology, nanoparticulate systems provide several advantages as compared with other delivery systems. A nanoparticle is defined as a particle that has a size range of approximately 1–100 nm, with properties that are not shared by non-nanoscale particles with the same chemical composition. Regarding the application in periodontitis, first, it is easier for nanoparticle carriers to access deeper into the site of tooth furcation and periodontal pocket regions under gum line, while it may be inaccessible for other delivery systems [21]. Second, frequency reduction of administration in the periodontal pockets by applying nanoparticles would enhance the therapeutic effects and reduce side effects [7]. Third, nanoparticles possess better stability in biological fluid and high dispersibility in an aqueous medium [7]. Sadat et al. prepared both PLGA and PEGylated PLGA nanoparticles by various methods, such as single and double solvent evaporation emulsion, ion pairing, and nanoprecipitation [67]. Antibacterial properties against *Aggregatibacter actinomycetemcomitans* (*A. actinomycetemcomitans*) showed that the encapsulation of minocyline into the polymeric nanoparticles improved the antibacterial efficiency by two folds, compared to that of the free drugs. This was possibly due to better penetration of the nanoparticles into bacterial cells and better delivery of minocyline to the site of action [67]. Besides encapsulation, drugs can also be doped onto the surface of polymeric nanoparticles due to the specific surface chemistry. A novel type of polymeric nanoparticles, PolymP-*n* active nanoparticles, was recently developed, with potential for periodontal regeneration [72]. Due to the surface chemistry of the nanoparticles, containing functional groups with sequences of anionic carboxylate (i.e. COO^-), it was possible to dope metal cations (in this case calcium, zinc and silver) and antibiotics (doxycycline), with potential antibacterial activity [73]. A multispecies periodontal biofilm was developed by using *Streptococcus oralis* (*S. oralis*), *Actinomyces naeslundii* (*A. naeslundii*), *Veillonella parvula* (*V. parvula*), *Fusobacterium nucleatum* (*F. nucleatum*), *P. gingivalis* and *A. actinomycetemcomitans* to investigate the antibacterial properties of polymeric PolymP-n active nanoparticles doped with different substances: zinc, calcium, silver and doxycycline [73]. A similar biofilm formation was observed, although reductions in bacterial viability were detected in biofilms in contact with the different nanoparticles, and were more pronounced with silver and doxycycline nanoparticles. PolymP-n nanoparticles with doxycycline resulted in unstructured biofilm formation and significantly lower colony units of the six species, compared with the other specimens and controls [73]. However, with the emergence and increase of microbial resistance to antibiotics, further studies should investigate not only antibiotic-free delivery systems but also antimicrobial peptides (AMPs) for treating periodontal infections. Bacterial flora is controlled initially by the innate immune system of oral epithelia, saliva and gingival crevicular fluid, which are rich with AMPs [74]. AMPs such as LL37 and β-defensins have demonstrated excellent antibacterial efficacy against periodontal pathogens [75]. Therefore, the existing and newly-identified AMPs may be promising for therapeutic uses in treating periodontal disease, and they may serve as templates for peptides and peptide-mimetics with improved therapeutic efficacy [74].

3. Antibacterial Polymeric Materials Against Periodontal Pathogens

Although polymers can serve as matrix materials holding the antibacterial agents for treatment of infectious disease, the development of polymers with antimicrobial activity themselves is also an important area of research. In addition, increasing antibiotic drug-resistance of microorganisms has drawn considerable attention toward the development of new types of antibacterial agents. Several antibacterial polymers are applied in infectious diseases caused by pathogenic microorganisms.

However, their antibacterial properties against periodontal pathogens or biofilms are rarely investigated [9,76].

Chitosan, a linear polycationic hetero polysaccharide copolymer, exhibits an excellent capacity of antimicrobial efficacy. The contact between negatively charged cell wall and positively charged chitosan can alter the cell wall permeability and eventually lead to the complete cell wall disruption and cell death. Molecular weight, concentration, and hydrophilic/hydrophobic characteristics of chitosan also play some role in antibacterial efficacy [77]. Chitosan showed antimicrobial activity against periodontal pathogens *P. gingivalis*, *A. actinomycetemcomitans* and *Prevotella intermedia* (*P. intermedia*) with quick and efficient bactericidal activity [78]. Similar excellent antibacterial activity of chitosan against *P. gingivalis* and *A. actinomycetemcomitans* was also reported by Arancibia et al. [79]. Furthermore, Sarasam et al. confirmed that chitosan-mediated antibacterial activity was contact-dependent; therefore, blending chitosan with other components such as polycaprolactone (PCL) compromised its antibacterial activity against *A. actinomycetemcomitans* [80]. The possible explanation is that the surface characteristics of chitosan, such as surface roughness and charge distribution, may be altered when blending with PCL, thereby decreasing the antibiotic performance.

Recent efforts developed a new class of antimicrobial agents, termed "structurally nanoengineered antimicrobial peptide polymers" (SNAPPs), as shown in Figure 1. They exhibited sub-µM activity against Gram-negative bacteria *Acinetobacter baumannii* (*A. baumannii*) [81]. It is possible that in addition to putative periodontal pathogens, non-oral bacterial species such as *A. baumannii* may also play a role in the etiopathogenesis of periodontal diseases [82]. The antibacterial activity of SNAPPs proceeds via a multimodal mechanism of bacterial cell death by outer membrane destabilization, unregulated ion movement across the cytoplasmic membrane and induction of the apoptotic-like death pathway [81]. Therefore, SNAPPs showed great promise as low-cost and effective antimicrobial agents in combating the growing threat of Gram-negative bacteria, which is prevalent in periodontitis.

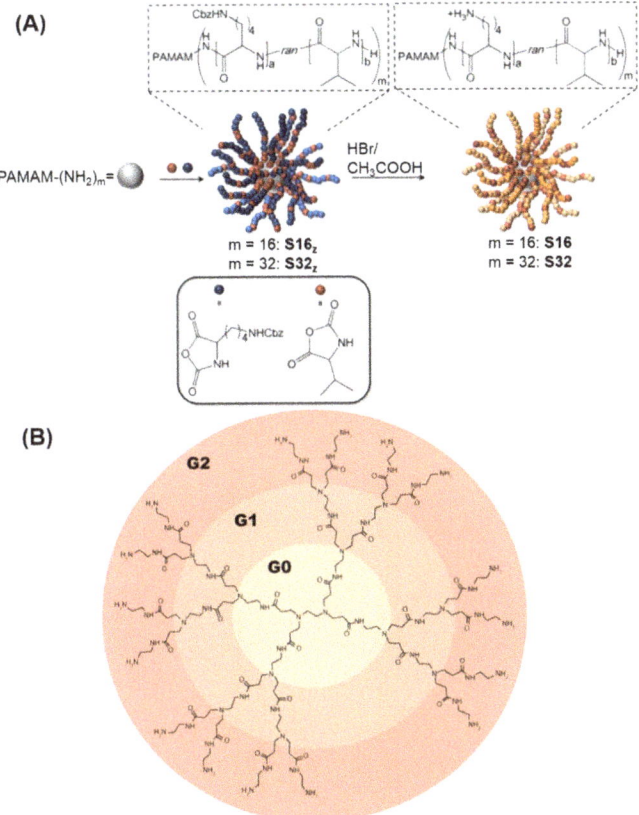

Figure 1. Synthesis of SNAPPs. (**A**) Synthesis of SNAPPs via ring-opening polymerization of lysine and valine N-carboxyanhydrides (NCAs) was initiated from the terminal amines of poly(amido amine) (PAMAM) dendrimers. Second- and third-generation PAMAM dendrimers in (**B**) with 16 and 32 peripheral primary amines were used to prepare 16- and 32-arm SNAPPs, respectively. Note that the number of initiating points on the figure does not reflect the actual number, which is 16 or 32. The number of repeat units for lysine and valine are a and b, respectively. (Reproduced with permission from [81]. Spinger Nature, 2016.)

4. Antibacterial Polymeric Membrane for GTR Inhibiting Periodontitis

GTR strategies are widely applied for periodontal tissue regeneration. Generally, a mechanical barrier membrane is established to create a protected space over bone defect and prevent the apical migration of the gingival epithelium. This facilitates the growth of periodontal ligament and bone tissue to selectively re-attach the root surface [12]. To enhance the bioactivity and adjust the degradation rates, polymeric materials such as collagen, chitosan, gelatin, silk fibroin, and synthetic polymers (PLGA, PCL and poly (ethylene glycol) (PEG)) are used to fabricate the GTR membranes.

Clinically, infection is a major reason for GTR failure [83]. Infection can be caused by either pathogen colonization at the wound site or foreign body response to the implant material [84]. Periodontal disease and GTR implant-related infections mainly result from anaerobic bacteria such as bacteroides species, fusobacteria, and clostridia. Hence, multifunctional GTR membranes were recently developed to not only possess barrier and tissue regenerative properties, but also exhibit antibacterial effects against periodontal pathogens.

Metronidazole (MET) is widely used to treat periodontitis in patients for whom mechanical debridement is not successful or possible [85]. Xue et al. developed MET-loaded electrospun PCL nanofiber membranes. A wide range (1–40 wt %) of MET was incorporated into the membrane. An in vitro antibacterial effect against F. nucleatum showed clear inhibition zones around the membranes. GTR membranes with 30 wt % MET showed excellent comprehensive properties. However, the release time of metronidazole was only a few days [86]. To sustain the drug release for a longer time, gelatin was added into PCL in the same electrospun system to form a PCL/gelatin nanofiber membrane [87]. As effective MET carriers, PCL/gelatin membranes with various contents of MNA showed an approximately 60% release of MET within one week. This was followed by a sustained release of up to three weeks, which was predominantly controlled by diffusion and gelatin degradation [87]. In addition, an efficient anti-infective GTR membrane was developed by doping drug-loaded clay nanotube into electrospun PCL/gelatin microfibers [88]. By combining the drug-loading capability of nanotubes and direct drug loading into electrospun microfiber matrix, composite membranes with a three-week sustained drug release capability were realized. This extended release prevents the colonization of F. nucleatum over period of three weeks [88]. This three-week prolonged drug release is considered to be an optimal treatment time period.

Bittino et al. fabricated a novel functionally-graded periodontal membrane containing MET with a spatially designed layer structure via sequential electrospinning [89]. As shown in Figure 2, the functionally-graded periodontal membrane consisted of a core layer (CL) and two functional surface layers (SLs) interfacing with bone (nano-hydroxyapatite, n-HAp) and epithelial (MET) tissues. This multi-layered electrospun GTR membranes had nano-sized hydroxyapatite for osteoconductive/inductive behavior, and metronidazole to combat periodontal pathogens. Other antibiotics such as amoxicillin, tetracycline, chlorhexidine and doxycycline were also incorporated into polymeric membrane with therapeutic properties [90–93]. Composite GTR membranes with polytetrafluoroethylene (ePTFE) and collagen were loaded with chlorhexidine and inhibited A. actinomycetemcomitans, allowing the attachment of periodontal ligament cells [92]. Similar results were obtained when amoxicillin and tetracycline were incorporated into GTR membranes [94].

Besides antibiotic addition, metal or metallic oxide such as silver, zinc, copper and zinc oxide nanoparticles were also incorporated into the GTR membranes. For example, zinc oxide (ZnO) nanoparticles not only introduced an antibacterial activity, but also improved the osteoconductivity of the periodontal membrane [12]. Nasajpour et al. developed a GTR membrane through electrospinning methods with a dispersed solution of ZnO within a polymeric carrier PCL. Incorporation of 0.5% (w/v) ZnO nanoparticles provided antibacterial effects against periodontal pathogens P. gingivalis, while supporting the viability and the osteodifferentiation of the seeded periodontal ligament stem cells, without negatively impacting their biocompatibility feature [12]. Zinc phosphate was also loaded into the GTR membrane by an immersion method. The zinc phosphate mineralized membranes possessed a strong antibacterial effect against A. actinomycetemcomitans [95]. A recent study developed a chitosan/polyurethane (CSP) nanofibrous membrane with silver nanoparticles (AgNPs) in the membrane [96]. The antibacterial effects of the membrane against P. gingivalis was maintained when the AgNP level was adjusted to be at a nontoxic level.

It was reported that high drug ionic strength and rapid solvent evaporation favored the presence of the drug on the membrane surface, which led to a high initial burst release, thereby avoiding and/or eliminating biofilm formation [97]. However, the high burst release and short release period could not effectively prevent bacterial infections. Hence, it is highly desirable to develop novel GTR membranes with sustained and controlled release of antibacterial agents, particularly for patients with a predisposition to such complications: smokers, patients with diabetes mellitus, etc. [98].

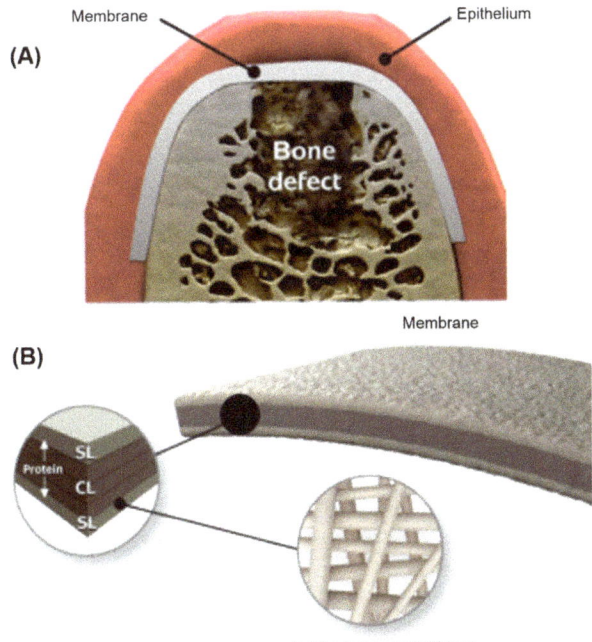

Figure 2. Schematic illustration of the spatially designed and functionally graded periodontal membrane. (**A**) Membrane placed in a guided bone regeneration scenario. (**B**) Details of the core layer (CL) and the functional surface layers (SLs) interfacing bone (n-HAp) and epithelial (MET) tissues. Note the chemical composition step-wise grading from the CL to SLs, i.e., polymer content decreased and protein content increased. (Reproduced with permission from [89]. Elsevier, 2011).

5. Antibacterial Polymeric Composites to Combat Periodontal Pathogens

To suppress oral biofilm/plaque buildup and increase the restoration's longevity, non-agent-leaching monomers are incorporated into dental polymers. Imazato et al. combined alkylpyridinium, a type of quaternary ammonium methacrylates (QAM), with a methacrylate, and synthesized a novel monomer, 12-methacryloyloxydodecylpyridinium bromide (MDPB) [99]. The QAM was chemically copolymerized with the resin by forming a covalent bonding with the polymer network [100,101]. While the quaternary ammonium group was responsible for the antibacterial activity of QAM, the methacrylate group allowed for the copolymerization with other conventional monomers. Therefore, the antibacterial QAM immobilized in the resin matrix was not released or lost over time, thus providing a durable antibacterial capability. The three likely mechanisms for bactericidal QAMs against microorganism were: (1) contact between negatively charged bacteria and positively charged QAMs leading to osmotic pressure; (2) diffusion through the cell wall and binding to the cytoplasmic membrane; and (3) disruption of the cytoplasmic membrane, releasing of cytoplasmic constituents, and cell death [102–104]. Several papers review the antibacterial monomers in dental resins [105–108], as well as studies on antibacterial functions against cariogenic bacteria and oral biofilms to inhibit dental caries [109–112]. Therefore, the present article focuses on new developments in antibacterial dental resins for root caries restorations with an emphasis on their antibacterial effects on periodontal pathogens.

Elderly people suffer more risks of root caries because of gingival recession and less saliva flow [113]. Periodontitis-related gingival recession often leads to more exposure of the root surfaces, which results in the increased risk of root caries. Root surfaces differ from enamel surfaces with a lower mineral content and a higher amount of organic materials [114]. Therefore, root caries lesions may occur on all exposed root surfaces but are mainly found in biofilm retention sites [114]. Root caries can be treated with a Class-V restoration, whose margins are often subgingival, which can hinder cleaning and provide pockets for bacterial growth, thus gradually resulting in the loss of the periodontal attachment of the tooth. Indeed, it is well-established that microbial biofilms are the primary etiological factor that causes periodontitis [5]. Recent research demonstrated that *P. gingivalis*, *P. intermedia* and *A. actinomycetemcomitans* are the three major bacterial species that contribute to periodontitis and peri-implantitis in subgingival plaque [115]. In the periodontal pockets, these bacteria can generate virulence factors that lead to the gradual loss of the supporting bone [115]. In addition, *Prevotella nigrescens* (*P. nigrescens*) is associated with both healthy and diseased conditions of the periodontium [116]. *F. nucleatum* is correlated with the progress in periodontitis [117] and can enhance the invasion into human gingival epithelial and endothelial cells by *P. gingivalis* [118]. Furthermore, *Enterococcus faecalis* (*E. faecalis*) is regarded as an endodontic pathogen and also detected in subgingival plaque and saliva of patients with chronic periodontal disease [119].

Therefore, these six species were selected in a recent study [120]. A polymeric composite for Class-V tooth cavity restorations was developed with therapeutic functions to combat these six species of pathogens related to the start and the exacerbation of periodontitis [120]. The polymeric matrix in the composite was composed of ethoxylated bisphenol A dimethacrylate (EBPADMA) and pyromellitic dianhydride glycerol dimethacrylate (PMGDM) at a 1:1 mass ratio (referred to as EBPM). A novel antibacterial monomer dimethylaminohexadecyl methacrylate (DMAHDM) was added at a mass ratio of 3%. DMAHDM incorporation did not compromise the mechanical properties of polymeric composite. The flexural strength of EBPM + 3% DMAHDM was similar to that of a commercial control composite that had no antibacterial effect [120]. Static single-species biofilms of six types of pathogens were used to evaluate the antibacterial effects of polymeric composites with DMAHDM incorporation. For all six species, incorporating 3% DMAHDM into EBPM composite decreased the biofilm CFU by several orders of magnitude, compared to the commercial control and the 0% DMAHDM group ($p < 0.05$). DMAHDM composite reduced the CFU of different bacterial species differently, some by slightly less than 3 log, others by more than 3 log (as shown in Figure 3) [120]. The killing efficacy of DMAHDM composite against the six species was: *E. faecalis* < *F. nucleatum* < *P. nigrescens* = *P. intermedia* < *A. actinomycetemcomitans* < *P. gingivalis*. Furthermore, the biomass and the polysaccharide production by biofilms were also reduced on the EBPM composite with 3% DMAHDM, compared to control composite [120].

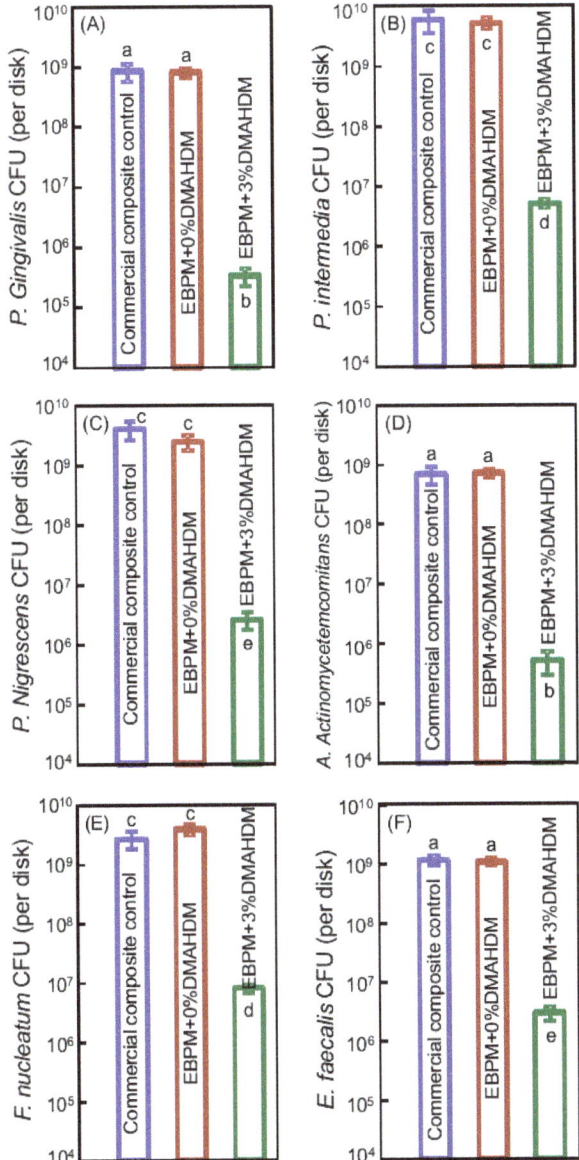

Figure 3. CFU counts of two-day biofilms on composites (mean ± SD; $n = 6$): (**A**) *P. gingivalis*; (**B**) *P. intermedia*; (**C**) *P. nigrescens*; (**D**) *A. actinomycetemcomitans*; (**E**) *F. nucleatum*; and (**F**) *E. faecalis*. Note the log scale for the y-axis. CFU counts on composite containing DMAHDM were nearly three orders of magnitude lower than composite without DMAHDM. Bars with dissimilar letters are significantly different from each other ($p < 0.05$). (Reproduced with permission from [120]. Elsevier, 2016.)

Salivary protein adsorption on the surface is required for pellicle formation and is a prerequisite for oral bacteria adherence [121]. Based on this mechanism, a protein-repellent composite was developed using 2-methacryloyloxyethyl phosphorylcholine (MPC). MPC is a methacrylate with a phospholipid polar group in the side chain [122]. MPC has strong protein-repellency, and has been incorporated into artificial blood vessels, hip joints, and microfluidic devices [123–125]. Several MPC-containing medical devices have won the approvals of the United States Food and Drug Administration, and have been used clinically [123,126]. A recent study developed a multifunctional polymeric dental composite containing bioactive agents (MPC for protein-repellency, and DMAHDM for anti-biofilm activity) to suppress periodontal pathogens [127]. These results showed that adding up to 3% MPC and 3% DMAHDM did not compromise the strength and elastic modulus, compared to the control. Representative live/dead images of two-day biofilms for the 5 × 4 full-factorial design are shown in Figure 4. Live bacteria were stained green, and bacteria with compromised membranes were stained red. For all four species periodontal biofilms (*P. gingivalis*, *P. intermedia*, *A. actinomycetemcomitans*, and *F. nucleatum*), the two control composites were covered by live bacteria. In contrast, composite with 3% MPC had much less bacterial adhesion. Composite with 3% DMAHDM had substantial dead bacteria. Composite with 3% DMAHDM + 3% MPC had much less bacterial adhesion, and the bacteria were mostly dead [127]. Dual agents of MPC + DMAHDM incorporation into polymeric composites exerted a much greater anti-biofilm activity against periodontal pathogens, than using MPC or DMAHDM alone. Therefore, the polymeric composite containing 3% DMAHDM and 3% MPC appeared to be the optimal composition. It showed a high potential for applications in Class-V restorations to inhibit periodontal biofilms, by reducing biofilm CFU by nearly four orders of magnitude for all the periodontitis-related pathogens examined in that study [127].

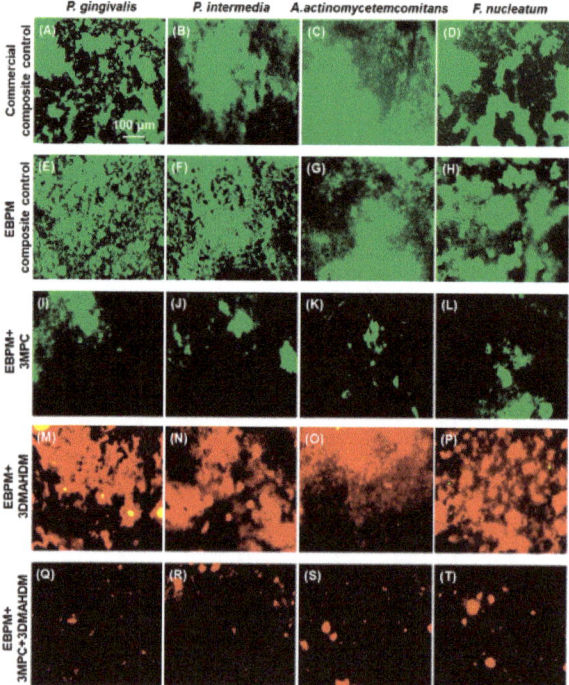

Figure 4. Representative live/dead staining images of two-day biofilms of four species of periodontal pathogens on the five composites: (**A–D**) Commercial composite control; (**E–H**) EBPM composite control; (**I–L**) EBPM + 3MPC; (**M–P**) EBPM + 3DMAHDM; and (**Q–T**) EBPM + 3DMAHDM + 3MPC. All images have the same scale bar as shown in (**A**). Live bacteria were stained green. Dead bacteria were stained red. Composites without DMAHDM had primarily live bacteria. EBPM + 3DMAHDM + 3MPC had much less bacterial adhesion, and the biofilms consisted of primarily dead bacteria. DMAHDM: dimethylaminohexadecyl methacrylate; MPC: 2-methacryloyloxyethyl phosphorylcholine (Reproduced with permission from [127]. Elsevier, 2016.)

Previous studies tested single species biofilms [128]. However, single species models are not representative of natural biofilms where multispecies communities are by far the most predominant [129]. The eradication of multispecies biofilms is more difficult to achieve than single species, as multispecies biofilms are more highly resistant to antimicrobial agents than single species [130]. Furthermore, the biofilm composition may influence the outcome of periodontitis treatments [131] and the killing efficacy of antibacterial agents [130].

Therefore, a recent study investigated the effects of the number of species (from 1 to 9) in the periodontal biofilm on the inhibition efficacy of the composite [132]. Moreover, the effect of dual agents (MPC + DMAHDM) versus single agent on the inhibition efficacy was investigated as a function of the number of species in the biofilm for the first time. Figure 5 illustrates the anti-biofilm strategy. The bioactive composite reduced protein adsorption by an order of magnitude and greatly reduced biofilm viability. It decreased the biofilm CFU by more than three orders of magnitude for all four types of periodontal biofilms (single-species, three-species, six-species, and nine-species biofilms), compared to the control composite. With increasing the biofilm species from 1 to 9, the antibacterial efficacy of DMAHDM composite decreased; the folds of CFU reduction decreased from 947 to 44 folds. In contrast, the DMAHDM+MPC composite maintained a CFU reduction folds of greater than 3000, showing a similarly high antibacterial potency from 1 to 9 species in the biofilms.

Therefore, DMAHDM composite was more effective in inhibiting single species biofilm; the inhibition efficacy decreased with increasing the number of species in the biofilms. Adding MPC into the DMAHDM composite increased the efficacy against multi-species biofilms, achieving nearly the same high efficacy against biofilms with 1–9 species. The novel nanocomposite containing dual agents (MPC + DMAHDM) with potent antibiofilm and protein-repellent functions is promising for Class-V restorations to treat root caries, inhibit periodontal pathogens, and protect the periodontal tissues.

To enhance the antibacterial efficacy, Xiao et al. incorporated nanoparticles of silver (NAg) into the aforementioned MPC + DMAHDM composites to inhibit pathogens such as *A. actinomycetemcomitans*, *F. nucleatum* and *P. gingivalis* [133]. There are several advantages for NAg incorporation into polymeric nanocomposite. (1) The small particle size of NAg (2.6 nm) yielded a relative high surface area to mass ratio, which enabled a small quantity of NAg to be sufficient for the composite to be strongly antibacterial. This avoided the need to use a high mass fraction of NAg and compromised the nanocomposite's mechanical properties and esthetics [134]. (2) Ag is known to have a superior biocompatibility and low toxicity to humans. (3) Resins containing NAg exhibited long-lasting antimicrobial properties. For example, a previous study demonstrated that NAg-containing resins showed antibacterial activity even after 12 months of water-aging [135]. (4) Ag have less possibility for causing bacterial resistance than antibiotics, which alleviates the drug-resistance concern [136]. (5) NAg is capable of long-distance killing of bacteria due to the release and diffusion of the Ag ions. This is expected to be useful to inhibit the suspended bacteria in the periodontal pockets away from the composite surface. Indeed, the combination of MPC, DMAHDM and NAg achieved the reduction in biofilm CFU by nearly five orders of magnitude, which is much greater than those achieved by previous antibacterial dental composites [120,127].

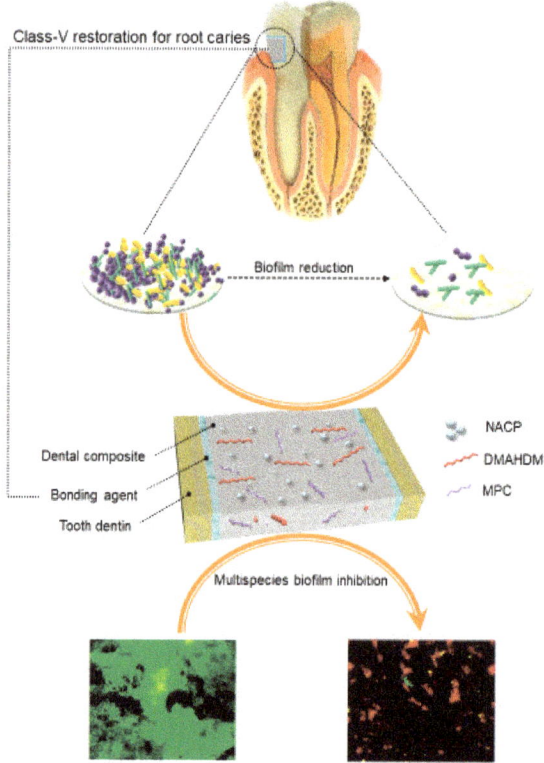

Figure 5. Antibacterial strategy using dual agents in dental composite. Dimethylaminohexadecyl methacrylate (DMAHDM) can inactivate periodontal pathogens by contact without leaching from resins. Methacryloyloxyethyl phosphorylcholine (MPC) can detach proteins, thereby hampering bacterial attachment. DMAHDM and MPC are both non-volatile, chemically stable and can sustain long-term antibacterial activity. DMAHDM: dimethylaminohexadecyl methacrylate; MPC: 2-methacryloyloxyethyl phosphorylcholine; NACP: nanoparticles of amorphous calcium phosphate (Revised and resubmitted to Dent. Mater. Ref [132].)

Glass ionomer materials have been widely used in Class-V restorations clinically due to their fluoride release, good biocompatibility with dental pulp tissues, and ability to bond to tooth structures. Fluoride release has a slight antimicrobial effect and a good remineralization effect. However, a previous study indicated that a commercial resin-modified glass ionomer cement was not potent enough to inhibit bacterial growth and biofilm formation [137]. In addition, for anterior teeth, cervical lesions need to be esthetic, which can be better satisfied with a resin composite. Therefore, the aforementioned polymeric dental composites are promising for Class-V restorations due to their strong antibacterial effects against periodontal pathogens.

6. Polymeric Bonding Agent Inhibiting Periodontal Pathogens

A dental bonding agent is used to bond restorations to teeth. A previous study developed a polymeric bonding agent with nanoparticles of amorphous calcium phosphate (NACP) and DMAHDM for tooth root caries restorations and endodontic applications [138]. A primer contained PMGDM and 2-hydroxyethyl methacrylate (HEMA) at a mass ratio 10:3, with 50% acetone solvent (all by mass ratio). The adhesive contained PMGDM, EBPADMA, 2-hydroxyethyl methacrylate (HEMA) and BisGMA at 45/40/10/5 mass ratio (referred to as PEHB) [135]. *P. gingivalis*, *P. intermedia*, *P. nigrescens*,

A. actinomycetemcomitans, *F. nucleatum* and *Parvimonas micra* (*P. micra*) were used to represent periodontal pathogens, and *Enterococcus faecium* (*E. faecium*) and *E. faecalis* were selected as endodontic pathogens. Therefore, eight types of single-species biofilms were formed on resins. Adding 5% DMAHDM and 30% NACP into the adhesive resin did not negatively affect the dentin bond strength. Biofilm CFU was reduced by nearly three orders of magnitude via the therapeutic resin. The inhibition efficacy via DMAHDM-containing resin was ranked as: *P. gingivalis* > *A. actinomycetemcomitans* > *P. intermedia* > *P. nigrescens* > *F. nucleatum* > *P. micra* > *E. faecalis* > *E. faecium*. Biofilm biomass, metabolic activity and polysaccharide were also greatly reduced via DMAHDM [138].

In addition, three bioactive agents (NACP for remineralization, MPC for protein-repellency, and DMAHDM for anti-biofilm activity) were combined into a polymeric bonding agent (PEHB) to suppress periodontal pathogens [139]. PEHB with 5% DMAHDM showed a strong antibacterial function and protein-repellent properties. The use of dual agents, 5% DMAHDM + 5% MPC, achieved a greater killing efficacy against *P. gingivalis* single-species biofilm than against multi-species biofilm. However, this novel polymeric bonding agents still showed great reduction in multispecies biofilm growth, metabolic activity and polysaccharide production, yielding three orders of magnitude in CFU reduction [139].

The mechanism of contact-inhibition implied that the polymer surface was separated from the overlaying biofilm by the presence of the salivary protein pellicles on the polymer surface. This would reduce the extent of contact, and hence result in the decreased contact-inhibition efficacy. Therefore, because of the protein-repellency of the MPC, it helped diminish protein coverage on the polymer surface, thus exposing more polymer surface with quaternary amine N^+ sites, thereby promoting the contact-inhibition ability. Therefore, the dual use of DMAHDM and MPC in the dental polymer could work synergistically to maximize the periodontal bacteria inhibition capability.

Besides the antibacterial agents, NACP were also incorporated in polymeric bonding agents [140–142]. While having little antibacterial activity, the NACP composite was "smart" and could greatly increase the Ca and P ion release at a cariogenic low pH, when such ions were most needed to inhibit caries [143]. Indeed, a previous study showed that an NACP nanocomposite successfully remineralized enamel lesions, and achieved an enamel lesion remineralization efficacy that was four-fold greater than that of a commercial fluoride-releasing control [144]. In addition, a previous study showed that NACP composite could be recharged repeatedly with Ca and P ions, which ensured that it could continuously release Ca and P ions to provide long-term remineralization [145]. In Class-V restorations, these Ca and P ions from the composite are expected to help remineralize tooth roots, reduce root sensitivity, neutralize biofilm acids, and protect the root structures.

Currently, several contemporary dental adhesives have been reported to possess a favorable "immediate" bond strength to enamel and dentin. However, the clinical longevity of the bonded restorations is still too short, mainly due to the degradation of the adhesive tooth-composite interface, especially for Class-V restorations with subgingival margins. First, in comparison with bonding composite resins to enamel, bonding to cervical dentin is less predictable due to the relatively low density and oblique orientation of dentinal tubules in cervical dentin in Class-V restoration [146]. Second, marginal openings are located most frequently at the dentin/cementum margins when Class-V cavities are restored with composite-based materials. Besides polymerization stress, forces that result from volumetric changes due to temperature fluctuations and non-uniform deformation of restoratives and the tooth substance during functional loading also repeatedly stress the restorative interface [147]. Third, the subgingival cavity is difficult to dry. The inadequate air drying could result in too much residual solvent in the adhesive and in the hybrid layer, which would reduce the bonding durability [148]. Therefore, advanced restorative techniques such as the incremental filling technique with the application of flowable materials as an intermediate layer are used to improve the marginal adaptation of composites to the dentin/cementum margin in Class-V restoration [147].

Investigation of the toxicity of the antimicrobial monomers is a prerequisite before their use in oral restorations. Imazato et al. indicated that the first QAM for dental application, MDPB, exhibited a low level of toxicity to human pulpal cells, similar to the diluent resin monomer triethyleneglycol dimethacrylate (TEGDMA) [101]. Although a previous study demonstrated that the increasing monomer concentration and increasing chain length of QAMs would increase the cytotoxicity, QAMs with chain lengths from 3 to 18 were shown to have less cytotoxicity than BisGMA [149]. At monomer concentrations of ≤ 2 µg/mL, all the tested QAMs with CL ≤ 16 had cytotoxicity matching that of HEMA and TEGDMA [149]. Clinically, a typical tooth cavity would use approximately 20 µg of the bonding agent. In the unrealistic worst-case scenario, assume that all 20 µg were leached out in one day [149]. Human saliva flow is approximately 1000–1500 mL/day [150]. This would yield a monomer concentration of 0.02 µg/mL, which would be acceptable for clinical applications.

7. Polymeric Materials for Antibacterial Photodynamic Therapy Against Periodontal Pathogens

Currently, mechanical debridement and antibiotic therapy are still the major approaches for periodontitis treatment. However, conventional tools can hardly reach deep periodontal pockets. The overuse of antibiotics could lead to drug-resistant bacteria. In the past decade, antibacterial photodynamic therapy (aPDT) gradually attracted the attention of researchers, and several studies on the efficient clearance of periodontal pathogens or biofilms using aPDT were reported [151,152]. aPDT is a promising antibacterial therapeutic approach for periodontal pathogens to make up for the aforementioned shortcomings. aPDT involves three components: photosensitizer (PS), light, and oxygen. For periodontal pathogens, PS should have properties of good biocompatibility, high selectivity, high solubility, light stability, high quantum yield of reactive oxygen species (ROS) generation having positive charge, and causing no staining on gingiva [153,154]. The ideal irradiation light should be at red to near-infrared wavelengths to obtain a deeper penetration. As shown in Figure 6, the mechanism of aPDT is that, after being excited by a specific wavelength of light, the PS converts energy or electrons to generate ROS in the presence of molecular ground triplet state oxygen, thus leading to bacterial cell death [155]. Generally, the bactericidal effect of aPDT can be attributed to oxidative damage, including DNA damage and cell membrane system damage (biofilm matrix destruction, lipid oxidation, cell surface damage, etc.) [156].

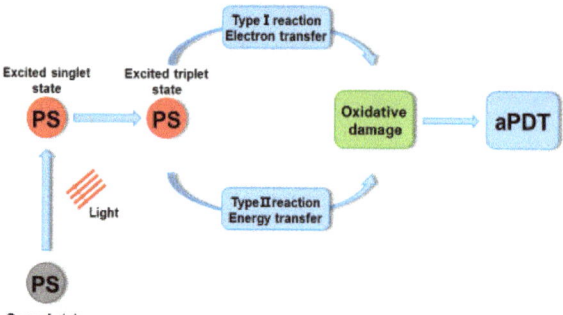

Figure 6. Schematic representation of mechanism of aPDT. Triggered by the light, ground state photosensitizer transfer into excited singlet state and triplet state. The triplet state can undergo type I (electron transfer) reaction and type II (energy transfer) reaction to produce singlet oxygen, which can cause oxidative damage.

Recently, attention has been paid to biodegradable polymeric materials in PDT studies due to their most remarkable properties of biocompatibility and low toxicity [157]. Regarding aPDT, application of polymeric materials carries several advantages: (1) increasing positive charge of PS and enhancing the binding between PS and bacteria; (2) reducing aggregation of PS and increasing its bioavailability; and (3) serving as a carrier or scaffold with good biocompatibility and biodegradability.

Periodontitis is a chronic infectious disease associated with Gram-negative bacteria. The cell envelope of Gram-negative bacteria consists of an outer membrane, a thinner peptidoglycan layer and a cytoplasmic membrane. Lipopolysaccharides (LPS) and the porins, the two main components of the outer membrane, have the membrane barrier protection to allow only certain molecules to pass through [158]. Negatively charged LPS molecules have a strong affinity for cations or cationic group. In contrast, anionic and neutral group cannot be up-taken by bacteria, which hinders the effective implementation of aPDT [159]. Thus, cationic PSs are considered to be used to overcome the initial difficulty in aPDT.

Figure 7 depicts different strategies of PS modification by polymers for bactericidal effect enhancement. In a recent study, compared with free methylene blue (MB) alone, MB-loaded PLGA cationic nanoparticles showed greater bactericidal effect on microorganisms in both planktonic and biofilm phase from human dental plaque samples collected from untreated patients with chronic periodontitis (Figure 7A) [160]. With a concentration of 50 mg/mL, exposure to red light for 5 min with a power density of 100 mW/cm^2, MB-loaded PLGA cationic nanoparticles reduced bacterial viability by approximately 60% from the planktonic PDT and 48% from the biofilm PDT [160]. In addition, the effect of this MB-NP-based aPDT as an adjunctive treatment combining with ultrasonic scaling (US) and scaling and root planning (SRP) showed a slightly better outcome than using US + SRP alone [161]. All clinical parameters including visible plaque and gingival bleeding indexes (GBI), bleeding on probing and probing pocket depth in both groups showed the greatest improvement one month later. However, US + SRP + aPDT showed a greater effect (28.82%) on GBI compared with US + SRP at three months [161]. Similarly, indocyanine green-loaded nanospheres coated with chitosan (ICG-Nano/c) was designed to cope with the clearance of P. gingivalis. ICG-Nano/c could adhere to the surface of P. gingivalis and significantly reduced the number of P. gingivalis by an order of 2 $\log_{10}$(96.71%) to 4 $\log_{10}$(99.99%) [162,163]. In addition, the strategy of intermittent irradiation with air cooling also improved therapeutic penetration and prevented tissue thermal damage [162]. This was probably because the PLGA provided positive charge and helped aPDT to produce a sustained effect on the periodontal lesions for a long time [164].

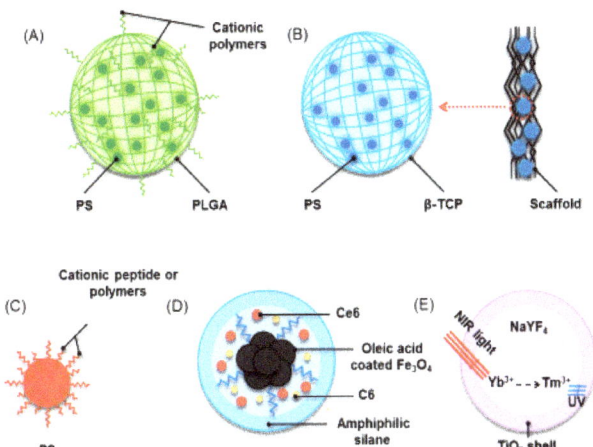

Figure 7. The various strategy of photosensitizer (PS) modification by polymeric materials to enhance bactericidal effect: (**A**) PS-loaded PLGA nanospheres with cationic polymers; (**B**) a scaffold or a carrier for PS; (**C**) PS binding to cationic peptide or polymers; (**D**) the structure of antibacterial multifunctional nanoparticles Fe$_3$O$_4$-silane@Ce6/C6; and (**E**) the structure of nanoparticles NaYF$_4$:Yb^{3+}, Tm^{3+}@TiO$_2$.

Recently, a chitosan-based hydrogel containing 0.5% hydroxypropyl methylcellulose and toluidine blue O with high adhesiveness was developed for the treatment of periodontitis [165]. Two major periodontal pathogens, *A. actinomycetemcomitans* and *P. gingivalis* biofilms, were used to evaluate the bactericidal effects. When the irradiation power was higher than 32.4 J·cm^{-2} using 630 nm light, a significant reduction in survival rate was observed in both single-species periodontal biofilms [165]. Furthermore, when the light dose was increased to 54 and 108 J·cm^{-2}, *A. actinomycetemcomitans* and *P. gingivalis* biofilms were completely eradicated, respectively [165]. Regarding periodontal regeneration, two in-situ curable biomaterials, BioM1 and BioM2, were developed as support for PS and had excellent mechanical and antimicrobial behaviors [15]. The BioM1 and BioM2 consisted of urethane dimethacrylate and a tri-armed oligoester-urethane methacrylate, respectively. The PS was composed of a mixture of β-tricalcium phosphate (β-TCP) microparticles and 20 wt % photosensitizer mTHPC (Figure 7B). The BioM2 + PS with a single laser-illumination (652 nm) caused total suppression of *P. gingivalis*, while BioM2 + PS with repeated irradiation reduced 3.1 log in CFU counts [15].

PS binding to various cationic peptide or polymers can enhance their loading into the bacterial cells and target periodontal pathogens (Figure 7C). It was confirmed that aPDT with chlorin e6 (Ce6) and BLC 1010 suppressed periodontopathogenic bacteria [166]. Ce6-(Lys)$_5$-OH (Ce6-5K) conjugate broadened the spectrum of activity against periodontal pathogens, compared to the pure Ce6. Ce6-5K showed a strong killing effect on almost all oral bacteria tested, and showed at least six logs of killing for periodontal pathogens including *P. gingivalis*, *A. actinomycetemcomitans*, and *B. forsythus* [167]. In addition, two types of polylysin-porphycene conjugates GlamTMPn and BOHTMPn were synthesized to assess the development of resistance in bacterial cells [168]. The combination of polylysin-porphycene conjugates and bacterial cells was quite stable and showed an extremely high photosensitivity on *F. nucleatum* with 60 s irradiation [168]. Considering the precise targeting of aPDT, LiDps genetic construct was dual functionalized with SnCe6 and biotin (KLFC-LiDps-B-SnCe6) for *A. actinomycetemcomitans* biofilm-targeting, producing light-activated membrane disruption [169]. Streptavidin was used to couple biotinylated dodecamer to a biotinylated anti-*A. actinomycetemcomitans* antibody, which increased the loading efficacy of photosensitizer onto the bacterial cells. Light-induced activity of the targeted photosensitizer reduced the viability of *A. actinomycetemcomitans* biofilm [169]. In addition, a Fotolon sensitizer, composed of Ce6 and polyvinylpyrrolidone (PVP), obtained over 99.9% reduction in CFU in twenty Gram-positive and thirty Gram-negative clinical anaerobic strains. The PVP increased the quantum yield and fluorescence lifetime of Ce6, which contributed to the dispersion of particles and increased its bioavailability [170].

In recent years, nanoparticle-based PDT has become a hot research field in both tumor treatment and antibacterial therapy [171–173]. Extensive efforts had been made on how to disturb the formation of biofilms, and enhance the delivery of PS and its combination with bacteria to improve bactericidal efficiency by using the nanoparticles in oral diseases [51,174,175].

For intra-pocket administration, a major disadvantage of traditional nanoparticles carrying PS agents is the low delivery efficiency due to the drainage of gingival crevicular fluid and high saliva fluid turnover. Therefore, efficient delivery and penetration of the antibacterial agent to the exact site of infection is still highly desirable. In addition, real-time monitoring of the drug consumption and distribution is another issue that should be taken into consideration. The unknown effective dose of therapeutic agents reaching the disease site is an important uncertainty, and often leads to over-dosing or insufficient dosing [176]. In a recent study, a novel type of multifunctional nanoparticles Fe$_3$O$_4$-silane@Ce6/C6 was developed to trigger the aPDT for periodontal therapy, as shown in Figure 7D [177]. Fe$_3$O$_4$ and PS molecules were encapsulated with amphiphilic silane, which formed the hydrophobic interspace between the alkyl chains of silane and the octadecyl groups of oleic acid being bonded on the surface of Fe$_3$O$_4$ NPs. The PS molecules were well dispersed inside the nanocomposites. The hydroxyl of silane stretched out to enhance the water solubility. In addition, to solve the real-time monitoring issue, dye Coumarin 6 (C6) hydrophobic organic molecules were also encapsulated together inside the hydrophobic environment of silane via the hydrophobic interaction, without increasing the particle size. Besides the imaging function with the efficient green emission of C6, another advantage in this design was the real-time aPDT monitoring function [177]. The C6 molecule was not sensitive to red light (630 nm wavelength) but could be co-excited with Ce6 by 405 nm wavelength. Therefore, by visual imaging monitoring of the ratio of the fluorescence of Ce6/C6, the aPDT effect (Ce6 consumption) and distribution profile in periodontal pockets could be monitored in real time. This facilitated the optimization of therapeutic doses and treatment time-windows. Figure 8 shows the real-time monitoring and magnetic targeting functions of the multifunctional nanoparticles. The in vitro antibacterial experiments showed that three single-species periodontitis-related biofilm survival was reduced by about 4–5 orders of magnitude after 3 min of irradiation by the 630 nm light (100 mW·cm^{-2}) [177]. Therefore, the multifunctional design has great potential for antibacterial applications to inhibit the occurrence and progression of periodontitis.

Visible light is usually used as the main light source to trigger the PS for periodontal therapy. Red light is used as the excited light source since it can penetrate deeper than violet, blue, green, or yellow lasers [178]. However, the limited penetration depth of visible light cannot reach deep periodontal pocket to disturb or clear the periodontal pathogens. There is a biological tissue window ranging from 700 nm to 1100 nm in the near-infrared (NIR) light. The excitation of NIR light provides a deeper penetration and lower autofluorescence, and reduces phototoxicity and photodamage side effects [179]. Titanium dioxide (TiO_2) is widely used as a catalyst because of its high stability and good photocatalytic activity. ROS produced by photocatalysis of TiO_2 has high bactericidal and sterilizing effects on oral pathogens [180]. However, one major concern about TiO_2 application is that it can only be activated by ultraviolet (UV) light due to its wide band gap energy of 3.2 eV. Furthermore, the irradiation of UV light may cause DNA damage and cell death. Recently, various upconversion nanoparticles (UCNs) have been developed to solve this problem and are applied widely in cancer therapy. However, little research has been performed on antimicrobial and bacteriostasis. Under near-infrared light irradiation, the UCN core converts the low energy NIR light to high energy UV light, which induces the photocatalysis activity of TiO_2 via an anti-Stokes emission process. Based on this mechanism, a recent study synthesized a core–shell structured $NaYF_4$:Yb^{3+}, Tm^{3+}@TiO_2 (TiO_2-UCNs) which was applied in aPDT for periodontal pathogens (Figure 7E). The UCN cores, $NaYF_4$:Yb^{3+}, Tm^{3+}, were synthesized by thermal decomposition in an oleic acid system [181]. Polyvinylpyrrolidone (PVP) was added for the modification of the surface of UCNs. Subsequently, titanium n-butoxide served as a titanium precursor to coat the TiO_2 shell on the surface of the UCNs under hydrothermal reactions. The results showed that TiO_2-UCNs had excellent antibacterial activity against periodontal pathogens including *P. gingivalis* and *F. nucleatum*. Reductions of 4–5 orders of magnitude in bacteria CFU were achieved in the light groups. At 4 h after the initial irradiation of 2.5 W·cm^{-2} for 5 min, the suspension of bacteria was almost cleared when the concentration of drugs was at 2 mM. Therefore, NIR-triggered aPDT is a promising approach for effective periodontitis treatment.

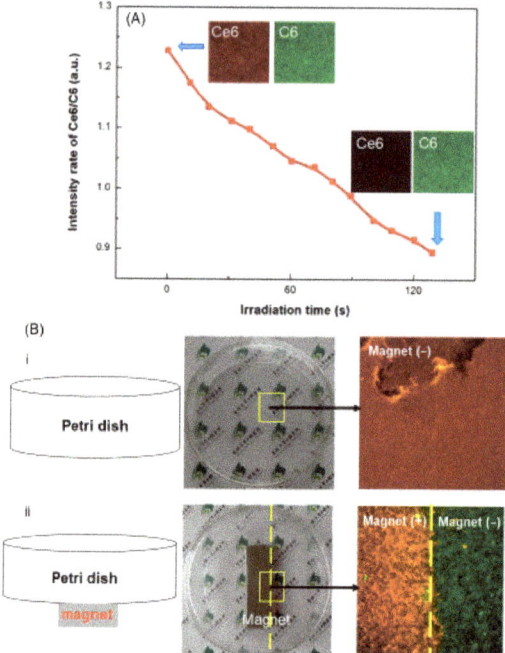

Figure 8. Real-time monitoring and magnetic targeting functions of multifunctional nanoparticles: (**A**) Ratio metric intensity of Ce6/C6 based on the grayscale value of the confocal images from different detection channels in the irradiation time 0–130 s. Inset: The first two and last two images for illustration of the Ce6 consumption. (**B**) Comparison of aPDT effect in the presence of Fe_3O_4-silane@Ce6/C6 magnetic nanoparticles (MNPs, 2.5 µM Ce6) with and without external magnetic field. (i) aPDT effect of Fe_3O_4-silane@Ce6/C6 MNPs without magnetic targeting: (Left) schematic diagram; (middle) photograph showed culture dish without the magnet; and (right) live/dead image in yellow pane. (ii) aPDT effect of Fe_3O_4-silane@Ce6/C6 MNPs with magnetic targeting: (Left) schematic diagram; (middle) photograph showed culture dish with the magnet; and (right) live/dead image in the yellow pane. Live bacteria were stained green. Dead bacteria were stained red. Samples without magnet showed primarily dead bacteria. Samples with magnet had primarily dead bacteria in the magnetic region. (Reproduced with permission from [177]. Elsevier, 2019.)

Despite of many publications on the use of aPDT to combat periodontal pathogens and biofilms, several problems remain. For instance, PS parameters, the strategy of surface modification and doses of PS, and irradiation intensity which determines the type and kinetics of bio-distribution and toxicity at the cellular and tissue level, should be strictly tested to ensure minimal toxicity. In addition, the efficient PS delivery, organ distribution, accumulation, retention, degradation, metabolism and clearance properties should be investigated at the organ level. It is essential for PS to enhance the selectivity of the pathogens without killing the benign microflora in oral environment. Another concern is that the irradiation intensity should be strictly and repeatedly tested before clinical application to avoid oxidative damage to the host cells. In addition, in vivo studies should be performed in animal models to confirm the feasibility for clinical applications. Further studies are needed to solve these problems for clinical application to be successful.

8. Conclusions

This article reviews cutting-edge research on antibacterial properties of novel polymeric materials against periodontal pathogens and oral biofilms. The focus was particularly on antibiotics delivery, functional GTR membrane, dental composite and bonding agents for decay restoration, and PS modification for aPDT enhancement. Due to increasing resistance development, there is a need to find delivery systems compatible with a diversity of antibacterial agents. Novel polymers offer meritorious opportunities and are compatible with a wide range of antibiotics to combat periodontitis. Endowing GTR membranes with antibacterial functions could not only benefit tissue regeneration, but also lower the risk of infection. In addition, the new generation of resins for Class-V restorations offers strong protein-repellent and antibacterial capabilities against periodontal biofilms, and is promising to improve a wide range of dental treatments. Furthermore, polymer modification of PS could increase the dispersion of PS and improve its bioavailability, thus enhancing the aPDT effects against periodontal pathogens. Therefore, the novel bioactive and therapeutic polymers have great potential for treating periodontal disease and other dental diseases.

Author Contributions: M.C., M.Q. and X.S. performed the experiments and data analyses. M.D.W. and L.A contributed to the experiments. B.D. and M.D.W. helped supervise students and researchers in the experiments. P.W. and M.A.M. provided discussions and advised on clinical relevance. H.H.K.X. and J.W. proposed the ideas and wrote the manuscript. C.L. and L.W. contributed to supervising the research and writing the paper.

Funding: This study was financially supported by Natural Science Foundation of China NSFC 81400487 (L.W.), 61775080 (B.D.), and 81671032 (J.W.); China Postdoctoral Science Foundation 2015M581405 and 2017T100213 (L.W.); "The 13th Five-Year Plan" Science Foundation of Education Board Jilin Province JJKH20180235KJ (L.W.); Health Department Research Projects in Jilin Province 2016Q032 (L.W.) and 20165074 (C.L.); a seed grant (H.X.) from the University of Maryland Baltimore; and a bridge fund (HX) from the University of Maryland School of Dentistry.

Acknowledgments: We thank Joseph M. Antonucci, Nancy J. Lin, Sheng Lin-Gibson, Laurence C. Chow, Ashraf F. Fouad, Jirun Sun and Grape J.Y. Xiao for discussions.

Conflicts of Interest: The authors declare no conflict of interest.

References

1. Bartold, P.M.; Van Dyke, T.E. Periodontitis: A host-mediated disruption of microbial homeostasis. Unlearning learned concepts. *Periodontol. 2000* **2013**, *62*, 203–217. [CrossRef] [PubMed]
2. Kassebaum, N.; Bernabé, E.; Dahiya, M.; Bhandari, B.; Murray, C.; Marcenes, W. Global burden of severe periodontitis in 1990–2010: A systematic review and meta-regression. *J. Dent. Res.* **2014**, *93*, 1045–1053. [CrossRef] [PubMed]
3. Albandar, J.; Brunelle, J.; Kingman, A. Destructive periodontal disease in adults 30 years of age and older in the United States, 1988–1994. *J. Periodontol.* **1999**, *70*, 13–29. [CrossRef] [PubMed]
4. Jin, L.; Armitage, G.; Klinge, B.; Lang, N.; Tonetti, M.; Williams, R. Global oral health inequalities: Task group—periodontal disease. *Adv. Dent. Res.* **2011**, *23*, 221–226. [CrossRef] [PubMed]
5. Ravald, N.; Johansson, C.S. Tooth loss in periodontally treated patients. A long–term study of periodontal disease and root caries. *J. Clin. Periodontol.* **2012**, *39*, 73–79. [CrossRef] [PubMed]
6. Prakasam, A.; Elavarasu, S.S.; Natarajan, R.K. Antibiotics in the management of aggressive periodontitis. *J. Pharm. Bioallied Sci.* **2012**, *4* (Suppl. 2), S252–S255. [CrossRef] [PubMed]
7. Jain, N.; Jain, G.K.; Javed, S.; Iqbal, Z.; Talegaonkar, S.; Ahmad, F.J.; Khar, R.K. Recent approaches for the treatment of periodontitis. *Drug Discov. Today* **2008**, *13*, 932–943. [CrossRef] [PubMed]
8. Malmsten, M. Antimicrobial and antiviral hydrogels. *Soft Mater.* **2011**, *7*, 8725–8736. [CrossRef]
9. Ikinci, G.; Şenel, S.; Akıncıbay, H.; Kaş, S.; Erciş, S.; Wilson, C.; Hıncal, A. Effect of chitosan on a periodontal pathogen Porphyromonas gingivalis. *Int. J. Pharm.* **2002**, *235*, 121–127. [CrossRef]
10. Hahnel, S.; Wieser, A.; Lang, R.; Rosentritt, M. Biofilm formation on the surface of modern implant abutment materials. *Clin. Oral Implant. Res.* **2014**, *26*, 1297–1301. [CrossRef]
11. Toledano-Osorio, M.; Babu, J.; Osorio, R.; Medina-Castillo, A.; García-Godoy, F.; Toledano, M. Modified Polymeric Nanoparticles Exert In vitro Antimicrobial Activity Against Oral Bacteria. *Materials* **2018**, *11*, 1013. [CrossRef] [PubMed]
12. Nasajpour, A.; Ansari, S.; Rinoldi, C.; Rad, A.S.; Aghaloo, T.; Shin, S.R.; Mishra, Y.K.; Adelung, R.; Swieszkowski, W.; Annabi, N. A multifunctional polymeric periodontal membrane with osteogenic and antibacterial characteristics. *Adv. Funct. Mater.* **2017**, *28*, 1703437. [CrossRef]

13. Saarani, N.N.; Jamuna-Thevi, K.; Shahab, N.; Hermawan, H.; Saidin, S. Antibacterial efficacy of triple-layered poly (lactic-co-glycolic acid)/nanoapatite/lauric acid guided bone regeneration membrane on periodontal bacteria. *Dent. Mater. J.* **2017**, *36*, 260–265. [CrossRef] [PubMed]
14. Shao, J.; Yu, N.; Kolwijck, E.; Wang, B.; Tan, K.W.; Jansen, J.A.; Walboomers, X.F.; Yang, F. Biological evaluation of silver nanoparticles incorporated into chitosan-based membranes. *Nanomedicine* **2017**, *12*, 2771–2785. [CrossRef] [PubMed]
15. Sigusch, B.; Dietsch, S.; Berg, A.; Voelpel, A.; Guellmar, A.; Rabe, U.; Schnabelrauch, M.; Steen, D.; Gitter, B.; Albrecht, V. Antimicrobial photodynamic active biomaterials for periodontal regeneration. *Dent. Mater.* **2018**, *34*, 1542–1554. [CrossRef] [PubMed]
16. Sela, M.N.; Babitski, E.; Steinberg, D.; Kohavi, D.; Rosen, G. Degradation of collagen-guided tissue regeneration membranes by proteolytic enzymes of Porphyromonas gingivalis and its inhibition by antibacterial agents. *Clin. Oral Implant. Res.* **2009**, *20*, 496–502. [CrossRef]
17. Munoz-Bonilla, A.; Fernández-García, M. Polymeric materials with antimicrobial activity. *Prog. Polym. Sci.* **2012**, *37*, 281–339. [CrossRef]
18. Li, S.; Dong, S.; Xu, W.; Tu, S.; Yan, L.; Zhao, C.; Ding, J.; Chen, X. Antibacterial Hydrogels. *Adv. Sci.* **2018**, *5*, 1700527. [CrossRef]
19. Chen, J.; Wang, F.; Liu, Q.; Du, J. Antibacterial polymeric nanostructures for biomedical applications. *Chem. Commun.* **2014**, *50*, 14482–14493. [CrossRef]
20. Joshi, D.; Garg, T.; Goyal, A.K.; Rath, G. Advanced drug delivery approaches against periodontitis. *Drug Deliv.* **2014**, *23*, 363–377. [CrossRef]
21. Pragati, S.; Ashok, S.; Kuldeep, S. Recent advances in periodontal drug delivery systems. *Int. J. Drug Deliv.* **2009**, *1*, 1–14.
22. Hau, H.; Rohanizadeh, R.; Ghadiri, M.; Chrzanowski, W. A mini-review on novel intraperiodontal pocket drug delivery materials for the treatment of periodontal diseases. *Drug Deliv. Transl. Res.* **2013**, *4*, 295–301. [CrossRef] [PubMed]
23. Bottino, M.C.; Thomas, V.; Schmidt, G.; Vohra, Y.K.; Chu, T.-M.G.; Kowolik, M.J.; Janowski, G.M. Recent advances in the development of GTR/GBR membranes for periodontal regeneration—A materials perspective. *Dent. Mater.* **2012**, *28*, 703–721. [CrossRef] [PubMed]
24. Gentile, P.; Chiono, V.; Tonda-Turo, C.; Ferreira, A.M.; Ciardelli, G. Polymeric membranes for guided bone regeneration. *Biotechnol. J.* **2011**, *6*, 1187–1197. [CrossRef] [PubMed]
25. Puppi, D.; Chiellini, F.; Piras, A.; Chiellini, E. Polymeric materials for bone and cartilage repair. *Prog. Polym. Sci.* **2010**, *35*, 403–440. [CrossRef]
26. Ferracane, J.L. Resin composite—State of the art. *Dent. Mater.* **2011**, *27*, 29–38. [CrossRef] [PubMed]
27. Breschi, L.; Mazzoni, A.; Ruggeri, A.; Cadenaro, M.; Di Lenarda, R.; Dorigo, E.D.S. Dental adhesion review: Aging and stability of the bonded interface. *Dent. Mater.* **2008**, *24*, 90–101. [CrossRef] [PubMed]
28. Spencer, P.; Ye, Q.; Park, J.; Topp, E.M.; Misra, A.; Marangos, O.; Wang, Y.; Bohaty, B.S.; Singh, V.; Sene, F. Adhesive/dentin interface: The weak link in the composite restoration. *Ann. Biomed. Eng.* **2010**, *38*, 1989–2003. [CrossRef]
29. Milward, P.J.; Adusei, G.O.; Lynch, C.D. Improving some selected properties of dental polyacid-modified composite resins. *Dent. Mater.* **2011**, *27*, 997–1002. [CrossRef]
30. Ilie, N.; Hilton, T.; Heintze, S.; Hickel, R.; Watts, D.; Silikas, N.; Stansbury, J.; Cadenaro, M.; Ferracane, J. Academy of Dental Materials guidance—Resin composites: Part I—Mechanical properties. *Dent. Mater.* **2017**, *33*, 880–894. [CrossRef]
31. Xu, X.; Ling, L.; Wang, R.; Burgess, J.O. Formulation and characterization of a novel fluoride-releasing dental composite. *Dent. Mater.* **2006**, *22*, 1014–1023. [CrossRef] [PubMed]
32. Ferracane, J.L. Placing dental composites—A stressful experience. *Oper. Dent.* **2008**, *33*, 247–257. [CrossRef] [PubMed]
33. Wei, Y.; Silikas, N.; Zhang, Z.; Watts, D.C. Hygroscopic dimensional changes of self-adhering and new resin-matrix composites during water sorption/desorption cycles. *Dent. Mater.* **2011**, *27*, 259–266. [CrossRef] [PubMed]
34. Huang, S.; Podgórski, M.; Zhang, X.; Sinha, J.; Claudino, M.; Stansbury, J.; Bowman, C. Dental restorative materials based on thiol-Michael photopolymerization. *J. Dent. Res.* **2018**, *97*, 530–536. [CrossRef] [PubMed]

35. Vallittu, P.K.; Boccaccini, A.R.; Hupa, L.; Watts, D.C. Bioactive dental materials—Do they exist and what does bioactivity mean? *Dent. Mater.* **2018**, *34*, 693–694. [CrossRef] [PubMed]
36. Kitagawa, H.; Miki-Oka, S.; Mayanagi, G.; Abiko, Y.; Takahashi, N.; Imazato, S. Inhibitory effect of resin composite containing S-PRG filler on Streptococcus mutans glucose metabolism. *J. Dent.* **2018**, *70*, 92–96. [CrossRef] [PubMed]
37. Hajishengallis, G. Periodontitis: From microbial immune subversion to systemic inflammation. *Nat. Rev. Immunol.* **2015**, *15*, 30–44. [CrossRef] [PubMed]
38. Zupančič, Š.; Preem, L.; Kristl, J.; Putriņš, M.; Tenson, T.; Kocbek, P.; Kogermann, K. Impact of PCL nanofiber mat structural properties on hydrophilic drug release and antibacterial activity on periodontal pathogens. *Eur. J. Pharm. Sci.* **2018**, *122*, 347–358. [CrossRef]
39. Joshi, D.; Garg, T.; K Goyal, A.; Rath, G. Development and characterization of novel medicated nanofibers against periodontitis. *Curr. Drug Deliv.* **2015**, *12*, 564–577. [CrossRef]
40. Monteiro, A.P.; Rocha, C.M.; Oliveira, M.F.; Gontijo, S.M.; Agudelo, R.R.; Sinisterra, R.D.; Cortés, M.E. Nanofibers containing tetracycline/β-cyclodextrin: Physico-chemical characterization and antimicrobial evaluation. *Carbohyd. Polym.* **2017**, *156*, 417–426. [CrossRef]
41. Reise, M.; Wyrwa, R.; Müller, U.; Zylinski, M.; Völpel, A.; Schnabelrauch, M.; Berg, A.; Jandt, K.D.; Watts, D.C.; Sigusch, B.W. Release of metronidazole from electrospun poly (L-lactide-co-D/L-lactide) fibers for local periodontitis treatment. *Dent. Mater.* **2012**, *28*, 179–188. [CrossRef] [PubMed]
42. Friesen, L.R.; Williams, K.B.; Krause, L.S.; Killoy, W.J. Controlled local delivery of tetracycline with polymer strips in the treatment of periodontitis. *J. Periodontol.* **2002**, *73*, 13–19. [CrossRef] [PubMed]
43. Ahmed, M.G.; Charyulu, R.N.; Harish, N.; Prabhu, P. Formulation and in-vitro evaluation of Chitosan films containing tetracycline for the treatment of periodontitis. *Asian J. Pharm.* **2009**, *3*, 113. [CrossRef]
44. Loo, S.C.J.; Tan, Z.Y.S.; Chow, Y.J.; Lin, S.L.I. Drug release from irradiated PLGA and PLLA multi-layered films. *J. Pharm. Sci.* **2010**, *99*, 3060–3071. [CrossRef]
45. Heller, J.; Barr, J.; Ng, S.; Shen, H.-R.; Schwach-Abdellaoui, K.; Gurny, R.; Vivien-Castioni, N.; Loup, P.; Baehni, P.; Mombelli, A. Development and applications of injectable poly (ortho esters) for pain control and periodontal treatment. *Biomaterials* **2002**, *23*, 4397–4404. [CrossRef]
46. Phaechamud, T.; Mahadlek, J.; Chuenbarn, T. In situ forming gel comprising bleached shellac loaded with antimicrobial drugs for periodontitis treatment. *Mater. Des.* **2016**, *89*, 294–303. [CrossRef]
47. Gjoseva, S.; Geskovski, N.; Sazdovska, S.D.; Popeski-Dimovski, R.; Petruševski, G.; Mladenovska, K.; Goracinova, K. Design and biological response of doxycycline loaded chitosan microparticles for periodontal disease treatment. *Carbohyd. Polym.* **2018**, *186*, 260–272. [CrossRef] [PubMed]
48. De Souza Ferreira, S.B.; de Assis Dias, B.R.; Obregón, C.S.; Gomes, C.C.; de Araújo Pereira, R.R.; Ribeiro Godoy, J.S.; Estivalet Svidzinski, T.I.; Bruschi, M.L. Microparticles containing propolis and metronidazole: In vitro characterization, release study and antimicrobial activity against periodontal pathogens. *Pharm. Dev. Technol.* **2013**, *19*, 173–180. [CrossRef] [PubMed]
49. Kilicarslan, M.; Gumustas, M.; Yildiz, S.; Baykara, T. Preparation and characterization of chitosan-based spray-dried microparticles for the delivery of clindamycin phosphate to periodontal pockets. *Curr. Drug Deliv.* **2014**, *11*, 98–111. [CrossRef] [PubMed]
50. Yao, W.; Xu, P.; Pang, Z.; Zhao, J.; Chai, Z.; Li, X.; Li, H.; Jiang, M.; Cheng, H.; Zhang, B. Local delivery of minocycline-loaded PEG-PLA nanoparticles for the enhanced treatment of periodontitis in dogs. *Int. J. Nanomed.* **2014**, *9*, 3963–3970.
51. Shrestha, A.; Hamblin, M.R.; Kishen, A. Photoactivated rose bengal functionalized chitosan nanoparticles produce antibacterial/biofilm activity and stabilize dentin-collagen. *Nanomed. Nanotechnol.* **2014**, *10*, 491–501. [CrossRef] [PubMed]
52. Ignjatović, N.; Wu, V.; Ajduković, Z.; Mihajilov-Krstev, T.; Uskoković, V.; Uskoković, D. Chitosan-PLGA polymer blends as coatings for hydroxyapatite nanoparticles and their effect on antimicrobial properties, osteoconductivity and regeneration of osseous tissues. *Mater. Sci. Eng. C* **2016**, *60*, 357–364. [CrossRef] [PubMed]
53. Di Turi, G.; Riggio, C.; Vittorio, O.; Marconcini, S.; Briguglio, F.; Funel, N.; Campani, D.; Barone, A.; Raffa, V.; Covani, U. Sub-Micrometric Liposomes as Drug Delivery Systems in the Treatment and Periodontitis. *Int. J. Immunopathol. Pharmacol.* **2012**, *25*, 657–670. [CrossRef] [PubMed]

54. Xu, X.; Wang, L.; Luo, Z.; Ni, Y.; Sun, H.; Gao, X.; Li, Y.; Zhang, S.; Li, Y.; Wei, S. Facile and Versatile Strategy for Construction of Anti-Inflammatory and Antibacterial Surfaces with Polydopamine-Mediated Liposomes Releasing Dexamethasone and Minocycline for Potential Implant Applications. *ACS Appl. Mater. Interfaces* **2017**, *9*, 43300–43314. [CrossRef] [PubMed]
55. Sundararaj, S.C.; Thomas, M.V.; Peyyala, R.; Dziubla, T.D.; Puleo, D.A. Design of a multiple drug delivery system directed at periodontitis. *Biomaterials* **2013**, *34*, 8835–8842. [CrossRef]
56. Gad, H.A.; El-Nabarawi, M.A.; El-Hady, S.S.A. Formulation and evaluation of PLA and PLGA in situ implants containing secnidazole and/or doxycycline for treatment of periodontitis. *AAPS PharmSciTech* **2008**, *9*, 878–884. [CrossRef]
57. Persson, G.R.; Salvi, G.E.; Heitz-Mayfield, L.J.; Lang, N.P. Antimicrobial therapy using a local drug delivery system (Arestin®) in the treatment of peri-implantitis. I: Microbiological outcomes. *Clin. Oral Implant. Res.* **2006**, *17*, 386–393. [CrossRef]
58. Ganguly, A.; Ian, C.K.; Sheshala, R.; Sahu, P.S.; Al-Waeli, H.; Meka, V.S. Application of diverse natural polymers in the design of oral gels for the treatment of periodontal diseases. *J. Mater. Sci. Mater. Med.* **2017**, *28*, 39. [CrossRef]
59. Garrett, S.; Johnson, L.; Drisko, C.H.; Adams, D.F.; Bandt, C.; Beiswanger, B.; Bogle, G.; Donly, K.; Hallmon, W.W.; Hancock, E.B. Two multi-center studies evaluating locally delivered doxycycline hyclate, placebo control, oral hygiene, and scaling and root planing in the treatment of periodontitis. *J. Periodontol.* **1999**, *70*, 490–503. [CrossRef]
60. Stoller, N.H.; Johnson, L.R.; Trapnell, S.; Harrold, C.Q.; Garrett, S. The pharmacokinetic profile of a biodegradable controlled-release delivery system containing doxycycline compared to systemically delivered doxycycline in gingival crevicular fluid, saliva, and serum. *J. Periodontol.* **1998**, *69*, 1085–1091. [CrossRef]
61. Yue, I.C.; Poff, J.; Cortés, M.A.E.; Sinisterra, R.D.; Faris, C.B.; Hildgen, P.; Langer, R.; Shastri, V.P. A novel polymeric chlorhexidine delivery device for the treatment of periodontal disease. *Biomaterials* **2004**, *25*, 3743–3750. [CrossRef] [PubMed]
62. Hirasawa, M.; Takada, K.; Makimura, M.; Otake, S. Improvement of periodontal status by green tea catechin using a local delivery system: A clinical pilot study. *J. Period. Res.* **2002**, *37*, 433–438. [CrossRef]
63. Yang, B.; Lv, W.; Deng, Y. Drug loaded poly (glycerol sebacate) as a local drug delivery system for the treatment of periodontal disease. *RSC Adv.* **2017**, *7*, 37426–37435. [CrossRef]
64. Rao, S.K.; Setty, S.; Acharya, A.B.; Thakur, S.L. Efficacy of locally-delivered doxycycline microspheres in chronic localized periodontitis and on Porphyromonas gingivalis. *J. Investig. Clin. Dent.* **2012**, *3*, 128–134. [CrossRef] [PubMed]
65. Grossi, S.G.; Goodson, J.M.; Gunsolley, J.C.; Otomo-Corgel, J.; Bland, P.S.; Doherty, F.; Comiskey, J. Mechanical therapy with adjunctive minocycline microspheres reduces red-complex bacteria in smokers. *J. Periodontol.* **2007**, *78*, 1741–1750. [CrossRef] [PubMed]
66. Wayakanon, K.; Thornhill, M.H.; Douglas, C.I.; Lewis, A.L.; Warren, N.J.; Pinnock, A.; Armes, S.P.; Battaglia, G.; Murdoch, C. Polymersome-mediated intracellular delivery of antibiotics to treat Porphyromonas gingivalis-infected oral epithelial cells. *FASEB J.* **2013**, *27*, 4455–4465. [CrossRef] [PubMed]
67. Kashi, T.S.J.; Eskandarion, S.; Esfandyari-Manesh, M.; Marashi, S.M.A.; Samadi, N.; Fatemi, S.M.; Atyabi, F.; Eshraghi, S.; Dinarvand, R. Improved drug loading and antibacterial activity of minocycline-loaded PLGA nanoparticles prepared by solid/oil/water ion pairing method. *Int. J. Nanomed.* **2012**, *7*, 221.
68. Moulari, B.; Lboutounne, H.; Chaumont, J.-P.; Guillaume, Y.; Millet, J.; Pellequer, Y. Potentiation of the bactericidal activity of Harungana madagascariensis Lam. ex Poir.(Hypericaceae) leaf extract against oral bacteria using poly (D,L-lactide-co-glycolide) nanoparticles: In vitro study. *Acta Odontol. Scand.* **2006**, *64*, 153–158. [CrossRef] [PubMed]
69. Garg, T.; Goyal, A.K. Medicated chewing gum: Patient compliance oral drug delivery system. *Drug Deliv. Lett.* **2014**, *4*, 72–78. [CrossRef]
70. Garg, T.; Goyal, A.K. Biomaterial-based scaffolds–current status and future directions. *Expert Opin. Drug Deliv.* **2014**, *11*, 767–789. [CrossRef]
71. Gentile, P.; Frongia, M.E.; Cardellach, M.; Miller, C.A.; Stafford, G.P.; Leggett, G.J.; Hatton, P.V. Functionalised nanoscale coatings using layer-by-layer assembly for imparting antibacterial properties to polylactide-co-glycolide surfaces. *Acta Biomater.* **2015**, *21*, 35–43. [CrossRef] [PubMed]

72. Osorio, R.; Alfonso-Rodríguez, C.A.; Medina-Castillo, A.L.; Alaminos, M.; Toledano, M. Bioactive polymeric nanoparticles for periodontal therapy. *PLoS ONE* **2016**, *11*, e0166217. [CrossRef] [PubMed]
73. Sánchez, M.; Toledano-Osorio, M.; Bueno, J.; Figuero, E.; Toledano, M.; Medina-Castillo, A.; Osorio, R.; Herrera, D.; Sanz, M. Antibacterial effects of polymeric PolymP-n Active nanoparticles. An in vitro biofilm study. *Dent. Mater.* **2019**, *35*, 156–168. [CrossRef] [PubMed]
74. Gorr, S.U.; Abdolhosseini, M. Antimicrobial peptides and periodontal disease. *J. Clin. Periodont.* **2011**, *38*, 126–141. [CrossRef] [PubMed]
75. Ouhara, K.; Komatsuzawa, H.; Yamada, S.; Shiba, H.; Fujiwara, T.; Ohara, M.; Sayama, K.; Hashimoto, K.; Kurihara, H.; Sugai, M. Susceptibilities of periodontopathogenic and cariogenic bacteria to antibacterial peptides, β-defensins and LL37, produced by human epithelial cells. *J. Antimicrob. Chemother.* **2005**, *55*, 888–896. [CrossRef] [PubMed]
76. Choi, B.-K.; Kim, K.-Y.; Yoo, Y.-J.; Oh, S.-J.; Choi, J.-H.; Kim, C.-Y. In vitro antimicrobial activity of a chitooligosaccharide mixture against Actinobacillus actinomycetemcomitans and Streptococcus mutans. *Int. J. Antimicrob. Agents* **2001**, *18*, 553–557. [CrossRef]
77. Jain, A.; Duvvuri, L.S.; Farah, S.; Beyth, N.; Domb, A.J.; Khan, W. Antimicrobial polymers. *Adv. Healthc. Mater.* **2014**, *3*, 1969–1985. [CrossRef]
78. Costa, E.; Silva, S.; Pina, C.; Tavaria, F.; Pintado, M. Evaluation and insights into chitosan antimicrobial activity against anaerobic oral pathogens. *Anaerobe* **2012**, *18*, 305–309. [CrossRef]
79. Arancibia, R.; Maturana, C.; Silva, D.; Tobar, N.; Tapia, C.; Salazar, J.; Martínez, J.; Smith, P. Effects of chitosan particles in periodontal pathogens and gingival fibroblasts. *J. Dent. Res.* **2013**, *92*, 740–745. [CrossRef]
80. Sarasam, A.R.; Brown, P.; Khajotia, S.S.; Dmytryk, J.J.; Madihally, S.V. Antibacterial activity of chitosan-based matrices on oral pathogens. *J. Mater. Sci-Mater. Med.* **2008**, *19*, 1083–1090. [CrossRef]
81. Lam, S.J.; O'Brien-Simpson, N.M.; Pantarat, N.; Sulistio, A.; Wong, E.H.; Chen, Y.-Y.; Lenzo, J.C.; Holden, J.A.; Blencowe, A.; Reynolds, E.C. Combating multidrug-resistant Gram-negative bacteria with structurally nanoengineered antimicrobial peptide polymers. *Nat. Microbiol.* **2016**, *1*, 16162. [CrossRef] [PubMed]
82. Da Silva-Boghossian, C.M.; do Souto, R.M.; Luiz, R.R.; Colombo, A.P.V. Association of red complex, A. actinomycetemcomitans and non-oral bacteria with periodontal diseases. *Arch. Oral Biol.* **2011**, *56*, 899–906. [CrossRef] [PubMed]
83. Coello, R.; Charlett, A.; Wilson, J.; Ward, V.; Pearson, A.; Borriello, P. Adverse impact of surgical site infections in English hospitals. *J. Hosp. Infect.* **2005**, *60*, 93–103. [CrossRef]
84. Campoccia, D.; Montanaro, L.; Arciola, C.R. A review of the clinical implications of anti-infective biomaterials and infection-resistant surfaces. *Biomaterials* **2013**, *34*, 8018–8029. [CrossRef] [PubMed]
85. Löfmark, S.; Edlund, C.; Nord, C.E. Metronidazole is still the drug of choice for treatment of anaerobic infections. *Clin. Infect. Dis.* **2010**, *50*, S16–S23. [CrossRef] [PubMed]
86. Xue, J.; He, M.; Niu, Y.; Liu, H.; Crawford, A.; Coates, P.; Chen, D.; Shi, R.; Zhang, L. Preparation and in vivo efficient anti-infection property of GTR/GBR implant made by metronidazole loaded electrospun polycaprolactone nanofiber membrane. *Int. J. Pharm.* **2014**, *475*, 566–577. [CrossRef]
87. Xue, J.; He, M.; Liu, H.; Niu, Y.; Crawford, A.; Coates, P.D.; Chen, D.; Shi, R.; Zhang, L. Drug loaded homogeneous electrospun PCL/gelatin hybrid nanofiber structures for anti-infective tissue regeneration membranes. *Biomaterials* **2014**, *35*, 9395–9405. [CrossRef]
88. Xue, J.; Niu, Y.; Gong, M.; Shi, R.; Chen, D.; Zhang, L.; Lvov, Y. Electrospun microfiber membranes embedded with drug-loaded clay nanotubes for sustained antimicrobial protection. *ACS Nano* **2015**, *9*, 1600–1612. [CrossRef]
89. Bottino, M.C.; Thomas, V.; Janowski, G.M. A novel spatially designed and functionally graded electrospun membrane for periodontal regeneration. *Acta Biomater.* **2011**, *7*, 216–224. [CrossRef]
90. Cheng, C.F.; Lee, Y.Y.; Chi, L.Y.; Chen, Y.T.; Hung, S.L.; Ling, L.J. Bacterial Penetration Through Antibiotic-Loaded Guided Tissue Regeneration Membranes. *J. Periodontol.* **2009**, *80*, 1471–1478. [CrossRef]
91. Park, Y.J.; Lee, Y.M.; Park, S.N.; Lee, J.Y.; Ku, Y.; Chung, C.P.; Lee, S.J. Enhanced guided bone regeneration by controlled tetracycline release from poly (L-lactide) barrier membranes. *J. Biomed. Mater. Res.* **2000**, *51*, 391–397. [CrossRef]
92. Chen, Y.-T.; Hung, S.-L.; Lin, L.-W.; Chi, L.-Y.; Ling, L.-J. Attachment of periodontal ligament cells to chlorhexidine-loaded guided tissue regeneration membranes. *J. Periodontol.* **2003**, *74*, 1652–1659. [CrossRef] [PubMed]

93. Rani, S.; Chandra, R.V.; Reddy, A.; Reddy, B.; Nagarajan, S.; Naveen, A. Evaluation of the Antibacterial Effect of Silver Nanoparticles on Guided Tissue Regeneration Membrane Colonization-An in vitro Study. *J. Int. Acad. Periodontol.* **2015**, *17*, 66–76. [PubMed]
94. Hung, S.L.; Lin, Y.W.; Chen, Y.T.; Ling, L.J. Attachment of periodontal ligament cells onto various antibiotics-loaded GTR membranes. *Int. J. Periodontics Restor. Dent.* **2005**, *25*, 265–275.
95. Chou, A.-H.; LeGeros, R.Z.; Chen, Z.; Li, Y. Antibacterial effect of zinc phosphate mineralized guided bone regeneration membranes. *Implant Dent.* **2007**, *16*, 89–100. [CrossRef]
96. Lee, D.; Lee, S.J.; Moon, J.-H.; Kim, J.H.; Heo, D.N.; Bang, J.B.; Lim, H.-N.; Kwon, I.K. Preparation of antibacterial chitosan membranes containing silver nanoparticles for dental barrier membrane applications. *J. Ind. Eng. Chem.* **2018**, *66*, 196–202. [CrossRef]
97. Zamani, M.; Morshed, M.; Varshosaz, J.; Jannesari, M. Controlled release of metronidazole benzoate from poly ε-caprolactone electrospun nanofibers for periodontal diseases. *Eur. J. Pharm. Biopharm.* **2010**, *75*, 179–185. [CrossRef] [PubMed]
98. Wang, J.; Wang, L.; Zhou, Z.; Lai, H.; Xu, P.; Liao, L.; Wei, J. Biodegradable polymer membranes applied in guided bone/tissue regeneration: A review. *Polymers* **2016**, *8*, 115. [CrossRef]
99. Imazato, S.; Torii, M.; Tsuchitani, Y.; McCabe, J.; Russell, R. Incorporation of bacterial inhibitor into resin composite. *J. Dent. Res.* **1994**, *73*, 1437–1443. [CrossRef]
100. Imazato, S. Antibacterial properties of resin composites and dentin bonding systems. *Dent. Mater.* **2003**, *19*, 449–457. [CrossRef]
101. Imazato, S.; Ebi, N.; Tarumi, H.; Russell, R.R.; Kaneko, T.; Ebisu, S. Bactericidal activity and cytotoxicity of antibacterial monomer MDPB. *Biomaterials* **1999**, *20*, 899–903. [CrossRef]
102. Xu, X.; Wang, Y.; Liao, S.; Wen, Z.T.; Fan, Y. Synthesis and characterization of antibacterial dental monomers and composites. *J. Bioimed. Mater. Res. A* **2012**, *100*, 1151–1162. [CrossRef] [PubMed]
103. Lu, G.; Wu, D.; Fu, R. Studies on the synthesis and antibacterial activities of polymeric quaternary ammonium salts from dimethylaminoethyl methacrylate. *React. Funct. Polym.* **2007**, *67*, 355–366. [CrossRef]
104. He, J.; Söderling, E.; Österblad, M.; Vallittu, P.K.; Lassila, L.V. Synthesis of methacrylate monomers with antibacterial effects against S. mutans. *Molecules* **2011**, *16*, 9755–9763. [CrossRef] [PubMed]
105. Cocco, A.R.; da Rosa, W.L.D.O.; da Silva, A.F.; Lund, R.G.; Piva, E. A systematic review about antibacterial monomers used in dental adhesive systems: Current status and further prospects. *Dent. Mater.* **2015**, *31*, 1345–1362. [CrossRef] [PubMed]
106. Imazato, S.; Ma, S.; Chen, J.; Xu, H.H.K. Therapeutic polymers for dental adhesives: Loading resins with bio-active components. *Dent. Mater.* **2014**, *30*, 97–104. [CrossRef]
107. Xue, Y.; Xiao, H.; Zhang, Y. Antimicrobial polymeric materials with quaternary ammonium and phosphonium salts. *Int. J. Mol. Sci.* **2015**, *16*, 3626–3655. [CrossRef]
108. Makvandi, P.; Jamaledin, R.; Jabbari, M.; Nikfarjam, N.; Borzacchiello, A. Antibacterial quaternary ammonium compounds in dental materials: A systematic review. *Dent. Mater.* **2018**, *34*, 851–867. [CrossRef]
109. Melo, M.A.; Guedes, S.F.; Xu, H.H.; Rodrigues, L.K. Nanotechnology-based restorative materials for dental caries management. *Trends Biotechnol.* **2013**, *31*, 459–467. [CrossRef]
110. Cheng, L.; Zhang, K.; Zhang, N.; Melo, M.; Weir, M.; Zhou, X.; Bai, Y.; Reynolds, M.; Xu, H. Developing a new generation of antimicrobial and bioactive dental resins. *J. Dent. Res.* **2017**, *96*, 855–863. [CrossRef]
111. Zhang, N.; Zhang, K.; Xie, X.; Dai, Z.; Zhao, Z.; Imazato, S.; Al-Dulaijan, Y.; Al-Qarni, F.; Weir, M.; Reynolds, M. Nanostructured Polymeric Materials with Protein-Repellent and Anti-Caries Properties for Dental Applications. *Nanomaterials* **2018**, *8*, 393. [CrossRef] [PubMed]
112. Zhang, K.; Baras, B.; Lynch, C.; Weir, M.; Melo, M.; Li, Y.; Reynolds, M.; Bai, Y.; Wang, L.; Wang, S. Developing a New Generation of Therapeutic Dental Polymers to Inhibit Oral Biofilms and Protect Teeth. *Materials* **2018**, *11*, 1747. [CrossRef]
113. Fure, S. Ten-year incidence of tooth loss and dental caries in elderly Swedish individuals. *Caries Res.* **2003**, *37*, 462–469. [CrossRef] [PubMed]
114. Heasman, P.A.; Ritchie, M.; Asuni, A.; Gavillet, E.; Simonsen, J.L.; Nyvad, B. Gingival recession and root caries in the ageing population: A critical evaluation of treatments. *J. Clin. Periodontol.* **2017**, *44*, S178–S193. [CrossRef] [PubMed]

115. Kumar, P.S.; Griffen, A.L.; Moeschberger, M.L.; Leys, E.J. Identification of candidate periodontal pathogens and beneficial species by quantitative 16S clonal analysis. *J. Clin. Microbiol.* **2005**, *43*, 3944–3955. [CrossRef] [PubMed]
116. Charalampakis, G.; Leonhardt, Å.; Rabe, P.; Dahlén, G. Clinical and microbiological characteristics of peri-implantitis cases: A retrospective multicentre study. *Clin. Oral Implant. Res.* **2012**, *23*, 1045–1054. [CrossRef] [PubMed]
117. Signat, B.; Roques, C.; Poulet, P.; Duffaut, D. Role of Fusobacterium nucleatum in periodontal health and disease. *Curr. Issues Mol. Biol.* **2011**, *13*, 25–36. [PubMed]
118. Saito, A.; Inagaki, S.; Kimizuka, R.; Okuda, K.; Hosaka, Y.; Nakagawa, T.; Ishihara, K. Fusobacterium nucleatum enhances invasion of human gingival epithelial and aortic endothelial cells by Porphyromonas gingivalis. *FEMS Immunol. Med. Microbiol.* **2008**, *54*, 349–355. [CrossRef] [PubMed]
119. Souto, R.; Colombo, A.P.V. Prevalence of Enterococcus faecalis in subgingival biofilm and saliva of subjects with chronic periodontal infection. *Arch. Oral Biol.* **2008**, *53*, 155–160. [CrossRef]
120. Wang, L.; Melo, M.A.; Weir, M.D.; Xie, X.; Reynolds, M.A.; Xu, H.H. Novel bioactive nanocomposite for Class-V restorations to inhibit periodontitis-related pathogens. *Dent. Mater.* **2016**, *33*, e351–e361. [CrossRef]
121. Periasamy, S.; Kolenbrander, P.E. Mutualistic biofilm communities develop with Porphyromonas gingivalis and initial, early, and late colonizers of enamel. *J. Bacteriol.* **2009**, *191*, 6804–6811. [CrossRef] [PubMed]
122. Lewis, A.L. Phosphorylcholine-based polymers and their use in the prevention of biofouling. *Colloids Surf. B* **2000**, *18*, 261–275. [CrossRef]
123. Kuiper, K.K.; Nordrehaug, J.E. Early mobilization after protamine reversal of heparin following implantation of phosphorylcholine-coated stents in totally occluded coronary arteries. *Am. J. Cardiol.* **2000**, *85*, 698–702. [CrossRef]
124. Moro, T.; Kawaguchi, H.; Ishihara, K.; Kyomoto, M.; Karita, T.; Ito, H.; Nakamura, K.; Takatori, Y. Wear resistance of artificial hip joints with poly (2-methacryloyloxyethyl phosphorylcholine) grafted polyethylene: Comparisons with the effect of polyethylene cross-linking and ceramic femoral heads. *Biomaterials* **2009**, *30*, 2995–3001. [CrossRef] [PubMed]
125. Sibarani, J.; Takai, M.; Ishihara, K. Surface modification on microfluidic devices with 2-methacryloyloxyethyl phosphorylcholine polymers for reducing unfavorable protein adsorption. *Colloids Surf. B* **2007**, *54*, 88–93. [CrossRef] [PubMed]
126. Lewis, A.; Tolhurst, L.; Stratford, P. Analysis of a phosphorylcholine-based polymer coating on a coronary stent pre-and post-implantation. *Biomaterials* **2002**, *23*, 1697–1706. [CrossRef]
127. Wang, L.; Xie, X.; Imazato, S.; Weir, M.D.; Reynolds, M.A.; Xu, H.H. A protein-repellent and antibacterial nanocomposite for Class-V restorations to inhibit periodontitis-related pathogens. *Mater. Sci. Eng. C* **2016**, *67*, 702–710. [CrossRef] [PubMed]
128. Kolenbrander, P.E.; Palmer, R.J., Jr.; Periasamy, S.; Jakubovics, N.S. Oral multispecies biofilm development and the key role of cell–cell distance. *Nat. Rev. Microbiol.* **2010**, *8*, 471–480. [CrossRef]
129. Hall-Stoodley, L.; Costerton, J.W.; Stoodley, P. Bacterial biofilms: From the natural environment to infectious diseases. *Nat. Rev. Microbiol.* **2004**, *2*, 95–108. [CrossRef]
130. Zollinger, L.; Schnyder, S.; Nietzsche, S.; Sculean, A.; Eick, S. In-vitro activity of taurolidine on single species and a multispecies population associated with periodontitis. *Anaerobe* **2015**, *23*, 18–23. [CrossRef]
131. Fujise, O.; Hamachi, T.; Inoue, K.; Miura, M.; Maeda, K. Microbiological markers for prediction and assessment of treatment outcome following non-surgical periodontal therapy. *J. Periodontol.* **2002**, *73*, 1253–1259. [CrossRef] [PubMed]
132. Wang, L.; Qi, M.; Weir, M.D.; Reynolds, M.A.; Li, C.; Zhou, C.; Xu., H.H.K. Effects of single species versus multi-species periodontal biofilms on the antibacterial efficacy of a novel bioactive Class-V nanocomposite. *Dent. Mater.* **2018**. submitted.
133. Xiao, S.; Liang, K.; Tay, F.R.; Weir, M.D.; Melo, M.A.S.; Wang, L.; Wu, Y.; Oates, T.W.; Ding, Y.; Xu, H.H.K. Novel multifunctional nanocomposite for root caries restorations to inhibit periodontitis-related pathogens. *J. Dent.* **2019**. [CrossRef] [PubMed]
134. Cheng, Y.J.; Zeiger, D.N.; Howarter, J.A.; Zhang, X.; Lin, N.J.; Antonucci, J.M.; Lin-Gibson, S. In situ formation of silver nanoparticles in photocrosslinking polymers. *J. Biomed. Mater. Res. B* **2011**, *97*, 124–131. [CrossRef] [PubMed]

135. Cheng, L.; Zhang, K.; Zhou, C.-C.; Weir, M.D.; Zhou, X.-D.; Xu, H.H. One-year water-ageing of calcium phosphate composite containing nano-silver and quaternary ammonium to inhibit biofilms. *Int. J. Oral Sci.* **2016**, *8*, 172–181. [CrossRef] [PubMed]
136. Percival, S.L.; Bowler, P.; Russell, D. Bacterial resistance to silver in wound care. *J. Hosp. Infect.* **2005**, *60*, 1–7. [CrossRef] [PubMed]
137. Zhang, N.; Zhang, K.; Melo, M.A.S.; Chen, C.; Fouad, A.F.; Bai, Y.; Xu, H.H. Novel protein-repellent and biofilm-repellent orthodontic cement containing 2-methacryloyloxyethyl phosphorylcholine. *J. Biomed. Mater. Res. B* **2016**, *104*, 949–959. [CrossRef]
138. Wang, L.; Xie, X.; Weir, M.D.; Fouad, A.F.; Zhao, L.; Xu, H.H. Effect of bioactive dental adhesive on periodontal and endodontic pathogens. *J. Mater. Sci. Mater. Med.* **2016**, *27*, 168. [CrossRef]
139. Wang, L.; Li, C.; Weir, M.D.; Zhang, K.; Zhou, Y.; Xu, H.H. Novel multifunctional dental bonding agent for class-V restorations to inhibit periodontal biofilms. *RSC Adv.* **2017**, *7*, 29004–29014. [CrossRef]
140. Melo, M.A.S.; Cheng, L.; Zhang, K.; Weir, M.D.; Rodrigues, L.K.A.; Xu, H.H. Novel dental adhesives containing nanoparticles of silver and amorphous calcium phosphate. *Dent. Mater.* **2013**, *29*, 199–210. [CrossRef]
141. Cheng, L.; Weir, M.D.; Xu, H.H.K.; Antonucci, J.M.; Kraigsley, A.M.; Lin, N.J.; Lin-Gibson, S.; Zhou, X. Antibacterial amorphous calcium phosphate nanocomposites with a quaternary ammonium dimethacrylate and silver nanoparticles. *Dent. Mater.* **2012**, *28*, 561–572. [CrossRef] [PubMed]
142. Al-Dulaijan, Y.A.; Cheng, L.; Weir, M.D.; Melo, M.A.S.; Liu, H.; Oates, T.W.; Wang, L.; Xu, H.H.K. Novel rechargeable calcium phosphate nanocomposite with antibacterial activity to suppress biofilm acids and dental caries. *J. Dent.* **2018**, *72*, 44–52. [CrossRef] [PubMed]
143. Xu, H.H.; Moreau, J.L.; Sun, L.; Chow, L.C. Nanocomposite containing amorphous calcium phosphate nanoparticles for caries inhibition. *Dent. Mater.* **2011**, *27*, 762–769. [CrossRef] [PubMed]
144. Weir, M.D.; Chow, L.C.; Xu, H.H.K. Remineralization of demineralized enamel via calcium phosphate nanocomposite. *J. Dent. Res.* **2012**, *91*, 979–984. [CrossRef] [PubMed]
145. Zhang, L.; Weir, M.D.; Chow, L.C.; Antonucci, J.M.; Chen, J.; Xu, H.H.K. Novel rechargeable calcium phosphate dental nanocomposite. *Dent. Mater.* **2016**, *32*, 285–293. [CrossRef] [PubMed]
146. Ferrari, M.; Cagidiaco, M.C.; Vichi, A.; Mannocci, F.; Mason, P.N.; Mjor, I.A. Bonding of all-porcelain crown: Structural characteristics of the substrate. *Dent. Mater.* **2001**, *17*, 156–164. [CrossRef]
147. Li, Q.; Jepsen, S.; Albers, H.K.; Eberhard, J. Flowable materials as an intermediate layer could improve the marginal and internal adaptation of composite restorations in Class-V-cavities. *Dent. Mater.* **2006**, *22*, 250–257. [CrossRef]
148. Brackett, M.G.; Dib, A.; Franco, G.; Estrada, B.E.; Brackett, W.W. Two-year clinical performance of Clearfil SE and Clearfil S3 in restoration of unabraded non-carious class V lesions. *Oper. Dent.* **2010**, *3*, 273–278. [CrossRef]
149. Li, F.; Weir, M.D.; Xu, H.H.K. Effects of quaternary ammonium chain length on antibacterialbonding agents. *J. Dent. Res.* **2013**, *92*, 932–938. [CrossRef]
150. Humphrey, S.P.; Williamson, R.T. A review of saliva: Normal composition, flow, and function. *J. Prosthet. Dent.* **2001**, *85*, 162–169. [CrossRef]
151. Goulart, R.d.C.; Bolean, M.; Paulino, T.d.P.; Thedei, G., Jr.; Souza, S.L.; Tedesco, A.C.; Ciancaglini, P. Photodynamic therapy in planktonic and biofilm cultures of Aggregatibacter actinomycetemcomitans. *Photomed. Laser Surg.* **2010**, *28*, S53–S60. [CrossRef] [PubMed]
152. Cieplik, F.; Tabenski, L.; Buchalla, W.; Maisch, T. Antimicrobial photodynamic therapy for inactivation of biofilms formed by oral key pathogens. *Front. Microbiol.* **2014**, *5*, 405. [CrossRef] [PubMed]
153. Raghavendra, M.; Koregol, A.; Bhola, S. Photodynamic therapy: A targeted therapy in periodontics. *Aust. Dent. J.* **2009**, *54*, S102–S109. [CrossRef] [PubMed]
154. Soukos, N.S.; Goodson, J.M. Photodynamic therapy in the control of oral biofilms. *Periodontol. 2000* **2011**, *54*, 143–166. [CrossRef] [PubMed]
155. Vatansever, F.; de Melo, W.C.; Avci, P.; Vecchio, D.; Sadasivam, M.; Gupta, A.; Chandran, R.; Karimi, M.; Parizotto, N.A.; Yin, R. Antimicrobial strategies centered around reactive oxygen species–bactericidal antibiotics, photodynamic therapy, and beyond. *FEMS Microbiol. Rev.* **2013**, *37*, 955–989. [CrossRef] [PubMed]

156. Hu, X.; Huang, Y.-Y.; Wang, Y.; Wang, X.; Hamblin, M.R. Antimicrobial photodynamic therapy to control clinically relevant biofilm infections. *Front. Microbiol.* **2018**, *9*, 1299. [CrossRef]
157. Kumari, A.; Yadav, S.K.; Yadav, S.C. Biodegradable polymeric nanoparticles based drug delivery systems. *Colloids Surf. B* **2010**, *75*, 1–18. [CrossRef]
158. Malik, Z.; Ladan, H.; Nitzan, Y. Photodynamic inactivation of Gram-negative bacteria: Problems and possible solutions. *J. Photochem. Photobiol. B* **1992**, *14*, 262–266. [CrossRef]
159. George, S.; Hamblin, M.R.; Kishen, A. Uptake pathways of anionic and cationic photosensitizers into bacteria. *Photochem. Photobiol. Sci.* **2009**, *8*, 788–795. [CrossRef]
160. Klepac-Ceraj, V.; Patel, N.; Song, X.; Holewa, C.; Patel, C.; Kent, R.; Amiji, M.M.; Soukos, N.S. Photodynamic effects of methylene blue-loaded polymeric nanoparticles on dental plaque bacteria. *Lasers Surg. Med.* **2011**, *43*, 600–606. [CrossRef]
161. De Freitas, L.M.; Calixto, G.M.F.; Chorilli, M.; JGiusti, J.S.M.; Bagnato, V.S.; Soukos, N.S.; Amiji, M.M.; Fontana, C.R. Polymeric nanoparticle-based photodynamic therapy for chronic periodontitis in vivo. *Int. J. Mol. Sci.* **2016**, *17*, 769. [CrossRef] [PubMed]
162. Sasaki, Y.; Hayashi, J.-I.; Fujimura, T.; Iwamura, Y.; Yamamoto, G.; Nishida, E.; Ohno, T.; Okada, K.; Yamamoto, H.; Kikuchi, T. New irradiation method with indocyanine green-loaded nanospheres for inactivating periodontal pathogens. *Int. J. Mol. Sci.* **2017**, *18*, 154. [CrossRef] [PubMed]
163. Nagahara, A.; Mitani, A.; Fukuda, M.; Yamamoto, H.; Tahara, K.; Morita, I.; Ting, C.C.; Watanabe, T.; Fujimura, T.; Osawa, K. Antimicrobial photodynamic therapy using a diode laser with a potential new photosensitizer, indocyanine green-loaded nanospheres, may be effective for the clearance of P orphyromonas gingivalis. *J. Period. Res.* **2013**, *48*, 591–599. [CrossRef] [PubMed]
164. Chen, F.-M.; An, Y.; Zhang, R.; Zhang, M. New insights into and novel applications of release technology for periodontal reconstructive therapies. *J. Control. Release* **2011**, *149*, 92–110. [CrossRef] [PubMed]
165. Peng, P.-C.; Hsieh, C.-M.; Chen, C.-P.; Tsai, T.; Chen, C.-T. Assessment of photodynamic inactivation against periodontal bacteria mediated by a chitosan hydrogel in a 3D gingival model. *Int. J. Mol. Sci.* **2016**, *17*, 1821. [CrossRef] [PubMed]
166. Pfitzner, A.; Sigusch, B.W.; Albrecht, V.; Glockmann, E. Killing of periodontopathogenic bacteria by photodynamic therapy. *J. Periodontol.* **2004**, *75*, 1343–1349. [CrossRef] [PubMed]
167. Rovaldi, C.; Pievsky, A.; Sole, N.; Friden, P.; Rothstein, D.; Spacciapoli, P. Photoactive porphyrin derivative with broad-spectrum activity against oral pathogens in vitro. *Antimicrob. Agents Chemother.* **2000**, *44*, 3364–3367. [CrossRef] [PubMed]
168. Lauro, F.M.; Pretto, P.; Covolo, L.; Jori, G.; Bertoloni, G. Photoinactivation of bacterial strains involved in periodontal diseases sensitized by porphycene–polylysine conjugates. *Photochem. Photobiol. Sci.* **2002**, *1*, 468–470. [CrossRef] [PubMed]
169. Suci, P.; Kang, S.; Gmür, R.; Douglas, T.; Young, M. Targeted delivery of a photosensitizer to Aggregatibacter actinomycetemcomitans biofilm. *Antimicrob. Agents Chemother.* **2010**, *54*, 2489–2496. [CrossRef] [PubMed]
170. Kizerwetter-Swida, M.; Binek, M. Selection of potentially probiotic Lactobacillus strains towards their inhibitory activity against poultry enteropathogenic bacteria. *Pol. J. Microbiol.* **2005**, *54*, 287–294. [PubMed]
171. Punjabi, A.; Wu, X.; Tokatli-Apollon, A.; El-Rifai, M.; Lee, H.; Zhang, Y.; Wang, C.; Liu, Z.; Chan, E.M.; Duan, C. Amplifying the red-emission of upconverting nanoparticles for biocompatible clinically used prodrug-induced photodynamic therapy. *ACS Nano* **2014**, *8*, 10621–10630. [CrossRef]
172. Tian, G.; Zhang, X.; Gu, Z.; Zhao, Y. Recent Advances in Upconversion Nanoparticles-Based Multifunctional Nanocomposites for Combined Cancer Therapy. *Adv. Mater.* **2015**, *27*, 7692–7712. [CrossRef] [PubMed]
173. Dong, K.; Ju, E.; Gao, N.; Wang, Z.; Ren, J.; Qu, X. Synergistic eradication of antibiotic-resistant bacteria based biofilms in vivo using a NIR-sensitive nanoplatform. *Chem. Commun.* **2016**, *52*, 5312–5315. [CrossRef] [PubMed]
174. Shrestha, A.; Kishen, A. Antibiofilm efficacy of photosensitizer-functionalized bioactive nanoparticles on multispecies biofilm. *J. Endodont.* **2014**, *40*, 1604–1610. [CrossRef] [PubMed]
175. Allaker, R.P.; Memarzadeh, K. Nanoparticles and the control of oral infections. *Int. J. Antimicrob. Agents* **2014**, *43*, 95–104. [CrossRef] [PubMed]
176. Dong, Z.; Feng, L.; Zhu, W.; Sun, X.; Gao, M.; Zhao, H.; Chao, Y.; Liu, Z. $CaCO_3$ nanoparticles as an ultra-sensitive tumor-pH-responsive nanoplatform enabling real-time drug release monitoring and cancer combination therapy. *Biomaterials* **2016**, *110*, 60–70. [CrossRef] [PubMed]

177. Sun, X.; Wang, L.; Lynch, C.D.; Sun, X.; Li, X.; Qi, M.; Ma, C.; Li, C.; Dong, B.; Zhou, Y.; et al. Nanoparticles having amphiphilic silane containing Chlorin e6 with strong anti-biofilm activity against periodontitis-related pathogens. *J. Dent.* **2019**. [CrossRef] [PubMed]
178. Ng, D.Y.; Chan, A.K.; Dalci, O.; Petocz, P.; Papadopoulou, A.K.; Darendeliler, M.A. A pilot study of laser energy transmission through bone and gingiva. *J. Am. Dent. Assoc.* **2018**, *149*, 704–711. [CrossRef] [PubMed]
179. Cui, S.; Yin, D.; Chen, Y.; Di, Y.; Chen, H.; Ma, Y.; Achilefu, S.; Gu, Y. In vivo targeted deep-tissue photodynamic therapy based on near-infrared light triggered upconversion nanoconstruct. *ACS Nano* **2012**, *7*, 676–688. [CrossRef] [PubMed]
180. Khan, S.T.; Al-Khedhairy, A.A.; Musarrat, J. ZnO and TiO$_2$ nanoparticles as novel antimicrobial agents for oral hygiene: A review. *J. Nanopart. Res.* **2015**, *17*, 276. [CrossRef]
181. Li, Z.; Zhang, Y. An efficient and user-friendly method for the synthesis of hexagonal-phase NaYF4: Yb, Er/Tm nanocrystals with controllable shape and upconversion fluorescence. *Nanotechnology* **2008**, *19*, 345606. [CrossRef] [PubMed]

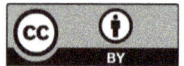

© 2019 by the authors. Licensee MDPI, Basel, Switzerland. This article is an open access article distributed under the terms and conditions of the Creative Commons Attribution (CC BY) license (http://creativecommons.org/licenses/by/4.0/).

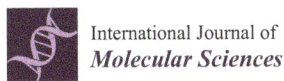

Article

Interaction of Halictine-Related Antimicrobial Peptides with Membrane Models

Markéta Pazderková [1,2], Petr Maloň [1], Vlastimil Zíma [1], Kateřina Hofbauerová [1], Vladimír Kopecký Jr. [1], Eva Kočišová [1], Tomáš Pazderka [1], Václav Čeřovský [2] and Lucie Bednárová [2,*]

[1] Institute of Physics, Faculty of Mathematics and Physics, Charles University, Ke Karlovu 5, 121 16 Prague 2, Czech Republic; pazderkova@karlov.mff.cuni.cz (M.P.); malonp@karlov.mff.cuni.cz (P.M.); vlastimil.zima@gmail.com (V.Z.); hofbauer@karlov.mff.cuni.cz (K.H.); kopecky@karlov.mff.cuni.cz (V.K.J.); kocisova@karlov.mff.cuni.cz (E.K.); tomas.pazderka@matfyz.cz (T.P.)

[2] Institute of Organic Chemistry and Biochemistry, v.v.i., Academy of Sciences of the Czech Republic, Flemingovo náměstí 2, 166 10 Prague 6, Czech Republic; cerovsky@uochb.cas.cz

* Correspondence: bednarova@uochb.cas.cz; Tel.: +420-220-183-593; Fax: +420-224-310-177

Received: 27 December 2018; Accepted: 28 January 2019; Published: 1 February 2019

Abstract: We have investigated structural changes of peptides related to antimicrobial peptide Halictine-1 (HAL-1) induced by interaction with various membrane-mimicking models with the aim to identify a mechanism of the peptide mode of action and to find a correlation between changes of primary/secondary structure and biological activity. Modifications in the HAL-1 amino acid sequence at particular positions, causing an increase of amphipathicity (Arg/Lys exchange), restricted mobility (insertion of Pro) and consequent changes in antimicrobial and hemolytic activity, led to different behavior towards model membranes. Secondary structure changes induced by peptide-membrane interaction were studied by circular dichroism, infrared spectroscopy, and fluorescence spectroscopy. The experimental results were complemented by molecular dynamics calculations. An α-helical structure has been found to be necessary but not completely sufficient for the HAL-1 peptides antimicrobial action. The role of alternative conformations (such as β-sheet, PPII or 3_{10}-helix) also seems to be important. A mechanism of the peptide mode of action probably involves formation of peptide assemblies (possibly membrane pores), which disrupt bacterial membrane and, consequently, allow membrane penetration.

Keywords: antibacterial peptides; halictine; circular dichroism; fluorescence; infrared spectroscopy

1. Introduction

Antimicrobial peptides (AMPs) are important participants in the initial response of immune systems and have been found in nearly all living organisms including bacteria, fungi, plants and animals [1–4]. Potentially, they offer alternatives to disease treatment as a replacement for common antibiotics, without disadvantages like resistance, allergies, etc. Many AMPs have been isolated and subsequently synthesized together with their analogs. Their antibacterial activities have been determined against Gram-negative and Gram-positive bacteria as well as against cancer cells [1,5–8]. A general lack of new antibiotics for the treatment of Gram-negative infections and a continuous increase in multi-drug resistance has recently caused a wave of interest in possible mechanisms of AMP action. One of the recognized effects is their ability to disrupt bacterial membranes *via* non-specific electrostatic interactions with the membrane lipid components [1]. There are two recognized common and important criteria for functionally active AMPs. These include a network of cationic charges and the ability to adopt an amphipathic structure, where hydrophobic and hydrophilic parts form oppositely oriented domains upon interaction with negatively charged bacterial membranes.

The possible mechanisms of AMP action fall into two basic categories: (1) formation of pores in bacterial membranes *via* transmembrane penetration (e.g., the barrel stave and toroidal pore models) or (2) disruption of membranes (e.g., the carpet and detergent models) [1,8–11]. These then lead to the breakdown of the transmembrane potential causing leakage of the cell contents and finally cell death. The physico-chemical concept of such antibacterial action has been discussed and particular attention has been paid to changes of the phase state of the membrane [12–14].

Quite importantly, AMPs exhibit high preference for bacterial over mammalian cells. This is probably associated with known significant differences between mammalian and bacterial cell membranes [5,6,12,15,16]. The type of mammalian cell membrane is represented by the plasma membrane of red blood cells. This membrane consists of about 60% phospholipids and 25% cholesterol. Distribution of phospholipids between outer and inner lipid leaflets of the bilayer is asymmetric with neutral phospholipids phosphatidylcholine and sphingomyelin exposed to the extracellular matrix. On the other hand, negatively charged lipids such as phosphatidylglycerol, diphosphatidylglycerol or cardiolipin and the zwitterionic phosphatidylethanolamine are the main constituents of the cytoplasmic membrane of both Gram-positive and Gram-negative bacteria (having an additional layer of peptidoglycan and an outer membrane layer composed mainly of lipopolysaccharides). In a simplified way, the AMPs are exposed to a neutral membrane surface in the case of mammalian cells and to a negatively charged surface in the case of bacteria.

Within the last decade, several original discoveries of AMPs isolated from the venom of *Hymenoptera* insects have been made and described by our collaborators [17–22]. Biological activities of these new AMPs have been determined and compared to the activities of their synthesized analogs to consider their eventual pharmacological application. Based on initial electronic circular dichroism (ECD) investigations, the peptides may undergo substantial structural changes in the presence of simple membrane-mimicking models such as 2,2,2-trifluoroethanol (TFE) and sodium dodecyl sulfate (SDS). Moreover, peptide structural behavior can be substantially affected by primary structure modifications. In our initial study of peptides related to Halictine-1 (HAL-1), a short linear AMP containing 12 amino acids isolated from the venom of the eusocial bee *Halictus sexcinctus*, we demonstrated that HAL-1 and its analogs are able to form amphipathic structures when in α-helical conformation [19]. A subsequent detailed spectroscopic study of the natural HAL-1 [23] resulted in a nontrivial picture involving not only a significant role of α-helical conformation but also an important role of other arrangements including random coil, β-structure and/or polyproline II (PPII) structures. Overall, the results presented overwhelming complexity and implied a need for additional, more detailed studies. Here, we focus in detail on physico-chemical properties and structure-activity relations of peptides related to HAL-1 including their geometries, conformation and dynamic behavior in various situations like in solutions, or in interaction with different membrane models. Conformational changes have been induced by an interaction with (a) TFE—an α-helix forming solvent [24], (b) SDS micelles—a very simple bacterial membrane model [25,26] and also by (c) liposomes of different phospholipid composition presented by a combination of various concentration mixtures of 1,2-dimyristoyl-*sn*-glycerol-3-phosphatidylcholine (PC) and 1,2-dimyristoyl-*sn*-glycero-3-phospho-(1'-*rac*-glycerol) (PG)—systems more accurately mimicking mammalian and bacterial membranes [25,26].

Inspired by the already presented analogues with specific sequence modifications and their known biological activities [19], here, we present a study of HAL-1 analogs (Table 1) with possible therapeutic potential (i.e., the analogs exhibiting potent activities against various pathogens while having substantially reduced hemolytic activity against red blood cells). Particularly, HAL-1/10 and HAL-1/20 analogs look promising for potential therapeutic applications because these peptides lack undesired hemolytic activities, while their antibacterial potencies, especially against *P. aeruginosa*, are higher than for natural HAL-1. A combined use of infrared (IR), circular dichroism (electronic (ECD) and vibrational (VCD)) and fluorescence spectroscopies allows us to obtain complex information about structural changes of the peptides upon interaction with model membranes. The set of IR, ECD, and fluorescence spectroscopy experiments performed at room temperature is complemented by time- and temperature-dependent ECD measurements, which allows us to distinguish and describe even subtle conformational changes of the peptides in interaction with membrane-mimicking environments, and by ECD and VCD study of a concentration dependency of HAL-1 analogs. Utilization of these experimental methods might help us to better understand the relation between the peptide primary/secondary structure changes and elucidate the mechanisms of the HAL-1 peptides action. A correlation between the peptide structural changes and biological activities can be also determined. The experimental data are compared to molecular dynamics (MD) simulations of HAL-1 in interaction with model membranes.

Table 1. Amino acid sequences, physico-chemical and biological properties (μ_H is the hydrophobic moment, and H represents the mean hydrophobicity, calculated according to [27]), of the studied antibacterial HAL-1 peptides. Data were taken from ref. [19]. Point mutations with respect to the natural HAL-1 peptide are underlined. The Schiffer–Edmundson wheel projection of the HAL-1 and its analogs is depicted below the table.

Acronym	Sequence	MW (Da)	Charge	μ_H	H	Antimicrobial Activity MIC (µM)				Hemolytic LC$_{50}$ (µM)
						B.[1]	S.[2]	E.[3]	P.[4]	
HAL-1	GMWSKILGHLIR	1408.9	+3	0.380	−0.004	0.8	7.7	3.8	45.0	82
HAL-1/2	GMWSKILGPLIR	1368.8	+3	0.361	+0.023	3.6	>100	30.0	>100	>200
HAL-1/6	GMWSKILGHLIK	1380.6	+3	0.323	+0.051	1.3	15.8	7.2	65.0	132
HAL-1/10	GMWKKILGKLIR	1440.9	+5	0.416	−0.133	0.8	15.0	2.3	13.1	>200
HAL-1/20	GKWSKILGKLIR	1396.9	+5	0.473	−0.176	1.7	21.7	2.3	28.3	>200

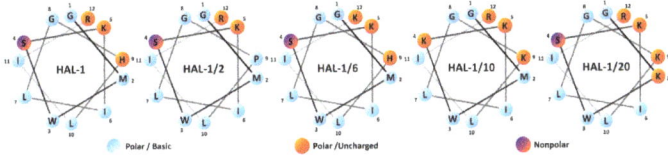

[1] *Bacillus subtilis*, [2] *Staphylococcus aureus*, [3] *Escherichia coli*, [4] *Pseudomonas aeruginosa*.

2. Results and Discussion

In our study, we investigate effects of changes in ionicity, hydrophobicity, flexibility and/or amphipathicity of the chosen peptides induced by an exchange of selected residues by Lys and Pro residues (see Table 1) on their structural behavior in membrane-mimicking environments represented by TFE, SDS micelles and phosphatidylcholine/phosphatidylglycerol-based liposomes. Based on the simple peptide structural prediction [28], the substitution of amino acids Ser4 and His9 (HAL-1/10), Met2 and His9 (HAL-1/20) or Arg12 (HAL-1/6) by Lys stabilizes the α-helical conformation, and the replacement of two amino acids by Lys (HAL-1/10 and HAL-1/20) improves the helical amphipathicity of the peptides (see Table 1). On the contrary, insertion of Pro9 (HAL-1/2) may cause structural irregularity, as Pro often breaks regular structures.

2.1. Structural Changes Followed by ECD

2.1.1. Structural Changes Due to the Presence of TFE and SDS

Native HAL-1 in the aqueous environment, as well as all HAL-1 analogs, show a predominantly unordered structure, characterized by a negative ECD band at ~198 nm [29] (Figure 1). Upon addition of TFE, ECD spectra undergo a shape change. Formation of double negative minima at ~205 and 222 nm indicates a gradual appearance of an α-helical component (an isodichroic point at 202 nm suggests a two-state conformational change) (not shown). According to the two-state model [30] (Table A1), the presence of 30% TFE (v/v) causes a ~20–30% increase in the α-helical content, depending slightly on the particular primary structure. In the presence of SDS, the spectral changes appear more complex (Figure 1). The process conditioned by SDS is contributed not only by unordered and α-helical conformations, but also by secondary structures like a β-sheet or PPII helix [31]. Interaction with various proportions of SDS occurs in several stages, and a simple process of the two-state equilibrium does not describe sufficiently all the observed structural changes (Tables A1 and A2). At low concentrations (less than 2 mM, i.e., below critical micelle concentration (cmc)) SDS causes an intensity decrease of ECD curves. In the case of HAL-1/6 (Arg12 replaced by Lys), this process causes even a sign flip. At low concentrations SDS does not act as a membrane model but serves as a denaturation agent [32], thus the ECD curves under such conditions offer two possible explanations: either the original unordered/PPII structure adopts a conformation with a higher β-sheet content, or it becomes a truly statistical random conformation due to an interaction with SDS molecules. These two structures can hardly be distinguished on the basis of ECD. Rather different spectral behavior is observed for the analog HAL-1/20, for which the formation of a positive band at 194 nm and negative bands at 208 and 222 nm typical for α-helical conformation is observed even for 0.16 mM SDS concentration (i.e., far below cmc). Moreover, the ECD bands at 194 and 222 nm exhibit, under these conditions, the highest spectral intensities. Formation of the α-helical conformation for HAL-1/20 below cmc could be due to the substitution of Met2 by Lys which favors interaction with anionic SDS molecules and increases the peptide polarity and amphipathicity (see Table 1) [27]. For all the analogs except for HAL-1/20, with the increase of SDS concentration above cmc (i.e., when SDS starts acting as a crude membrane model) [33], we observe a pronounced increase of the α-helical content (formation of negative maxima at 208 and 222 nm and an increase of overall spectral intensity; Figure 1). For these peptides, additional spectral changes appear with a further increase of SDS concentration above 8 mM. At first the negative maximum at 208 nm shifts to 205 nm with the preserved band intensity, and the intensity of the negative maximum at 222 nm discernibly decreases. Then, an overall ECD intensity decreases and the maxima at 205 nm and 222 nm shift to 206 nm and 219 nm, respectively. This could be due to an additional formation of 3_{10}-helix, PPII or β-structure [34]. For HAL-1/20 such spectral changes are observed for SDS concentration above 4 mM SDS.

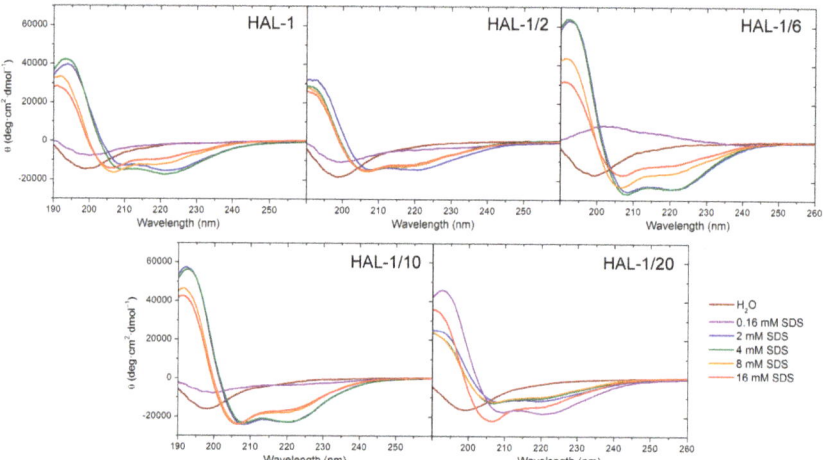

Figure 1. ECD spectra of HAL-1 and its analogs (0.125 mg/mL) in aqueous solution and in the presence of SDS (0.16, 2, 4, 8, and 16 mM).

The numerical ECD analysis confirms these qualitative findings (Table A1). As for HAL-1, for HAL-1/6 and HAL-1/10 the maximal α-helical content is achieved in 2 mM SDS while for HAL-1/20, it is maximal in 0.16 mM SDS. For SDS concentration above 4 mM, numerical analysis indicates a slight decrease of the α-helical and unordered structure content and a subtle increase of β-structures (β-sheet and β-turn) for all the peptides except for HAL-1/20. For 16 mM SDS, the α-helical structure still dominates at the expense of other structures (Table A2). As expected, the substitution of His9 by Pro in HAL-1/2 decreases the ability of the peptide to form an α-helix (the α-helical fraction does not exceed 50%). However, the numerical ECD data analysis, even with included PPII and the 3_{10}-helical structure, can provide only a rough estimation of observed spectral changes depending on the available reference set [35–38].

We have previously suggested that, for natural HAL-1, additional spectral changes in the presence of SDS could originate in an alternation of the PPII structure content [23]. In order to recognize the PPII structure in ECD spectra of HAL-1 analogs in SDS solution, we have combined differential ECD spectra with ECD spectra of the thermal denaturation (Figures 2 and 3) [31,39,40]. For all the studied peptides, differential ECD spectra indicate that a temporary increase of the α-helical content is followed by an additional structural reorganization—probably either a PPII structure formation or a decrease of a β-sheet content characterized by a positive band at ~225 nm, whose intensity increases with increasing SDS concentration (Figure 2). HAL-1/2 undergoes these changes only moderately, probably due to the presence of Pro residue, which may cause conformational stiffness. The temperature-dependent ECD spectra of HAL-1 analogs exhibit similar features. At low temperature (5 °C) they show the negative band at ~199 nm and the weaker positive band at ~220 nm (Figure 3). With a temperature increase, both of these bands decrease in intensity. An isodichroic point at ~210 nm indicates a two-state transition with decreasing PPII structure content [31,39]. At low temperature (5 °C), distinct spectral intensities of the analogs' ECD curves indicate differences in peptide structural arrangement. While HAL-1/10 seems to have the highest portion of PPII structure and higher flexibility, HAL-1/20 appears to possess the highest fraction of unordered structure and less flexibility in its arrangement. Principal component analysis (PCA) indicates that thermal denaturation of the peptides probably leads to an increase of the β-structure content at the expense of decreasing percentage of unordered and/or PPII conformations [39] (Figure A1). Higher temperature seems to have similar effects on the peptides' secondary structure if SDS acts as a denaturant (i.e., below cmc). The observed trends support the assumption that PPII conformation allows the polypeptide chain to switch easily to an α-helical or β-sheet and β-turn conformation [31,39].

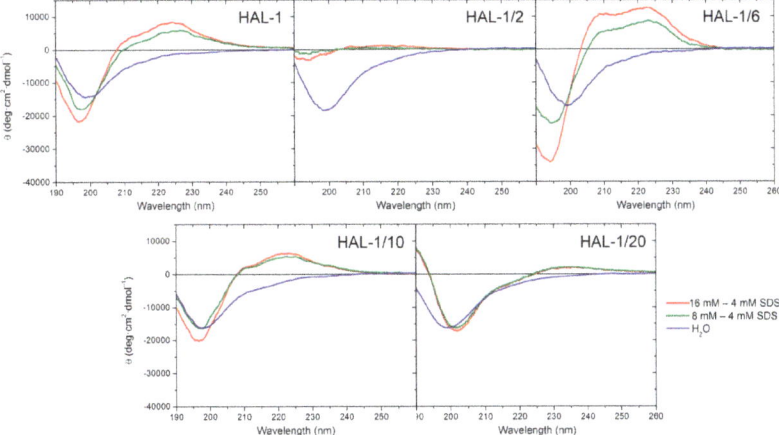

Figure 2. Difference of ECD spectra of HAL-1 and its analogs (0.125 mg/mL) in 8 mM SDS and in 16 mM SDS. ECD spectrum of the sample with the highest α-helical content in SDS solution (4 mM SDS peptide solution for HAL-1/2, HAL-1/6, HAL-1/10, and 0.16 mM SDS peptide solution for HAL-1/20 is taken as a reference). ECD spectra of the peptides in aqueous solution are depicted for comparison.

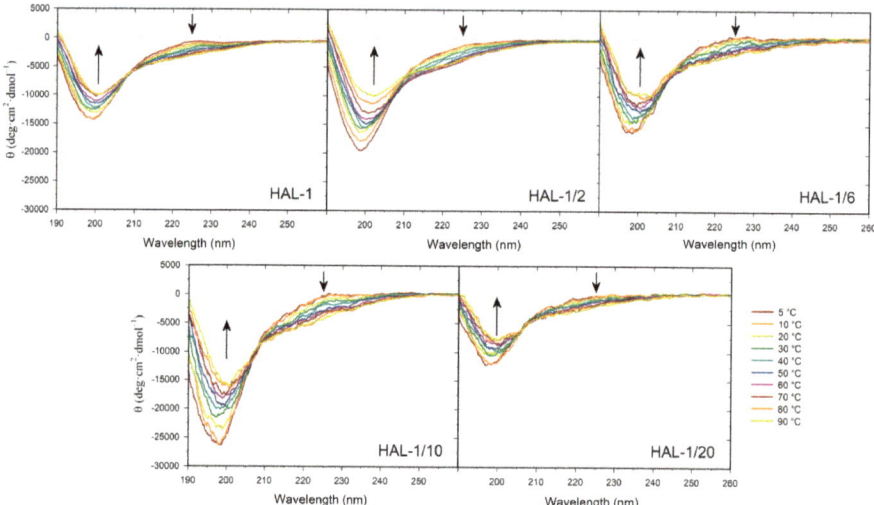

Figure 3. Thermal dependence of ECD spectra of HAL-1 and its analogs (0.125 mg/mL) in aqueous solution. The arrows show the direction of spectral changes with temperature increase from 5 to 90 °C (with a step of 10 °C).

2.1.2. Structural Changes Due to the Presence of LUVs

Neutral large unilamellar vesicles (LUVs) composed of PC were used as simple models of mammalian membranes. Similar to the natural HAL-1 [23], only subtle structural changes are observed in the ECD spectra of all the HAL-1 analogs upon addition of PC-based LUVs (Figure 4, Table A3). Slight conformational changes observed for HAL-1/2 and HAL-1/20 (Figure 4) likely correspond to an increase of β-sheet proportion. For HAL-1 and in part also for HAL-1/6, an α-helical structure can be induced when very high lipid/peptide (L/P) ratios (~600) are used (not shown). However, under such conditions, thorough analysis of ECD data is rather difficult due the limitations of ECD experiments (at high lipid concentrations, ECD spectra may be obscured due to light scattering on liposome molecules). The ability of all HAL-1 peptides to form the α-helical structure is enhanced in the presence of negatively charged PG-containing LUVs, representing a simple bacterial membrane model. Similar to HAL-1, for the proline-containing analog HAL-1/2, this enhancement is maximized with liposomes containing the highest fraction of PG (PC/PG = 1:4). For the other analogs, the maximal α-helical content is observed for the liposomes having the same fraction of PC and PG (PC/PG = 1:1) while an additional formation of β-structure occurs in the presence of the liposomes with the highest fraction of PG (PC/PG = 1:4) (Table A3). In order to obtain additional information about the structural stability of the peptides in the presence of PC/PG liposomes (composed of PC/PG in the 1:4 ratio), a time dependence of ECD spectra in the 280-min time interval has been studied for HAL-1 and its analogs HAL-1/2, HAL-1/6 and HAL-1/20 (Figure 5). The most pronounced spectral changes with time have been observed for HAL-1/20. This peptide shows the highest tendency to form a β-structure immediately upon interaction with PC/PG liposomes. A portion of the α-helical structure increases with time to a similar degree as for HAL-1/2. Following the PCA results (Figure A2), this structural change is compensated by a continuous β-structure content decrease. The structural behavior of HAL-1 seems to be comparable to HAL-1/6, with relatively small structural changes represented by a slight increase of the α-helical content. As expected, only minor structural changes are observed for HAL-1/2 (Figure 5).

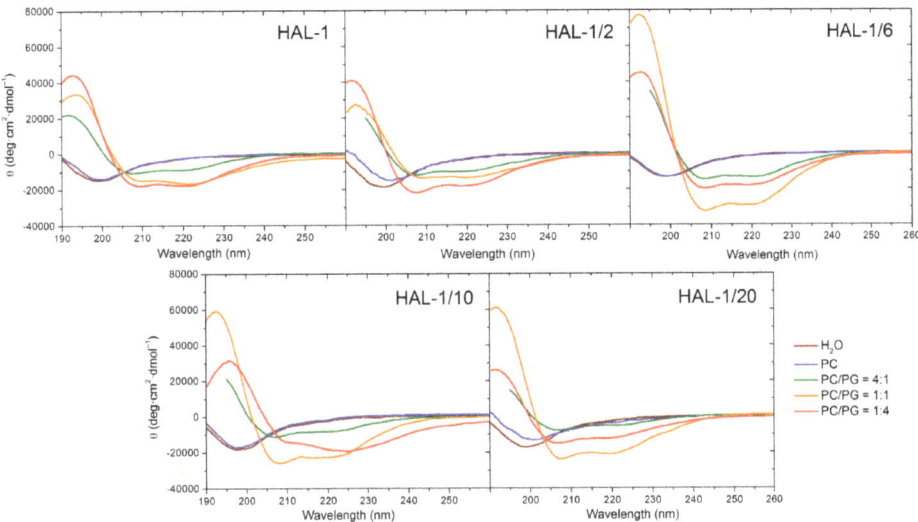

Figure 4. ECD spectra of HAL-1 and its analogs (0.125 mg/mL) in aqueous solution and in the presence of LUVs (L/P = 20) prepared from PC and PC/PG mixtures: 4:1, 1:1 and 1:4.

Since the liposomes composed of PC/PG in various ratios roughly simulate bacterial and mammalian membranes, an attempt can be made to correlate the secondary structure changes inferred from the experimental ECD spectra with the peptide biological properties. The observed very limited interactions of HAL-1 analogs with the mammalian membrane (PC-based) models seem to correlate with their low (or none) hemolytic activities. Rather hemolytic analogs HAL-1 and HAL-1/6 show some reduced tendency to form the α-helical structure but such conformational change is induced only by a significant increase in lipid concentration. This is probably caused by the fact that the peptide activity against mammalian cells is much lower (~10–100×) than against bacterial cells, and the peptide propensity to interact with mammalian membrane model is therefore notably reduced. Behavior of the HAL-1 peptides towards PG-containing LUVs is very different. According to our data, all the HAL-1 analogs show a tendency to become α-helical upon this interaction. As the highest α-helical fraction is observed for HAL-1/6, which is less active than the native HAL-1, it seems that biological activities of the peptides are not solely determined by their propensity for forming an α-helical structure. The spectral changes observed for the HAL-1 analogs in interaction with liposomes of various PC/PG compositions indicate that, similar to the peptide behavior in the presence of SDS micelles (see above), an additional formation of β-structure and/or PPII conformation cannot be excluded and could be also important for their biological activities.

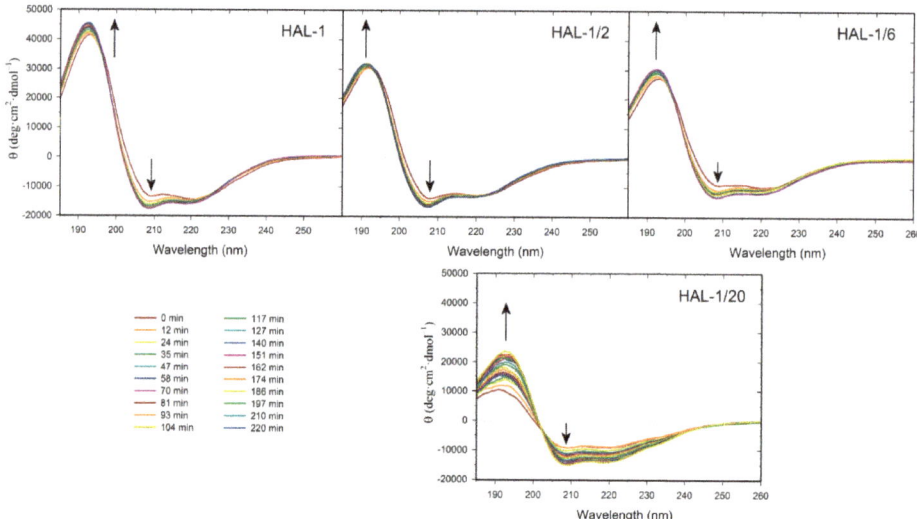

Figure 5. Time dependence of ECD spectra of HAL-1 and its analogs (0.125 mg/mL) in PC/PG = 1:4 mixtures (L/P = 20), measured within a 280-min time interval after the sample preparation with a 12-min step. The arrows show the direction of spectral changes with time.

2.2. Structural Changes Followed by Infrared Spectroscopy

IR spectroscopy is sensitive to the β-sheet and β-turn structure and its combination with ECD may provide further conformational details. IR experiments can be carried out in aqueous solution (H_2O or D_2O), and the structure assignment is based on band positions within the amide I region (1600–1700 cm^{-1}). For the peptides measured in H_2O, it is usually difficult to distinguish between the α-helical and disordered structures because the corresponding amide I bands can occur in the same spectral range. This problem may be partially solved using hydrogen/deuterium exchange, which significantly reduces the α-helix and disordered structure amide I band overlaps [41]. For the natural HAL-1 measured in H_2O, the amide I band positioned at ~1646 cm^{-1} indicates that the peptide is mainly in a random coil conformation [42] with a minor contribution of β-turns (a shoulder at ~1682 cm^{-1}) [43]. Such assignment is confirmed by the IR measurements in D_2O, where a band at ~1641 cm^{-1} (Figure 6, Table A4) can be again assigned to the random coil structure and bands at ~1658 and 1675 cm^{-1} to β-turns [41]. Upon addition of TFE (10–50% v/v), IR spectra of HAL-1 exhibit a blue shift of the amide I band from ~1646 to ~1656 cm^{-1} (Figure 6, Table A4), suggesting a secondary structure change from the random coil to the α-helical structure [42,43]. An additional band at ~1630 cm^{-1} suggests an occurrence of a β-sheet structure, and a band at ~1621 cm^{-1} indicates formation of intermolecular hydrogen bonds, typical for peptide aggregation [42,44]. The band at ~1683 cm^{-1}, due to the β-turn structure, remains at the same position. A similar spectral shift of the band at ~1645 cm^{-1} to 1657 cm^{-1} indicating a conformational change from the random coil to the α-helical structure is observed in the IR spectra of HAL-1 interacting with SDS (2–8 mM). In 8 mM SDS, the presence of a shoulder at ~1686 cm^{-1} together with a spectral band at ~1631 cm^{-1} suggests formation of the β-sheet structure [23,41]. Spectral shift of the band at ~1646 to 1657 cm^{-1} can be interpreted in terms of a formation of the α-helical structure. This assumption is confirmed by an analogous measurement of the same concentration dependence in D_2O (Figure 6, Table A4) where the main spectral component shifts from 1641 cm^{-1} (a disordered structure) in D_2O to ~1650 cm^{-1} (an α-helical structure [42]) in SDS at a concentration above cmc (8 mM). The high-frequency component at ~1682 cm^{-1} downshifts to 1676 cm^{-1}, most probably due to a β-sheet structure formation [42].

These findings are in agreement with the results of ECD analysis, showing that, besides the α-helical structure, the β-sheet structure is also present.

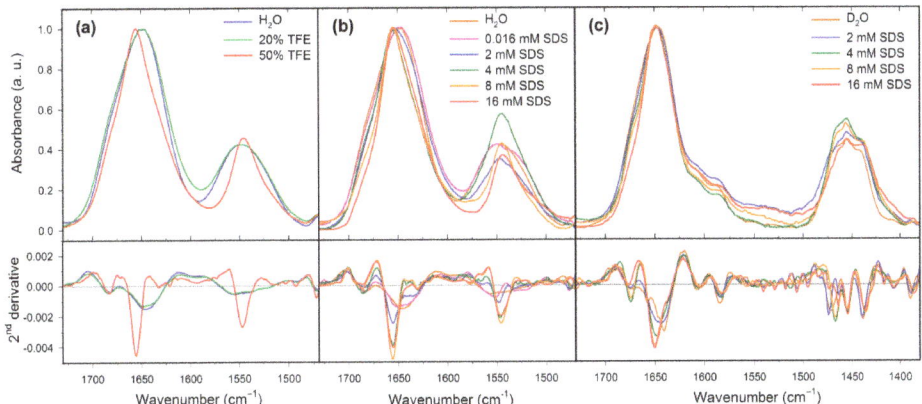

Figure 6. IR spectra (**top**) and their second derivatives (**bottom**) of HAL-1 (10 mg/mL) in (**a**) the presence of TFE (0%, 20%, and 50%); (**b**) of SDS/H$_2$O solution (0.016, 2, 4, 8, and 16 mM SDS). (**c**) of SDS/D$_2$O solution (2, 4, 8, and 16 mM SDS).

IR spectrum of HAL-1/2 in H$_2$O is dominated by a band at ~1648 cm^{-1} due to the presence of a random coil structure. An additional band at ~1684 cm^{-1} and a shoulder at ~1636 cm^{-1} indicate a minor portion of β-turn and β-sheet conformation [42]. Upon addition of SDS, the band at 1648 cm^{-1} diminishes and a dominant component at ~1655 cm^{-1} shows prevailing α-helical structures. Addition of SDS again seems to cause a change in the β-structure arrangement, as in 8 mM SDS, there are only two corresponding bands at ~1686 and 1639 cm^{-1}. Formation of a low-frequency band at ~1623 cm^{-1} indicates a partial peptide aggregation. Similar to HAL-1, IR spectrum of HAL-1/6 in water (Figure 7) is dominated by an amide I band at ~1646 cm^{-1} indicating prevailing random coil structure, and a lower-intensity component at ~1682 cm^{-1} assigned to β-turns [42]. Upon addition of SDS, the main amide I component shifts to ~1655 cm^{-1} (in 8 mM SDS), again hinting at a transition from a random coil to an α-helical structure. This process is accompanied by diminishing of the β-turn band at ~1682 cm^{-1} and formation of a band at ~1694 cm^{-1}, implying a conformational change from the β-turn to β-sheet conformation [42]. IR spectrum of HAL-1/10 (Figure 7, Table A4) in H$_2$O has the main feature at ~1643 cm^{-1} which can be assigned either to the random coil, or the β-sheet structure [41,42]. As for HAL-1, a lower-intensity band at ~1681 cm^{-1} suggests the presence of β-turns [42]. Conformational behavior of HAL-1/10 upon addition of SDS is practically the same as for HAL-1/6 (not shown). While the IR spectrum of HAL-1/20 (Figure 7, Table A4) in H$_2$O is (similar to HAL-1/10) dominated by a band at ~1642 cm^{-1} due to either random coil, or β-sheet structure [41,42], a shoulder at ~1656 cm^{-1} indicates, in this case, a minor contribution of the α-helical structure [42]. Upon addition of SDS, the band at ~1642 cm^{-1} diminishes and a new band at ~1651 cm^{-1} is formed, indicating a conformational change to α-helical and/or random coil structure. The higher-frequency component, which shifts to ~1659 cm^{-1}, can be assigned to a 3$_{10}$-helix [45]. In addition, we observe a new band at ~1692 cm^{-1}, reflecting the β-sheet structure formation [42].

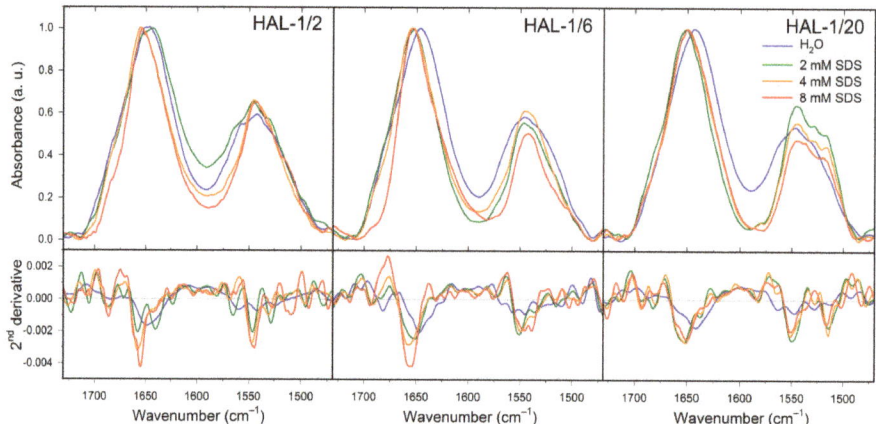

Figure 7. IR spectra (**top**) and their second derivatives (**bottom**) of HAL-1/2, HAL-1/6 and HAL-1/20 (10 mg/mL) in the presence of SDS (0, 2, 4, and 8 mM).

We have already shown that the secondary structure of HAL-1 in interaction with LUVs depends on LUV composition [23]. In the presence of neutral PC-based liposomes (a model of a mammalian membrane [1]), the dominant amide I band shifts to ~1652 cm^{-1} probably due to the simultaneous presence of a random coil and an α-helical structure. Bands at ~1686 and 1619 cm^{-1} relate to the formation of β-turns and β-sheet aggregates (Table A3). With an increasing fraction of negatively charged PG in the liposomes, the β-aggregates (the band at ~1619 cm^{-1}) almost disappear and the α-helical structure content increases (formation of a band at ~1655 cm^{-1}) with a continuous diminishing of the β-turn content (the band at ~1686 cm^{-1}). IR spectra of HAL-1/2 (Figure 8, Table A4) display a notable spectral shift of the amide I band (from ~1648 to 1656 cm^{-1}) already in the presence of neutral PC-based liposomes indicating a conformational change from an unordered to the α-helical structure. The highest α-helical fraction is observed for HAL-1/2 interacting with negatively charged liposomes composed of PC/PG in a 1:4 ratio. An increase in α-helical structure content is accompanied by diminishing of the β-sheet bands (at ~1640 and 1690 cm^{-1}) and also some minor changes in the β-turn arrangement (a slight shift of the band at ~1685 cm^{-1} to 1681 cm^{-1}). Similar to HAL-1/2, the formation of a band at ~1657 cm^{-1}, indicating an increase in the α-helical structure content, is observed also for HAL-1/6 upon addition of neutral PC-based liposomes (Figure 8). An additional band at ~1639 cm^{-1} is probably due to the β-sheet structure formation.

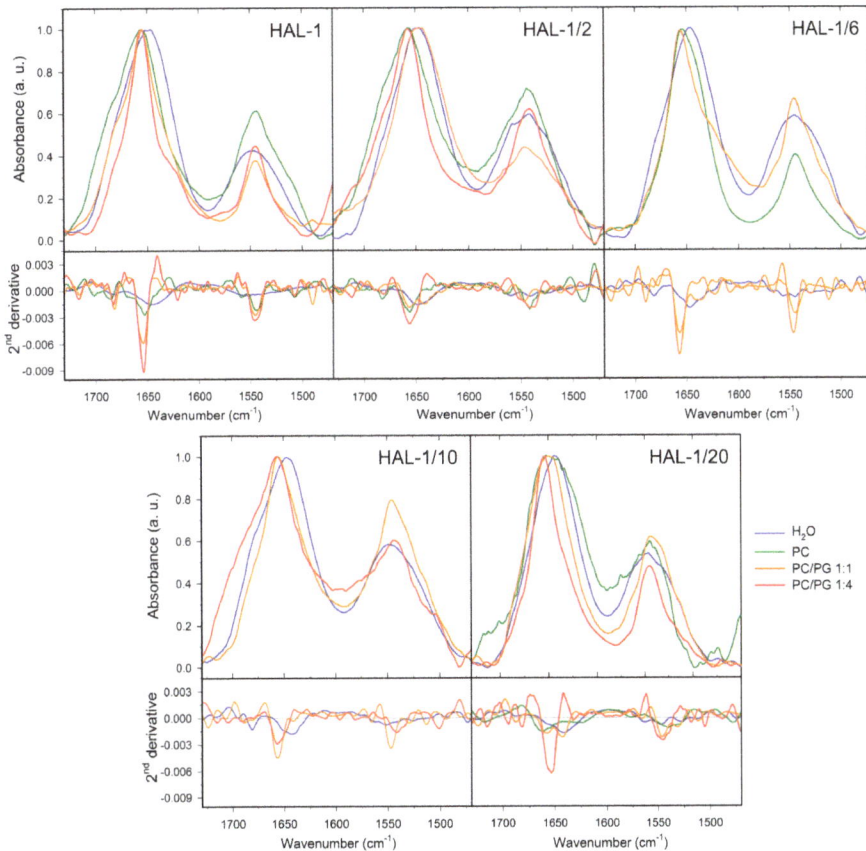

Figure 8. IR spectra (**top**) and their second derivatives (**bottom**) of HAL-1 and its analogs (10 mg/mL) in the presence of LUVs having different composition: in aqueous solution and in the presence of LUVs prepared from PC and PC/PG mixtures: 1:1 and 1:4.

For HAL-1/10 in the presence of LUVs, with an increasing fraction of PG in the liposomes, we observe diminishing of the band at ~1643 cm^{-1} and formation of a band at ~1656 cm^{-1}, indicating again a transition from β-sheet and/or random coil structure to α-helical structure. This process is accompanied by diminishing of the band at ~1681 cm^{-1} assigned to β-turns and formation of a band at ~1690 cm^{-1} probably due to β-sheet structure occurrence [41,42] (Figure 8, Table A4). FTIR spectra of HAL-1/20 in the presence of neutral PC-based liposomes indicate the formation of β-sheet aggregates (band at ~1626 cm^{-1}). A dominant spectral component at ~1663 cm^{-1} can be probably assigned to the 3$_{10}$-helical structure. These two spectral features disappear with an increasing fraction of PG in the liposomes and we observe formation of a band due to the α-helical structure (positioned at ~1658 and 1654 cm^{-1} in the presence of liposomes composed of PC/PG in the 1:1 and 1:4 ratio, respectively). For this analog, bands assigned to the β-sheet (at ~1634 and 1694 cm^{-1}) and β-turn structures (at ~1681 cm^{-1}) can be observed even in the presence of liposomes with the highest PG fraction (PC/PG in the 1:4 ratio).

IR spectroscopy confirms induced conformational change from the random coil to the α-helical structure in the biologically active HAL-1 analogs upon interaction with the bacterial membrane models and complements ECD results by providing information about the β-structure formation. Based on the results of IR analysis, spectral changes in ECD curves observed for the peptides interacting with SDS in concentration far above cmc and for PG-containing LUVs are probably due to changes in the β-sheet content. Behavior of HAL-1 peptides towards LUVs reveals (a) in accordance with biological data, the most active natural HAL-1 shows the lowest tendency to form β-aggregates and the β-sheet structure upon interaction with PG-containing LUVs; (b) contrary to the ECD results, all HAL-1 analogs adopt some portion of the α-helical structure already in the presence of neutral liposomes (representing a crude model of mammalian cells, against which the peptides have no or very low activity). This rather surprising conformational behavior could be caused by different experimental conditions used for the measurements of IR and ECD spectra (IR experiments require ~100× higher peptide concentration than ECD measurements, see experimental conditions for ECD and IR measurements in the Materials and Methods section). It seems that under such conditions, the peptides tend to form specific assemblies, adopting a conformation with a high α-helical content.

2.3. Concentration Dependence Measurements

In order to clarify the discrepancy between the results of the peptide conformational analyses obtained by ECD and IR, we have complemented our study by a measurement of concentration dependencies of ECD spectra of the HAL-1 peptides (Figure 9). Our ECD data indicate that with increasing peptide concentration, the unordered/PPII conformation changes to a partially α-helical conformation for all the studied analogs except for HAL-1/2, which seems to form β-aggregates when its concentration reaches 100 mg/mL. In order to determine the peptide conformational change induced by its high concentration more specifically, we have performed measurements of VCD spectra of the peptides (Figure 10) using the highest peptide concentration studied by ECD (i.e., 100 mg/mL). VCD measurements supported the results of ECD analysis, confirming that at high peptide concentration, HAL-1 and its analogs HAL-1/6, HAL-1/10, and HAL-1/20 spontaneously form the α-helical structure, indicated by a negative/positive VCD couplet in the amide I region [46–48]. On the contrary, the HAL-1/2 analog (Figure 10b) seems to undergo a distinct conformational change, forming highly organized β-sheet aggregates (β-sheet fibrils) characterized by an intense five-peak VCD signal with the ($-/-/+/-/-$) sign pattern in the amide I and II region [49–51]. Interestingly, a tendency to form the α-helical structure at high peptide concentration is common for all the HAL-1 analogs except for HAL-1/2, which exhibits the most reduced biological activity. It is therefore possible that for the peptide biological action, formation of specific assemblies with a high α-helical content might be also important.

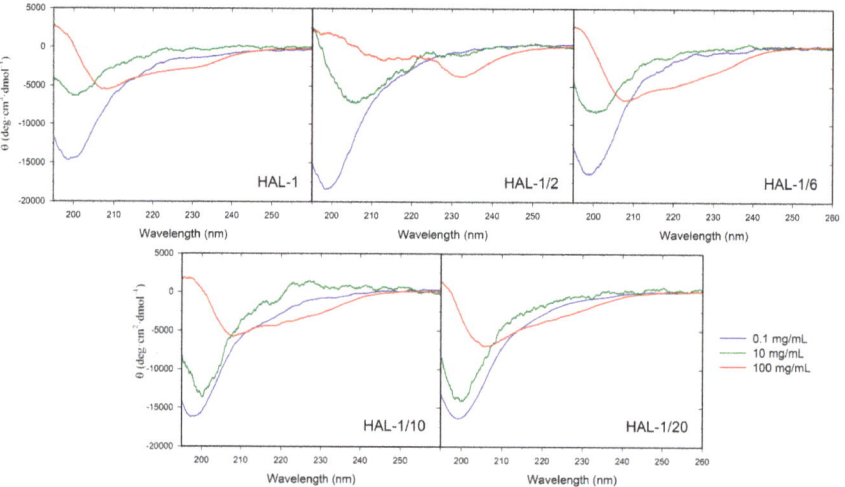

Figure 9. Concentration dependence of ECD spectra of HAL-1 and its analogs: 0.1, 10, 100 mg/mL.

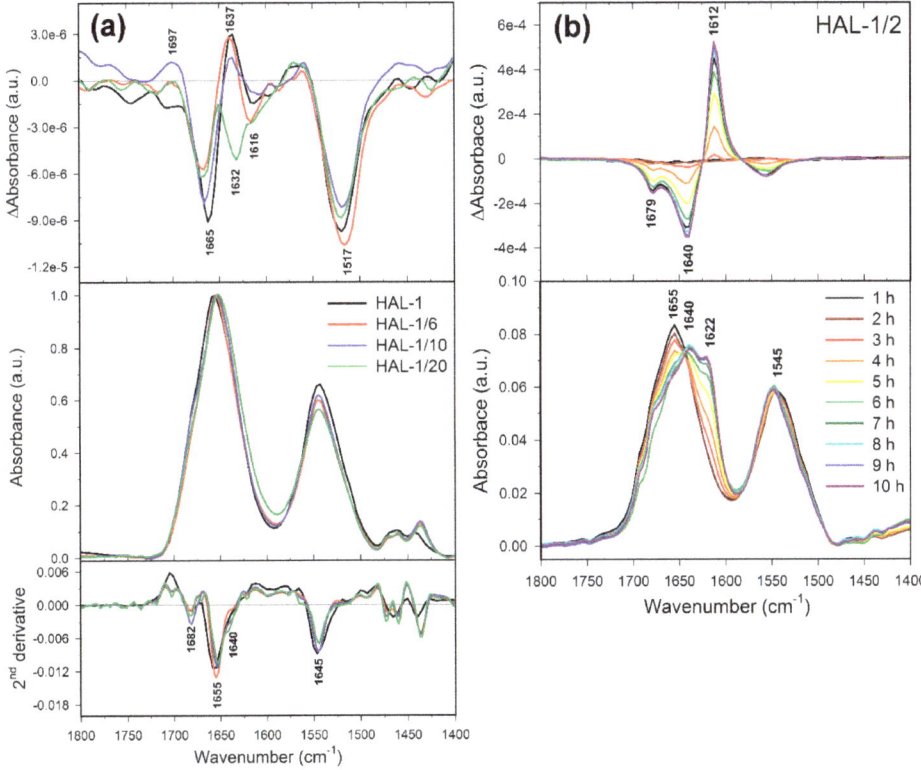

Figure 10. (**a**) VCD (**top**)/IR (**middle**)/second derivatives of IR spectra (**bottom**) of HAL-1, HAL-1/6, HAL-1/10, and HAL-1/20 in aqueous solution for samples in the 100 mg/mL concentration; (**b**) time dependence (1–10 h after preparation) of VCD (**top**) and IR spectra (**bottom**) of HAL-1/2 in aqueous solution for the sample in the 100 mg/mL concentration.

2.4. Structural Changes Followed by Fluorescence Spectroscopy

Participation of the tryptophan residue in the interaction of HAL-1 peptides with SDS and LUVs can be monitored selectively on the basis of fluorescence spectra. The observed fluorescence signals are assigned to the Trp3 residue. In aqueous solutions, the peptides exhibit fluorescence maxima at 360 nm (HAL-1), 356 nm (HAL-1/2), 361 nm (HAL-1/6) and 359 nm (HAL-1/20) (Table 2), i.e., the typical values for Trp residue in a hydrophilic environment. Upon interaction with LUVs, these maxima shift to about 330 nm (Table 2) indicating that tryptophan is not fully immersed in the lipophilic part of the liposome, but it is still in a close proximity of liposome phosphate heads [52]. In the case of HAL-1/2, the fluorescence maximum shifts only to 350 nm. Hence, it is probable that HAL-1/2 while interacting with LUVs, does not incorporate itself into the liposome despite the fact that parallel ECD experiments indicate a formation of some α-helical secondary structure. This result confirms our assumption that the α-helix formation is an important but not a sufficient condition for the efficient functioning of our AMPs. This conclusion is further supported by the results shown by HAL-1/6. Although HAL-1/6 readily interacts with LUVs by forming the α-helical structure, its biological activity is smaller than the activity of the natural HAL-1. Fluorescence spectroscopy shows that HAL-1 peptides are attached to the membrane surface with little penetration, indicating that the HAL-1 peptide mode of action probably involves either (a) dissolving the membrane in a detergent-like manner (the carpet model) or (b) formation of toroidal-type trans-membrane pores (lined both by peptide molecules and phospholipid headgroups) [53].

Table 2. Tryptophan fluorescence maxima of HAL-1 and its analogs (0.125 mg/mL—identical as for the ECD experiments) in aqueous solution and in the presence of LUVs (L/P = 20).

Solution	HAL-1	HAL-1/2	HAL-1/6	HAL-1/20
Water	360 nm	356 nm	361 nm	359 nm
PC	356 nm	362 nm	356 nm	359 nm
PC/PG (1:1)	331 nm	350 nm	336 nm	333 nm

2.5. Molecular Dynamics

As follows from the fluorescence spectroscopy measurements, HAL-1 peptides seem to bind to the outer leaflet of our model membranes. In order to better understand the mechanism of peptide-membrane interaction, we performed MD simulations of HAL-1 in water and in the presence of PC and PG-based model membranes. According to our results, HAL-1 in water is in a random coil conformation (Figure 11). When in the vicinity of a PC containing membrane, HAL-1 does not immerse into the membrane and it seems to have no defined orientation with regards to the membrane. HAL-1 does not change its structure and it still adopts a random coil conformation. The result of this simulation might seem rather surprising: Although the peptide exhibits hemolytic activity, we do not observe any peptide-membrane interaction. However, as follows from our spectroscopic results (see Section 2.3), HAL-1 structural behavior is concentration dependent and it is therefore probable that for its full activity, it is necessary to exceed a certain peptide threshold concentration. Under such conditions, the peptide might form specific assemblies (e.g., pores) that would allow for the peptide-membrane interaction [54].

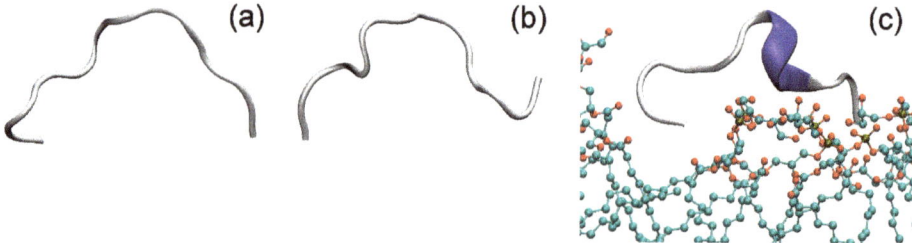

Figure 11. Molecular mechanic simulation of HAL-1 peptide (**a**) in water, (**b**) in the presence of PC and (**c**) PG model membrane.

When put into interaction with the PG based membrane, HAL-1 is anchored to the membrane by the terminal amino acid Arg. The peptide does not penetrate into the membrane and for the simulation time (110 ns) it stays in the vicinity of the membrane (Figure 11), which is in agreement with the fluorescence spectroscopy results, showing that tryptophan is in close proximity to the liposome phosphate heads (see Section 2.4). Based on the MD simulations, HAL-1 in a bacterial membrane-mimicking environment adopts mostly a 3_{10}-helical structure with a minor portion of the β-turn structure (Figure 11). Such a result does not contradict the ECD and IR data (suggesting under such conditions, formation of the α-helical conformation), as it was shown that the 3_{10}-helix is an important intermediate along the α-helix folding/unfolding pathway [55].

Based on the results of our spectroscopic investigation and MD simulations, we suggest a mechanism of HAL-1 interaction with model membranes: HAL-1 as a cationic peptide is mostly attracted to the negatively charged leaflets of the PG based model membranes, adopting predominantly a 3_{10}-helical conformation—an intermediate conformation and/or a precursor of the α-helical structure [55]. Since the peptide in such conformation already adopts an amphipathic structure, formation of peptide assemblies (most probably membrane pores), where the peptides are predominantly in the α-helical conformation, seems favorable. However, for the formation of such assemblies, it is necessary to exceed a specific threshold concentration of the peptide in a close proximity or in an immediate contact with the membrane. The proposed mechanisms of action are inspired by the molecular mechanisms of cooperativity of antibacterial peptides proposed by Huang et al. [54,56], and correspond to the mechanism and dynamics of AMP channel formation monitored *in situ*, where at least a three-step procedure of AMP insertion was suggested and the importance of the peptide–peptide interaction was demonstrated [57]. Several steps need to be taken to confirm this hypothesis: (1) It would be beneficial to perform more profound MD simulations of all HAL-1 analogs interacting with membranes of different composition. A peptide concentration dependency should be studied, investigating two or more peptides that interact on a membrane surface; (2) this computational study should be complemented by experiments allowing detailed study of peptide orientation with respect to the membrane such as oriented ECD [54], surface-enhanced infrared absorption spectroscopy [57], or oriented solid-state NMR measurements [58]. This will be a matter of further investigation.

3. Materials and Methods

3.1. Materials

The phospholipids, PC, and PG (sodium salt), were purchased from Avanti Polar Lipids (Alabaster, AL, USA). TFE was purchased from Merck (Darmstadt, Germany) and SDS from Sigma (Darmstadt, Germany). The peptides (see Table 1) were prepared by the standard procedures of solid phase peptide synthesis [19]. All the peptides were delivered as TFA salts (with TFA counterions bonded to the free amino termini and side chains of positively charged amino acids). For the natural HAL-1, it was possible to remove TFA counterions using a standard procedure [59] as there was a sufficient amount of the sample available.

3.2. Preparation of Vesicles

The phospholipids PC, PG or their mixtures (at 1:4, 1:1 or 4:1 molar ratios) were dissolved in chloroform/methanol (3:1) mixture and dried under vacuum. The dry lipid layer was hydrated with distilled water and gently stirred. LUVs with an approximate diameter of 0.1 μm were formed by extrusion through polycarbonate membranes (pore size 0.1 μm, a total of 30 passages through the membrane) using Mini-Extruder (Avanti Polar Lipids, Alabaster, AL, USA). The temperature of the lipid suspension was kept above the phase transition temperature T_m of the lipid with the highest T_m within the whole hydration and extrusion process. A liposome size of 0.1 μm was selected in order to avoid artifacts due to light scattering (especially in ECD experiments). The shapes and sizes of liposomes were checked by cryo-electron microscopy. Liposome stabilities and size distributions were verified by light scattering using Zetasizer Nano (Malvern Panalytical, Malvern, UK).

3.3. Electronic Circular Dichroism

ECD experiments were carried out on J-815 spectropolarimeter (Jasco, Tsukuba, Japan) equipped with the Peltier type temperature control system PTC-423S/L. The spectra were collected from 180 to 300 nm at room temperature in 0.1 cm quartz cells (0.125 mg/mL peptide concentration, 2 scans, 0.5 nm steps, 20 nm/min speed, 8 s time constant, 1 nm spectral bandwidth). For the measurements in high liposome concentration (L/P concentration ratio higher than 100), the cell with 0.02 cm path length and appropriate experimental conditions (5 nm/min speed, 32 s response time and 1 nm bandwidth) were used. After baseline subtraction, the final data were expressed as molar ellipticities θ (deg·cm^2·dmol^{-1}) per residue. All samples were prepared by dilutions of a stock peptide solution (1 mg/mL) to a final peptide concentration 0.125 mg/mL, followed by adding an appropriate aliquot of TFE (final TFE concentration 10–50% *v/v*), SDS (stock solution 32 mM, final SDS concentration 0.016–16 mM, i.e., below and above cmc; cmc ≈ 4 mM for the SDS-peptides solution [60]), or LUVs (stock solution

200 mg/mL). SDS measurements below and above cmc enable investigating the effects of SDS acting both as (a) a denaturation agent (below cmc) and (b) a simple membrane model (above cmc).

Concentration dependence was measured for all the peptides at the given concentrations: 0.1, 10, and 100 mg/mL. The spectra were collected from 180 to 300 nm at room temperature in 0.1 cm quartz cells for the 0.1 mg/mL peptide concentration, and in 6 µm homemade CaF_2 cells for 10 mg/mL and 100 mg/mL peptide concentration with the following setup: 2 scans, 0.5 nm steps, 20 nm/min speed, 8 s time constant, 1 nm spectral bandwidth. The α-helical fraction was calculated using a two-state model [30,61]. For the more detailed analysis of secondary structure, we used the CDPro software package [36,62].

3.4. Principle Component Analysis

Analysis of temperature- and time-dependent ECD spectra was performed using principal component analysis (PCA) based on a singular value decomposition algorithm applied to reduce spectral series $\{Y_i(\nu), i = 1, \ldots, n\}$ to their lowest dimension without the loss of spectroscopic information. Each spectrum of the matrix $Y_i(\nu)$ can be unambiguously expressed as:

$$Y_i(\nu) = \sum_{j=1}^{M} V_{ij} W_j S_j(\nu) \qquad (1)$$

where W_j is the diagonal matrix of singular values, $S(\nu)$ corresponds to the matrix of the orthonormal subspectra (eigenvectors) and V_{ij} is the unitary square matrix of coefficients (representing the influence strength of the subspectrum S_j). M represents a number of independent "spectral species", distinct from the spectral noise, found in the analyzed data set. The number of independent subspectra can be estimated from residual errors or from singular values. A detailed explanation of PCA can be found in [63]. The calculation of PCA was done using our own software programmed in Matlab™ (MathWorks®, Natick, MA, USA).

3.5. Infrared Spectroscopy

IR spectra in the transmission mode were recorded on Nicolet 6700 spectrometer (Thermo Fisher Scientific, Waltham, MA, USA) using standard mid-IR source, KBr beamsplitter and DTGS detector (2 cm^{-1} spectral resolution, Happ–Genzel apodization function, 2000 scans) in the 4000–1000 cm^{-1} spectral range. The cell compartment was purged by dry nitrogen during all the measurements. Aqueous solutions (10 mg/mL peptide concentration) were measured at room temperature in homemade CaF_2 cells with 6 µm path length (cell volume 1 µL). In our experiments involving peptide-membrane interaction, the L/P was always equal to 8 (LUVs stock solution 200 mg/mL). Numerical data treatment was carried out using Grams/AI software (Thermo Electron, Waltham, MA, USA). The spectral contribution of water was eliminated using a standard algorithm [64]. The IR signal of phospholipids was subtracted from spectra of peptide/phospholipid mixtures. Subsequently, the spectrum of water vapors was subtracted and the baseline was linearly corrected. Final IR spectra were normalized to amide I intensity maxima. The IR spectra of HAL-1 analogs were obtained by additional subtraction of trifluoroacetate signals, which were present due to a standard cleavage from the resin by TFA [65]. Such subtraction was not needed for the natural HAL-1 as for this peptide, the TFA counterions were successfully removed (see Section 3.1). The secondary structure analysis [41] was aided using second derivatives Savitzky–Golay algorithm (Grams/AI software, Thermo Electron, Waltham, MA, USA) and a band fitting procedure (Gaussian–Lorentzian band shape—OMNIC Thermo Fisher Scientific, Waltham, MA, USA).

3.6. Vibrational Circular Dichroism

VCD spectra were measured on a dual source [66] and dual photo-elastic modulator [67] VCD spectrometer ChiralIR-2X™ (BioTools, Jupiter, FL, USA) at room temperature in CaF_2–BioCell™ with

6 μm path length (BioTools, Jupiter, FL, USA). The data were collected for ~12 h (12 blocks of 6000 scans each at 8 cm^{-1} resolution). The spectra were processed in Grams/AI software (Thermo Electron, Waltham, MA, USA). Solvent scans were subtracted as background. Baseline was corrected using a linear function. The spectra were smoothed with a second-order Savitzky-Golay filter using a 9 point window and normalized to amide I maxima in the corresponding IR spectra.

3.7. Fluorescence Spectroscopy

Steady-state fluorescence spectra were measured on Fluoromax Z (Jobin-Yvon, Chilly-Mazarin, France) fluorimeter in a 10 mm quartz cell. Excitation at 280 nm was used to induce fluorescence of the tryptophan residue. The emission was collected from 300 to 450 nm with the 1.5 s integration time. The emission and excitation slits were chosen as 2 nm. The peptide concentration of 0.125 mg/mL was chosen identical as for the ECD experiments in order to maintain mutual compatibility. At this low concentration, there is no danger of Trp residues self-quenching. L/P = 20 was used for all the fluorescence measurements (2 mg/mL lipid concentration).

3.8. Molecular Dynamics

An all-atom structure model of the peptides was created using the tLEaP program from the AmberTools (San Francisco, CA, USA) [68] suite and the force field Amber FF99SB [69] PC and PG membrane models were created using program VMD [70] and its membrane plugin. PC and PG parameters were generated using programs Antechamber and Parmchk from the AmberTools suite. In total, three systems were created, a peptide in water and the peptide with PC and PG membranes. Each system was solvated in TIP3P water and neutralized using K$^+$ and Cl$^-$ ions. The initial equilibration of systems was performed using NAMD 2.9 [71] with a time step of 1 fs and rigid bonds in water molecules using Settle algorithm [72]. Systems were minimized for 1000 steps, warmed to 310 K and equilibrated for 1 ps. The system without a membrane was simulated for 10 ps, and the systems with membranes were simulated for 110 ps.

4. Conclusions

The combined use of the methods of molecular spectroscopy (ECD, IR absorption, VCD and fluorescence spectroscopy) together with MD simulations allowed us to follow secondary structure changes of HAL-1 and its analogs induced by an interaction with artificial membrane models. On the basis of the obtained results, formation of the α-helical structure appears important for the activity of the HAL-1 peptides. However, peptide biological activities seem to be determined not only by their propensity to form the α-helical structure. Additional factors like the ability of the peptides to adopt alternative conformations (such as β-sheet, PPII conformation or 3$_{10}$-helix) cannot be excluded and have to be considered for their biological activity as well. For biologically active analogs, the concentration-dependence ECD measurements together with VCD data suggest a possible formation of peptide assemblies high in α-helical content (most probably membrane pores), which might enable membrane penetration. Following our spectroscopic results, we can propose that HAL-1 structural behavior is concentration dependent and for its full activity, certain peptide threshold concentration should be exceeded. Under such conditions, the peptides might form specific assemblies (e.g., pores) that would allow for the peptide-membrane interaction and complete their task as antimicrobial agents.

Author Contributions: Conceptualization, M.P. and L.B.; methodology, M.P., V.Z., L.B.; software, V.Z. and V.K.J.; formal analysis, M.P., K.H., V.K.J. and L.B.; investigation, M.P., V.Z., K.H., V.K.J., E.K., T.P. and L.B.; resources, E.K. and V.Č.; writing—original draft preparation, M.P., P.M. and L.B.; writing—review and editing, M.P., K.H., V.K.J., E.K., T.P. and L.B.; visualization, M.P., V.Z., K.H., V.K.J. and L.B.; supervision, L.B.; project administration, V.K.J. and L.B.; funding acquisition, V.K.J. and L.B.

Funding: This research was funded by the Czech Science Foundation, grant number 208/10/0376 and by Research Projects RVO, grant number 61388963.

Acknowledgments: We would like to thank Rina K. Dukor (BioTools, USA) for allowing us to measure VCD spectra in their facility and to Jan Bednár (Institute de Biologie Structurale, France) for performing cryo-electron microscopy measurements of liposomes.

Conflicts of Interest: The authors declare no conflict of interest. The funders had no role in the design of the study; in the collection, analyses, or interpretation of data; in the writing of the manuscript, or in the decision to publish the results.

Abbreviations

AMPs	Antimicrobial peptides
cmc	Critical micelle concentration
ECD	Electronic circular dichroism
HAL	Halictine
IR	Infrared
L/P	Lipid/peptide ratio
LUV	Large unilamellar vesicle
MD	Molecular dynamics
PC	1,2-Dimyristoyl-sn-glycerol-3-phosphatidylcholine
PCA	Principal component analysis
PG	1,2-Dimyristoyl-sn-glycero-3-phospho-(1'-rac-glycerol)
PPII	Polyproline II
SDS	Sodium dodecyl sulfate
TFE	2,2,2-Trifluoroethanol
VCD	Vibrational circular dichroism

Appendix A

Table A1. Helical fraction for HAL-1 and its analogs in aqueous solution and in the presence of TFE (concentration expressed in volume percent (v/v)) and SDS (in mM) calculated using a two-state model from ECD spectra [30,61].

Solution	Hal-1	Hal-1/2	Hal-1/6	Hal-1/10	Hal-1/20
Water	14%	14%	13%	15%	15%
TFE 30%	32%	32%	37%	36%	36%
TFE 50%	32%	32%	40%	42%	36%
SDS 0.016 mM	13%	13%	3%	14%	14%
SDS 0.16 mM	14%	14%	3%	18%	52%
SDS 2 mM	46%	46%	66%	63%	36%
SDS 4 mM	51%	51%	46%	63%	32%
SDS 8 mM	37%	37%	46%	50%	31%
SDS 16 mM	31%	31%	36%	36%	42%

Table A2. Estimation of the secondary structure content calculated from ECD spectra using the CDPro package [62,73] for HAL-1 and its analogs in aqueous solution, and in the presence of SDS.

Structure	Sodium Dodecyl Sulfate						
	0 mM	0.016 mM	0.16 mM	2 mM	4 mM	8 mM	16 mM
HAL-1							
α-helix	12%	12%	14%	61%	61%	53%	53%
β-sheet	50%	50%	44%	6%	6%	10%	10%
β-turn	16%	16%	16%	12%	12%	17%	17%
Other	22%	22%	26%	22%	22%	21%	21%

Table A2. *Cont.*

HAL-1/2								
α-helix	12%	11%	14%	14%	47%	47%	44%	
β-sheet	53%	54%	45%	44%	13%	13%	15%	
β-turn	16%	16%	16%	16%	18%	18%	18%	
Other	19%	19%	25%	25%	22%	22%	24%	
HAL-1/6								
α-helix	12%	13%	11%	82%	85%	70%	60%	
β-sheet	52%	42%	37%	2%	2%	4%	9%	
β-turn	16%	16%	14%	9%	9%	14%	19%	
Other	20%	29%	38%	6%	4%	11%	14%	
HAL-1/10								
α-helix	11%	12%	13%	80%	79%	72%	70%	
β-sheet	52%	51%	43%	2%	2%	4%	5%	
β-turn	16%	16%	16%	10%	10%	14%	15%	
Other	21%	21%	27%	8%	9%	10%	10%	
HAL-1/20								
α-helix	12%	13%	66%	42%	39%	37%	60%	
β-sheet	52%	42%	5%	13%	17%	18%	18%	
β-turn	16%	13%	12%	17%	18%	18%	17%	
Other	20%	32%	18%	28%	27%	27%	15%	

Table A3. Estimation of the secondary structure content calculated from ECD spectra using the CDPro package [62,73] for HAL-1 and its analogs in aqueous solution, and in the presence of LUVs.

Structure	0 mM	LUV				
		PC (L/P = 20)	PC (L/P = 100)	PC/PG (4:1) (L/P = 20)	PC/PG (1:1) (L/P = 20)	PC/PG (1:4) (L/P = 20)
HAL-1						
α-helix	12%	12%	18%	35%	45%	61%
β-sheet	50%	51%	38%	17%	10%	7%
β-turn	16%	16%	18%	18%	17%	12%
Other	22%	21%	26%	30%	22%	21%
HAL-1/2						
α-helix	11%	11%	17%	37%	47%	69%
β-sheet	53%	53%	40%	17%	10%	5%
β-turn	16%	16%	18%	17%	16%	14%
Other	19%	21%	25%	29%	28%	13%
HAL-1/6						
α-helix	12%	12%	14%	60%	79%	60%
β-sheet	52%	50%	45%	7%	1%	6%
β-turn	16%	16%	17%	8%	5%	12%
Other	20%	22%	24%	25%	14%	21%
HAL-1/10						
α-helix	11%	12%	13%	35%	69%	36%
β-sheet	52%	52%	51%	18%	3%	38%
β-turn	16%	16%	17%	17%	9%	14%
Other	21%	20%	19%	30%	7%	13%
HAL-1/20						
α-helix	12%	12%	14%	25%	80%	46%
β-sheet	52%	50%	46%	24%	2%	13%
β-turn	16%	16%	17%	18%	10%	18%
Other	20%	21%	22%	34%	7%	24%

Table A4. Estimation of the secondary structure content from IR spectra, using a bandfitting procedure for HAL-1 and its analogs in aqueous solution (H_2O and D_2O), in the presence of SDS, TFE, and LUVs. The numbers in parentheses correspond to percentages of each fitted band in the amide I region.

Solvent	Amide I (cm^{-1})	Second Derivative Decomposition of Amide I (cm^{-1})						
		aggregate	β-sheet	α-helix	3$_{10}$-helix	coil	β-turn	β-sheet
HAL-1								
H_2O	1646	—	—	—	—	1648 (88)	1683 (12)	—
D_2O	1647	—	—	—	—	1642 (69)	1667 (31)	—
TFE	1655	—	1633 (26)	1656 (63)	—	—	1680 (11)	—
SDS 8 mM/H_2O	1655	1621 (12)	1635 (16)	1656 (63)	—	—	1682 (9)	—
SDS 8 mM/D_2O	1649	—	—	1649 (95)	—	—	1676 (5)	—
PC	1656	1619 (5)	—	1656 (63)	—	—	1688 (33)	—
PC/PG 1:1	1655	—	1634 (29)	1656 (52)	—	—	1680 (19)	—
PC/PG 1:4	1656	—	1633 (6)	1655 (58)	—	—	1678 (36)	—
HAL-1/2								
H_2O	1649	—	1637 (29)	—	—	1650 (56)	1684 (14)	—
SDS 8 mM/H_2O	1655	—	1635 (38)	1657 (58)	—	—	1685 (4)	—
PC	1657	—	1642 (32)	1657 (32)	—	—	1680 (35)	—
PC/PG 1:1	1647	1628 (34)	1642 (28)	1658 (24)	—	—	1676 (13)	—
PC/PG 1:4	1657	—	1632 (15)	1656 (43)	—	—	1680 (41)	—
HAL-1/6								
H_2O	1646	—	—	—	—	1647 (92)	1682 (8)	—
SDS 8 mM/H_2O	1654	1629 (29)	—	1655 (69)	—	—	—	1695 (2)
PC	1654	1621 (7)	1639 (29)	1657 (59)	—	—	1680 (5)	—
PC/PG 1:1	1656	1626 (9)	1642 (18)	1657 (62)	—	—	1682 (11)	—
HAL-1/10								
H_2O	1647	—	—	—	—	1647 (82)	1681 (18)	—
PC/PG 1:1	1655	1625 (12)	1640 (21)	1657 (57)	—	—	1681 (10)	—
PC/PG 1:4	1656	—	—	1656 (80)	—	—	1688 (20)	—
HAL-1/20								
H_2O	1644	—	1643 (93)	—	—	—	1676 (7)	—
SDS 8 mM/H_2O	1650	1629 (9)	—	1653 (83)	—	—	1685 (9)	—
PC	1649	1625 (36)	1639 (13)	1654 (28)	—	—	1685 (22)	—
PC/PG 1:1	1650	1628 (29)	1642 (16)	1659 (49)	—	—	1685 (6)	—
PC/PG 1:4	1654	1621 (19)	1634 (14)	1655 (43)	—	—	1678 (24)	—

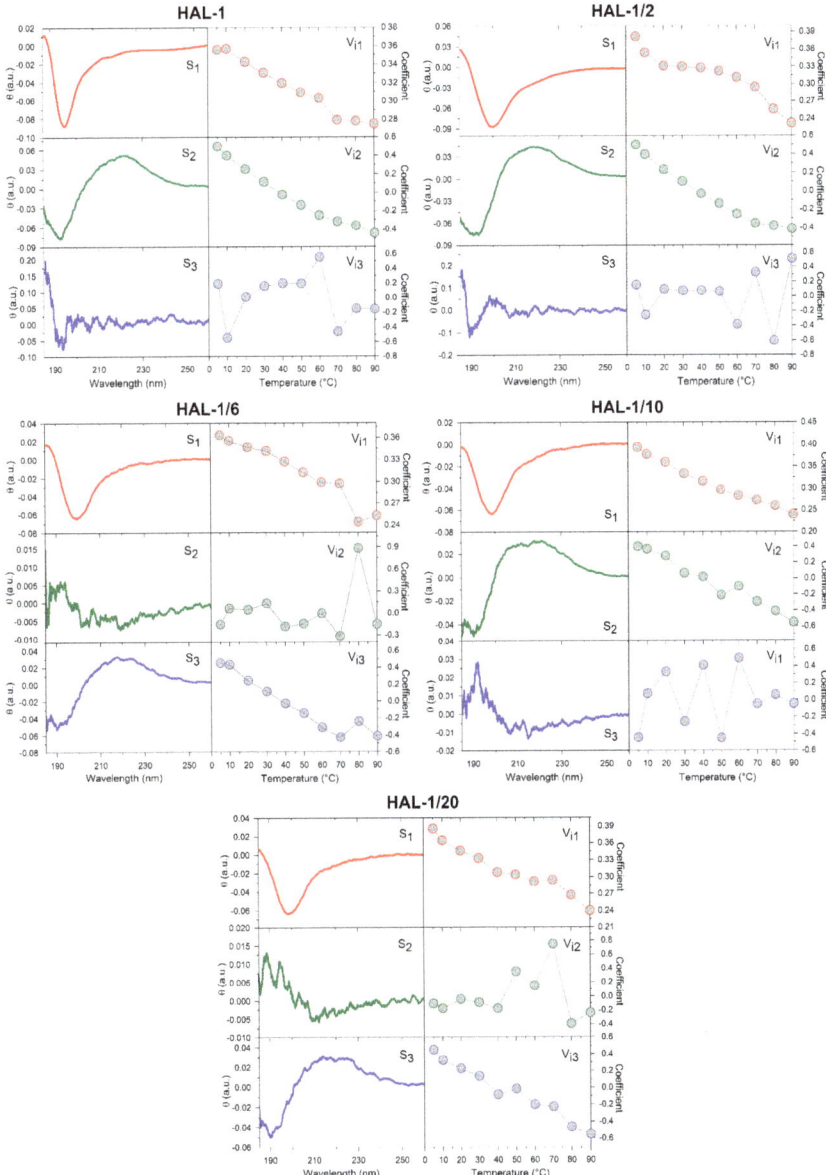

Figure A1. PCA results applied to the set of thermal dependence of ECD spectra (from 5 to 90 °C) of HAL-1 and its analogs. S_j represents the three most significant subspectra, and V_{ij} represents the appropriate coefficients indicating the relative contribution of the corresponding subspectrum.

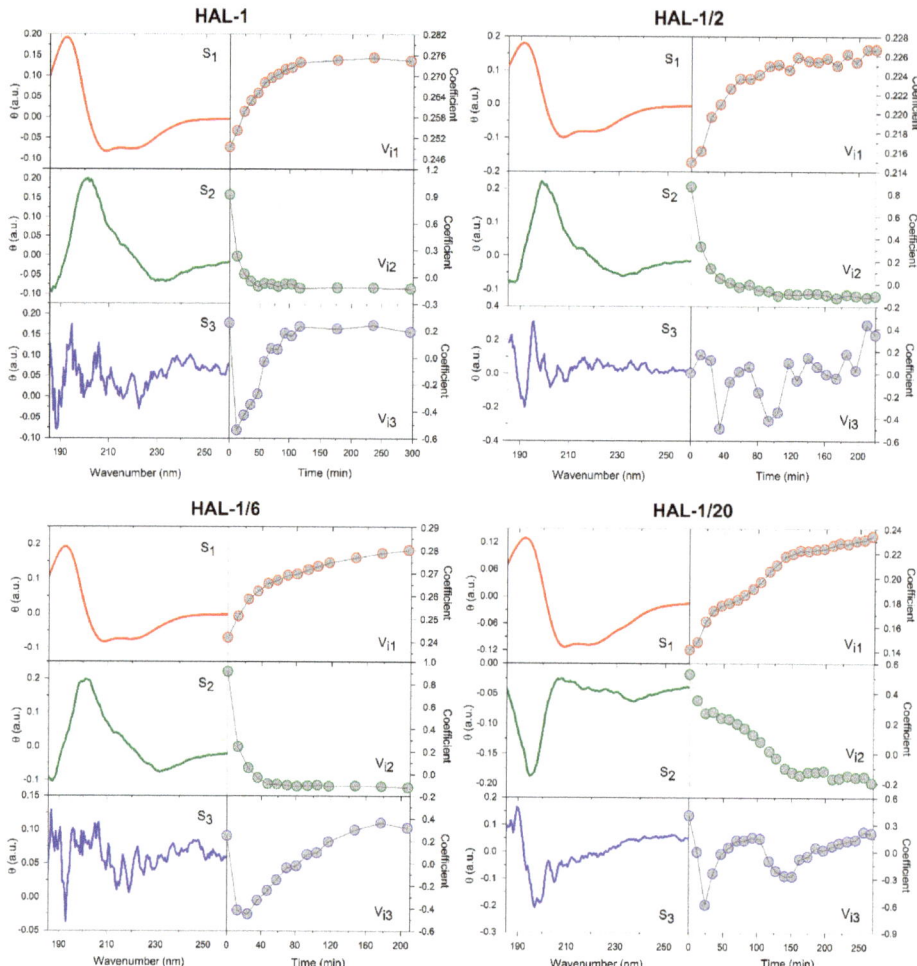

Figure A2. PCA results applied to the set of time dependence of ECD spectra of HAL-1 and its analogs in PC/PG = 1:4 mixtures measured within a 220 min time interval after the sample preparation with a 12-min time step. S_j represents the three most significant subspectra and V_{ij} represents the appropriate coefficients indicating the relative contribution of the corresponding subspectrum.

References

1. Phoenix, D.A.; Dennison, S.R.; Harris, F. *Antibacterial Peptides*; Wiley-VCH: Weinheim, Germany, 2013; ISBN 978-3-527-33263-2.
2. Brogden, K.A. Antimicrobial peptides: Pore formers or metabolic inhibitors in bacteria? *Nat. Rev. Microbiol.* **2005**, *3*, 238–250. [CrossRef] [PubMed]
3. Fjell, C.D.; Hiss, J.A.; Hancock, R.E.; Schneider, G. Designing antimicrobial peptides: Form follows function. *Nat. Rev. Drug Discov.* **2012**, *11*, 37–51. [CrossRef] [PubMed]
4. Zasloff, M. Antimicrobial peptides of multicellular organisms. *Nature* **2002**, *415*, 389–395. [CrossRef] [PubMed]
5. Hancock, R.E.; Diamond, G. The role of cationic antimicrobial peptides in innate host defences. *Trends Microbiol.* **2000**, *8*, 402–410. [CrossRef]

6. Hancock, R.E.; Scott, M.G. The role of antimicrobial peptides in animal defenses. *Proc. Natl. Acad. Sci. USA* **2000**, *97*, 8856–8861. [CrossRef] [PubMed]
7. Hoskin, D.W.; Ramamoorthy, A. Studies on anticancer activities of antimicrobial peptides. *Biochim. Biophys. Acta* **2008**, *1778*, 357–375. [CrossRef] [PubMed]
8. Papo, N.; Shai, Y. Host defense peptides as new weapons in cancer treatment. *Cell. Mol. Life Sci.* **2005**, *62*, 784–790. [CrossRef]
9. Papo, N.; Shai, Y. Can we predict biological activity of antimicrobial peptides from their interactions with model phospholipid membranes? *Peptides* **2003**, *24*, 1693–1703. [CrossRef]
10. Teixeira, V.; Feio, M.J.; Bastos, M. Role of lipids in the interaction of antimicrobial peptides with membranes. *Prog. Lipid Res.* **2012**, *51*, 149–177. [CrossRef]
11. Yount, N.Y.; Yeaman, M.R. Multidimensional signatures in antimicrobial peptides. *Proc. Natl. Acad. Sci. USA* **2004**, *101*, 7363–7368. [CrossRef]
12. Epand, R.M.; Epand, R.F. Domains in bacterial membranes and the action of antimicrobial agents. *Mol. Biosyst.* **2009**, *5*, 580–587. [CrossRef] [PubMed]
13. Epand, R.M.; Epand, R.F.; Arnusch, C.J.; Papahadjopoulos-Sternberg, B.; Wang, G.; Shai, Y. Lipid clustering by three homologous arginine-rich antimicrobial peptides is insensitive to amino acid arrangement and induced secondary structure. *Biochim. Biophys. Acta* **2010**, 1272–1280. [CrossRef] [PubMed]
14. Wimley, W.C.; Hristova, K. Antimicrobial peptides: Successes, challenges and unanswered questions. *J. Membr. Biol.* **2011**, *239*, 27–34. [CrossRef] [PubMed]
15. Blondelle, S.E.; Lohner, K.; Aguilar, M.I. Lipid-induced conformation and lipid-binding properties of cytolytic and antimicrobial peptides: Determination and biological specificity. *Biochim. Biophys. Acta* **1999**, *1462*, 89–108. [CrossRef]
16. Epand, R.F.; Mor, A.; Epand, R.M. Lipid complexes with cationic peptides and OAKs; their role in antimicrobial action and in the delivery of antimicrobial agents. *Cell. Mol. Life Sci.* **2011**, *68*, 2177–2188. [CrossRef]
17. Čeřovský, V.; Buděšínský, M.; Hovorka, O.; Cvačka, J.; Voburka, Z.; Slaninová, J.; Borovičková, L.; Fučík, V.; Bednárová, L.; Votruba, I.; et al. Lasioglossins: Three novel antimicrobial peptides from the venom of the eusocial bee *Lasioglossum laticeps* (Hymenoptera: Halictidae). *ChemBioChem* **2009**, *10*, 2089–2099. [CrossRef]
18. Čeřovský, V.; Slaninová, J.; Fučík, V.; Monincová, L.; Bednárová, L.; Maloň, P.; Stokrová, J. Lucifensin, a novel insect defensin of medicinal maggots: Synthesis and structural study. *ChemBioChem* **2011**, *12*, 1352–1361. [CrossRef]
19. Monincová, L.; Buděšínský, M.; Slaninová, J.; Hovorka, O.; Cvačka, J.; Voburka, Z.; Fučík, V.; Borovičková, L.; Bednárová, L.; Straka, J.; et al. Novel antimicrobial peptides from the venom of the eusocial bee *Halictus sexcinctus* (Hymenoptera: Halictidae) and their analogs. *Amino Acids* **2010**, *39*, 763–775. [CrossRef]
20. Čujová, S.; Bednárová, L.; Slaninová, J.; Straka, J.; Čeřovský, V. Interaction of a novel antimicrobial peptide isolated from the venom of solitary bee *Colletes daviesanus* with phospholipid vesicles and *Escherichia coli* cells. *J. Pept. Sci.* **2014**, *20*, 885–895. [CrossRef]
21. Stanchev, S.; Zawada, Z.; Monincová, L.; Bednárová, L.; Slaninová, J.; Fučík, V.; Čeřovský, V. Synthesis of lucifensin by native chemical ligation and characteristics of its isomer having different disulfide bridge pattern. *J. Pept. Sci.* **2014**, *20*, 725–735. [CrossRef]
22. Nešuta, O.; Hexnerová, R.; Buděšínský, M.; Slaninová, J.; Bednárová, L.; Hadravová, R.; Straka, J.; Veverka, V.; Čeřovský, V. Antimicrobial peptide from the wild bee *Hylaeus signatus* venom and its analogues: Structure-activity study and synergistic effect with antibiotics. *J. Nat. Prod.* **2016**, *79*, 1073–1083. [CrossRef] [PubMed]
23. Pazderková, M.; Kočišová, E.; Pazderka, T.; Maloň, P.; Kopecký, V.; Monincová, L.; Čeřovský, V.; Bednárová, L. Antimicrobial peptide from the eusocial bee *Halictus sexcinctus* interacting with model membranes. In *Advances in Biomedical Spectroscopy*; Marques, M.P., Batista de Carvalho, L.A.E., Haris, P.I., Eds.; IOE Press: Amsterdam, The Netherlands, 2013; Volume 7, pp. 79–83. ISBN 978-1-61499-183-0.
24. Myers, J.K.; Pace, C.N.; Scholtz, J.M. Trifluoroethanol effects on helix propensity and electrostatic interactions in the helical peptide from ribonuclease T-1. *Protein Sci.* **1998**, *7*, 383–388. [CrossRef] [PubMed]
25. Warschawski, D.E.; Arnold, A.A.; Beaugrand, M.; Gravel, A.; Chartrand, É.; Marcotte, I. Choosing membrane mimetics for NMR structural studies of transmembrane proteins. *Biochim. Biophys. Acta* **2011**, *1808*, 1957–1974. [CrossRef] [PubMed]

26. Strandberg, E.; Tiltak, D.; Ehni, S.; Wadhwani, P.; Ulrich, A.S. Lipid shape is a key factor for membrane interactions of amphipathic helical peptides. *Biochim. Biophys. Acta* **2012**, *1818*, 1764–1776. [CrossRef]
27. Eisenberg, D.; Weiss, R.M.; Terwilliger, T.C. The helical hydrophobic moment: A measure of the amphiphilicity of a helix. *Nature* **1982**, *277*, 371–374. [CrossRef]
28. Thévenet, P.; Shen, Y.; Maupetit, J.; Guyon, F.; Derreumaux, P.; Tufféry, P. PEP-FOLD: An updated de novo structure prediction server for both linear and disulfide bonded cyclic peptides. *Nucleic Acids Res.* **2012**, *40*, W288–W293. [CrossRef] [PubMed]
29. Sreerama, N.; Woody, R.W. Estimation of protein secondary structure from circular dichroism spectra: Comparison of CONTIN, SELCON, and CDSSTR methods with an expanded reference set. *Anal. Biochem.* **2000**, *287*, 252–260. [CrossRef] [PubMed]
30. Backlund, B.; Wikander, G.; Peeters, T.L.; Gräslund, A. Induction of secondary structure in the peptide hormone motilin by interaction with phospholipid vesicles. *Biochim. Biophys. Acta* **1994**, *1190*, 337–344. [CrossRef]
31. Drake, A.F.; Siligardi, G.; Gibbons, W.A. Reassessment of the electronic circular dichroism criteria for random coil conformations of poly(L-lysine) and the implications for protein folding and denaturation studies. *Biophys. Chem.* **1988**, *31*, 143–146. [CrossRef]
32. Wimmer, R.; Andersen, K.K.; Vad, B.; Davidsen, M.; Mølgaard, S.; Nesgaard, L.W.; Kristensen, H.H.; Otzen, D.E. Versatile interactions of the antimicrobial peptide Novispirin with detergents and lipids. *Biochemistry* **2006**, *45*, 481–497. [CrossRef] [PubMed]
33. Seddon, A.M.; Curnow, P.; Booth, P.J. Membrane proteins, lipids and detergents: Not just a soap opera. *Biochim. Biophys. Acta* **2004**, *1666*, 105–117. [CrossRef] [PubMed]
34. Berova, N.; Polavarapu, P.L.; Nakanishi, K.; Woody, R.W. *Comprehensive Chiroptical Spectroscopy Applications in Stereochemical Analysis of Synthetic Compounds, Natural Products and Biomolecules*; John Wiley & Sons: Hoboken, NJ, USA, 2012; ISBN 978-1-118-01292-5.
35. Abdul-Gader, A.; Miles, A.J.; Wallace, B.A. A reference dataset for the analyses of membrane protein secondary structures and transmembrane residues using circular dichroism spectroscopy. *Bioinformatics* **2011**, *27*, 1630–1636. [CrossRef] [PubMed]
36. Sreerama, N.; Woody, R.W. Poly(Pro)II helices in globular proteins: Identification and circular dichroic analysis. *Biochemistry* **1994**, *33*, 10022–10025. [CrossRef] [PubMed]
37. Whitmore, L.; Woollett, B.; Miles, A.J.; Janes, R.W.; Wallace, B.A. The protein circular dichroism data bank, a Web-based site for access to circular dichroism spectroscopic data. *Structure* **2010**, *18*, 1267–1269. [CrossRef] [PubMed]
38. Johnson, W.C. Analyzing protein circular dichroism spectra for accurate secondary structures. *Proteins* **1999**, *35*, 307–312. [CrossRef]
39. Bochicchio, B.; Tamburro, A.M. Polyproline II structure in proteins: Identification by chiroptical spectroscopies, stability, and functions. *Chirality* **2002**, *14*, 782–792. [CrossRef] [PubMed]
40. Lopes, J.L.S.; Miles, A.J.; Whitmore, L.; Wallace, B.A. Distinct circular dichroism spectroscopic signatures of polyproline II and unordered secondary structures: Applications in secondary structure analyses. *Protein Sci.* **2014**, *23*, 1765–1772. [CrossRef] [PubMed]
41. Barth, A. Infrared spectroscopy of proteins. *Biochim. Biophys. Acta* **2007**, *1767*, 1073–1101. [CrossRef]
42. Yang, H.; Yang, S.; Kong, J.; Dong, A.; Yu, S. Obtaining information about protein secondary structures in aqueous solution using Fourier transform IR spectroscopy. *Nat. Protoc.* **2015**, *10*, 382–396. [CrossRef]
43. Tesař, A.; Kopecký Jr., V.; Kočišová, E.; Bednárová, L. Dynamics of lipid layers with/without bounded antimicrobial peptide halictine-1. *Vibrat. Spectrosc.* **2017**, *93*, 42–51. [CrossRef]
44. Miller, L.M.; Bourassa, M.W.; Smith, R.J. FTIR spectroscopic imaging of protein aggregation in living cells. *Biochim. Biophys. Acta* **2013**, *1828*, 2339–2346. [CrossRef] [PubMed]
45. Jackson, M.; Mantsch, H.H. The use and misuse of FTIR spectroscopy in the determination of protein structure. *Crit. Rev. Biochem. Mol. Biol.* **1995**, *30*, 95–120. [CrossRef] [PubMed]
46. Keiderling, T.A.; Silva, R.A.; Yoder, G.; Dukor, R.K. Vibrational circular dichroism spectroscopy of selected oligopeptide conformations. *Bioorg. Med. Chem.* **1999**, *7*, 133–141. [CrossRef]
47. Keiderling, T.A. Protein and peptide secondary structure and conformational determination with vibrational circular dichroism. *Curr. Opin. Chem. Biol.* **2002**, *6*, 682–688. [CrossRef]

48. Ma, S.; Freedman, T.B.; Dukor, R.K.; Nafie, L.A. Near-infrared and mid-infrared Fourier transform vibrational circular dichroism of proteins in aqueous solution. *Appl. Spectrosc.* **2010**, *64*, 615–626. [CrossRef] [PubMed]
49. Ma, S.; Cao, X.; Mak, M.; Sadik, A.; Walkner, C.; Freedman, T.B.; Lednev, I.K.; Dukor, R.K.; Nafie, L.A. Vibrational circular dichroism shows unusual sensitivity to protein fibril formation and development in solution. *J. Am. Chem. Soc.* **2007**, *129*, 12364–12365. [CrossRef] [PubMed]
50. Kurouski, D.; Lombardi, R.A.; Dukor, R.K.; Lednev, I.K.; Nafie, L.A. Direct observation and pH control of reversed supramolecular chirality in insulin fibrils by vibrational circular dichroism. *Chem. Commun.* **2010**, *46*, 7154–7156. [CrossRef] [PubMed]
51. Measey, T.J.; Schweitzer-Stenner, R. Vibrational circular dichroism as a probe of fibrillogenesis: The origin of the anomalous intensity enhancement of amyloid-like fibrils. *J. Am. Chem. Soc.* **2011**, *133*, 1066–1076. [CrossRef]
52. Krishnakumar, S.S.; London, E. Effect of sequence hydrophobicity and bilayer width upon the minimum length required for the formation of transmembrane helices in membranes. *J. Mol. Biol.* **2007**, *374*, 671–687. [CrossRef]
53. Zeth, K. Structure and mechanism of human antimicrobial peptide dermcidin and its antimicrobial potential. In *Microbial Pathogens and Strategies for Combating Them: Science, Technology and Education*; Méndez-Vilas, A., Ed.; Formatex Research Center: Badajoz, Spain, 2013; Volume 2, pp. 1333–1342. ISBN 978-84-942134-0-3.
54. Huang, H.W. Molecular mechanism of antimicrobial peptides: The origin of cooperativity. *Biochim. Biophys. Acta* **2006**, *1758*, 1292–1302. [CrossRef]
55. Millhauser, G.L. Views of helical peptides: A proposal for the position of 3_{10}-helix along the thermodynamic folding pathway. *Biochemistry* **1995**, *34*, 3873–3877. [CrossRef] [PubMed]
56. Leontiadou, H.; Mark, A.E.; Marrink, S.J. Antimicrobial peptides in action. *J. Am. Chem. Soc.* **2006**, *128*, 12156–12161. [CrossRef] [PubMed]
57. Forbrig, E.; Staffa, J.K.; Salewski, J.; Mroginski, M.A.; Hildebrandt, P.; Kozuch, J. Monitoring the orientational changes of Alamethicin during incorporation into bilayer lipid membranes. *Langmuir* **2018**, *34*, 2373–2385. [CrossRef] [PubMed]
58. Reißer, S.; Strandberg, E.; Steinbrecher, T.; Elstner, M.; Ulrich, A.S. Best of two worlds? How MD simulations of amphiphilic helical peptides in membranes can complement data from oriented solid-state NMR. *J. Chem. Theory Comput.* **2018**, *14*, 6002–6014. [CrossRef] [PubMed]
59. Andruschenko, V.; Vogel, H.J.; Prenner, E.J. Optimization of the hydrochloric acid concentration used for trifluoroacetate removal from synthetic peptides. *J. Pept. Sci.* **2007**, *13*, 37–43. [CrossRef] [PubMed]
60. Mukerjee, P.; Mysels, K.J. *Critical Micelle Concentration of Aqueous Surfactant Systems*; NSRDS-NBS 36; U.S. Department of Commerce: Washington, DC, USA, 1971.
61. Rohl, C.; Baldwin, R.L. Deciphering rules of helix stability in peptides. *Methods Enzymol.* **1998**, *296*, 1–26. [CrossRef]
62. Sreerama, N.; Woody, R.W. Computation and analysis of protein circular dichroism spectra. *Methods Enzymol.* **2004**, *383*, 318–351. [CrossRef]
63. Malinowski, E.R. *Factor Analysis in Chemistry*, 3rd ed.; Wiley: Chichester, UK, 2002; ISBN 0-471-13479-1.
64. Dousseau, F.; Therrien, M.; Pézolet, M. On the spectral subtraction of water from the FT-IR spectra of aqueous solutions of proteins. *Appl. Spectrosc.* **1989**, *43*, 538–542. [CrossRef]
65. Roux, S.; Zékri, E.; Rousseau, B.; Paternostre, M.; Cintrat, J.C.; Fay, N. Elimination and exchange of trifluoroacetate counter-ion from cationic peptides: A critical evaluation of different approaches. *J. Pept. Sci.* **2008**, *14*, 354–359. [CrossRef]
66. Nafie, L.A.; Buijs, H.; Rilling, A.; Cao, X.; Dukor, R.K. Dual source Fourier transform polarization modulation spectroscopy: An improved method for the measurement of circular and linear dichroism. *Appl. Spectrosc.* **2004**, *58*, 647–654. [CrossRef]
67. Nafie, L.A. Dual polarization modulation: Real-time, spectral multiplex separation of circular dichroism from linear birefringence spectral intensities. *Appl. Spectrosc.* **2000**, *54*, 1634–1645. [CrossRef]
68. Case, D.A.; Darden, T.A.; Cheatham, T.E., III; Simmerling, C.L.; Wang, J.; Duke, R.E.; Luo, R.; Walker, R.C.; Zhang, W.; Merz, K.M.; et al. *AMBER 11*; University of California: San Francisco, CA, USA, 2010.

69. Hornak, V.; Abel, R.; Okur, A.; Strockbine, B.; Roitberg, A.; Simmerling, C. Comparison of multiple Amber force fields and development of improved protein backbone parameters. *Proteins* **2006**, *65*, 712–725. [CrossRef] [PubMed]
70. Humphrey, W.; Dalke, A.; Schulten, K. VMD: Visual Molecular Dynamics. *J. Mol. Graph.* **1996**, *14*, 33–38. [CrossRef]
71. Phillips, J.C.; Braun, R.; Wang, W.; Gumbart, J.; Tajkhorshid, E.; Villa, E.; Chipot, C.; Skeel, R.D.; Kalé, L.; Schulten, K. Scalable molecular dynamics with NAMD. *J. Comput. Chem.* **2005**, *26*, 1781–1802. [CrossRef] [PubMed]
72. Miyamoto, S.; Kollman, P.A.; Settle, K. An analytical version of the SHAKE and RATTLE algorithm for rigid water models. *J. Comput. Chem.* **1992**, *13*, 952–962. [CrossRef]
73. Sreerama, N.; Woody, R.W. On the analysis of membrane protein circular dichroism spectra. *Protein Sci.* **2004**, *13*, 100–112. [CrossRef] [PubMed]

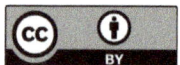

© 2019 by the authors. Licensee MDPI, Basel, Switzerland. This article is an open access article distributed under the terms and conditions of the Creative Commons Attribution (CC BY) license (http://creativecommons.org/licenses/by/4.0/).

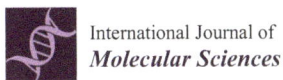

Article

Antibacterial and Antibiofilm Activity and Mode of Action of Magainin 2 against Drug-Resistant *Acinetobacter baumannii*

Min Kyung Kim [1], Na Hee Kang [1], Su Jin Ko [1], Jonggwan Park [2], Eunji Park [1], Dong Won Shin [3], Seo Hyun Kim [3], Seung A. Lee [3], Ji In Lee [3], Seung Hyun Lee [3], Eun Gi Ha [3], Seung Hun Jeon [3] and Yoonkyung Park [1,4,*]

1. Department of Biomedical Science, Chosun University, Gwangju 61452, Korea; charm5964@naver.com (M.K.K.); govlgovl_2414@hanmail.net (N.H.K.); ksj920708@hanmail.net (S.J.K.); fhhhhgfh@naver.com (E.P.)
2. Department of Bioinformatics, Kongju National University, Kongju 38065, Korea; for_quality@naver.com
3. Jangseong High School, Jeollanamdo 57216, Korea; dkatlf6017@naver.com (D.W.S.); twinpearl@naver.com (S.H.K.); iceone256325@naver.com (S.A.L.); jiin1839@gmail.com (J.I.L.); dltmdzus4001@naver.com (S.H.L.); dwar77@naver.com (E.G.H.); bioman255@naver.com (S.H.J.)
4. Research Center for Proteineous Materials, Chosun University, Gwangju 61452, Korea
* Correspondence: y_k_park@chosun.ac.kr; Tel.: +82-62-230-6854; Fax: +82-62-225-6758

Received: 6 September 2018; Accepted: 28 September 2018; Published: 5 October 2018

Abstract: Antimicrobial peptides (AMPs) are promising therapeutic agents for treating antibiotic-resistant bacterial infections. Previous studies showed that magainin 2 (isolated from African clawed fogs *Xenopus laevis*) has antimicrobial activity against gram-positive and gram-negative bacteria. The present study was conducted to investigate the antibacterial activity of magainin 2 against *Acinetobacter baumannii*. Magainin 2 showed excellent antibacterial activity against *A. baumannii* strains and high stability at physiological salt concentrations. This peptide was not cytotoxic towards HaCaT cells and showed no hemolytic activity. Biofilm inhibition and elimination were significantly induced in all *A. baumannii* strains exposed to magainin 2. We confirmed the mechanism of magainin 2 on the bacterial outer and inner membranes. Collectively, these results suggest that magainin 2 is an effective antimicrobial and antibiofilm agent against *A. baumannii* strains.

Keywords: *Acinetobacter baumannii*; multidrug-resistant; antimicrobial peptide; antibiofilm activity; physiological salt

1. Introduction

The use of antibiotics for treating infections has resulted in the emergence of resistant strains [1]. New antibiotic-resistant strains are becoming a problem worldwide because conventional antibiotics cannot be administered. A recent report using data from the Infectious Diseases Society of America and hospital-based surveillance research refers to the pathogens as "ESKAPE" [2,3]. The ESKAPE pathogens include *Enterococcus faecium*, *Staphylococcus aureus*, *Klebsiella pneumoniae*, *Acinetobacter*, *Pseudomonas aeruginosa*, and *Enterobacter* species [4]. The ability of these bacteria groups to withstand antibiotic treatment is a major cause of hospital infections worldwide [5]. Notably, *Acinetobacter baumannii* has been reported as one of the most serious ESKAPE organisms resistant to antibiotics [6].

Acinetobacter baumannii, a gram-negative bacterium, is an opportunistic bacterial pathogen and has a high morbidity and mortality, especially in intensive care units with high pathogen infections. Infectious diseases include urinary tract infection [7], meningitis [8], skin infection [9], bacteremia [10], and pneumonia [11]. Many strains causing infection show resistance to antibiotics such as aminoglycosides, fluoroquinolones, colistin, β-lactams, and tetracyclines [12,13]. Also, *A. baumannii* is prone to biofilm formation and their ability to increase resistance to antibiotics.

Biofilm is a microbial aggregate formed by cells and cells that attach to each other and become embedded in a matrix of self-generated extracellular polymeric substances [14]. Biofilms can form on various abiotic surfaces including glass, polystyrene, and surgical instruments. They can also attach to tissues that are easily exposed to bacterial infections and cause problems [15]. Therefore, new drugs are needed to effectively treat antibiotic-resistant bacteria and biofilm-related infections. Antimicrobial peptides (AMPs) are excellent candidates for developing therapeutic agents.

AMPs are an essential component of innate immunity in host organisms, including animals, insects, plants, and humans [16]. Human host defense antimicrobial peptides are a major component of innate immunity and play an important role in preventing microbial infection and these peptides expressed in the skin, eyes, ears, and various tissues [17]. Among them, Defensins, LL-37 and Histatins are important to prevent oral cavity [18–20]. These molecules are amphipathic peptides typically composed of 12–50 amino acids and show antimicrobial activity against a broad spectrum of microorganisms including gram-positive and gram-negative bacteria, fungi, viruses, and cancer cells. These peptides contain arginine and lysine, which are positively charged and important in their mechanism of action [21]. In general, the bacterial membrane contains a higher content of negatively charged phospholipids compared to mammalian cells, enabling the positively charged peptide to bind more strongly with bacterial cells through electrostatic interactions. This destabilizes or disrupts the bacterial membrane and intracellular processes, leading to microorganism death.

Frog skin is the most abundant source of antimicrobial peptides [22] and secretes major peptides such as esculentin [23], temporin [24] and magainin [25] to protect against microbial invasion. AMPs and its analogue peptides detected in the skin of many frogs exhibit strong antimicrobial activity against antibiotic-resistant bacteria. We previously investigated magainin 2 (GIGKFLHSAKKFGKAFVGEIMNS), an antimicrobial peptide consisting of 23 amino acids isolated from the skin of the African clawed frog *Xenopus laevis* [25]. This peptide has been reported to exhibit broad antibacterial activity against gram-positive and gram-negative bacteria and anti-cancer activity against certain tumor cell lines [26,27].

In this study, we examined the antimicrobial activity of magainin 2 against *A. baumannii* strains and its toxicity towards mammalian cells. We also confirmed that the antibacterial activity of the peptide was maintained even under high-salt conditions. Next, we investigated the activity in a biofilm model, which is closely related to bacterial resistance. The mechanism of action of the peptide was confirmed by membrane-related experiments using N-phenyl-1-naphthylamine (NPN) and 3,3'-dipropylthiadicarbocyanine iodide (DiSC$_3$-5). Our results suggest that magainin 2 can be used as an effective treatment for *A. baumannii* infections.

2. Results

2.1. Peptide Synthesis

The magainin 2 sequence, observed molecular weight, hydrophobicity, hydrophobic moment, and net charge are summarized in Table 1. Magainin 2 is an antimicrobial peptide consisting of 23 amino acids with hydrophobic content, hydrophobic moment, and net charge of 0.373, 0.475, and 3, respectively. The wheel diagram and three-dimensional structure analysis predicted that the peptide contains hydrophobic residues (yellow circles) and forms an α-helix structure (Figure 1).

Table 1. Amino acid sequence and properties of magainin 2.

Name	Sequence	Molecular Mass (Da)	H	μH	Net Charge
Magainin 2	GIGKFLHSAKKFGKAFVGEIMNS-NH$_2$	2465.9	0.373	0.475	+3

H: Hydrophobicity; μH: Hydrophobic moment.

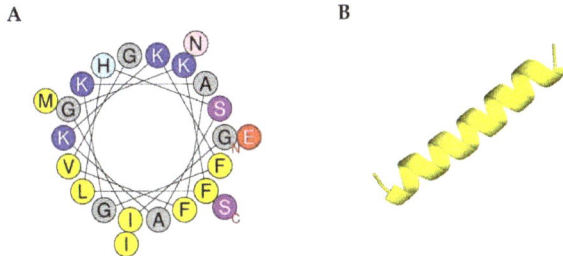

Figure 1. Structure analysis of magainin 2. (**A**) Helical wheel diagram of the peptide. The projection was obtained from http://heliquest.ipmc.cnrs.fr/cgibn/ComputParam.py. Positively charged residues are represented in blue, while hydrophobic residues are shown as yellow circles. The N-terminal and C-terminal parts are represented in red letters "N" and "C". (**B**) Three-dimensional structure of magainin 2.

2.2. Circular Dichroism Measurements

Based on the predicted results shown in Figure 1B; we measured the secondary structure of magainin 2 by circular dichroism (CD) spectroscopy. Structure analysis of magainin 2 was performed in various concentrations of trifluoroethanol (TFE) and sodium dodecyl sulfate (SDS) solutions (Figure 2). In 10 mM sodium phosphate buffer; the CD spectra of the peptide displayed a random coil. However; the peptide adopted a typical α-helical conformation with increasing TFE and SDS concentrations. The calculated α-helical contents of the peptide are shown in Table 2. As the TFE and SDS concentration increased; the α-helical contents increased from 6.4% to 50.8% and from 21.8% to 33.3%; respectively. These results demonstrate that magainin 2 forms a strong α-helix structure.

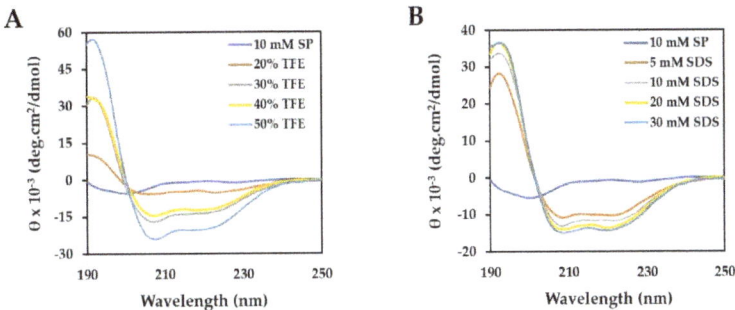

Figure 2. Circular dichroism (CD) spectra of magainin 2. (**A**) The peptide was measured in TFE, which mimics the hydrophobic environment of the microbial membrane and (**B**) SDS, which mimics the negatively charged prokaryotic membrane environment.

Table 2. Mean residual ellipticity at 222 nm ($[\theta]_{222}$) and percent α-helical contents of magainin 2 in various solutions.

	Buffer	TFE				SDS			
	10 mM SP	20%	30%	40%	50%	5 mM	10 mM	20 mM	30 mM
$[\theta]_{222}$	−700.8	−5128.3	−13,207.4	−11,989	−19,749.5	−10,184.8	−11,782	−13,227.2	−13,974.2
% α-helix	RC	6.4	30.9	27.2	50.8	21.8	26.6	31.0	33.3

10 mM SP: 10 mM Sodium Phosphate buffer, pH 7.2.

2.3. Antimicrobial Assay

The antimicrobial activity of the peptides against *A. baumannii* strains are summarized in Table 3. We compared the antibacterial effect of magainin 2 with those of melittin, buforin 2, ciprofloxacin, and gentamicin. Magainin 2 showed strong antibacterial activity with minimum inhibitory concentrations (MICs) of 4 and 2 µM against the standard strain (Korea Collection for Type Cultures (KCTC) 2508) and drug-resistant strains, respectively. This is similar to the MIC of melittin, which is known to have strong antibacterial activity. The activity of buforin 2 was 8-fold lower, ranging from 8 to 16 µM. Antibiotics showed activity against drug-resistant strains at 128 µM. Particularly, gentamicin showed low antibacterial activity with an MIC of 256 µM.

Table 3. Minimum inhibitory concentration (MIC) of peptides and conventional agents against *Acinetobacter baumannii* strains.

Microorganisms	Minimum Inhibitory Concentration (µM)				
	Magainin 2	Buforin 2	Melittin	Ciprofloxacin	Gentamicin
A. baumannii KCTC 2508	4	8	2	2	4
A. baumannii 244752	2	8	2	256	>256
A. baumannii 409081	2	8	1	>256	>256
A. baumannii 719705	2	8	2	128	>256
A. baumannii 892199	2	16	2	256	>256
A. baumannii 907233	2	16	2	128	>256

2.4. Cytotoxicity Assay

Hemolysis and cell viability assays were conducted to measure the toxicity of the peptides in mammalian cells. As shown in Figure 3A, melittin, a positive control peptide, induced more than 50% hemolysis at concentrations of 1–2 µM. In contrast, magainin 2-treated cells showed no hemolysis at 64 µM. We confirmed the cytotoxicity of magainin 2 in HaCaT cells. The curve in Figure 3B shows that high concentrations of magainin 2 exhibited low cytotoxicity of 0%, while melittin exhibited 100% toxicity at 2 µM. These results confirm that magainin 2 is not toxic to cells.

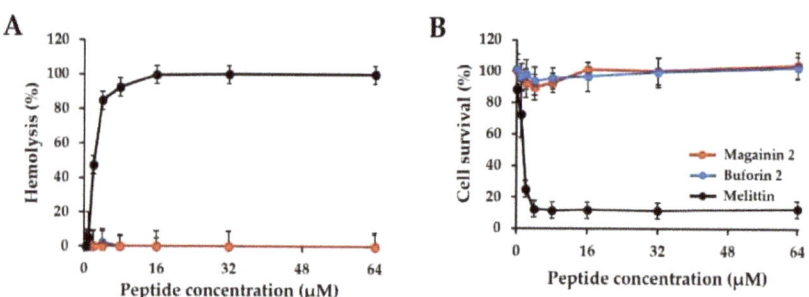

Figure 3. Cytotoxicity and hemolytic activity of magainin 2. (**A**) Hemolytic activity of peptides against mouse red blood cells (RBCs). (**B**) Cytotoxicity of peptides against HaCaT cells.

2.5. Biofilm Inhibition Assay

To investigate whether magainin 2 can inhibit biofilm formation, the degree of biofilm formation by *A. baumannii* strains was confirmed in Mueller-Hinton broth (MHB) supplemented with glucose. As shown in Figure 4A, all strains formed biofilms and the *A. baumannii* 907233 strain had a biofilm mass of 3 at OD 595 nm. Compared to *A. baumannii* KCTC 2508 in the crystal violet staining assay, *A. baumannii* 907233 showed a 57.6% higher biofilm mass after 24 h of incubation (Figure 4A). The ability of magainin 2 and antibiotics (ciprofloxacin, gentamicin) to prevent biofilm formation was compared.

Magainin 2 and antibiotics inhibited the biofilm formation of *A. baumannii* KCTC 2508 at concentrations of 2–8 µM, whereas buforin 2 showed inhibition at 64 µM. In resistant strains, magainin 2 inhibited biofilm formation at a low concentration of 4 µM, while the antibiotics did not exhibit biofilm formation inhibition activity until 32 µM (Figure 4B). The biofilm biomass was determined using the green dye SYTO9 and detected with the EVOS AUTO2 fluorescence microscope. *Acinetobacter baumannii* 907233 formed biofilm showing strong green fluorescence (Figure 5). Following treatment of the biofilm with magainin 2, SYTO9 fluorescence decreased in a concentration-dependent manner, while this was not observed following treatment with the other antibiotics. This data shows that magainin 2 has strong antibiofilm activity against drug-resistant *A. baumannii*.

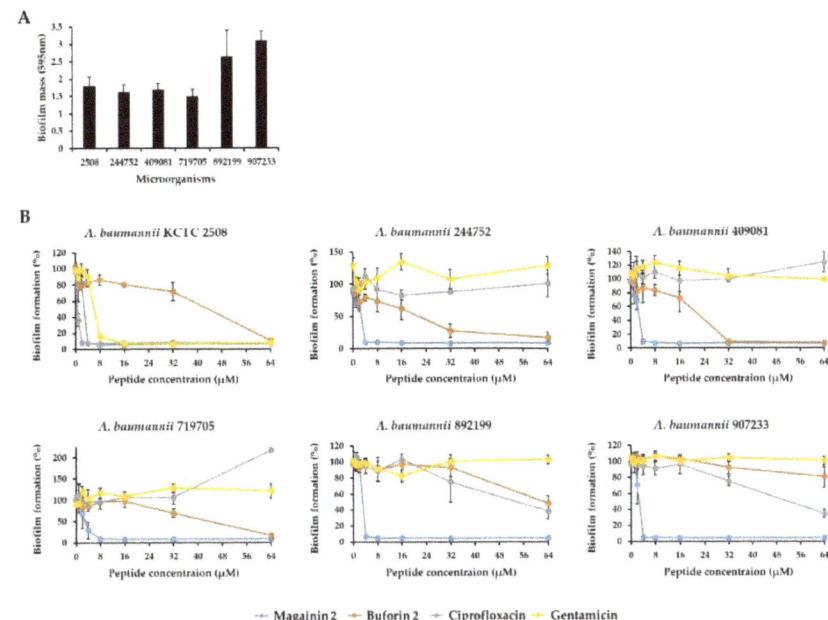

Figure 4. Effect of *Acinetobacter baumannii* biofilm formation by magainin 2. (**A**) Quantitative measurements of biofilm formation using crystal violet staining. (**B**) Inhibitory effect of peptides on biofilm formation. Antibiotics (ciprofloxacin and gentamicin) and buforin 2 were used as controls.

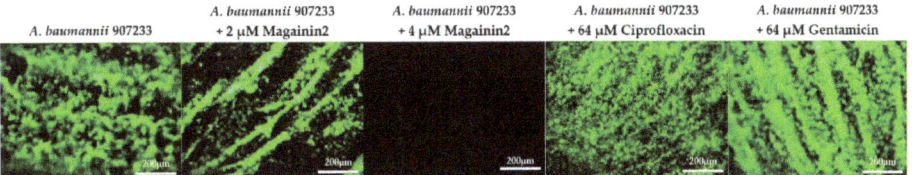

Figure 5. EVOS2 images of *Acinetobacter baumannii* biofilm stained with SYTO9 dye (green fluorescence).

2.6. Biofilm Reduction Assay

The biofilm reduction activity of magainin 2 was confirmed against *A. baumannii* 907233, which easily forms biofilm. Figure 6 shows the effect of the peptide and antibiotics on biofilm formed for 24 h. In the crystal violet staining assay, *A. baumannii* 907233 showed strong staining after incubation for 24 h (Figure 6B). Antibacterial treatment with magainin 2 and ciprofloxacin exhibited similar abilities to eradicate biofilm formation. The biofilm inhibition rates of magainin 2 were 33.3%, 53.4%, and 66.2% at 128, 192, and 256 µM, respectively. In contrast, gentamicin showed no biofilm inhibition effects at 256 µM (Figure 6A). Next, the biofilm was observed using SYTO9 (green dye). After 24 h, the biofilm stained with SYTO9 showed strong green fluorescence. The fluorescence was low in the presence of 256 µM magainin 2, indicating that it effectively disrupted the biofilm. Gentamicin showed no decrease in biofilm (Figure 6C). These results suggest that magainin 2 not only inhibits but also effectively eliminates biofilm.

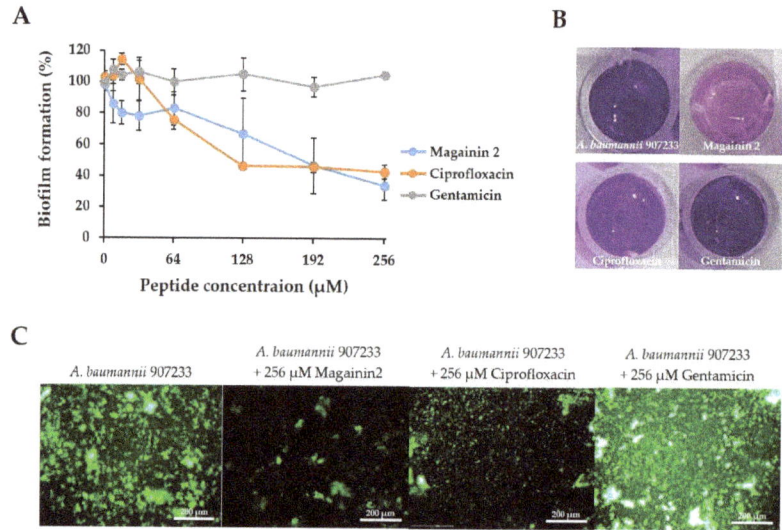

Figure 6. Biofilm reduction assay. (**A**) Degree of biofilm removal by magainin 2, ciprofloxacin, and gentamicin using crystal violet staining. (**B**) Image of removed biofilm after treatment with 256 µM of peptide and antibiotics. (**C**) SYTO9-stained biofilm image.

2.7. Salt Sensitivity Assay

To investigate the effects of salts on antimicrobial activity, antimicrobial activity was measured at a physiological salt concentration (Table 4). As shown in Table 3, magainin 2 exhibited similar stability in the presence of physiological salts compared to buforin 2. The MIC values of *A. baumannii* KCTC 2508 and *A. baumannii* 907233 strain were 4 and 2 µM, respectively. In the presence of NaCl and $FeCl_3$, magainin 2 activity was nearly maintained in both strains. In contrast, magainin 2 activity was slightly reduced to 8 µM in the presence of $MgCl_2$.

Table 4. MIC values of peptides in the presence of physiological salts.

Salt	Concentration	*A. baumannii* KCTC 2508		*A. baumannii* 907233	
		Magainin 2	Buforin 2	Magainin 2	Buforin 2
NaCl	50 mM	4	16	2	32
	100 mM	4	32	4	>32
	150 mM	4	>32	4	>32
$MgCl_2$	0.5 mM	4	16	4	>32
	1 mM	8	32	8	>32
	2 mM	8	>32	8	>32
$FeCl_3$	2 µM	4	4	2	16
	4 µM	4	4	2	16
	8 µM	4	4	2	16

2.8. Mechanism of Action Of Magainin 2

To investigate the mechanism of magainin 2 activity towards drug-resistant bacteria, *A. baumannii* 907233 was used, while *A. baumannii* KCTC 2508 as a control strain. First, the outer membrane permeability of *A. baumannii* 907233 following treatment with magainin 2 was examined using NPN dye (hydrophobic fluorescent dye, exhibits fluorescence intensity in a hydrophobic environment). The bacterial outer membrane was disrupted, and the hydrophobic part of the membrane was exposed, after which NPN reacted to show fluorescence. As shown in Figure 7A,B, the intensity increased in a concentration-dependent manner, indicating that magainin 2 acts on the outer membrane. For *A. baumannii* KCTC 2508, the fluorescence intensity rapidly increased to 268, 246, and 209 within 2 min at 4×, 2×, and 1× MIC, respectively. In contrast, fluorescence increased to approximately 80 in *A. baumannii* 907233.

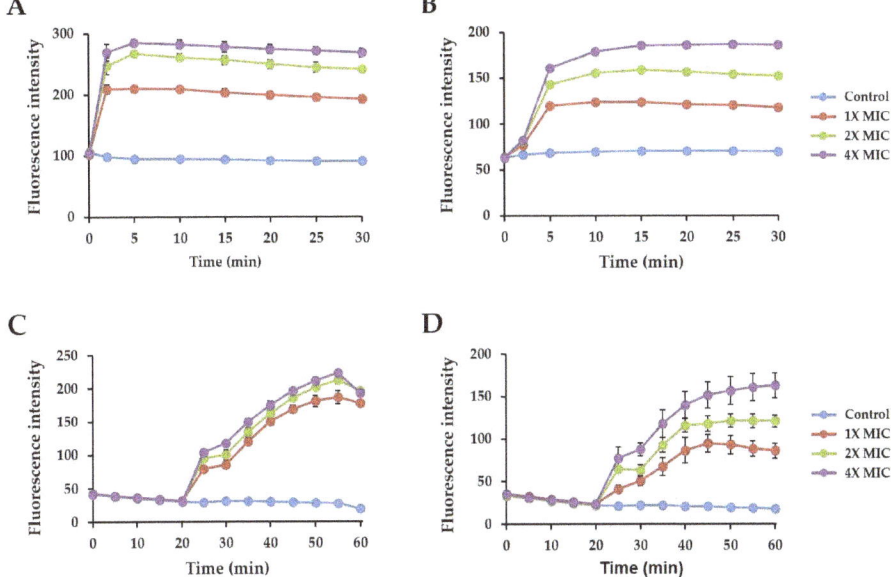

Figure 7. Magainin 2 mechanism of action. (**A,B**) The outer membrane permeability of magainin 2 was measured using NPN dye. (**C,D**) Depolarization of cytoplasmic membrane induced by magainin 2, determined using the membrane potential-sensitive fluorescent dye DisC$_3$-5. (**A,C**: *Acinetobacter baumannii* KCTC 2508, **B,D**: *Acinetobacter baumannii* 907233).

The ability to depolarize the *A. baumannii* 907233 inner membrane in the presence of magainin 2 was further confirmed using DiSC$_3$-5. DiSC$_3$-5 is a dye that accumulates in the cytoplasmic membrane of bacteria; the dye is released when the bacteria membrane is affected by the peptide. As shown in Figure 7C,D, addition of magainin 2 resulted in increased fluorescence in a dose-dependent manner, indicating the ability of magainin 2 to depolarize the membrane. The fluorescence intensity of *A. baumannii* KCTC 2508 was higher than that of *A. baumannii* 907233 strain and decreased at 60 min after peptide treatment. These results suggest that magainin 2 affects the inner membranes of both *A. baumannii* KCTC 2508 and 907233.

3. Discussion

Bacterial infections are among the major causes of death worldwide [28]. Conventional antibiotics were effectively used to treat pathogenic infections for half a century, but the emergence of antibiotic-resistant bacteria has made these infections difficult to treat [29,30]. Generally, long-term exposure to antibiotics leads to resistance. Antibiotics function against proteins that are essential to bacteria cells, and mutations in bacterial proteins cause antibiotic resistance. Bacteria can also transform antibiotics and make them inefficient by producing specific enzymes. Thus, an antibacterial with a new mechanism of action differing from existing antibiotics is urgently needed. Antimicrobial peptides have distinctive mechanisms and are emerging as new therapeutic agents.

AMPs are classified according to their α-helical, β-sheet, and random coil structures; the α-helical structure is the most common [31]. The predicted magainin 2 structure was confirmed by CD spectroscopy to be a-helical in the bacteria membrane, mimicking the surrounding environment, and appeared as a random coil structure in an aqueous environment. In increasing concentrations of SDS and TFE, the percent of a-helix content of magainin 2 also increased. This suggests that the α-helical structure enabled magainin 2 to interact with the bacterial membrane, which is related to its mechanism of action [32].

Because bacteria isolated from hospital patients are resistant to antibiotics, treatment of *A. baumannii* infection is becoming increasingly difficult [33]. Therefore, the activity of magainin 2 towards bacteria isolated from patients was evaluated. Magainin 2 exhibited lower antibacterial activity against drug-resistant *A. baumannii* than that observed against the susceptible *A. baumannii* (KCTC 2508) and exhibited more potent activity than antibiotics (ciprofloxacin and gentamicin). Thus, magainin 2 is a more effective therapeutic agent than antibiotics, which are not resistant to AMPs. Additionally, magainin 2 is not toxic to mammalian cells.

Biofilms are important for the survival of bacteria in the environment, and biofilm formation has been correlated with drug-resistance and several virulence factors [34,35]. The antibiotic resistance of biofilms is significantly higher than that of planktonic bacteria [36,37]. These biofilm-related infections are more difficult to control and can lead to death. *Acinetobacter baumannii* is a pathogen that commonly forms biofilm [38,39]. We analyzed the biofilm formation of *A. baumannii* strains treated with a peptide. Peptides and antibiotics showed similar abilities to inhibit biofilm formation by susceptible *A. baumannii*. However, in the five resistant strains, magainin 2 showed higher antibiofilm activity than antibiotics at low concentrations. These results suggest that magainin 2 exerts strong antibiofilm activity against drug-resistant *A. baumannii*. Furthermore, we evaluated the efficacy of magainin 2 on *A. baumannii* within established biofilms. Removing biofilms formed by pathogenic microorganisms is difficult. We found that magainin 2 was more effective than antibiotics towards removing formed biofilms. Thus, magainin 2 may be effective for treating biofilm-related infectious diseases.

The antimicrobial activity of most AMPs is strongly inhibited by presence of high ionic concentrations, which is a disadvantage as therapeutic agents in the serum or other body fluids [40]. For example, the activity of human β-defensins is influenced by NaCl in the airway surface liquid of cystic fibrosis patients [41]. In the presence of NaCl, $MgCl_2$, and $FeCl_3$ at concentrations similar to those in human bodily fluids, the activity of magainin 2 was maintained. These results demonstrate that magainin 2 is stable in high-salt environments, which did not affect the killing mechanism. Combined with previous toxicity data, this peptide may be useful for therapeutic applications in a physiological environment.

AMPs, which have cationic peptides, bind to the negatively charged bacterial membrane through electrostatic interactions [42]. Peptides can disrupt the membrane after binding or enter the membrane to form pores. Pore-forming mechanisms include models of "barrel-stave", "carpet", and "toroidal-pore" [42,43]. In a previous study, magainin 2 was shown to bind to the anionic lipid bilayers of the bacterial membrane via electrostatic attractions and form a pore, which eventually destroyed the membrane [44]. The peptide was suggested to form toroidal pores ~80 Å diameter in DMPC/DMPG liposomes [45]. Thus, we investigated the mechanism of magainin 2 against *A. baumannii* strains in this study.

To determine the mechanism of action against *A. baumannii* strains, we used NPN and $DiSC_3$-5 dyes. First, damage to the bacterial outer membrane was monitored by measuring the fluorescence intensity of NPN. Magainin 2 induced an increase in fluorescence in both stains. Compared to the drug-resistant strain, the response of susceptible *A. baumannii* was faster. Depolarization of the bacterial cytoplasmic membrane was monitored by measuring the fluorescence intensity of $DiSC_3$-5. Consistent with the results of the NPN test, the fluorescence intensity decreased at 55 min, indicating that magainin 2 rapidly affected the susceptible *A. baumannii*. Collectively, magainin 2 has an α-helical structure, which can associate with the *A. baumannii* membrane and uses a mechanism in which both the outer and inner membranes are affected.

4. Materials and Methods

4.1. Materials

SDS, trifluoroethanol (TFE), 3-(4,5-dimethylthiazol-2-yl)-2,5-diphenyltetrazolium bromide (MTT), dimethyl sulfoxide (DMSO), N-phenyl-1-naphthylamine (NPN), 3,3′-dipropylthiadicarbocyanine iodide ($DiSC_3$-5), ciprofloxacin, and gentamicin were purchased from Sigma-Aldrich (St. Louis, MO, USA). Dulbecco's Modified Eagle's medium (DMEM), fetal bovine serum (FBS), and Dulbecco's Phosphate Buffered Saline (DPBS) were obtained from Welgene (Daegu, Korea).

4.2. Microorganisms and Mouse Red Blood Cells

Acinetobacter baumannii KCTC 2508 was obtained from the KCTC. Other *Acinetobacter baumannii* 244752, 409081, 719705, 892199, and 907233 were antibiotic-resistant bacteria isolated from patients at Eulji University Hospital (Seoul, Korea). The study protocol was reviewed and approved by the institutional review board of Eulji Hospital (No. EMCS 2016). All patients gave their informed consent to participate in this study or the informed consent process was waived in accordance with the decision of the ethics committee of each hospital. The mouse used in this study was carried out in strict accordance with the recommendations in the Guide for the Care and Use of Laboratory Animals of the National Institutes of Health, and approved by the Committee on the Ethics of Animal Experiments (CIACUC2017-S0042; Chosun University, Gwangju, South Korea).

4.3. Peptide Synthesis and Sequence Analysis

The peptides were synthesized using the solid-phase-9-fluorenylmethoxycarbonyl method as reported previously [46] on a Rink amide 4-methylbenzhydrylamine resin using a Liberty microwave peptide synthesizer (CEM, Matthews, NY, USA). The purity and molecular weight of the peptide was confirmed by reversed-phase high-performance liquid chromatography and matrix-assisted laser desorption ionization-time of flight mass spectrometry. Projections of the predicted three-dimensional structures were constructed online using the Mobyle@RPBS bioinformatics portal (http://mobyle.rpbs.univ-paris-diderot.fr/cgi-bin/portal.py#welcome), whereas the HeliQuest site (http://heliquest.ipmc.cnrs.fr) was used to create helical wheel diagrams and determine the relative hydrophobic moments of the peptides.

4.4. Circular Dichroism Measurements

CD measurements were performed on a JASCO 810 spectropolarimeter (Jasco, Tokyo, Japan) using a 0.1-cm path length rectangular quartz cell [47]. The peptide structure was evaluated in various solutions. The solutions were prepared at a 40 μM peptide concentration in 10 mM sodium phosphate buffer, pH 7.2, to mimic an aqueous environment, TFE (20%, 30%, 40%, and 50% TFE) to mimic the hydrophobic environment of the microbial membrane, and SDS (5, 10, 20, and 30 mM SDS) as a negatively charged prokaryotic membrane-comparable environment. The spectra were recorded between 190 and 250 nm. The percent of α-helix content was calculated as follows:

$$\% \ \alpha\text{-helix} = -100 \ ([\theta]_{222} + 3000)/33{,}000$$

4.5. Antimicrobial Activity Assay

The MIC of peptides was determined by the standard micro-dilution method [48] in 96-well microtiter plates. Briefly, A. baumannii strains were cultured in MHB media and prepared at 2×10^5 colony-forming units per milliliter (CFU/mL). The peptides were serially diluted to concentrations between 1 and 32 µM in 10 mM sodium phosphate buffer in a 96-well plate. The bacteria were mixed with serially diluted peptide in the 96-well plate and incubated at 37°C for 18–24 h. The absorbance of the sample at 600 nm was measured using a microplate reader and repeated three times.

4.6. Hemolysis Assay

The hemolytic activity of peptides was evaluated using mouse red blood cells (RBCs). RBCs were washed three times with PBS (Phosphate Buffered Saline) until the supernatant was clear. The peptides were diluted to 64 µM and added to a 96-well plate. RBCs were added at a final concentration of 8% (v/v). After incubation for 1 h, the plate was centrifuged for 10 min and the absorbance of the supernatant was measured at 414 nm. The percentage of hemolysis was calculated using the following formula:

$$\text{Hemolysis (\%)} = (A_{414} \text{ of peptide} - A_{414} \text{ of PBS}) / (A_{414} \text{ of Triton} - A_{414} \text{ of PBS}) \times 100$$

RBCs suspended in PBS and 1% Triton X-100 represented zero hemolysis and 100% hemolysis, respectively.

4.7. Cytotoxicity Assay

The MTT assay was conducted to measure the cytotoxicity of the peptides towards HaCaT cells. HaCaT cells were cultured in DMEM supplemented with 1% penicillin and 10% FBS at 37 °C with CO_2. Briefly, a total of 2×10^4 cells/well were seeded into a 96-well plate, which was incubated overnight. Peptides serially diluted with DMEM at 0–64 µM were added to each well and reacted for 23 h. Next, 10 µL of 5 mg/mL MTT was added to each well, followed by incubation for 1 h. The supernatants were removed and dissolved by adding DMSO. Absorbance was measured at 570 nm [49]. The control was DMEM media without peptide. Cytotoxicity was calculated using the following formula:

$$\text{Cytotoxicity (\%)} = 100 - [(A_{570} \text{ of peptide treated cells} / A_{570} \text{ of control}) \times 100]$$

4.8. Biofilm Inhibition Assay

To investigate the inhibitory effect of peptide on biofilm formation, A. baumannii strains were cultured in MHB [50]. Bacteria were diluted to 5×10^5 CFU/mL in MHB supplemented with 0.2% glucose, and then 90 µL of the bacterial suspension was mixed with 10 µL of the peptide in a 96-well plate for 24 h. The supernatant was then carefully removed, and the formed biofilm was fixed with 100% methanol for 10 min. After removing the methanol, the biofilms were stained with 0.1% crystal violet for 30 min. The plates were then washed with distilled water three times. Finally, the biofilms were completely dissolved in 95% ethanol and absorbance was measured at 595 nm using a Versa-Max microplate ELISA reader (Molecular Devices, Sunnyvale, CA, USA).

4.9. Biofilm Eradication Assay

To measure the removal effect of the formed biofilms, 100 µL aliquots of A. baumannii 907233 (5×10^5 CFU/mL) were incubated in MHB with 0.2% glucose and incubated for 24 h. The culture medium was removed, and the wells were carefully washed with PBS to remove planktonic bacteria. Peptide or antibiotics were added at up to 256 µM in MHB supplemented with 0.2% glucose for 24 h. The biofilms were stained with crystal violet for 30 min, washed three times with PBS, and dissolved in 95% ethanol.

4.10. Visualization of Biofilms

To visualize the inhibition and elimination effect of the peptide on the biofilm, SYTO9 dye was used [51]. The formed *A. baumannii* 907233 biofilm was fixed with 100% methanol and stained with SYTO9 dye for 30 min in the dark. Images were obtained using an EVOS FL Auto 2 fluorescence microscope (Invitrogen, Carlsbad, CA, USA).

4.11. Salts Sensitivity Assay

Acinetobacter baumannii KCTC 2508 and *A. baumannii* 907233 strains were diluted to 2×10^5 CFU/mL in MHB media. The peptide was serially diluted from 0 to 32 µM in the presence of physiological salts. The final concentrations of physiological salts were as follows: 50, 100, 150 mM NaCl, 0.5, 1, 2 mM $MgCl_2$, and 2, 4, 8 µM $FeCl_3$. After these treatments, the procedures were same as used for the MIC assay described above.

4.12. Mechanism of Action Analysis

Outer membrane permeabilization assay. Permeation of the bacterial outer membrane by the peptide was measured by conducting a 1-*N*-phenylnaphthylamine (NPN) uptake assay [52]. *Acinetobacter baumannii* KCTC 2508 and *A. baumannii* 907233 strains were cultured in MHB, washed, and suspended to 0.25 at OD 600 nm in 5 mM HEPES buffer. Each strain was mixed with NPN to a final concentration of 10 µM. Next, 50 µL of peptide (1×, 2×, or 4× MIC) was added to the mixture in a 96-well plate. The relative fluorescence intensity was measured over time using a Spectramax M3 spectrophotometer (Molecular Devices) at 420 nm.

Cytoplasmic membrane depolarization assay. The membrane potential-sensitive dye $DiSC_3$-5 was used to measure cytoplasmic membrane depolarization [53]. *Acinetobacter baumannii* KCTC 2508 and *A. baumannii* 907233 strains were cultured in MHB and washed three times with 5 mM HEPES (pH 7.3) containing 20 mM glucose. The bacteria were resuspended to 0.05 at OD 600 in buffer (5 mM HEPES, 20 mM glucose, and 100 mM KCl) and incubated with 1 µM $DiSC_3$-5. The fluorescence was stabilized for 1 h and the peptides were added to the mixture. The fluorescence was measured using a Spectramax M3 spectrophotometer with excitation at 622 nm and emission at 670 nm.

5. Conclusions

In this study, we confirmed that magainin 2 has an α-helix structure and showed strong antibacterial activity against *A. baumannii* including multidrug-resistant strains. Magainin 2 is not toxic towards mammalian cells and maintained its stability and excellent antibacterial activity in a biologically relevant salt environment. Magainin 2 is also effective for treating infections by inhibiting or eliminating biofilm formation. The mechanism of action of standard and drug-resistant strains is that magainin 2 acts on both the outer and inner membranes. Taken together, magainin 2 may be useful as a new antibacterial and antibiofilm agent.

Author Contributions: Data curation, S.J.K., D.W.S., S.H.K., S.A.L., J.I.L., S.H.L., E.G.H. and S.H.J.; Formal analysis, N.H.K., J.P. and E.P.; Supervision, Y.P.; Writing—original draft, M.K.K.

Funding: This work was supported by a National Research Foundation of Korea (NRF) grant funded by the Korean Government (No. 2016R1A2A1A05005440, NRF-2017M3A9E4077206), Global Research Laboratory (GRL) Grant (No. NRF-2014K1A1A2064460), and Institute for Information & communications Technology Promotion (IITP) grant funded by the Korea government (MSIT) (No. 2017-0-01714, Development of Antimicrobial Peptide using Deep Learning).

Conflicts of Interest: The authors declare no conflict of interest.

References

1. Laxminarayan, R.; Duse, A.; Wattal, C.; Zaidi, A.K.; Wertheim, H.F.; Sumpradit, N.; Vlieghe, E.; Hara, G.L.; Gould, I.M.; Goossens, H.; et al. Antibiotic Resistance-the Need for Global Solutions. *Lancet Infect. Dis.* **2013**, *13*, 1057–1098. [CrossRef]
2. Rice, L.B. Federal Funding for the Study of Antimicrobial Resistance in Nosocomial Pathogens: No Eskape. *J. Infect. Dis.* **2008**, *197*, 1079–1081. [CrossRef] [PubMed]
3. Boucher, H.W.; Talbot, G.H.; Bradley, J.S.; Edwards, J.E.; Gilbert, D.; Rice, L.B.; Scheld, M.; Spellberg, B.; Bartlett, J. Bad Bugs, No Drugs: No Eskape! An Update from the Infectious Diseases Society of America. *Clin. Infect. Dis.* **2009**, *48*, 1–12. [CrossRef] [PubMed]
4. Rice, L.B. Progress and Challenges in Implementing the Research on Eskape Pathogens. *Infect. Control Hosp. Epidemiol.* **2010**, *31* (Suppl. 1), S7–S10. [CrossRef] [PubMed]
5. Santajit, S.; Indrawattana, N. Mechanisms of Antimicrobial Resistance in Eskape Pathogens. *Biomed. Res. Int.* **2016**, *2016*, 2475067. [CrossRef] [PubMed]
6. Kwon, J.; Mistry, T.; Ren, J.; Johnson, M.E.; Mehboob, S. A Novel Series of Enoyl Reductase Inhibitors Targeting the Eskape Pathogens, Staphylococcus Aureus and Acinetobacter Baumannii. *Bioorg. Med. Chem.* **2018**, *26*, 65–76. [CrossRef] [PubMed]
7. Jimenez-Guerra, G.; Heras-Canas, V.; Gutierrez-Soto, M.; Aznarte-Padial, M.d.; Exposito-Ruiz, M.; Navarro-Mari, J.M.; Gutierrez-Fernandez, J. Urinary Tract Infection by Acinetobacter Baumannii and Pseudomonas Aeruginosa: Evolution of Antimicrobial Resistance and Therapeutic Alternatives. *J. Med. Microbiol.* **2018**. [CrossRef] [PubMed]
8. Kim, B.N.; Peleg, A.Y.; Lodise, T.P.; Lipman, J.; Li, J.; Nation, R.; Paterson, D.L. Management of Meningitis Due to Antibiotic-Resistant Acinetobacter Species. *Lancet Infect. Dis.* **2009**, *9*, 245–255. [CrossRef]
9. Guerrero, D.M.; Perez, F.; Conger, N.G.; Solomkin, J.S.; Adams, M.D.; Rather, P.N.; Bonomo, R.A. Acinetobacter Baumannii-Associated Skin and Soft Tissue Infections: Recognizing a Broadening Spectrum of Disease. *Surg. Infect.* **2010**, *11*, 49–57. [CrossRef] [PubMed]
10. Cisneros, J.M.; Rodriguez-Bano, J. Nosocomial Bacteremia Due to Acinetobacter Baumannii: Epidemiology, Clinical Features and Treatment. *Clin. Microbiol. Infect.* **2002**, *8*, 687–693. [CrossRef] [PubMed]
11. Maragakis, L.L.; Perl, T.M. Acinetobacter Baumannii: Epidemiology, Antimicrobial Resistance, and Treatment Options. *Clin. Infect. Dis.* **2008**, *46*, 1254–1263. [CrossRef] [PubMed]
12. Peleg, A.Y.; Seifert, H.; Paterson, D.L. Acinetobacter Baumannii: Emergence of a Successful Pathogen. *Clin Microbiol. Rev.* **2008**, *21*, 538–582. [CrossRef] [PubMed]
13. Fair, R.J.; Tor, Y. Antibiotics and Bacterial Resistance in the 21st Century. *Perspect. Med. Chem.* **2014**, *6*, 25–64. [CrossRef] [PubMed]
14. Hall-Stoodley, L.; Costerton, J.W.; Stoodley, P. Bacterial Biofilms: From the Natural Environment to Infectious Diseases. *Nat. Rev. Microbiol.* **2004**, *2*, 95–108. [CrossRef] [PubMed]
15. Jamal, M.; Ahmad, W.; Andleeb, S.; Jalil, F.; Imran, M.; Nawaz, M.A.; Hussain, T.; Ali, M.; Rafiq, M.; Kamil, M.A. Bacterial Biofilm and Associated Infections. *J. Chin. Med. Assoc.* **2018**, *81*, 7–11. [CrossRef] [PubMed]
16. Zhang, L.; Gallo, R.L. Antimicrobial Peptides. *Curr. Biol.* **2016**, *26*, R14–R19. [CrossRef] [PubMed]
17. Khurshid, Z.; Najeeb, S.; Mali, M.; Moin, S.F.; Raza, S.Q.; Zohaib, S.; Sefat, F.; Zafar, M.S. Histatin peptides: Pharmacological functions and their applications in dentistry. *Saudi Pharm. J.* **2017**, *25*, 25–31. [CrossRef] [PubMed]
18. Khurshid, Z.; Naseem, M.; Sheikh, Z.; Najeeb, S.; Shahab, S.; Zafar, M.S. Oral antimicrobial peptides: Types and role in the oral cavity. *Saudi Pharm. J.* **2016**, *24*, 515–524. [CrossRef] [PubMed]
19. Khurshid, Z.; Naseem, M.; Yahya I Asiri, F.; Mali, M.; Sannam Khan, R.; Sahibzada, H.A.; Zafar, M.S.; Faraz Moin, S.; Khan, E. Significance and Diagnostic Role of Antimicrobial Cathelicidins (LL-37) Peptides in Oral Health. *Biomolecules* **2017**, *7*, 80. [CrossRef] [PubMed]
20. Khurshid, Z.; Zafar, M.S.; Naseem, M.; Khan, R.S.; Najeeb, S. Human Oral Defensins Antimicrobial Peptides: A Future Promising Antimicrobial Drug. *Curr. Pharm. Des.* **2018**, *24*, 1130–1137. [CrossRef] [PubMed]
21. Jiang, Z.; Vasil, A.I.; Hale, J.D.; Hancock, R.E.W.; Vasil, M.L.; Hodges, R.S. Effects of Net Charge and the Number of Positively Charged Residues on the Biological Activity of Amphipathic A-Helical Cationic Antimicrobial Peptides. *Biopolymers* **2008**, *90*, 369–383. [CrossRef] [PubMed]

22. Ladram, A.; Nicolas, P. Antimicrobial Peptides from Frog Skin: Biodiversity and Therapeutic Promises. *Front. Biosci.* **2016**, *21*, 1341–1371. [CrossRef]
23. Simmaco, M.; Mignogna, G.; Barra, D.; Bossa, F. Novel Antimicrobial Peptides from Skin Secretion of the European Frog Rana Esculenta. *FEBS Lett.* **1993**, *324*, 159–161. [CrossRef]
24. Simmaco, M.; Mignogna, G.; Canofeni, S.; Miele, R.; Mangoni, M.L.; Barra, D. Temporins, Antimicrobial Peptides from the European Red Frog Rana Temporaria. *Eur. J. Biochem.* **1996**, *242*, 788–792. [CrossRef] [PubMed]
25. Zasloff, M. Magainins, a Class of Antimicrobial Peptides from Xenopus Skin: Isolation, Characterization of Two Active Forms, and Partial Cdna Sequence of a Precursor. *Proc. Natl. Acad. Sci. USA* **1987**, *84*, 5449–5453. [CrossRef] [PubMed]
26. Baker, M.A.; Maloy, W.L.; Zasloff, M.; Jacob, L.S. Anticancer Efficacy of Magainin2 and Analogue Peptides. *Cancer Res.* **1993**, *53*, 3052–3057. [PubMed]
27. Hoskin, D.W.; Ramamoorthy, A. Studies on Anticancer Activities of Antimicrobial Peptides. *Biochim. Biophys. Acta* **2008**, *1778*, 357–375. [CrossRef] [PubMed]
28. Fauci, A.S. Infectious Diseases: Considerations for the 21st Century. *Clin. Infect. Dis.* **2001**, *32*, 675–685. [CrossRef] [PubMed]
29. Fernebro, J. Fighting Bacterial Infections-Future Treatment Options. *Drug Resist. Updates* **2011**, *14*, 125–139. [CrossRef] [PubMed]
30. Thabit, A.K.; Crandon, J.L.; Nicolau, D.P. Antimicrobial Resistance: Impact on Clinical and Economic Outcomes and the Need for New Antimicrobials. *Expert Opin. Pharmacother.* **2015**, *16*, 159–177. [CrossRef] [PubMed]
31. Nguyen, L.T.; Haney, E.F.; Vogel, H.J. The Expanding Scope of Antimicrobial Peptide Structures and Their Modes of Action. *Trends Biotechnol.* **2011**, *29*, 464–472. [CrossRef] [PubMed]
32. Roccatano, D.; Colombo, G.; Fioroni, M.; Mark, A.E. Mechanism by Which 2,2,2-Trifluoroethanol/Water Mixtures Stabilize Secondary-Structure Formation in Peptides: A Molecular Dynamics Study. *Proc. Natl. Acad. Sci. USA* **2002**, *99*, 12179–12184. [CrossRef] [PubMed]
33. Del Mar Tomas, M.; Cartelle, M.; Pertega, S.; Beceiro, A.; Llinares, P.; Canle, D.; Molina, F.; Villanueva, R.; Cisneros, J.M.; Bou, G. Hospital Outbreak Caused by a Carbapenem-Resistant Strain of Acinetobacter Baumannii: Patient Prognosis and Risk-Factors for Colonisation and Infection. *Clin. Microbiol. Infect.* **2005**, *11*, 540–546. [CrossRef] [PubMed]
34. Qi, L.; Li, H.; Zhang, C.; Liang, B.; Li, J.; Wang, L.; Du, X.; Liu, X.; Qiu, S.; Song, H. Relationship between Antibiotic Resistance, Biofilm Formation, and Biofilm-Specific Resistance in Acinetobacter Baumannii. *Front. Microbiol.* **2016**, *7*, 483. [CrossRef] [PubMed]
35. Rao, R.S.; Karthika, R.U.; Singh, S.P.; Shashikala, P.; Kanungo, R.; Jayachandran, S.; Prashanth, K. Correlation between Biofilm Production and Multiple Drug Resistance in Imipenem Resistant Clinical Isolates of Acinetobacter Baumannii. *Indian J. Med. Microbiol.* **2008**, *26*, 333–337. [PubMed]
36. Babapour, E.; Haddadi, A.; Mirnejad, R.; Angaji, S.; Amirmozafari, N. Biofilm Formation in Clinical Isolates of Nosocomial Acinetobacter Baumannii and Its Relationship with Multidrug Resistance. *Asian Pac. J. Trop. Biomed.* **2016**, *6*, 528–533. [CrossRef]
37. Wang, L.; Wang, L. Acinetobacter Baumannii Biofilm Resistance Mechanisms and Prevention and Control of Progress. *Discuss. Clin. Cases* **2016**, *3*, 22–26. [CrossRef]
38. Gaddy, J.A.; Actis, L.A. Regulation of Acinetobacter Baumannii Biofilm Formation. *Future Microbiol.* **2009**, *4*, 273–278. [CrossRef] [PubMed]
39. Longo, F.; Vuotto, C.; Donelli, G. Biofilm Formation in Acinetobacter Baumannii. *New Microbiol.* **2014**, *37*, 119–127. [PubMed]
40. Huang, J.; Hao, D.; Chen, Y.; Xu, Y.; Tan, J.; Huang, Y.; Li, F.; Chen, Y. Inhibitory Effects and Mechanisms of Physiological Conditions on the Activity of Enantiomeric Forms of an Alpha-Helical Antibacterial Peptide against Bacteria. *Peptides* **2011**, *32*, 1488–1495. [CrossRef] [PubMed]
41. Goldman, M.J.; Anderson, G.M.; Stolzenberg, E.D.; Kari, U.P.; Zasloff, M.; Wilson, J.M. Human Beta-Defensin-1 Is a Salt-Sensitive Antibiotic in Lung That Is Inactivated in Cystic Fibrosis. *Cell* **1997**, *88*, 553–560. [CrossRef]
42. Jean-François, F.; Elezgaray, J.; Berson, P.; Vacher, P.; Dufourc, E.J. Pore Formation Induced by an Antimicrobial Peptide: Electrostatic Effects. *Biophys. J.* **2008**, *95*, 5748–5756. [CrossRef] [PubMed]

43. Brogden, K.A. Antimicrobial Peptides: Pore Formers or Metabolic Inhibitors in Bacteria? *Nat. Rev. Microbiol.* **2005**, *3*, 238–250. [CrossRef] [PubMed]
44. Tamba, Y.; Yamazaki, M. Magainin 2-Induced Pore Formation in the Lipid Membranes Depends on Its Concentration in the Membrane Interface. *J. Phys. Chem. B* **2009**, *113*, 4846–4852. [CrossRef] [PubMed]
45. Han, M.; Mei, Y.; Khant, H.; Ludtke, S.J. Characterization of Antibiotic Peptide Pores Using Cryo-Em and Comparison to Neutron Scattering. *Biophys. J.* **2009**, *97*, 164–172. [CrossRef] [PubMed]
46. Fields, G.B.; Noble, R.L. Solid Phase Peptide Synthesis Utilizing 9-Fluorenylmethoxycarbonyl Amino Acids. *Int. J. Pept. Protein Res.* **1990**, *35*, 161–214. [CrossRef] [PubMed]
47. Lee, J.K.; Park, S.C.; Hahm, K.S.; Park, Y. A Helix-Pxxp-Helix Peptide with Antibacterial Activity without Cytotoxicity against Mdrpa-Infected Mice. *Biomaterials* **2014**, *35*, 1025–1039. [CrossRef] [PubMed]
48. Lee, D.G.; Kim, H.N.; Park, Y.; Kim, H.K.; Choi, B.H.; Choi, C.; Hahm, K. Design of Novel Analogue Peptides with Potent Antibiotic Activity Based on the Antimicrobial Peptide, Hp (2–20), Derived from N-Terminus of Helicobacter Pylori Ribosomal Protein L1. *Biochim. Biophys. Acta* **2002**, *1598*, 185–194. [CrossRef]
49. Cho, E.; Lee, J.; Park, E.; Seo, C.H.; Luchian, T.; Park, Y. Antitumor Activity of Hpa3p through Ripk3-Dependent Regulated Necrotic Cell Death in Colon Cancer. *Oncotarget* **2018**, *9*, 7902–7917. [CrossRef] [PubMed]
50. Kim, M.K.; Kang, H.K.; Ko, S.J.; Hong, M.J.; Bang, J.K.; Seo, C.H.; Park, Y. Mechanisms Driving the Antibacterial and Antibiofilm Properties of Hp1404 and Its Analogue Peptides against Multidrug-Resistant Pseudomonas Aeruginosa. *Sci. Rep.* **2018**, *8*, 1763. [CrossRef] [PubMed]
51. Rasamiravaka, T.; Vandeputte, O.M.; Pottier, L.; Huet, J.; Rabemanantsoa, C.; Kiendrebeogo, M.; Andriantsimahavandy, A.; Rasamindrakotroka, A.; Stevigny, C.; Duez, P.; el Jaziri, M. Pseudomonas Aeruginosa Biofilm Formation and Persistence, along with the Production of Quorum Sensing-Dependent Virulence Factors, Are Disrupted by a Triterpenoid Coumarate Ester Isolated from Dalbergia Trichocarpa, a Tropical Legume. *PLoS ONE* **2015**, *10*, e0132791. [CrossRef] [PubMed]
52. Yan, J.; Wang, K.; Dang, W.; Chen, R.; Xie, J.; Zhang, B.; Song, J.; Wang, R. Two Hits Are Better Than One: Membrane-Active and DNA Binding-Related Double-Action Mechanism of Nk-18, a Novel Antimicrobial Peptide Derived from Mammalian Nk-Lysin. *Antimicrob. Agents Chemother.* **2013**, *57*, 220–228. [CrossRef] [PubMed]
53. Nagant, C.; Pitts, B.; Nazmi, K.; Vandenbranden, M.; Bolscher, J.G.; Stewart, P.S.; Dehaye, J.P. Identification of Peptides Derived from the Human Antimicrobial Peptide Ll-37 Active against Biofilms Formed by Pseudomonas Aeruginosa Using a Library of Truncated Fragments. *Antimicrob. Agents Chemother.* **2012**, *56*, 5698–5708. [CrossRef] [PubMed]

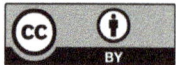

© 2018 by the authors. Licensee MDPI, Basel, Switzerland. This article is an open access article distributed under the terms and conditions of the Creative Commons Attribution (CC BY) license (http://creativecommons.org/licenses/by/4.0/).

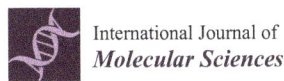

Article

Antibacterial Activities of Lipopeptide $(C_{10})_2$-KKKK-NH$_2$ Applied Alone and in Combination with Lens Liquids to Fight Biofilms Formed on Polystyrene Surfaces and Contact Lenses

Malgorzata Anna Paduszynska [1,*], Magdalena Maciejewska [1,2], Katarzyna Ewa Greber [3], Wieslaw Sawicki [3] and Wojciech Kamysz [1]

1. Department of Inorganic Chemistry, Faculty of Pharmacy, Medical University of Gdansk, 80-416 Gdansk, Poland; maciejewska.kj@gmail.com (M.M.); kamysz@gumed.edu.pl (W.K.)
2. Pharmaceutical Laboratory Avena Sp.z o.o., 86-031 Osielsko, Poland
3. Department of Physical Chemistry, Faculty of Pharmacy, Medical University of Gdansk, 80-416 Gdansk, Poland; greber@gumed.edu.pl (K.E.G.); wsawicki@gumed.edu.pl (W.S.)
* Correspondence: mdawgul@gumed.edu.pl; Tel.: +48-691-930-090; Fax: +48-58-349-1624

Received: 11 December 2018; Accepted: 14 January 2019; Published: 17 January 2019

Abstract: The widespread use of biomaterials such as contact lenses is associated with the development of biofilm-related infections which are very difficult to manage with standard therapies. The formation of bacterial biofilms on the surface of biomaterials is associated with increased antibiotic resistance. Owing to their promising antimicrobial potential, lipopeptides are being intensively investigated as novel antimicrobials. However, due to the relatively high toxicity exhibited by numerous compounds, a lot of attention is being paid to designing new lipopeptides with optimal biological activities. The principal aim of this study was to evaluate the potential ophthalmic application of lipopeptide $(C_{10})_2$-KKKK-NH$_2$. This lipopeptide was synthesized according to Fmoc chemistry using the solid-phase method. The antibiofilm activities of the lipopeptide, antibiotics used in ocular infections, and commercially available lens liquids were determined using the broth dilution method on polystyrene 96-well plates and contact lenses. Resazurin was applied as the cell-viability reagent. The effectiveness of the commercially available lens liquids supplemented with the lipopeptide was evaluated using the same method and materials. $(C_{10})_2$-KKKK-NH$_2$ exhibited stronger anti-biofilm properties compared to those of the tested conventional antimicrobials and showed the ability to enhance the activity of lens liquids at relatively low concentrations (4–32 mg/L). Estimation of the eye irritation potential of the lipopeptide using Toxtree software 2.6.13 suggests that the compound could be safely applied on the human eye. The results of performed experiments encourage further studies on $(C_{10})_2$-KKKK-NH$_2$ and its potential application in the prophylaxis of contact lens-related eye infections.

Keywords: lipopeptides; biofilm; persister cells; ocular infections; biofilm on contact lenses

1. Introduction

Nowadays, the alarming growth and spread of antibiotic-resistant microorganisms is such a serious problem that it threatens the achievements of modern medicine [1]. Moreover, microorganisms form biofilms on the surface of biomaterials or human tissues that are up 1000 times more resistant to standard antibiotic therapy compared to their planktonic counterparts [2,3]. The continuing rise in antibiotic and multi-drug resistant as well as biofilm-related bacterial infections is a major global medical health issue and is associated with the failure of clinical treatment, the limitation of antibiotic use, and increased morbidity, mortality, and healthcare costs. All these factors significantly impact the world economy and, therefore, a new generation of antimicrobial compounds is required [4,5].

Cationic antimicrobial peptides (AMPs) are promising alternatives to conventional antibiotics, due to their unique mechanism of action that reduces the risk of bacteria developing resistance to them, and also because of their ability to inhibit multi-drug resistant bacterial biofilms [6,7]. AMPs, as part of the innate immune system, naturally occur in many parts of the human body. For instance, LL-37, defensins and psoriasin, as part of tear fluid, form an important part of the innate defense system in the human eye [8]. LL-37 is an intensively studied human AMP with confirmed anti-biofilm activity [9,10] that has provided a foundation on which to design numerous peptides to fight bacterial biofilm [11,12]. Natural AMPs, as well as their derivatives, have been investigated with regard to their potential ophthalmic use [13,14], including topical application [15,16], incorporation into contact lenses (CLs) [17,18], and as preservative agents in CL solution [14,19] and corneal storage media [20]. However, despite the promising results obtained with AMPs, their broad spectrum of antimicrobial activity and their low risk of resistance development, the application of these compounds in therapy is limited due to their potential toxicity, allergenicity, enzymatic degradation, poor stability in vivo, and high costs of production [21–26].

The research on features determining the antimicrobial activity of AMPs have yielded essential information for the design of novel, highly effective compounds with optimized biological properties that can also be produced at lower cost compared to their natural antimicrobial counterparts. Numerous studies focus on evaluating and designing shorter analogs, creating multimeric AMP-based sequences and developing peptidomimetics which can imitate the bactericidal mechanism of action.

A successful approach to modulating the activity and bioavailability of peptides is the acylation of cationic peptides with fatty acid. It has been shown that the introduction of D-amino acid or non-peptide residues significantly improves the antimicrobial spectrum activity of cationic peptides and determines a higher resistance to proteolytic degradation [27,28]. Simple modification, such as the acylation of short cationic residue, has resulted in short synthetic lipopeptides, a particularly promising group of compounds exhibiting a strong and broad spectrum of antimicrobial activity. They are composed of short positively-charged peptide chains conjugated with a fatty acid that provides amphipathicity. Those two features determine the surface-active properties of the compounds and allow them to electrostatically interact with a negatively-charged microbial membrane, leading to a rapid-kill drug-resistant pathogen [29]. The compounds are cost-effective and less time-consuming to produce in comparison with native AMPs.

So far, research has allowed numerous short lipopeptides endowed with high antibacterial as well as antifungal activity to be identified [21,30–32]. These lipopeptides have also been found to be effective against biofilms and multi-drug resistant bacteria [33]. However, their practical use in ophthalmology remains limited. Two critical issues are their potential toxicity or allergenicity [31,34]. These issues are especially important in the case of such a delicate and sensitive structure like the human eye and, therefore, a great deal of attention is being paid to optimizing the biological activities of lipopeptides.

In previous studies, we identified very a promising compound—$(C_{10})_2$-KKKK-NH$_2$—which exhibits strong antibacterial activities and low toxicity towards human cells in vitro [35,36]. In this study we have further investigated the antimicrobial activity of this compound with regard to its potential application in ophthalmology, and pre-evaluated its irritation potential via computational methods which have proved to be very useful in predicting and describing the properties of the compound [37–39].

2. Results

2.1. Activity of the Lipopeptide and Conventional Antibiotics against Biofilms Formed on Polystyrene

The tested compounds exhibited diverse antibiofilm activities towards various bacterial species. The durability of the antimicrobial effect after the withdrawal of the active compound varied significantly depending on the applied compound and the tested strain. In many cases, the removal of the antibiotic caused partial or even full renewal of bacterial biofilms.

Structures formed by *Staphylococcus epidermidis* (SE) on the surface of 96-well plates turned out to be sensitive to all tested compounds (Figure 1, Table 1). The application of solutions of ciprofloxacin significantly reduced the metabolic activity of cells in the pre-grown structures. The antibiotic used at a range of concentrations from 1–8 mg/L caused a ca. 70–80% decrease in the metabolic activity of cultured bacteria, while concentrations of 16 mg/L and higher resulted in the reduction of metabolic activity to 10% and lower in comparison to the positive control. Additional incubation in the pure medium after the removal of solutions of ciprofloxacin (1–128 mg/L) caused an increase in the metabolic activity of the bacteria (Table 1). Only the concentration of 256 mg/L of the antibiotic created a permanent antibiofilm effect.

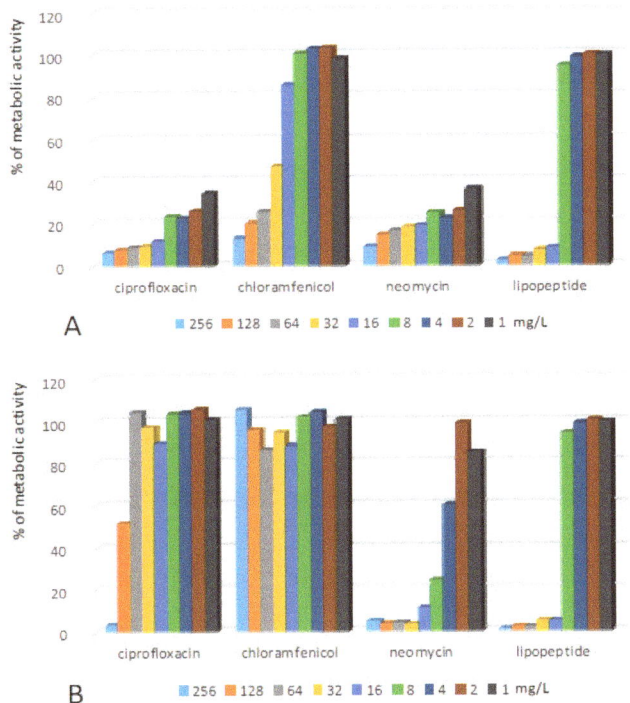

Figure 1. Activity of the lipopeptide and conventional antimicrobials applied at concentrations of 1–256 mg/L against SE biofilms formed on polystyrene (**A**) results read after 24 h exposure to compounds; and (**B**) results read after the withdrawal of compounds and an additional 24 h of incubation in MHB II. The results are presented as the percentage of metabolic activity in comparison to positive (100%) and negative (0%) controls; RSD ≤ 15%.

Table 1. Activities of conventional antimicrobials and the lipopeptide—$(C_{10})_2$-KKKK-NH$_2$ against bacterial biofilms formed on polystyrene plates presented as MBEC—minimum biofilm eradication concentration (mg/L); MBEC 90—the lowest concentration which allowed to reduce the metabolic activity of bacteria by at least $90 \pm 5\%$; MBEC 90 II – the lowest concentration which resulted in permanent reduction of metabolic activity by at last $90 \pm 5\%$; MBEC 50—the lowest concentration which allowed to reduce the metabolic activity by at least $50 \pm 5\%$; MBEC 50 II—the lowest concentration resulted in permanent reduction of the metabolic activity by at least $50 \pm 5\%$.

Compound	MBEC 90	MBEC II 90	MBEC 50	MBEC II 50
Staphylococcus epidermidis				
Ciprofloxacin	16	256	≤1	128
Chloramphenicol	256	>256	32	>256
Neomycin	16	16	≤1	8
Lipopeptide	16	16	16	16
Staphylococcus aureus				
Ciprofloxacin	>256	>256	16	128
Chloramphenicol	>256	>256	128	>256
Neomycin	64	64	4	64
Lipopeptide	32	32	8	16
Enterococcus feacalis				
Ciprofloxacin	>256	>256	64	256
Chloramphenicol	>256	>256	32	>256
Neomycin	>256	>256	64	>256
Lipopeptide	32	32	16	32
Escherichia coli				
Ciprofloxacin	32	32	≤1	≤1
Chloramphenicol	16	>256	8	>256
Neomycin	>256	>256	8	>256
Lipopeptide	64	64	64	64
Pseudomonas aeruginosa				
Ciprofloxacin	≤1	32	≤1	16
Chloramphenicol	128	>256	4	256
Neomycin	64	>256	8	128
Lipopeptide	256	>256	64	64

Similar antibiofilm activity against SE was presented by neomycin. However, in the case of this antibiotic, the effect remained after its withdrawal and additional incubation. Chloramphenicol exhibited rather low antibiofilm potential. In the first antibiofilm assay, the compound reduced the metabolic activity of bacteria to ca. 12, 20, and 25% once applied at concentrations of 256, 128, and 64 mg/L respectively. The activity was removed totally in the second assay—the metabolic activity of bacteria in all the samples after exposure and the subsequent withdrawal of chloramphenicol increased significantly. Lipopeptide $(C_{10})_2$-KKKK-NH$_2$ turned out to be very active against SE biofilm. Application at concentrations of 16–256 mg/L caused the metabolic activity of bacterial cells to reduce to ca. 5%. This was the strongest reduction of metabolic activity of SE cells observed in this assay. Moreover, the effect remained after additional incubation in the pure medium after the withdrawal of the lipopeptide.

Staphylococcus aureus (SA) cultured on polystyrene plates turned out to be less sensitive in comparison to SE (Figure 2, Table 1). The difference in susceptibility is especially visible in the case of conventional antibiotics. Ciprofloxacin reduced the metabolic activity of SA to less than 20% when applied at the highest tested concentration and to ca. 30% when applied at concentrations of 128–164 mg/L. The antibiofilm effect was permanent only at the two highest concentrations (Table 1). The removal of the antibiotic SA in the sample treated with a concentration of 64 mg/L increased metabolic activity to ca. 70% of the positive control. Neomycin exhibited some higher and more permanent activity. However, the reduction of metabolic activity was not as significant as in the case of SE. The most potent antistaphylococcal agent was the lipopeptide. The compound caused a reduction in the metabolic activity of SA cells by over 90% when applied at concentrations of 32 mg/L and higher. The exposure to the lipopeptide caused a permanent antibiofilm effect—metabolic activity did not increase after the compound was replaced with pure MHB II. As in the case of SE, chloramphenicol was the least promising agent. The metabolic activity of SA was reduced by half only after the application of the compound at concentrations of 128–256 mg/L and increased significantly after the withdrawal of the antibiotic.

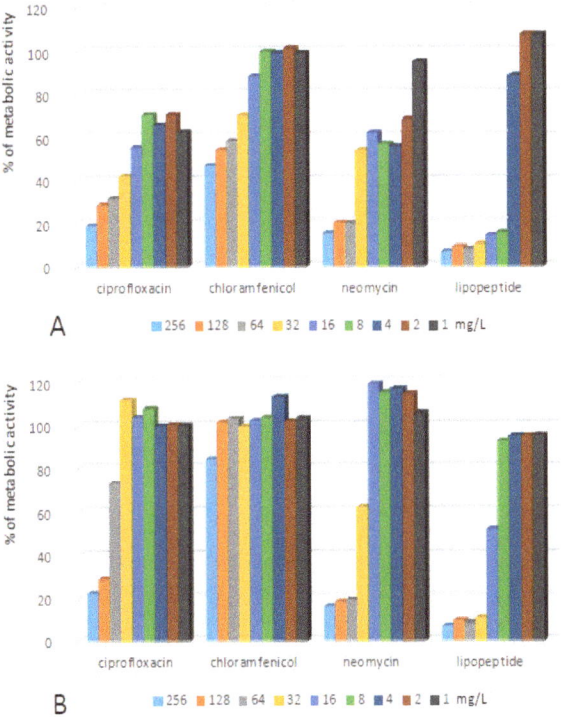

Figure 2. Activity of the lipopeptide and conventional antimicrobials applied at concentrations of 1–256 mg/L against SA biofilms formed on polystyrene (**A**) results read after 24 h exposure to compounds; and (**B**) results read after the withdrawal of compounds and an additional 24 h of incubation in MHB II. The results are presented as the percentage of metabolic activity in comparison to positive (100%) and negative (0%) controls; RSD ≤ 15%.

Biofilms formed by *Enterococcus feacalis* (EF) turned out to be the most resistant to conventional antimicrobials (Figure 3, Table 1). Application of all three compounds at the highest concentrations resulted in a reduction of metabolic activity in biofilms to ca. 35% of initial populations. After the withdrawal of antibiotics, the effect remained for ciprofloxacin, while the removal of chloramphenicol and neomycin resulted in the complete renewal of the metabolic activity of bacteria. The lipopeptide exhibited the ability to permanently eradicate the biofilm at concentrations of 32–256 mg/L. In both antibiofilm assays, a reduction of the metabolic activity of EF to less than 10% of the positive control was observed.

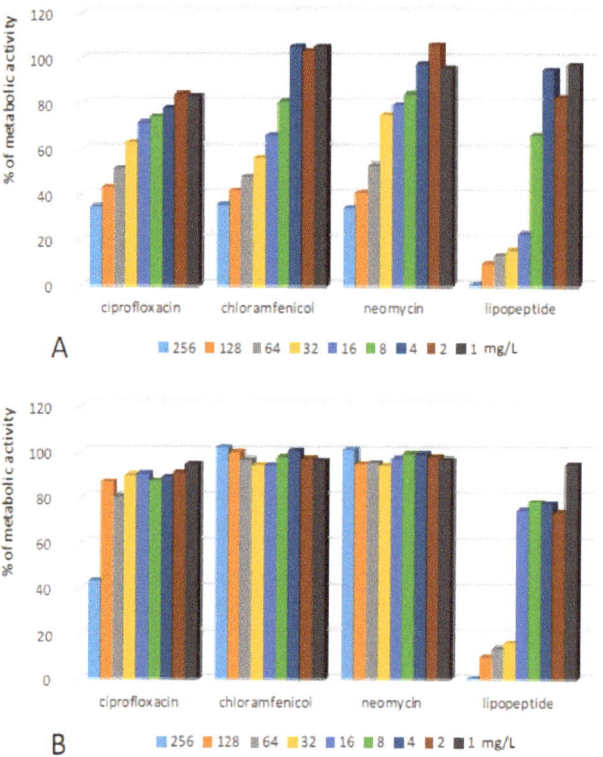

Figure 3. Activity of the lipopeptide and conventional antimicrobials applied at concentrations of 1–256 mg/L against EF biofilms formed on polystyrene (**A**) results read after 24 h exposure to compounds; and (**B**) results read after the withdrawal of compounds and an additional 24 h of incubation in MHB II. The results are presented as the percentage of metabolic activity in comparison to positive (100%) and negative (0%) controls; RSD $\leq$ 15%.

Some higher concentrations of the lipopeptide were required to fight structures formed by *Escherichia coli* (EC) (Figure 4, Table 1). This effect was observed after application of the lipopeptide at concentrations of 64 mg/L and higher. However, the reduction of metabolism was also very high and did not deteriorate after the withdrawal of the compound. A similar effect was observed after the exposure of EC biofilms to ciprofloxacin at concentrations of 32–256 mg/L. Treatment with lower concentrations reduced metabolic activity by 75 to 85%, however, after removal of the antibiotic, a certain increase of metabolic activity was observed. Chloramphenicol, as well as neomycin, also exhibited rather high effectiveness towards EC biofilms; however, the bacterial populations were able to fully restore their metabolic activity when the compounds were removed from the environment.

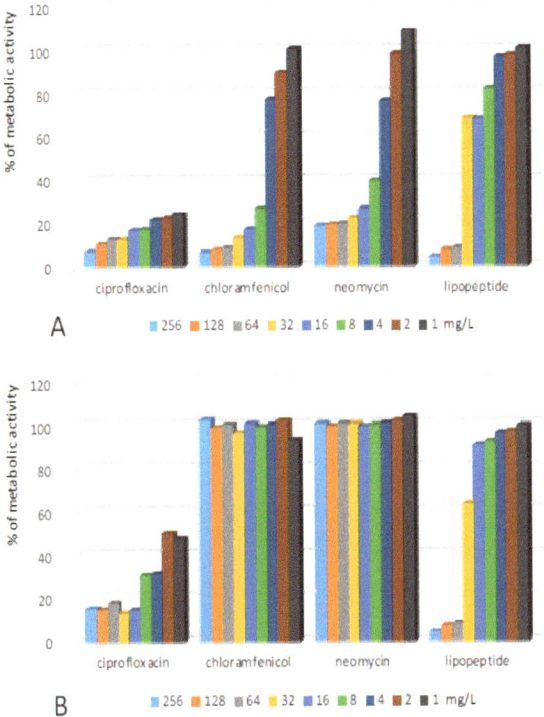

Figure 4. Activity of the lipopeptide and conventional antimicrobials applied at concentrations of 1–256 mg/L against EC biofilms formed on polystyrene (**A**) results read after 24 h exposure to compounds; and (**B**) results read after the withdrawal of compounds and additional 24 h of incubation in MHB II. The results are presented as the percentage of metabolic activity in comparison to positive (100%) and negative (0%) controls; RSD ≤ 15%.

Pseudomonas aeruginosa (PA) formed a biofilm which exhibited the highest resistance towards the lipopeptide (Figure 5, Table 1). The compound reduced the metabolic activity of bacteria to 10% only when applied at a concentration of 256 mg/L. Unfortunately, the bacteria repopulated and gained 40% of the metabolic activity of the positive control after the removal of the lipopeptide. Application of lower concentrations resulted in a 50% decrease of bacterial metabolism which did not increase after the withdrawal of the compound. Ciprofloxacin was highly active against PA—it reduced the metabolic activity of bacteria by more than 90% even at the lowest applied concentrations. Further incubation in the medium without antibiotics caused a certain renewal of metabolic activity within the biofilm, but only in wells treated with the antibiotic applied at concentrations lower than 32 mg/L. Exposure of the PA biofilm to chloramphenicol at concentrations of 128–256 and 32–64 mg/L resulted in the reduction of the metabolic activities of bacteria by ca. 90% and 70%, respectively. The incubation of PA after replacing solutions of chloramphenicol with MHB II resulted in a significant increase in metabolism. Interestingly, pretreating the biofilm with the compound at concentrations lower than 32 mg/L resulted in a significant promotion of biofilm growth. Very similar results were obtained for neomycin. The compound reduced metabolic activity by over 90% at concentrations of 64–256 mg/L and 75% after the exposure of PA to the compound at a concentration of 32 mg/L. Removal of the antibiotic resulted in a significant increase of PA metabolism. As in the case of chloramphenicol, pretreatment of a PA biofilm with concentrations lower than 32 mg/L caused the enhanced metabolism of bacteria in comparison to the positive control.

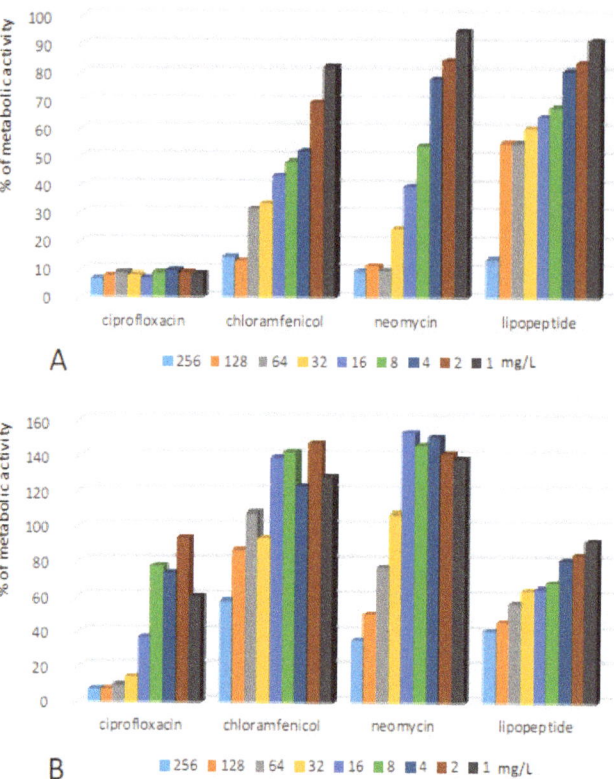

Figure 5. Activity of the lipopeptide and conventional antimicrobials applied at concentrations of 1–256 mg/L against PA biofilms formed on polystyrene (**A**) results read after 24 h exposure to compounds; and (**B**) results read after the withdrawal of compounds and additional 24 h of incubation in MHB II). The results are presented as the percentage of metabolic activity in comparison to positive (100%) and negative (0%) controls; RSD ≤ 15%.

2.2. Activity of Lipopeptide and CL Solutions against Biofilms Formed on CLs

Commercially-available lens liquids proved to be highly active against biofilms formed on CLs. They reduced the metabolism of bacteria cultured on CLs by at least 90% for the vast majority of tested strains. Both liquids A and B caused a reduction of bacterial metabolism to 10% of the positive control (or lower) for SA, SE, EF, and EC, while only liquid A demonstrated this activity against PA. The application of the lipopeptide dissolved in PBS allowed biofilms formed by all tested strains to be removed from the CLs. The highest effectiveness was observed for SE and EF. After exposure to the lipopeptide at a concentration of 8 mg/L, the metabolic activity of bacteria reduced by at least 90%. For such a significant decrease of metabolism of SA cells, the application of the lipopeptide at a concentration of 16 mg/L was needed. The most difficult cultures to eliminate with lipopeptide solutions were EC and PA—to reduce the metabolic activity of these strains by more than 90%, a concentration of 32 mg/L of lipopeptide were required (Figure 6).

These very promising results were obtained when the exposure to CL liquids and solutions of lipopeptide lasted until the reading of results. Once the CL liquids were removed and the CLs were further incubated in MHB II, the metabolic activities of bacterial populations of the majority of strains were nearly fully renewed. The antibacterial effect of CL solutions remained only for SE, while for liquid A and the EF strain, biofilm growth increased. Some better, but also not fully satisfying, results were obtained for the lipopeptide. It permanently removed SA and SE biofilms from CLs once applied at a concentration of 16 mg/L. For Gram-negative strains, the bacterial populations regrew to a high extent (PA was fully restored, EC to ca. 50%) after the removal of the lipopeptide at all tested concentrations. Similarly as in the case of CL solution A, treating EF with the lipopeptide promoted bacterial growth.

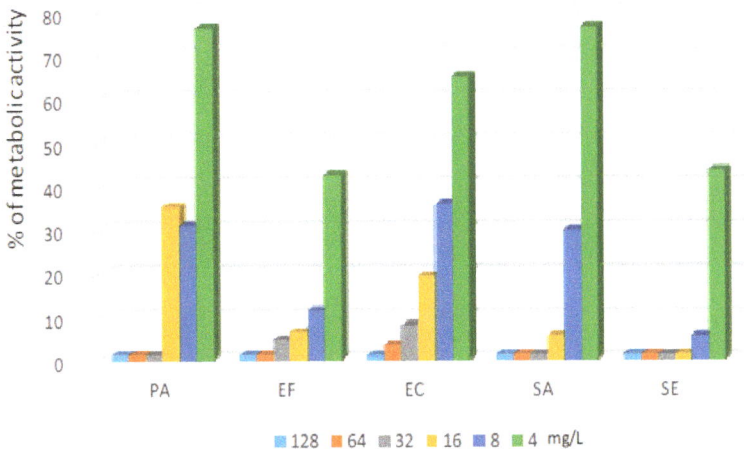

Figure 6. Activity of the lipopeptide applied at concentrations 4–128 mg/L against biofilms formed on CLs. The results are presented as the percentage of metabolic activity in comparison to positive (100%) and negative (0%) controls; RSD $\leq$ 20%.

2.3. Antibiofilm Activity of the Lipopeptide Applied in Combination with CL Liquids

2.3.1. Biofilms Formed on Polystyrene Surfaces

In this assay we found that the supplementation of CL solutions with lipopeptide positively influenced their antibacterial activity (Figure 7). This was especially noticeable for liquid B, which demonstrated lower effectiveness in comparison to liquid A. The latter caused the reduction of metabolic activity of bacteria by more than 90% for almost all tested strains, but supplementation with the lipopeptide resulted in an even higher decrease of microbial metabolism. Exposure of PA biofilms to liquid A reduced biofilm metabolism to ca. 15% of the positive control, while supplementation with the lipopeptide at a very low concentration (1 mg/L) caused further reduction in bacterial metabolic activity - to 5% of positive control.

Liquid B applied alone caused only partial reduction of bacterial metabolic activity for the majority of strains. Its supplementation with the lipopeptide at a concentration of 4–8 mg/L reduced the biofilms of SE, SA, EC, and EF by at least 90%. The PA biofilm was not affected by liquid B at all. Its combination with the lipopeptide at concentrations of 128 and 64 mg/L reduced the bacterial metabolism to ca. 4 and 20%, respectively.

The lipopeptide applied alone was highly active against biofilms formed by SA and SE at concentrations of 32 and 16 mg/L, respectively. Application of the same concentration of the lipopeptide reduced metabolic activity in the EF biofilm by ca. 95%. Gram-negative strains cultured on polystyrene surfaces turned out to be much less sensitive to the lipopeptide, which caused partial reduction of bacterial metabolism. For PA, we observed medium antibacterial activity only at the highest concentration—128 mg/L.

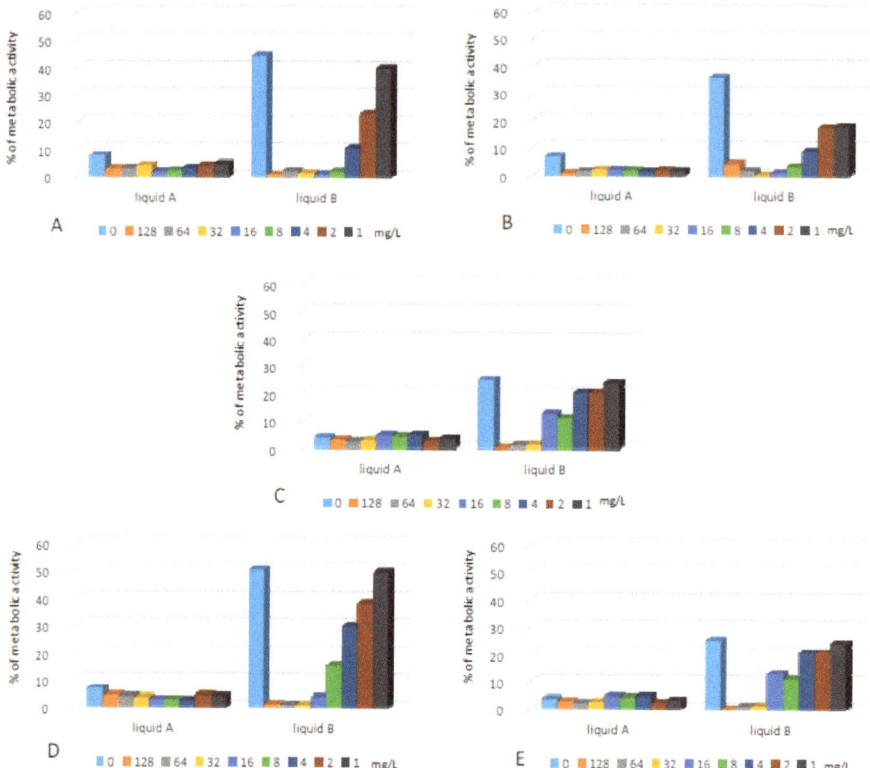

Figure 7. Activity of CL liquids alone and supplemented with the lipopeptide applied at concentrations of 1–128 mg/L against biofilms formed on polystyrene plates by: (**A**) SE; (**B**) SA; (**C**) EF; (**D**) EC; and (**E**) PA. The results are presented as the percentage of metabolic activity in comparison to positive (100%) and negative (0%) controls; RSD ≤ 15%.

2.3.2. Biofilms Formed on CLs

As described in Section 2.2, the antibacterial effect of CL solutions as well as the lipopeptide applied alone does not last once the agents are replaced with MHB II. Supplementation of CL solutions with the lipopeptide significantly improved their antibiofilm activity, which remained after the withdrawal of active agents (Figure 8). The synergistic effect was especially noticeable for PA, EC and EF. When the CL solutions or lipopeptide were applied alone against EC and PA biofilms, the metabolic activities of bacteria were partially or fully restored. Supplementation of both liquids with the lipopeptide at a concentration of 4 mg/L reduced bacterial metabolism to ca. 2%. A permanent and sufficient activity against PA was obtained after the application of liquid B with the lipopeptide at a concentration of 32 mg/L. To nearly totally remove (metabolic activities ca. 1–2%) the EF biofilms from the surface of CLs, liquids A and B were supplemented with the lipopeptide at concentrations of 16 and 32 mg/L, respectively. SA was permanently eliminated from CLs once the lipopeptide was added at concentrations of 8 and 4 mg/L to liquid A and B, respectively. Despite the fact that SE biofilms were susceptible to the agents when applied alone, we also noticed a synergistic effect between the lipopeptide and CL solutions.

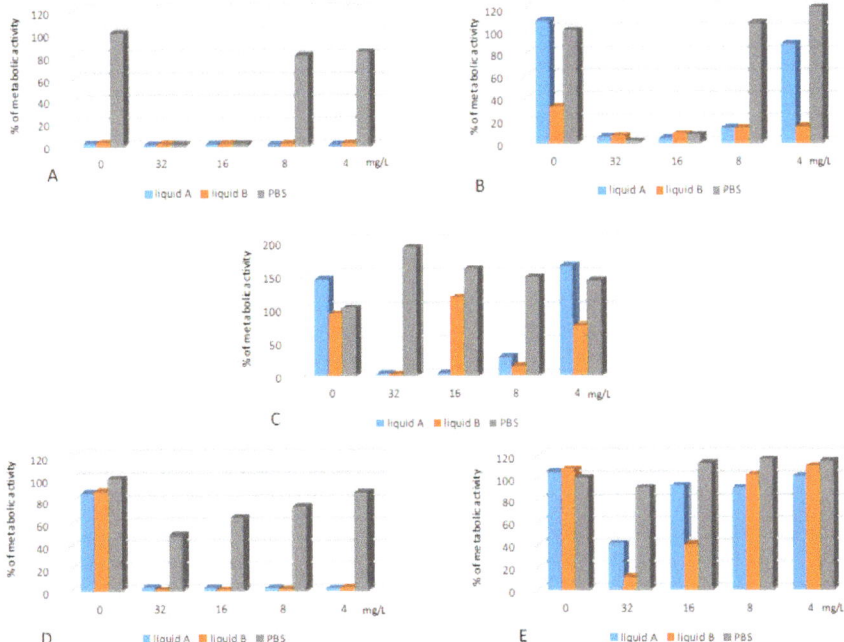

Figure 8. Activity of CL liquids alone and supplemented with the lipopeptide applied at concentrations of 4–32 mg/L against biofilms formed on CL by: (**A**) SE; (**B**) SA; (**C**) EF; (**D**) EC; and (**E**) PA. The results are presented as the percentage of metabolic activity in comparison to positive (100%) and negative (0%) controls; RSD ≤ 20%.

2.4. Eye Corrosion

Obtained result suggested that target structures do not show eye irritation properties as well as do not cause skin corrosion.

3. Discussion

The handling of CLs after insufficient hand washing, CL storage cases and solutions may be potential sources of contamination causing the development of CL-associated infections, which are relatively rare, but can pose severe vision-threatening complications [40–43]. Due to the development of bacterial resistance as well as the existence of bacteria in the form of biofilms, the standard means of prevention and treatment of ocular infections are not always sufficient. Numerous AMPs and their derivatives have been investigated as potential alternatives to conventional antibiotics, as well as disinfecting solutions.

The topical application of a cecropin-melittin hybrid was effective in a pseudomonas keratitis model in rabbits [16]. Another hybrid (protamine-melittin) peptide—melimine—was successfully evaluated as an antimicrobial CL coating for the prevention of contact lens-induced acute red eye (CLARE) in the PA guinea pig model [17] and contact lens-induced peripheral ulcer (CLPU) in the rabbit model [18]. CLs coated with the peptide were also tested in a human clinical trial, where they demonstrated broad spectrum, high antimicrobial activity and turned out to be safe for use [44]. A derivative of melimine—mel4—was recently successfully applied as an antimicrobial coating for silicone hydrogel CLs [45].

Peptide Shiva-11—a synthetic analogue of cecropin—was found to be effective against PA, SE, and SA as antibacterial agent in CL solutions [46]. In another study, the peptide demonstrated a wide range of antimicrobial activity against pathogens isolated from a human suffering from ocular infections [14]. Another analogue of cecropin—D5C—exhibited the ability to enhance the effectiveness of commercially-available disinfecting solutions [19]. The lipopeptide used in our study also demonstrated the potential to enhance the antimicrobial activity of commercial CL solutions.

For our study, we chose the CL liquids which were the most effective in our previous work [47]. As in the previous work, the application of liquid A eliminated at least 90% of living cells of all strains cultured on CL. Liquid B was effective against the majority of strains except PA. When applied alone, the lipopeptide demonstrated high activity against Gram-positive bacteria and some lower activity against Gram-negative strains.

A further assay revealed that the above activities do not last if the CL solutions, and in some cases also the solutions of lipopeptide, are removed from the environment. This suggests that a certain population of microbial cells survived the exposure to tested solutions and repopulated after the removal of these solutions. Further evaluation should be performed in order to determine if the remaining cells can be identified as persister cells. Persister cells are considered to be responsible for the resistance of biofilm to antimicrobial agents. They constitute a small population of microbial cells which exist in the presence of antibiotics, have low metabolic activity and do not grow. They are believed to be responsible for the return of infections after the withdrawal of antibiotic treatment [48]. It has not been determined if the repopulation of biofilms in the study was the result of the presence of persisters or regular cells protected by exopolysaccharide (EPS) or other resistance mechanisms. Therefore, the results are interpreted as permanent/non-permanent antimicrobial activity.

The obtained results revealed that the antimicrobial effect of CL solutions was permanent only in the case of SE, while the lipopeptide turned out to be active only against staphylococci. Interestingly, exposure of EF to the lipopeptide resulted in the promotion of biofilm growth on CLs after the solution was replaced with MHB II. This may be explained by the defense mechanism of bacteria. Biofilm formation is described as a mechanism developed by bacteria in order to avoid the action of human AMPs in a human body [49–51]. In order to assess if there is synergistic activity between CL solutions and the lipopeptide, bacterial biofilms cultured on polystyrene were exposed to CL solutions supplemented with the compound. We observed a positive influence of lipopeptide supplementation on the effectiveness of applied CL solutions against all tested strains, and due to this, an assay with CLs was performed. As expected, the supplementation of CL liquids with the lipopeptide achieved permanent disinfection of CLs. For staphylococci and EC, this was observed after usage of the lipopeptide at a concentration of 4 mg/L, while for EF some higher concentrations were necessary. For PA, only usage of liquid B with the lipopeptide at 32 mg/L gave satisfying results.

PA was also the most difficult strain to eliminate from the surface of CL in the previous study, in which we investigated amphibian peptides and short lipopeptides containing hexadecanoic acid according to their potential application as CL solution additives [47]. The results of performed antimicrobial assays were also very promising. However, due to high toxicity towards human keratinocytes in vitro, the ocular applications of lipopeptides with hexadecanoic acid are not worth further consideration [31,36]. In contrast to those lipopeptides, the compound with two residues of decanoic acid does not exhibit toxicity towards human cells in vitro at its microbiologically-active concentrations [35,36]. The results obtained in the present study revealed that the lipopeptide enhances the activity of commercial CL solutions at concentrations much lower than the ones identified as toxic to both human keratinocytes and erythrocytes. Moreover, according to the results obtained by the computational method, the compound is expected not to irritate the human eye. This needs to be confirmed with experimental methods, but data collected so far suggest that $(C_{10})_2$-KKKK-NH$_2$ might be a promising antibacterial additive to CL solutions.

The results obtained in assays on polystyrene plates demonstrated that the compound could also be worth further consideration as an alternative to antibiotic therapy of biofilm-related infections. In previous studies we confirmed the high antibiofilm activities of lipopeptides containing hexadecanoic acid [21,52]. However, due to high toxicity in vitro, the compounds should not be further considered for administration other than topical skin application [31,36]. $(C_{10})_2$-KKKK-NH$_2$ demonstrates the ability to eradicate a bacterial biofilm at slightly higher concentrations in comparison to lipopeptides with hexadecanoic acid. However, for the majority of strains, the active concentrations were identified as safe to human cells. Moreover, the results obtained for the lipopeptide in the case of Gram-positive bacteria are much more satisfying in comparison to those obtained for conventional antimicrobials. The compound demonstrated the ability to permanently eliminate the living bacterial cells of EF, SA, and SE once applied at concentrations of 32 (EF, SA) and 16 (SE) mg/L, which are below the concentrations identified as toxic to human cells. For SE, similar results were obtained for neomycin: the antibiotic was also active at a concentration of 16 mg/L. However, the reduction of bacterial metabolism was not as significant as was demonstrated by the lipopeptide. The antibiotic was also active against SA, but at some higher concentration in comparison to the lipopeptide. The remaining conventional antimicrobials exhibited certain activity in the first assay, however after the withdrawal of compounds, the bacteria repopulated to a high extent. EF cultured on polystyrene plates turned out to be not sensitive to the action of all conventional antibiotics. The number of living cells reduced somewhat at higher concentrations (64–256 mg/L), but after the removal of antibiotics, the bacteria repopulated almost completely. Based on these results, we can expect the clinical failure of application of these compounds for biofilm-related infections. Even in the case of a positive effect of therapy, a return of infection can be expected after the treatment is completed.

Difficulties in the elimination of SA and EF biofilms with ciprofloxacin have previously been reported [53]. Ciprofloxacin exhibited much higher activity against Gram-negative bacteria, which was to be expected as the infections caused by EC are the main therapeutic indications for the application of this antimicrobial. The structures were permanently removed from polystyrene after application of the compound at a concentration of 16 mg/L, while to eradicate PA a concentration of 32 mg/L was sufficient. The lipopeptide demonstrated the activity at a concentration of 64 mg/L in the case of EC, but full elimination of PA was not achieved at the tested range of concentrations: even after application of the peptide at 256 mg/L, the bacterial population regrew significantly (to 40%). Chloramphenicol and neomycin showed rather weak activity against EC and PA biofilms, moreover the bacteria repopulated to a high extent after the withdrawal of compounds, even after exposure to their highest concentrations. The obtained results suggest that for biofilm-associated infections, ciprofloxacin can be recommended for Gram-negative infections and neomycin is expected to be effective against staphylococcal infections, while chloramphenicol is ineffective in the fight against biofilms of all tested strains. The lipopeptide shows high activity against biofilms formed by Gram-positive bacteria and is definitely worth further testing in this regard. Its concentrations that were active against biofilms are only a few times higher in comparison to the previously determined minimum inhibitory concentrations [35], while for conventional antimicrobials, concentrations at least 50–100 times higher in comparison to MICs are needed to eradicate biofilms [21,52].

According to the literature, the mechanisms responsible for biofilm resistance/persistence include the protection of microbial cells by the presence of EPS, changes in gene expression, the slowing down of metabolism and the presence of persister cells [54,55]. Promising results obtained for lipopeptides can be explained by their mechanism of action, based on interactions with microbial cell membranes, which allows slow- or even non-growing bacteria to act. Moreover, the small size of the molecules as well as their surfactant activity probably facilitates their penetration through EPS.

The recalcitrance to eradication by antibiotics is described as a characteristic feature of the bacteria in biofilms. Even after exposure to high doses of an antimicrobial, a fraction of cells can survive and repopulate once the antibiotic is withdrawn, leading to secondary infection [56]. According to the obtained results, this is not to be expected after treatment with the lipopeptide as the compound seems to eliminate all the bacteria within the biofilm. It was previously reported that small molecules and AMPs demonstrate the ability to kill persister cells [57].

The excellent antimicrobial activity was previously reported for many lipopeptides. This, along with the relatively low production costs, has encouraged many research groups to study their antimicrobial activities and design molecules with optimal properties. C_{16}-KK-NH$_2$ is one of such extensively studied compounds. As mentioned, the lipopeptide exhibits broad spectrum, high antimicrobial activity, including antibiotic-resistant strains as well as biofilm-associated bacteria [21,58], but also demonstrates high toxicity towards human cells at very low concentrations [36]. Other derivatives of hexadecanoic acid containing short-sequence peptides with alanine, glycine, leucine and lysine have demonstrated strong activity against SA strains [59]. Lipopeptides containing tryptophan and ornithine residues combined with capric, caproic, caprylic, lauric, myristic, and palmitic acids, and combinations of lauric acid with short sequences composed of ornithine and cysteine exhibited similar activities [21,60].

There is no doubt that lipopeptides are a very interesting alternative for the therapy of biofilm-related or drug-resistant microbial infections. The main limitation is their high toxicity resulting from their non-specific mechanism of action. The compounds disrupt the membranes of red blood cells when the cells are exposed to the compounds at concentrations close to their minimum inhibitory concentrations [61,62]. Therefore, the need to design new molecules with optimal properties is very urgent. $(C_{10})_2$-KKKK-NH$_2$ is an example of a successfully designed and synthesized novel compound based on AMPs.

4. Materials and Methods

4.1. Bacterial Strains and Culture Conditions

Bacterial strains were obtained from the Polish Collection of Microorganisms (Polish Academy of Science, Wroclaw, Poland). Three Gram-positive and two Gram-negative strains linked with CL-related infections were chosen for the study (*Staphylococus aureus* ATCC 6538, *Staphylococcus epidermidis* ATCC 14990, *Pseudomonas aeruginosa* ATCC 9027, *Escherichia coli* ATCC 25922, and *Enterococcus faecalis* ATCC 29212). The bacteria were cultured in a Mueller Hinton Broth II (MHB, Biocorp, Warsaw, Poland) overnight, under aerobic conditions at 37 °C. After incubation, the liquid cultures were centrifuged (2500 rpm for 10 min) and washed with phosphoric buffer (PBS, AppliChem, Darmstadt, Germany) three times and resuspended in fresh MHB II for inoculums appropriate for the performed assays.

4.2. Antimicrobials and CL Liquids

Ciprofloxacin, chloramphenicol and neomycin (sulfate) were purchased from Sigma-Aldrich, (St. Louis, MO, USA). Lipopeptide $(C_{10})_2$-KKKK-NH$_2$ was synthesized in the Department of Physical Chemistry (Medical University of Gdansk, Gdansk, Poland) according to the previously described protocol [62]. Two commercially-available popular CL solutions with the following compositions were tested:

A: Citrate, Tetronic 1304, aminomethylpropanol, sodium chloride, boric acid, sorbitol, disodium edetate, Polyquad (Polyquaternium) 0.001%, Aldox (myristamidopropyl dimethylamine) 0.0005%.

B: Boric Acid, disodium edetate, sodium borate, sodium chloride, DYMED (polyaminopropyl biguanide) 0.0001%, HYDRANATE (hydroxyalkylphosphonate) 0.03%, Poloxamine 1%.

4.3. Activity of Lipopeptide and Antibiotics against Biofilms Formed on 96-Well Plates

Bacterial suspensions were added to 96-well plates (Kartell, Noviglio, Italy) at initial inoculums of ca. 5×10^8 CFU/mL and incubated under aerobic conditions with shaking (120 rpm) at 37 °C for 24 h. After this time, the wells were washed three times with PBS, and fresh medium supplemented with the lipopeptide and antibiotics was added. The bacterial cultures were exposed to graded concentrations (range 1–256 mg/mL) of antimicrobials in MHB II for 24 h (aerobic conditions, 120 rpm shaking, 37 °C). After exposure, the wells were washed three times with PBS and a solution of resazurin (Sigma Aldrich, St. Louis, MO, USA) in MHB II (0.01%) was added. This cell viability reagent is metabolized by bacterial dehydrogenases upon contact with living cells. As a result, the blue dye is reduced to a pink resorufin. After 1.5 h of incubation, the absorbance was measured at 570 and 600 nm using a microplate reader (Thermo Fisher Scientific, Waltham, MA, USA). The results are presented as a % of living cells (metabolic activity) compared to the positive control (sample with bacteria suspended in pure MHBII) and negative control (pure MHB II), which were taken as 100% and 0%, respectively. The metabolic activity of bacteria in the samples was measured according to the following formula:

Metabolic activity (%) = (ΔAbs of sample − ΔAbs of negative control)/(ΔAbs of positive control − ΔAbs of negative control);

ΔAbs = absorbance at 570 nm − absorbance at 600 nm;

The presented results are the means of nine results obtained on three different days.

4.4. Activity of Lipopeptide and Antibiotics against Biofilms Formed on 96-Well Plates after the Withdrawal of the Applied Antimicrobial

This assay was a continuation of assay 4.3 and was performed in order to assess the durability of the antibiofilm effect. The procedure was conducted as described in Section 4.3, with the difference that after exposure to antimicrobials, the wells were washed three times with PBS and pure MHB II was added. The samples were incubated for another 24 h (aerobic conditions, 120 rpm shaking, 37 °C). Then the medium was replaced with resazurin in MHB II (0.01%). The absorbance was measured at the same wave lengths and metabolic activity was calculated according to the formula given in Section 4.3. The presented results are means of nine results obtained on three different days.

4.5. Activity of Lipopeptide and CL Liquids against Biofilms Formed on CLs

Bacterial biofilms were cultured on commercially available CLs (1-Day Acuvue Moist, containing Etafilcon A, obtained from Johnson and Johnson Vision Care, Jacksonville, FL, USA). The CLs were placed in polystyrene 24-well plates (Orange Scientific, Braine-l'Alleud, Belgium) in bacterial suspensions in MHB II at initial inoculums of ca. 5×10^8 CFU/mL. After 24 h of incubation (aerobic conditions, 120 rpm shaking, 37 °C), all of the CLs were rinsed three times with PBS. The lenses were then transferred into new wells with CL liquids and solutions of the lipopeptide in PBS at graded concentrations (range 4–64 mg/mL) and incubated again for 24 h at 37 °C. After incubation, resazurin was added (final concentration per sample = 0.01%) and absorbance was measured as in the assays 4.3 and 4.4. Positive controls contained CLs with bacterial biofilms placed in pure PBS, while sterile CLs incubated in MHB II replaced with PBS served as negative controls. The experiments were performed in triplicate on three different days.

4.6. Antibiofilm Activity of the Lipopeptide Applied in Combination with Commercially-Available Lens Liquids

4.6.1. The Effect of the Lipopeptide on the Effectiveness of the Lens Liquids against Biofilms Formed on 96-Well Polystyrene Plates

The bacteria were cultured as described in Section 4.3 and afterwards exposed to graded concentrations (range 128mg/mL) of the lipopeptide dissolved in PBS and the CL solutions. The assay was also performed for the samples where biofilms were exposed to CL liquids without the lipopeptide. Positive controls (100%) were wells with pre-grown biofilms where the MHB II was replaced with pure PBS, while negative controls were wells with pure MHB II (also replaced with PBS). After 24 h of incubation (aerobic conditions, 120 rpm shaking, 37 °C), the solutions were replaced with resazurin in MHB II and the results were read and presented as described in Section 4.3.

4.6.2. Activity of the Lipopeptide, Lens Liquids and Their Combinations against Biofilms Formed on CLs after Withdrawal of the Antimicrobial Solution

Biofilms on CLs were grown as described in Section 4.5 and exposed to graded concentrations of the lipopeptide dissolved in CL solutions and PBS. The assay was also performed for the samples where biofilms on CLs were exposed to pure CL solutions. Positive controls (100%) were biofilms on CLs in PBS, while negative controls were CLs previously incubated in pure MHB II replaced for the exposure time with PBS. After 24 h of exposure (aerobic conditions, 120 rpm shaking, 37 °C) all the solutions were removed, replaced with MHB II and the samples were incubated for another 24 h. Resazurin was then added in order to visualize the results. The results were read, calculated, and presented as in the previously-described sections.

4.7. Eye Irritation Calculation Assay

The eye irritation of investigated structures was calculated using Toxtree software 2.6.13 (free and available on the web site http://toxtree.sourceforge.net/) based on the "Estimates eye irritation and corrosion potential by physicochemical property ranges and structural rules" algorithm implemented into a decision tree [63].

Author Contributions: M.A.P. designed the study, performed the experiments, analysed the data and wrote the paper, M.M. wrote the paper and helped with data analysis and preparation of the manuscript for publication, K.E.G. designed the lipopeptide and performed its synthesis and purification, W.S. helped with preparation of the manuscript for publication, W.K. contributed materials and analysis tools and helped with preparation of the manuscript for publication.

Funding: This research was supported by a young researchers' fund from the Medical University of Gdansk (Project No. 01-0373/08/508).

Conflicts of Interest: The authors declare no conflict of interest.

Abbreviations

AMP	Antimicrobial peptide
CL	Contact lens
EC	*Escherichia coli*
EF	*Enterococcus faecalis*
MHB II	Mueller Hinton Broth II
SA	*Staphylococcus aureus*
SE	*Staphylococcus epidermidis*
PA	*Pseudomonas aeruginosa*
PBS	Phosphoric buffer

References

1. Nischal, P.M. First global report on antimicrobial resistance released by the WHO. *Natl. Med. J. India* **2014**, *27*, 241. [PubMed]
2. Peters, B.M.; Jabra-Rizk, M.A.; O'May, G.A.; Costerton, J.W.; Shirtliff, M.E. Polymicrobial interactions: Impact on pathogenesis and human disease. *Clin. Microbiol. Rev.* **2012**, *25*, 193–213. [CrossRef] [PubMed]
3. Stewart, P.S.; Costerton, J.W. Antibiotic resistance of bacteria in biofilms. *Lancet* **2001**, *358*, 135–138. [CrossRef]
4. van Duin, D.; Paterson, D.L. Multidrug-Resistant Bacteria in the Community: Trends and Lessons Learned. *Infect. Dis. Clin. N. Am.* **2016**, *30*, 377–390. [CrossRef] [PubMed]
5. Frieri, M.; Kumar, K.; Boutin, A. Antibiotic resistance. *J. Infect. Public Health* **2017**, *10*, 369–378. [PubMed]
6. Gill, E.E.; Franco, O.L.; Hancock, R.E. Antibiotic adjuvants: Diverse strategies for controlling drug-resistant pathogens. *Chem. Biol. Drug Des.* **2015**, *85*, 56–78. [CrossRef]
7. Adermann, K.; Hoffmann, R.; Otvos, L. IMAP 2012: Antimicrobial peptides to combat (multi)drug-resistant pathogens. *Protein Pept. Lett.* **2014**, *21*, 319–320. [CrossRef]
8. Zhou, L.; Huang, L.Q.; Beuerman, R.W.; Grigg, M.E.; Li, S.F.; Chew, F.T.; Ang, L.; Stern, M.E.; Tan, D. Proteomic analysis of human tears: Defensin expression after ocular surface surgery. *J. Proteome Res.* **2004**, *3*, 410–416. [CrossRef]
9. Kolar, S.S.; McDermott, A.M. Role of host-defence peptides in eye diseases. *Cell. Mol. Life Sci.* **2011**, *68*, 2201–2213. [CrossRef]
10. Hell, E.; Giske, C.G.; Nelson, A.; Romling, U.; Marchini, G. Human cathelicidin peptide LL37 inhibits both attachment capability and biofilm formation of Staphylococcus epidermidis. *Lett. Appl. Microbiol.* **2010**, *50*, 211–215. [CrossRef]

11. Haney, E.F.; Mansour, S.C.; Hancock, R.E. Antimicrobial Peptides: An Introduction. *Methods Mol. Biol.* **2017**, *1548*, 3–22. [PubMed]
12. Ansari, J.M.; Abraham, N.M.; Massaro, J.; Murphy, K.; Smith-Carpenter, J.; Fikrig, E. Anti-Biofilm Activity of a Self-Aggregating Peptide against Streptococcus mutans. *Front. Microbiol.* **2017**, *8*, 488. [CrossRef] [PubMed]
13. Silva, N.C.; Sarmento, B.; Pintado, M. The importance of antimicrobial peptides and their potential for therapeutic use in ophthalmology. *Int. J. Antimicrob. Agents* **2013**, *41*, 5–10. [CrossRef] [PubMed]
14. Gunshefski, L.; Mannis, M.J.; Cullor, J.S.; Schwab, I.R.; Jaynes, J.; Smith, W.L.; Mabry, E.; Murphy, C.J. In vitro antimicrobial activity of Shiva-11 against ocular pathogens. *Cornea* **1994**, *13*, 237–242. [CrossRef] [PubMed]
15. Mannis, M.J. The use of antimicrobial peptides in ophthalmology: An experimental study in corneal preservation and the management of bacterial keratitis. *Trans. Am. Ophthalmol. Soc.* **2002**, *100*, 243–271. [PubMed]
16. Nos-Barbera, S.; Portoles, M.; Morilla, A.; Ubach, J.; Andreu, D.; Paterson, C.A. Effect of hybrid peptides of cecropin A and melittin in an experimental model of bacterial keratitis. *Cornea* **1997**, *16*, 101–106. [CrossRef] [PubMed]
17. Willcox, M.D.; Hume, E.B.; Aliwarga, Y.; Kumar, N.; Cole, N. A novel cationic-peptide coating for the prevention of microbial colonization on contact lenses. *J. Appl. Microbiol.* **2008**, *105*, 1817–1825. [CrossRef] [PubMed]
18. Cole, N.; Hume, E.B.; Vijay, A.K.; Sankaridurg, P.; Kumar, N.; Willcox, M.D. In vivo performance of melimine as an antimicrobial coating for contact lenses in models of CLARE and CLPU. *Investig. Ophthalmol. Vis. Sci.* **2010**, *51*, 390–395. [CrossRef]
19. Sousa, L.B.; Mannis, M.J.; Schwab, I.R.; Cullor, J.; Hosotani, H.; Smith, W.; Jaynes, J. The use of synthetic Cecropin (D5C) in disinfecting contact lens solutions. *CLAO J.* **1996**, *22*, 114–117.
20. Schwab, I.R.; Dries, D.; Cullor, J.; Smith, W.; Mannis, M.; Reid, T.; Murphy, C.J. Corneal storage medium preservation with defensins. *Cornea* **1992**, *11*, 370–375. [CrossRef]
21. Dawgul, M.; Baranska-Rybak, W.; Kamysz, E.; Karafova, A.; Nowicki, R.; Kamysz, W. Activity of short lipopeptides and conventional antimicrobials against planktonic cells and biofilms formed by clinical strains of Staphylococcus aureus. *Future Med. Chem.* **2012**, *4*, 1541–1551. [CrossRef] [PubMed]
22. Bandurska, K.; Berdowska, A.; Barczynska-Felusiak, R.; Krupa, P. Unique features of human cathelicidin LL-37. *Biofactors* **2015**, *41*, 289–300. [CrossRef] [PubMed]
23. Falagas, M.E.; Kasiakou, S.K. Toxicity of polymyxins: A systematic review of the evidence from old and recent studies. *Crit. Care* **2006**, *10*, R27. [CrossRef] [PubMed]
24. Vlieghe, P.; Lisowski, V.; Martinez, J.; Khrestchatisky, M. Synthetic therapeutic peptides: Science and market. *Drug Discov. Today* **2010**, *15*, 40–56. [CrossRef]
25. Fosgerau, K.; Hoffmann, T. Peptide therapeutics: Current status and future directions. *Drug Discov. Today* **2015**, *20*, 122–128. [CrossRef]
26. Giuliani, A.; Rinaldi, A.C. Beyond natural antimicrobial peptides: Multimeric peptides and other peptidomimetic approaches. *Cell. Mol. Life Sci.* **2011**, *68*, 2255–2266. [CrossRef]
27. Straus, S.K.; Hancock, R.E. Mode of action of the new antibiotic for Gram-positive pathogens daptomycin: Comparison with cationic antimicrobial peptides and lipopeptides. *Biochim. Biophys. Acta* **2006**, *1758*, 1215–1223. [CrossRef]
28. Mangoni, M.L.; Shai, Y. Short native antimicrobial peptides and engineered ultrashort lipopeptides: Similarities and differences in cell specificities and modes of action. *Cell. Mol. Life Sci.* **2011**, *68*, 2267–2280. [CrossRef]
29. Laverty, G.; Gorman, S.P.; Gilmore, B.F. The potential of antimicrobial peptides as biocides. *Int. J. Mol. Sci.* **2011**, *12*, 6566–6596. [CrossRef]
30. Jaskiewicz, M.; Neubauer, D.; Kamysz, W. Comparative Study on Antistaphylococcal Activity of Lipopeptides in Various Culture Media. *Antibiotics* **2017**, *6*, 15. [CrossRef]
31. Baranska-Rybak, W.; Pikula, M.; Dawgul, M.; Kamysz, W.; Trzonkowski, P.; Roszkiewicz, J. Safety profile of antimicrobial peptides: Camel, citropin, protegrin, temporin a and lipopeptide on HaCaT keratinocytes. *Acta Pol. Pharm.* **2013**, *70*, 795–801. [PubMed]
32. Catiau, L.; Traisnel, J.; Delval-Dubois, V.; Chihib, N.E.; Guillochon, D.; Nedjar-Arroume, N. Minimal antimicrobial peptidic sequence from hemoglobin alpha-chain: KYR. *Peptides* **2011**, *32*, 633–638. [CrossRef] [PubMed]

33. Vallon-Eberhard, A.; Makovitzki, A.; Beauvais, A.; Latge, J.P.; Jung, S.; Shai, Y. Efficient clearance of Aspergillus fumigatus in murine lungs by an ultrashort antimicrobial lipopeptide, palmitoyl-lys-ala-DAla-lys. *Antimicrob. Agents Chemother.* **2008**, *52*, 3118–3126. [CrossRef] [PubMed]
34. Pikula, M.; Zielinski, M.; Specjalski, K.; Baranska-Rybak, W.; Dawgul, M.; Langa, P.; Jassem, E.; Kamysz, W.; Trzonkowski, P. In Vitro Evaluation of the Allergic Potential of Antibacterial Peptides: Camel and Citropin. *Chem. Biol. Drug Des.* **2016**, *87*, 562–568. [CrossRef] [PubMed]
35. Greber, K.E.; Dawgul, M.; Kamysz, W.; Sawicki, W.; Lukasiak, J. Biological and surface-active properties of double-chain cationic amino acid-based surfactants. *Amino Acids* **2014**, *46*, 1893–1898. [CrossRef] [PubMed]
36. Dawgul, M.A.; Greber, K.E.; Bartoszewska, S.; Baranska-Rybak, W.; Sawicki, W.; Kamysz, W. In Vitro Evaluation of Cytotoxicity and Permeation Study on Lysine- and Arginine-Based Lipopeptides with Proven Antimicrobial Activity. *Molecules* **2017**, *22*, 2173. [CrossRef] [PubMed]
37. Greber, K.E.; Ciura, K.; Belka, M.; Kawczak, P.; Nowakowska, J.; Baczek, T.; Sawicki, W. Characterization of antimicrobial and hemolytic properties of short synthetic cationic lipopeptides based on QSAR/QSTR approach. *Amino Acids* **2018**, *50*, 479–485. [CrossRef]
38. Greber, K.E.; Zielinska, J.; Nierzwicki, L.; Ciura, K.; Kawczak, P.; Nowakowska, J.; Baczek, T.; Sawicki, W. Are the short cationic lipopeptides bacterial membrane disruptors? Structure-Activity Relationship and molecular dynamic evaluation. *Biochim. Biophys. Acta Biomembr.* **2019**, *1861*, 93–99. [CrossRef]
39. Ciura, K.; Belka, M.; Kawczak, P.; Baczek, T.; Markuszewski, M.J.; Nowakowska, J. Combined computational-experimental approach to predict blood-brain barrier (BBB) permeation based on "green" salting-out thin layer chromatography supported by simple molecular descriptors. *J. Pharm. Biomed. Anal.* **2017**, *143*, 214–221. [CrossRef]
40. McDermott, A.M. The role of antimicrobial peptides at the ocular surface. *Ophthalmic Res.* **2009**, *41*, 60–75. [CrossRef]
41. Szczotka-Flynn, L.B.; Bajaksouzian, S.; Jacobs, M.R.; Rimm, A. Risk factors for contact lens bacterial contamination during continuous wear. *Optom. Vis. Sci.* **2009**, *86*, 1216–1226. [CrossRef] [PubMed]
42. Szczotka-Flynn, L.; Lass, J.H.; Sethi, A.; Debanne, S.; Benetz, B.A.; Albright, M.; Gillespie, B.; Kuo, J.; Jacobs, M.R.; Rimm, A. Risk factors for corneal infiltrative events during continuous wear of silicone hydrogel contact lenses. *Investig. Ophthalmol. Vis. Sci.* **2010**, *51*, 5421–5430. [CrossRef] [PubMed]
43. Szczotka-Flynn, L.; Debanne, S.M.; Cheruvu, V.K.; Long, B.; Dillehay, S.; Barr, J.; Bergenske, P.; Donshik, P.; Secor, G.; Yoakum, J. Predictive factors for corneal infiltrates with continuous wear of silicone hydrogel contact lenses. *Arch. Ophthalmol.* **2007**, *125*, 488–492. [CrossRef] [PubMed]
44. Dutta, D.; Ozkan, J.; Willcox, M.D. Biocompatibility of antimicrobial melimine lenses: Rabbit and human studies. *Optom. Vis. Sci.* **2014**, *91*, 570–581. [CrossRef]
45. Dutta, D.; Kamphuis, B.; Ozcelik, B.; Thissen, H.; Pinarbasi, R.; Kumar, N.; Willcox, M.D.P. Development of Silicone Hydrogel Antimicrobial Contact Lenses with Mel4 Peptide Coating. *Optom. Vis. Sci.* **2018**, *95*, 937–946. [CrossRef] [PubMed]
46. Mannis, M.J.; Cullor, J. The use of synthetic cecropin (Shiva-11) in preservative-free timolol and contact lens solutions. *Invest. Ophthalmol. Vis. Sci.* **1993**, *34*, 859.
47. Maciejewska, M.; Bauer, M.; Neubauer, D.; Kamysz, W.; Dawgul, M. Influence of Amphibian Antimicrobial Peptides and Short Lipopeptides on Bacterial Biofilms Formed on Contact Lenses. *Materials* **2016**, *9*, 873. [CrossRef]
48. Keren, I.; Kaldalu, N.; Spoering, A.; Wang, Y.; Lewis, K. Persister cells and tolerance to antimicrobials. *FEMS Microbiol. Lett.* **2004**, *230*, 13–18. [CrossRef]
49. Kostakioti, M.; Hadjifrangiskou, M.; Hultgren, S.J. Bacterial biofilms: Development, dispersal, and therapeutic strategies in the dawn of the postantibiotic era. *Cold Spring Harb. Perspect. Med.* **2013**, *3*, a010306. [CrossRef]
50. Jorge, P.; Grzywacz, D.; Kamysz, W.; Lourenco, A.; Pereira, M.O. Searching for new strategies against biofilm infections: Colistin-AMP combinations against Pseudomonas aeruginosa and Staphylococcus aureus single- and double-species biofilms. *PLoS ONE* **2017**, *12*, e0174654. [CrossRef]
51. Bormann, N.; Koliszak, A.; Kasper, S.; Schoen, L.; Hilpert, K.; Volkmer, R.; Kikhney, J.; Wildemann, B. A short artificial antimicrobial peptide shows potential to prevent or treat bone infections. *Sci. Rep.* **2017**, *7*, 1506. [CrossRef] [PubMed]

52. Dawgul, M.; Maciejewska, M.; Jaskiewicz, M.; Karafova, A.; Kamysz, W. Antimicrobial peptides as potential tool to fight bacterial biofilm. *Acta. Pol. Pharm.* **2014**, *71*, 39–47. [PubMed]
53. Cruz, C.D.; Shah, S.; Tammela, P. Defining conditions for biofilm inhibition and eradication assays for Gram-positive clinical reference strains. *BMC Microbiol.* **2018**, *18*, 173. [CrossRef] [PubMed]
54. Shapiro, J.A.; Nguyen, V.L.; Chamberlain, N.R. Evidence for persisters in Staphylococcus epidermidis RP62a planktonic cultures and biofilms. *J. Med. Microbiol.* **2011**, *60*, 950–960. [CrossRef] [PubMed]
55. Potera, C. ANTIBIOTIC RESISTANCE: Biofilm Dispersing Agent Rejuvenates Older Antibiotics. *Environ. Health Perspect.* **2010**, *118*, A288. [CrossRef]
56. Fisher, R.A.; Gollan, B.; Helaine, S. Persistent bacterial infections and persister cells. *Nat. Rev. Microbiol.* **2017**, *15*, 453–464. [CrossRef] [PubMed]
57. Schmidt, N.W.; Deshayes, S.; Hawker, S.; Blacker, A.; Kasko, A.M.; Wong, G.C. Engineering persister-specific antibiotics with synergistic antimicrobial functions. *ACS Nano* **2014**, *8*, 8786–8793. [CrossRef]
58. Kamysz, W.; Silvestri, C.; Cirioni, O.; Giacometti, A.; Licci, A.; Della Vittoria, A.; Okroj, M.; Scalise, G. In vitro activities of the lipopeptides palmitoyl (Pal)-Lys-Lys-NH(2) and Pal-Lys-Lys alone and in combination with antimicrobial agents against multiresistant gram-positive cocci. *Antimicrob. Agents Chemother.* **2007**, *51*, 354–358. [CrossRef]
59. Serrano, G.N.; Zhanel, G.G.; Schweizer, F. Antibacterial activity of ultrashort cationic lipo-beta-peptides. *Antimicrob. Agents Chemother.* **2009**, *53*, 2215–2217. [CrossRef]
60. Laverty, G.; McLaughlin, M.; Shaw, C.; Gorman, S.P.; Gilmore, B.F. Antimicrobial activity of short, synthetic cationic lipopeptides. *Chem. Biol. Drug Des.* **2010**, *75*, 563–569. [CrossRef]
61. Shai, Y.; Makovitzky, A.; Avrahami, D. Host defense peptides and lipopeptides: Modes of action and potential candidates for the treatment of bacterial and fungal infections. *Curr. Protein Pept. Sci.* **2006**, *7*, 479–486. [CrossRef] [PubMed]
62. Greber, K.E.; Dawgul, M.; Kamysz, W.; Sawicki, W. Cationic Net Charge and Counter Ion Type as Antimicrobial Activity Determinant Factors of Short Lipopeptides. *Front. Microbiol.* **2017**, *8*, 123. [CrossRef] [PubMed]
63. Gerner, I.; Liebsch, M.; Spielmann, H. Assessment of the eye irritating properties of chemicals by applying alternatives to the Draize rabbit eye test: The use of QSARs and in vitro tests for the classification of eye irritation. *Altern. Lab. Anim.* **2005**, *33*, 215–237. [PubMed]

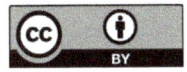

© 2019 by the authors. Licensee MDPI, Basel, Switzerland. This article is an open access article distributed under the terms and conditions of the Creative Commons Attribution (CC BY) license (http://creativecommons.org/licenses/by/4.0/).

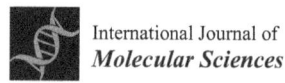

Article

Functionalized Polymeric Materials with Bio-Derived Antimicrobial Peptides for "Active" Packaging

Bruna Agrillo [1], Marco Balestrieri [2], Marta Gogliettino [2], Gianna Palmieri [2,*], Rosalba Moretta [3], Yolande T.R. Proroga [4], Ilaria Rea [3], Alessandra Cornacchia [5], Federico Capuano [4], Giorgio Smaldone [6] and Luca De Stefano [3]

1. Materias S.r.l., Corso N. Protopisani, 80146 Napoli, Italy; bruna.agrillo@ibbr.cnr.it
2. Institute of Biosciences and BioResources, National Research Council (CNR-IBBR), 80131 Napoli, Italy; marco.balestrieri@ibbr.cnr.it (M.B.); marta.gogliettino@ibbr.cnr.it (M.G.)
3. Institute for Microelectronics and Microsystems, National Research Council (CNR-IMM), 80131 Napoli, Italy; rosalba.moretta@na.imm.cnr.it (R.M.); ilaria.rea@na.imm.cnr.it (I.R.); luca.destefano@na.imm.cnr.it (L.D.S.)
4. Department of Food Microbiology, Istituto Zooprofilattico Sperimentale del Mezzogiorno, 80055 Portici, Italy; proroga.yolande@izsmportici.it (Y.T.R.P.); federico.capuano@cert.izsmportici.it (F.C.)
5. National Reference Laboratory for Listeria monocytogenes, Istituto Zooprofilattico Sperimentale dell'Abruzzo e del Molise, 64100 Teramo, Italy; a.cornacchia@izs.it
6. Department of Agricultural Science, University of Naples "Federico II", 80055 Portici, Italy; giorgio.smaldone@unina.it
* Correspondence: gianna.palmieri@ibbr.cnr.it; Tel.: +39-081-613-2711

Received: 20 December 2018; Accepted: 28 January 2019; Published: 30 January 2019

Abstract: Food packaging is not only a simple protective barrier, but a real "active" component, which is expected to preserve food quality, safety and shelf-life. Therefore, the materials used for packaging production should show peculiar features and properties. Specifically, antimicrobial packaging has recently gained great attention with respect to both social and economic impacts. In this paper, the results obtained by using a polymer material functionalized by a small synthetic peptide as "active" packaging are reported. The surface of Polyethylene Terephthalate (PET), one of the most commonly used plastic materials in food packaging, was plasma-activated and covalently bio-conjugated to a bactenecin-derivative peptide named 1018K6, previously characterized in terms of antimicrobial and antibiofilm activities. The immobilization of the peptide occurred at a high yield and no release was observed under different environmental conditions. Moreover, preliminary data clearly demonstrated that the "active" packaging was able to significantly reduce the total bacterial count together with yeast and mold spoilage in food-dairy products. Finally, the functionalized-PET polymer showed stronger efficiency in inhibiting biofilm growth, using a *Listeria monocytogenes* strain isolated from food products. The use of these "active" materials would greatly decrease the risk of pathogen development and increase the shelf-life in the food industry, showing a real potential against a panel of microorganisms upon exposure to fresh and stored products, high chemical stability and re-use possibility.

Keywords: active packaging; antimicrobial peptides; food shelf-life; foodborne pathogens; plastic materials

1. Introduction

Today, food preservation, quality maintenance and safety are considered the major growing concerns in the food industry. Food products can undergo different processes of contamination, which lead to loss of colour, texture and nutritive values, allowing the growth of pathogenic microorganisms and deterioration of the quality of the products, making them non-edible. Food contamination can occur with its exposure to the environment during slaughtering, food processing, packaging, transportation or distribution. In addition, one of the main problems in the food industry is represented by the presence of biofilms, which are considered a serious public health risk. A biofilm is a functional consortium of microorganisms formed principally by exopolysaccharides that can exist on all types of surfaces in food plants ranging from plastic, glass, metal, wood, to food products. For these reasons, biofilms enhance the persistence of several foodborne pathogens on product contact surfaces due to their special structure, and so they are more resistant to antimicrobial agents. Current conventional methods for maintaining food quality and safety over time during drying, freezing, heating or salting have not found to satisfy consumers as recontamination may often occur, rendering the food unpalatable.

Another relevant issue concerning the food industry is the need to feed an ever-increasing global population, which makes it obligatory to reduce the millions of tons of avoidable perishable waste along the food supply chain. In this context, a considerable share of these losses is caused by non-optimal chain processes and management. Shelf-life is defined as the time span under defined storage conditions within which foods remain acceptable for human consumption in terms of safety, nutritional attributes and sensory properties [1]. Unappealing foods and the uncertain safety of food items have been reported as the main causes for discarding food products among consumers and retailers. Indeed, about 15% of perishable foods are actually wasted at retail stores due to damage and spoilage [2]. Consequently, prolonging the shelf-life of food products, ensuring their quality, safety, and integrity, is a crucial aspect to minimize food waste.

All these concerns demand a need for more effective food quality systems for food protection, preservation, and transport to consumers in a wholesome form. Therefore, today, the food industry is more interested in exploring innovative and alternative solutions to presently used methods. In this context, antimicrobial packaging represents a novel strategy to suppress the activities of targeted microorganisms that can contaminate the food products and then strongly affect their shelf-life. One strategy to achieve this goal is to use active materials projected *"ad hoc"* to kill harmful microorganisms or to inhibit their growth on their surface or in the surrounding environments. In this respect, antimicrobial polymers present several advantages because of their high tunability in terms of physico-chemical properties, efficacy, resistance, and prolonged lifetime. However, in spite of the large developments in the preparation and structure-property relationship of this class of antimicrobial polymers, very few of them are practically suitable to solve food-related problems [3]. In this context, plastics are the most commonly used materials for packaging applications because of low-cost, ease of processing and the availability of abundant resources for their production. Indeed, during the last few years, several studies have been focused on the incorporation of antimicrobial peptides (AMPs) into polymeric materials through covalent or physical binding [4,5]. AMPs are essential components of innate immunity [6], contributing to the first line of defence against infections [7,8] and are actually the most promising antimicrobial compounds, mainly because of their broad spectrum of action, high selectivity toward bacterial cells and low risk to promote resistance. The AMP family comprises peptides, which are usually short and amphipathic molecules with a high number of basic residues and a strong tendency to assume prevalently α-helix conformations, which are important to explicate their antimicrobial functions including also antibiofilm activity [9–12]. Amphiphilic AMPs with net positive charge have the capacity to tune their secondary structure upon interacting with the lipid tails inside the membrane, enhancing the membrane rupture activity of these peptides [13]. One of the most studied AMPs, is the innate defence regulator peptide-1018 (IDR-1018), a 12-mer cationic compound (VRLIVAVRIWRR-NH2), derived from the bovine host-defense peptide (HDP) bactenecin, found in the bovine neutrophil granules and belonging to the cathelicidin family [10–12,14,15]. Recently, a new 1018-derivative antimicrobial peptide, named 1018K6, in which the alanine is replaced with a lysine residue (VRLIV**K**VRIWRR-NH2), was designed and characterized [16,17]. This single point mutation was revealed to have a strong impact on the conformational status of 1018K6, inducing an increased propensity to assume an α-helix structure in the membrane-mimetic models such as micellar solutions of SDS [16,17]. Furthermore, 1018K6 was revealed to be able to retain its structural integrity better than the cognate IDR-1018 under a wide range of pH and temperature conditions for prolonged incubation times. In addition, 1018K6 exhibited a significant bactericidal/antibiofilm activity specifically against L. *monocytogenes* isolates from food-products and food-processing environments [16,17].

Actually, wet and dry procedures can be used to link peptides to polymer surfaces [18,19], although it is not trivial to functionalize them with AMPs as they can completely lose their antimicrobial activity, once bound on the surface. Cold plasma is considered an emerging novel technology industrially used for activation of polymer surfaces, which exhibit reactive -COOH* and -OH* groups that rapidly interact with the free $-NH_2$ and -COOH in the peptide sequence. The resulting functionalized surfaces are very stable and can be used in solution under a wide range of pHs and salt conditions [20].

The aim of this study was to develop a new class of packaging materials, functionalized with the bactericidal peptide 1018K6 by cold plasma technology, able to inhibit the biofilm formation of L. *monocytogenes* and to significantly reduce the Aerobic Plate Count (APC) and yeast and mold spoilage of food dairy products.

2. Results and Discussion

2.1. Activation of PET Polymer by 1018K6

Currently, the packaging sector accounts for over 40% of the total worldwide plastic consumption [21,22]. The essential properties for packaging materials are determined by the physical and chemical characteristics of the products, as well as by the external conditions under which the product is stored/transported [21]. As plastics have a wide range of properties which can be tailored according to the specific requirements, they are the most attractive materials for packaging applications.

In this work, polyethylene terephthalate (PET), one of the most common packaging materials accounting for more than 90% of the total volume of plastics used, was functionalized with the already characterized AMP, 1018K6. As the PET surfaces appeared to be hydrophobic, i.e., water contact angle greater than 90°, it was impossible to perform the functionalization by incubating them with the antibacterial peptide 1018K6 in aqueous solutions. Therefore, a possible approach was to pre-activate the PET surfaces by using the radio frequency cold plasma technique and oxygen as gas, which induces the formation of reactive -COOH* and -OH* groups [23], allowing the covalent binding with the peptide, as sketched in Figure 1.

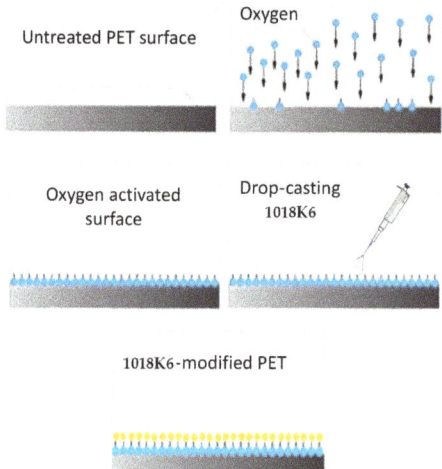

Figure 1. Process diagram for the modification of the PET surface by activation with radiofrequency cold plasma using oxygen as gas and coupling of the synthetic peptide 1018K6 with antibacterial properties.

In this experimental procedure, PET disks were taken directly from the container, used for the preservation of fresh dairy products, specifically buffalo mozzarella cheese, and provided by the customer. To assess quantitatively the PET surface wettability induced by oxygen plasma activation and peptide functionalization, WCA (water contact angle) measurements were carried out on PET samples acquiring the images after 30 sec, before and after treatments (Figure 2).

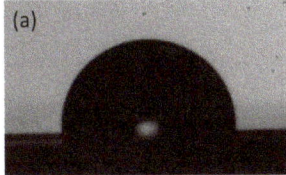  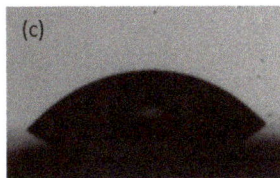

Figure 2. WCA measured on pristine PET (**a**), oxygen plasma activated-PET (**b**) and 1018K6-functionalized PET (**c**). The measurements were performed on five samples in duplicate.

Firstly, the WCA value of the pristine PET disks was equal to $98 \pm 3°$ (Figure 2a). Upon oxygen plasma treatment, the WCA profiles of PET membranes shifted to lower values, indicating that a higher degree of surface hydrophilicity was achieved. Specifically, the change in the surface wettability was quantified, carrying out the measurements at different exposure times (T) and RF powers and varying the concentration and the partial pressure (P) of the oxygen (O_2). The obtained results demonstrated that, already at 50 W and 10 sec of exposure time, the PET surface became less hydrophobic and more hydrophilic (WCA = $56 \pm 5°$), as shown in Figure 2b. However, no variations were observed in WCA values by changing the oxygen pressure and concentration parameters. On the contrary, it should be noted that when high values of RF power (RF = 300 W) and long exposure times (T = 100–300 sec) were applied, a macroscopic change in the roughness of the PET surface was detectable, indicative of the beginning of a material degradation process. This behaviour suggested that the cold radio frequency plasma treatment was not suitable for PET materials under the aforementioned operating conditions. Generally, the surface of the pristine PET was hydrophobic due to the presence of aliphatic carbonaceous chains. Hence, the plasma treatment induced the formation of extremely reactive radical groups that interrupted the carbon chains and reduced the inborn hydrophobicity of the material, making it more hydrophilic and able to interact strongly with water molecules [24]. Immediately after plasma exposure, the pre-treated PET samples were incubated for a minimum of 8 h in an aqueous solution of 1018K6 peptide, using samples not subjected to radio frequency cold plasma treatment as controls. The PET exposure to the peptide solution favoured the coupling between the peptide chemical groups (typically -COOH and –NH_2) and the generated reactive groups (-COOH*, -OH*) on PET, which were not passivated by the atmospheric water. The coupling of the peptide on the polymeric surface resulted in a further modification of the wettability as revealed by the WCA value (WCA = $36 \pm 2°$), due to the hydrophilic nature of the chemical groups of the amino acid residues along the peptide sequence (Figure 2c). On the other hand, PET control samples not pre-treated by radio frequency cold plasma and incubated for 24 h in aqueous solution containing 1018K6, clearly showed a negligible non-specific adsorption of the peptide on the PET surface.

In order to confirm the 1018K6-PET linkage, the Fourier Transform InfraRed spectroscopy (FTIR) was carried out under inert (N2) atmosphere. The FTIR spectra of the control samples before radio frequency cold plasma treatment displayed different main peaks corresponding to the C-C, C-H, C-O groups of the polymer and to the –OH groups of the water adsorbed on the polymer surface after the incubations (Figure 3a).

After the plasma treatment, a relevant increase of the –OH group peaks in the FTIR spectra was observed (Figure 3b), consistent with the improvement of the surface wettability quantified by WCA measurements [25,26]. Next, the functionalization of the activated PET samples with 1018K6 was responsible for the appearance, in the FTIR spectra, of the characteristic absorption signals of a peptide, including the Amide I and Amide II bands (Figure 3c). These bands arise from the peptide bonds that link the amino acids (O=C-NH) in the 1018K6 sequence. Specifically, the absorption associated with the Amide I band, which was observed in the 1650–1560 cm^{-1} interval, produced the stretching vibrations of the C=O bond of the amide, whilst the absorption associated with the Amide II band showed in the 1580–1490 cm^{-1} interval, led primarily to bending vibrations of the N—H bond (Figure 3c). Therefore, the FTIR analyses validated the successful bio-conjugation of 1018K6 peptide on the plasma-activated PET surface, in complete agreement with WCA characterization.

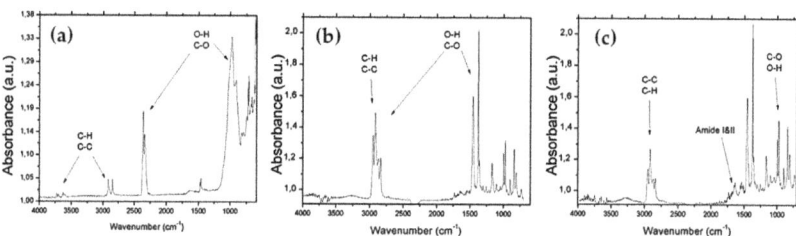

Figure 3. FTIR spectrum of the PET sample before radiofrequency cold plasma treatment (**a**); after plasma treatment (**b**); after 1018K6 bio-conjugation (**c**).

2.2. Immobilization Yield and Leakage of 1018K6 from PET Polymer

One of the most important factors in fabricating antimicrobial packaging is to immobilize on a polymeric surface the functional compounds without losing their activity. Therefore, to keep them active, it is necessary to immobilize the peptides in a way that preserves their folded structural integrity. Firstly, to obtain stable and active packaging, it is crucial to regulate the peptide surface concentration which depends on the binding strategy used, as it can strongly affect the efficiency of peptide immobilization. Therefore, the immobilization yield of different 1018K6 concentrations on the PET surface after the coupling reaction was indirectly estimated by Reverse-Phase High-Performance Liquid Chromatography (RP-HPLC). In this experiment, once the conjugation reaction was completed, the supernatant solutions were recovered after 24 h incubation and analysed by RP-HPLC, evaluating the peak area of the peptide not bound to the polimeric surface. Consequently, by knowing the initial peptide concentration, the quantity of the peptide attached to the PET surface was indirectly determined by comparing the peak area. The data obtained from these analyses showed that the coupling reaction yield varied from 50% using a starting peptide concentration of 25 µM, to 25% per 100 µM. The representative chromatograms obtained for 1018K6 50 µM initial concentration, and used to calculate the immobilization yield, are reported in Figure 4. The coupling yields were validated by a six-point calibration curve, which was constructed utilizing known 1018K6 concentrations, and the number of peptide molecules capable of binding to the polymeric surface was determined via interpolation (Figure 4 insert). Based on the yield data, the surface coverage on the polymer was found to be approximately 6.4 nmol/cm^2 per 25 µM peptide concentration, 9.3 nmol/cm^2 per 50 µM and 8.3 nmol/cm^2 per 100 µM, thus demonstrating that the surface coverage was clearly concentration-dependent (Figure 5).

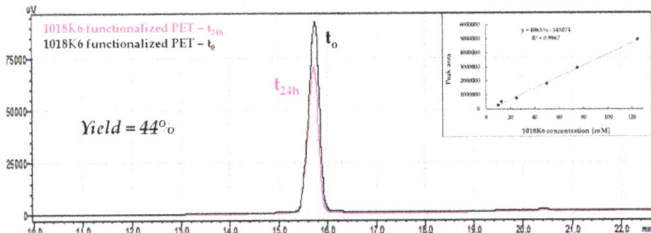

Figure 4. Immobilization yield (%) of 1018K6 on PET surface determined by reverse-phase HPLC chromatography on a C18 column after the coulping reaction (24 h). Pre-activated PET surfaces by plasma were incubated for 24 h with 1018K6 (50 µM) in PBS pH 7.0. The solutions recovered after incubation were further analysed. The peptide solution placed in contact with the pre-activated surface at time 0 ($t = 0$) was used as control. The chromatograms are representative of three independent experiments. **Insert**: Calibration curve of the C18 column obtained using different 1018K6 concentrations.

The Holliday model was used to assess the peptide concentration effects on the coverage density and to estimate the concentration value producing the best immobilization yield [27]. As shown in the dose-response experiments (Figure 5), the most suitable coupling condition to improve the immobilization yield was obtained with a peptide concentration of 71 µM, but 50 µM was selected to perform the further experiments as this value represents a better compromise between the functionalization yield and the peptide costs.

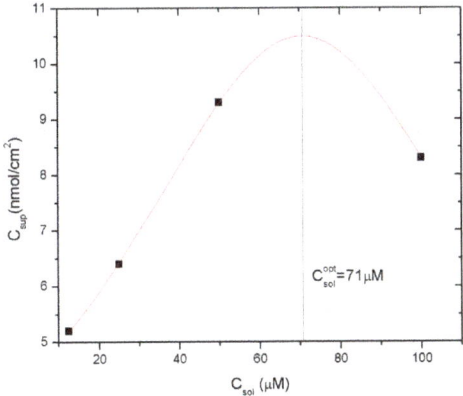

Figure 5. Immobilization yield expressed as nmol of bound 1018K6 per cm² of PET surface as function of peptide concentration. The dose-response curve has been built by using the Holliday model. Data are expressed as means ± standard deviations. Standard deviation values lower than 5% are not shown.

The production process of antimicrobial active packaging, which is able to guarantee the quality, the safety and prolong the shelf-life of food products, requires an efficient immobilization procedure that permits a stable conjugation of AMP on the polymers, avoiding the release of the immobilized active compound after contact with foods or liquids. Fresh dairy products, such as mozzarella cheese, an Italian traditional cheese packaged in saline brine, are ready-to-eat foods having a very short shelf-life of about 3 or 4 days, because they are easily contaminated by undesirable microorganisms.

In this context, the release of 1018K6 from the functionalized PET into mozzarella cheese brine during 24 h of incubation at 4 °C was analysed by RP-HPLC, using the free 1018K6 as control. As shown in Figure 6a, no peptide-release process occurred from the functionalized polymeric support. The same results were obtained after 24 h incubation in pure water at 4 °C (Figure 6b) and at 25 °C suggesting that the peptide was stably coupled on the polymer. In addition, no leakage of 1018K6 was detectable even after prolonged incubations (until to 72 h) under all the conditions explored. The high stability of the peptide-PET bond is important because in this way the peptide-PET system does not require the related EFSA (European Food Safety Authority) standards.

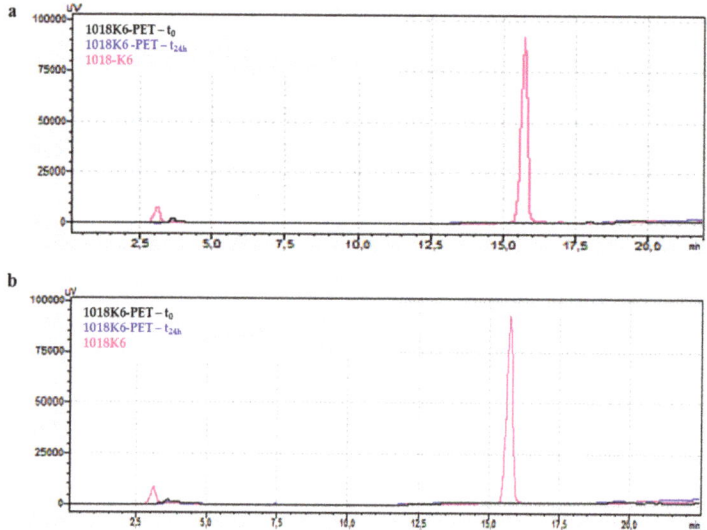

Figure 6. Release analysis of 1018K6 from functionalized PET performed by reverse-phase HPLC chromatography on a C18 column after 24 h incubation at 4 °C in mozzarella brine (**a**) or pure water (**b**). After incubation, the solutions were recovered and injected on C18. The solution in contact with 1018K6-PET at time 0 (t = 0) and 1018K6 peptide (50 µM) were used as controls.

However, as far as the cytotoxicity of the free 1018K6, preliminary tests clearly indicated that the peptide is not toxic against different fibroblast cell lines at the concentrations used in the bactericidal assays [16], thus suggesting that there is no potential risk for human health associated with the use of 1018K6 in the food industry.

2.3. Effect of 1018K6 Functionalized PETs on Mozzarella Cheese

Microbial contamination, causing approximately one-fourth of the world's food supply loss, has become an enormous economic and ethical problem worldwide [28]. Specifically, fresh dairy products stored in packaging, such as mozzarella cheese, are characterized by reduced shelf-life, which diminishes their commercial value because they are an excellent growth medium for a wide range of troublesome spoilage microorganisms including aerobic mesophiles, yeasts and molds [29].

Hence, it is very important and advantageous for the food industry to extend the shelf-life of mozzarella cheese, which is a good source of protein, vitamins and minerals, and to spread the distribution of this traditional product beyond the market borders.

In this context, the efficacy of 1018K6 functionalized PETs in preventing the growth of spoilage microorganisms in mozzarella was analysed at a preliminary shorter storage time. In a first set of experiments, with the aim to set up the optimal experimental conditions minimizing peptide consumption, PET disks of 3 cm diameter (surface of 7 cm^2) were functionalized with 1018K6 and incubated with 3 ml of the conditioning brine in the presence of small slices of mozzarella (about 10 g of weight) in Petri dishes. Sliced mozzarella in the presence of brine with non-modified PETs disks was used as controls. As shown in Table 1, the Aerobic Plate Count (APC), and the yeast and mold counts of the samples exposed to 1018K6-PETs significantly decreased during the storage period (24 h) compared to the control samples. In a second set of experiments, a scale up of the previous procedure was applied in order to evaluate the effectiveness of 1018K6-PETs in slowing down the growth of the spoilage microorganisms under the storage conditions. Specifically, the effects of 1018K6-PET disks (10 cm diameter, 78 cm^2) were studied directly in the package as distributed on the market, which contained two balls of fresh mozzarella (about 25 g each) and 30 mL brine. Control samples were prepared in an identical way, using non-modified PET disks. Results demonstrated that, in one day of storage, mozzarella packaged in the presence of 1018K6-PETs had the lowest bacterial counts with respect to that incubated in conditioning brine with non-modified PETs, in which microbes were able to proliferate (Table 1). In addition, a significant reduction in yeasts and molds count was also observed in the samples with the modified PETs during the storage. Therefore, the projected 1018K6 active packaging could have potential applications in the food market, aiming to ensure and increase the quality and safety of the food products by preventing the growth of spoilage and/or pathogenic microorganisms and promoting a shelf-life extension.

Table 1. Effects of 1018K6-PETs treatment on mozzarella cheese.

Disk Diameter	Microorganisms	PET Disk in Brine + Mozzarella Cheese	1018K6-PET Disk in Brine + Mozzarella Cheese	Inhibition of Growth (% Value)
3 cm	APC	311 ± 29 CFU/mL	11 ± 2 CFU/mL	97%
	Yeasts and Molds	700 ± 75 CFU/mL	280 ± 25 CFU/mL	60%
10 cm	APC	173 ± 21 CFU/mL	44 ± 7 CFU/mL	75%
	Yeasts and Molds	406 ± 37 CFU/mL	137 ± 23 CFU/mL	67%

Further studies will be necessary in order to assess the ability of 1018K6-PETs to affect the APC and the total yeast and mold at prolonged storage times.

2.4. Inhibition of Listeria Biofilm Formation

Cross-contamination of pathogenic and spoilage microorganisms from food contact surfaces remains a significant challenge in the safety, quality and security of food supply chain. Indeed, some pathogenic and food spoilage bacteria can form biofilms, which represent one of the main sources of food contamination and foodborne disease outbreaks. To address this challenge, there is an unmet need to develop novel antimicrobial materials able to inhibit and treat biofilms in the food processing industry. Specifically, the use of natural preservatives to inhibit growth of serious pathogens such as *L. monocytogenes* is of great interest as it is considered an important worldwide public health problem [30]. *L. monocytogenes* is one of the most dangerous human food pathogens that causes listeriosis. Foods considered as high-risk sources of listeriosis include meat and dairy products, which are ready-to-eat, require refrigeration and are stored for extended time periods. Listeria can persist within food processing environments, due to its ability to grow at wide-ranging temperatures and pH and to form biofilms [31,32].

In this context, the ability of 1018K6-PETs to prevent biofilm formation was assessed against an *L. monocytogenes* strain isolated from dairy products, by the crystal violet staining method [17]. As shown in Figure 7, the biofilm formation on 1018K6-PETs was significantly reduced (75%), compared to the control sample (non-functionalized PETs), indicating a strong anti-adhesion capability of the 1018K6-tethered surfaces against *L. monocytogenes*.

Therefore, packaging films containing 1018K6 peptide can pose a potential solution to reduce spoilage.

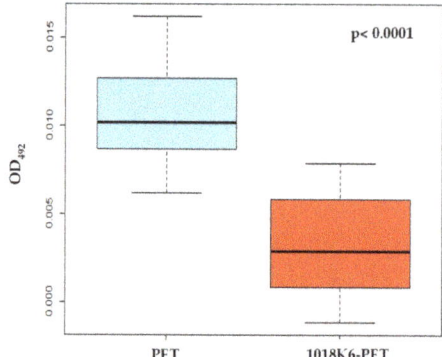

Figure 7. Boxplot of the inhibition activity of the biofilm production of *Listeria monocytogenes* by PET and 1018K6-PET. Average OD measurements of crystal violet-stained biofilms are shown with error bars representing the standard deviation.

3. Materials and Methods

3.1. Plasma Treatment

Plasma treatment was performed using a Reactive Ion Etching (RIE) model PLASMA Plus 80 machine (Oxford Instruments, Abingdon, Oxfordshire, UK). The following process parameters were changed: exposure time [T] (10-20-30-50-100-300 sec); molecular oxygen concentration [O2] (10-50-100 sccm); partial gas pressure [P] (0.1–0.5 atm); power of radio frequency generator [RF] (50-100-300 W).

3.2. Water Contact Angle Measurements

The sessile drop technique was used for water contact angle (WCA) measurements on a First Ten Angstroms FTA 1000 C Class coupled with drop shape analysis software under static conditions. A 10-µL drop was deposited on the sample surface, and the image was recorded after 30 sec. Results of WCA are expressed as mean ± standard deviation (s.d.) of at least three measurements on the same sample in three independent experiments (i.e., at least nine measurements for each result).

3.3. Fourier Transform Infrared Spectroscopy

The Fourier transform infrared spectra of all samples were obtained using a Nicolet Continuum XL (Thermo Scientific, Waltham, MA, USA) microscope in the wavenumber region of 4000−650 cm^{-1} with a resolution of 4 cm^{-1}. The FITR measurements were performed using a micro-ATR (Attenuated Total Reflection) module under inert (N_2) atmosphere.

3.4. Peptide Bio-conjugation

Polymer samples treated by cold plasma were incubated in aqueous solution of 1018K6 (50 µM) in PBS (10 mM), pH 7.0, for 24 h at 25 °C. After incubation, the solutions containing the peptide not bound to the polymer were removed and the functionalized PETs were extensively washed in water and DMSO in order to completely eliminate traces of unbound peptide before performing surface characterization by WCA, FTIR and the release experiments. The PET containers used in all the analyses were kindly provided by the dairy "Mini Caseificio Costanzo s.r.l." located in Lusciano (Caserta, Italy).

3.5. Functionalization Yield Analysis of Polymers

Functionalization yield analysis of 1018K6-modified PETs was performed by using a reverse-phase high-performance liquid chromatography (RP-HPLC) system (Waldbronn, Germany). Once functionalization was completed, the supernatant solutions were recovered after 24 h and analyzed to calculate the amount of the peptide not attached to the polymeric surfaces. For the analyses, 200 µL of the samples were injected over a µBondapak C18 reverse-phase column (3.9 mm × 300 mm, Waters Corp., Milford, MA, USA) connected to a HPLC system (Shimadzu, Milan, Italy) using a linear gradient of 0.1% TFA in acetonitrile from 5 to 95%. A reference solution was prepared with the initial peptide concentration used for the functionalization under the same reaction conditions and run in parallel. Therefore, by knowing the added peptide (reference solution), the amount of peptide not bound to the polymers (expressed as a percentage) was determined by comparing the peak area. A calibration curve of the C18 column using different 1018K6 concentrations was built. All measurements were performed in triplicate in three different preparations.

3.6. Release Test

The release of 1018K6 from the functionalized polymers was examined by the reverse-phase high-performance liquid chromatography (RP-HPLC) system using a µBondapak C18 column (3.9 × 300 mm, Waters) and a linear gradient of 5–95% acetonitrile in 0.1% TFA, at a flow rate of 1 mL/min. A volume of 1 mL of pure water or mozzarella cheese brine was poured onto the functionalized polymers, incubated for 24 h at 4 °C and then loaded onto the RP column. The solutions in contact with the functionalized polymers at time t = 0 were used as control samples and were run in parallel. The same experiments were conducted in the presence of the non-functionalized polymers. All measurements were performed in triplicate on three different preparations.

3.7. Shelf-life Testing on Mozzarella Cheese

The 1018K6-functionalized PETs were cut into disks of 3 cm diameter (surface of 7 cm^2) and immersed in 3 mL mozzarella cheese brine in 5-cm Petri dishes that contained small slices of mozzarella (about 10 g of weight), which were directly placed on the activated PET disks. Non-functionalized PETs were used as a control. The samples were incubated for 24 h at 25 °C. Therefore, the mozzarella cheese brine was plated on PCA plates to quantify the APC (Aerobic Plate Count), which was performed according to ISO 4833-1 procedure. Specifically, 1 mL of cheese brine was diluted in 9 mL diluent (0.1% peptone and 0.8% sodium chloride, biomerieux- France), and scalar dilutions of sample up to 10^{-5} were set up. Then, 1 mL of brine and 1 mL of each subsequent dilution were seeded by inclusion in PCA plates (Plate Count Agar-Biolife-Italy) which were incubated at 30 ± 1 °C for 72 h. Plates with no more than 300 colonies were considered for the colony count. The presence of yeasts and molds was tested, according to ISO 21527-1, analyzing 1 mL of cheese brine, diluted in 9 mL diluent (0.1% peptone and 0.8% sodium chloride, biomerieux- France) and performing scalar dilutions up to 10^{-5}. Then, 0.1 mL of each dilution was seeded on Dichloran Rose Bengal Chloramphenicol Agar plates (DRBC - Italian Biolife), which were incubated at 25 ± 1 °C for 5 days for the colony count. Plates with no more than 150 colonies were considered. The same analyses were performed using 1018K6-PET disks of 10 cm diameter (78 cm^2), immersed in the package containing two balls of fresh mozzarella (about 25 g each) and 30 mL brine. The samples were incubated for 24 h at 25 °C. The analyses were performed in triplicate on three different preparations, and the data were expressed as means ± s.d.

3.8. Anti-adhesion Activity Assay

L. monocytogenes cultures, isolated from dairy products, were prepared to inoculate BHI broth (Brain Heart Infusion, Sigma-Aldrich, St. Louis, Missouri, USA) at 37 °C up to a logarithmic phase of growth. After the incubation, 10 ml of bacterial suspension at a concentration of 5×10^6 in growth broths was centrifuged, and the cell pellet was washed in PBS pH 7.3 (Thermo Fisher Scientific Inc.,

Waltham, MA, USA) and diluted in BHI broth to reach the useful concentration to obtain biofilm formation. The assays were conducted using PET disks as the food contact surface. PETs were placed into 12-well tissue culture plates (Falcon, Thermo Fisher Scientific Inc., Waltham, MA, USA), with a flat bottom and lid. After washing in sterile ultrapure water, the PETs were incubated in ethanol ($\geq$ 99.8%) for 10 min under gentle shaking and were then washed in sterile ultrapure water, dried and packaged. In each experiment set, 600 µL of the standardized inoculum in the presence of 1018K6- PETs or non-functionalized PETs was added to 12-well tissue culture plates. BHI broth was used as negative control, and the plates were incubated at 37 °C for 72 h under the static condition. Cell counting of *L. monocytogenes*, in agreement with the ISO 11290-2:98 (ISO 11290-2: 1998/Amd 1, 2004) method, was performed to assess the concentration and purity of the standardized inoculum. After incubation, PETs were washed three times with PBS pH 7.3 and placed in a new plate to dry. At the end of the fixing phase, 1 mL of 0.2% Crystal Violet (Panreac Quimica SAU, Barcelona, Spain) in 95% ethanol was added to each well to stain the PETs. After gentle shaking for 15 min, the PETs were washed three times with sterile water and were then transferred into a new plate to dry at 37 °C. The quantitative analysis of biofilm production was performed by adding 1 mL of 33% acetic acid to destain the PETs, and 200 µL of each solution was transferred to a microtiter plate to measure the level (OD492) of the crystal violet. Anti-adhesion assay was performed in triplicate on three independent sets of experiments. OD492 values were compared through non-parametric analysis of variance (Kruskal-Wallis test), followed by multiple comparisons using Dunn test pairs (with Bonferroni correction) ($p < 0.05$). Statistical analyses were performed using Microsoft®Excel 2000/XLSTAT©-Pro.

4. Conclusions

Adding new functionalities to food packaging is a key issue in the production of the next generation of active materials. In this context, polymers represent good candidates as their production, use and disposal/recovery are well established at very low costs. Among the main useful packaging materials, PET is one of the most widely employed worldwide in the food industry.

The results of this study demonstrated that PET material can be efficiently and quickly pre-activated by the cold oxygen plasma technique, which represents an industrial scalable technology, in order to promote the functionalization with 1018K6, a peptide showing potent antibacterial and anti-adhesion properties, and to obtain antimicrobial packaging. 1018K6-PETs were tested under real conditions, using samples of mozzarella cheese, and it was found that APC, yeast and mold counts of the samples stored in the presence of modified polymers were strongly reduced during the first 24 h, thus demonstrating the 1018K6 was still active and preserved its antimicrobial abilities upon polymer surface immobilization. Moreover, 1018K6-PET was very effective against the formation of *Listeria* biofilms, a non-trivial result since not all antimicrobial agents are able to combat bacterial biofilms.

This work represents a preliminary study, which provides a starting point to develop a new PET-based system, functionalized with a biologically-derived AMP, which can have potential as antimicrobial packaging, providing an innovative and breakthrough technology in food applications, due to its comparable cost, small peptide dimension, effective antimicrobial activity, polymer characteristics and environmental friendliness. However, further investigations will be required to establish whether the projected antimicrobial-polymers may find industrial uses and whether they will be effective to improve the safety and extend the shelf-life of food products.

5. Patents

International Patent, Application No: PCT/EP2018/069304 Publication Date: 16/07/2018. Antimicrobial peptides. BALESTRIERI Marco, PALMIERI Gianna, CAPUANO Federico, DE STEFANO Luca et al.

Author Contributions: Conceptualization, M.B., G.P., M.G. and L.D.S.; methodology, B.A., A.C., Y.T.R.P., R.M.; validation, Y.T.R.P., R.M. and A.C.; investigation, B.A., A.C., Y.T.R.P. and R.M.; resources, G.P. and F.C.; data curation, L.D.S. and M.G.; writing—original draft preparation, M.B., G.P., M.G., I.R. and L.D.S.; writing—review and editing, M.B., G.P., M.G., I.R. and L.D.S.; supervision, G.P., M.G. and L.D.S.; cytotoxicity tests, G.S.

Funding: This research was funded by the "Packaging innovativi a base di pEptidi antimicRobici per la SIcurezza Alimentare" (PERSIA) project, grant number POR FESR CAMPANIA 2014/2020 n. B63D18000530007 and the "Sviluppo di metodologie innovative per ridurre il rischio di malattie trasmesse da alimenti in prodotti della filiera ittica" Ricerca Corrente 2016 project, grant number IZS ME 01/16 RC.

Acknowledgments: The authors gratefully acknowledge the dairy "Mini Caseificio Costanzo s.r.l." located in Lusciano (Caserta, Italy) that provided the PET containers necessary for the reported analyses.

Conflicts of Interest: The authors declare no conflict of interest.

References

1. Corradini, M.G. Shelf life of food products: From open labeling to real-time measurements. *Annu. Rev. Food Sci. Technol.* **2018**, *9*, 251–269. [CrossRef] [PubMed]
2. Ferguson, M.; Katzenberg, M.E. Information sharing to improve retail product freshness of perishables. *Prod. Oper. Manag.* **2006**, *15*, 57–73.
3. Munoz-Bonilla, A.; Fernandez-Garcia, M. Polymeric materials with antimicrobial activity. *Prog. Polym. Sci.* **2012**, *37*, 281–339. [CrossRef]
4. Sobczak, M.; Dębek, C.; Olędzka, E.; Kozłowski, R. Polymeric systems of antimicrobial peptides—Strategies and potential applications. *Molecules* **2013**, *18*, 14122–14137. [CrossRef] [PubMed]
5. Irkin, R.; Esmer, O.K. Novel food packaging systems with natural antimicrobial agents. *J. Food Sci. Technol.* **2015**, *52*, 6095–6111. [CrossRef]
6. De Smet, K.; Contreras, R. Human antimicrobial peptides: Defensins, cathelicidins and histatins. *Biotechnol. Lett.* **2005**, *27*, 1337–1347. [CrossRef]
7. Bals, R. Epithelial antimicrobial peptides in host defense against infection. *Respir. Res.* **2000**, *1*, 141–150. [CrossRef]
8. Henzler Wildman, K.A.; Lee, D.K.; Ramamoorthy, A. Mechanism of lipid bilayer disruption by the human antimicrobial peptide, LL-37. *Biochemistry* **2003**, *42*, 6545–6558. [CrossRef]
9. Amer, L.S.; Bishop, B.M.; van Hoek, M.L. Antimicrobial and antibiofilm activity of cathelicidins and short, synthetic peptides against Francisella. *Biochem. Biophys. Res. Commun.* **2010**, *396*, 246–251. [CrossRef]
10. De la Fuente-Núñez, C.; Korolik, V.; Bains, M.; Nguyen, U.; Breidenstein, E.B.; Horsman, S.; Lewenza, S.; Burrows, L.; Hancock, R.E. Inhibition of bacterial biofilm formation and swarming motility by a small synthetic cationic peptide. *Antimicrob. Agents Chemother.* **2012**, *56*, 2696–2704. [CrossRef]
11. De la Fuente-Núñez, C.; Reffuveille, F.; Haney, E.F.; Straus, S.K.; Hancock, R.E. Broad-spectrum anti-biofilm peptide that targets a cellular stress response. *PLoS Pathog.* **2014**, *10*, e1004152. [CrossRef] [PubMed]
12. Overhage, J.; Campisano, A.; Bains, M.; Torfs, E.C.; Rehm, B.H.; Hancock, R.E. Human host defense peptide LL-37 prevents bacterial biofilm formation. *Infect. Immun.* **2008**, *76*, 4176–4182. [CrossRef] [PubMed]
13. Wang, G.; Li, X.; Wang, Z. APD3: The antimicrobial peptide database as a tool for research and education. *Nucleic Acids Res.* **2016**, *44*, D1087–D1093. [CrossRef] [PubMed]
14. Pompilio, A.; Scocchi, M.; Pomponio, S.; Guida, F.; Di Primio, A.; Fiscarelli, E.; Gennaro, R.; Di Bonaventura, G. Antibacterial and anti-biofilm effects of cathelicidin peptides against pathogens isolated from cystic fibrosis patients. *Peptides* **2011**, *32*, 1807–1814. [CrossRef] [PubMed]
15. Reffuveille, F.; de la Fuente-Núñez, C.; Mansour, S.; Hancock, R.E.W. A broad spectrum anti-biofilm peptide enhances antibiotic action against bacterial biofilms. *Antimicrob. Agents Chemother.* **2014**, *58*, 5363–5371. [CrossRef] [PubMed]
16. Palmieri, G.; Balestrieri, M.; Capuano, F.; Proroga, Y.T.R.; Pomilio, F.; Centorame, P.; Riccio, A.; Marrone, R.; Anastasio, A. Bactericidal and antibiofilm activity of bactenecin-derivative peptides against the food-pathogen *Listeria monocytogenes*: New perspectives for food processing industry. *Int. J. Food. Microbiol.* **2018**, *279*, 33–42. [CrossRef]
17. Palmieri, G.; Balestrieri, M.; Proroga, Y.T.R.; Falcigno, L.; Facchiano, A.; Riccio, A.; Capuano, F.; Marrone, R.; Neglia, G.; Anastasio, A. New antimicrobial peptides against foodborne pathogens: From in silico design to experimental evidence. *Food Chem.* **2016**, *211*, 546–554. [CrossRef]

18. Holmberg, K.V.; Abdolhosseini, M.; Li, Y.; Chen, X.; Gorr, S.-U.; Aparicio, C. Bio-inspired stable antimicrobial peptide coatings for dental applications. *Acta Biomater.* **2013**, *9*, 8224–8231. [CrossRef]
19. Hamley, I.W. PEG−Peptide Conjugates. *Biomacromolecules* **2014**, *15*, 1543–1559. [CrossRef]
20. Jordá-Vilaplana, A.; Fombuena, V.; García-García, D.; Samper, M.D.; Sánchez-Nácher, L. Surface modification of polylactic acid (PLA) by air atmospheric plasma treatment. *Eur. Polym. J.* **2014**, *58*, 23–33. [CrossRef]
21. Silvestre, C.; Duraccio, D.; Cimmino, S. Food packaging based on polymer nanomaterials. *Prog. Polym. Sci.* **2011**, *36*, 1766–1782. [CrossRef]
22. Alavi, S.; Thomas, S.; Sandeep, K.P.; Kalarikkal, N.; Varghese, J.; Yaragalla, S. *Polymers for Packaging Applications*, 1st ed.; CRC Press: Boca Raton, FL, USA, 2014; 486p.
23. Pankaj, S.K.; Bueno-Ferrer, C.; Misra, N.N.; Milosavljevic, V.; O'Donnel, C.P.; Bourke, P.; Keener, K.M.; Cullen, P.J. Applications of cold plasma technology in food packaging. *Trends Food Sci. Technol.* **2014**, *35*, 5–17. [CrossRef]
24. De Stefano, L.; Rotiroti, L.; De Tommasi, E.; Rea, I.; Rendina, I.; Canciello, M.; Maglio, G.; Palumbo, R. Hybrid polymer-porous silicon photonic crystals for optical sensing. *J. App. Phys.* **2009**, *106*, 023109. [CrossRef]
25. Socrates, G. *Infrared and Raman Characteristic Group Frequencies*, 3rd ed.; John Wiley & Sons Ltd.: New York, NY, USA, 1994.
26. De Stefano, L.; Oliviero, G.; Amato, J.; Borbone, N.; Piccialli, G.; Mayol, L.; Rendina, I.; Terracciano, M.; Rea, I. Aminosilane functionalizations of mesoporous oxidized silicon for oligonucleotide synthesis and detection. *J. R. Soc. Interface* **2013**, *10*, 20130160. [CrossRef] [PubMed]
27. Holliday, R. Plant population and crop yield. *Nature* **1960**, *186*, 22–24. [CrossRef]
28. Huis in't Veld, J.H.J. Microbial and biochemical spoilage of foods: An overview. *Int. J. Food Microbiol.* **1998**, *33*, 1–18. [CrossRef]
29. Losito, F.; Arienzo, A.; Bottini, G.; Priolisi, F.R.; Mari, A.; Antonini, G. Microbiological safety and quality of Mozzarella cheese assessed by the microbiological survey method. *J. Dairy Sci.* **2014**, *97*, 46–55. [CrossRef] [PubMed]
30. Bondi, M.; Lauková, A.; de Niederhausern, S.; Messi, P.; Papadopoulou, C. Natural Preservatives to Improve Food Quality and Safety. *J. Food Qual.* **2017**, *2017*. [CrossRef]
31. Beresford, M.R.; Andrew, P.W.; Shama, G. *Listeria monocytogenes* adheres to many materials found in food-processing environments. *J. Appl. Microbiol.* **2001**, *90*, 1000–1005. [CrossRef]
32. Wong, A.C.L. Biofilms in Food Processing Environments. *J. Dairy Sci.* **1998**, *81*, 2765–2770. [CrossRef]

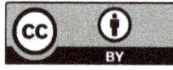

© 2019 by the authors. Licensee MDPI, Basel, Switzerland. This article is an open access article distributed under the terms and conditions of the Creative Commons Attribution (CC BY) license (http://creativecommons.org/licenses/by/4.0/).

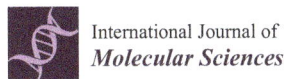

Article

Antibiofilm Activity of Polyamide 11 Modified with Thermally Stable Polymeric Biocide Polyhexamethylene Guanidine 2-Naphtalenesulfonate

Olena Moshynets [1,*], Jean-François Bardeau [2], Oksana Tarasyuk [3], Stanislav Makhno [4], Tetiana Cherniavska [4], Oleg Dzhuzha [3], Geert Potters [5,6] and Sergiy Rogalsky [3,*]

1 Institute of Molecular Biology and Genetics of NAS of Ukraine, 03143 Kyiv, Ukraine
2 Institut des Molécules et Matériaux du Mans, UMR CNRS 6283, Université du Mans, 72085 Le Mans, France; jean-francois.bardeau@univ-lemans.fr
3 V. P. Kukhar Institute of Bioorganic Chemistry and Petrochemistry of NAS of Ukraine, 02160 Kyiv, Ukraine; oksanatarasyuk@bigmir.net (O.T.); dzhuzha.oleg@gmail.com (O.D.)
4 Chuiko Institute of Surface Chemistry of NAS of Ukraine, 03680 Kyiv, Ukraine; stmax@ukr.net (S.M.); t-cherniavska@ukr.net (T.C.)
5 Antwerp Maritime Academy, Noordkasteel Oost 6, 2030 Antwerp, Belgium; geert.potters@hzs.be
6 University of Antwerp, Groenenborgerlaan 171, 2020 Antwerp, Belgium
* Correspondence: moshynets@gmail.com (O.M.); sergey.rogalsky@gmail.com (S.R.); Tel.: +38-044-5594622 (S.R.)

Received: 9 December 2018; Accepted: 8 January 2019; Published: 16 January 2019

Abstract: The choice of efficient antimicrobial additives for polyamide resins is very difficult because of their high processing temperatures of up to 300 °C. In this study, a new, thermally stable polymeric biocide, polyhexamethylene guanidine 2-naphtalenesulfonate (PHMG-NS), was synthesised. According to thermogravimetric analysis, PHMG-NS has a thermal degradation point of 357 °C, confirming its potential use in joint melt processing with polyamide resins. Polyamide 11 (PA-11) films containing 5, 7 and 10 wt% of PHMG-NS were prepared by compression molding and subsequently characterised by FTIR spectroscopy. The surface properties were evaluated both by contact angle, and contactless induction. The incorporation of 10 wt% of PHMG-NS into PA-11 films was found to increase the positive surface charge density by almost two orders of magnitude. PA-11/PHMG-NS composites were found to have a thermal decomposition point at about 400 °C. Mechanical testing showed no change of the tensile strength of polyamide films containing PHMG-NS up to 7 wt%. Antibiofilm activity against the opportunistic bacteria *Staphylococcus aureus* and *Escherichia coli* was demonstrated for films containing 7 or 10 wt% of PHMG-NS, through a local biocide effect possibly based on an influence on the bacterial eDNA. The biocide hardly leached from the PA-11 matrix into water, at a rate of less than 1% from its total content for 21 days.

Keywords: polyamide 11; antibacterial; polymeric biocide; thermal stability; biofilm

1. Introduction

Produced from a renewable source, polyamide 11 (PA-11) is a unique thermoplastic polymer with excellent functional properties, combining high ductility and mechanical strength, dimensional stability, low density, excellent abrasion and fatigue resistance, a low friction coefficient, high barrier properties and resistance to many types of chemicals. Many industries around the world (automotive, transport, textile, oil and gas, wire and cables, and electronics) have been using PA-11 for decades [1]. PA-11 powder coatings were developed to protect metal parts from corrosion, particularly for the protection of steel in the fluid transfer industry, for example in pipes and fittings in water treatment plants, water/hydrocarbon transportation pipelines, transport and building constructions, medical equipment, office furniture, and many other appliances [2].

It is known that the surface of polyamide plastics can be colonised rapidly by bacteria, fungi and algae, especially in a humid environment, which is then followed by the formation of biofilms/fouling. Moreover, the emerging biofilm causes contamination, staining, odours and eventually deterioration of the mechanical properties of the plastic because of the degradation of the polymer, utilising the carbon in the course of development as a nutrient [3–5]. Biofilm formation starts with the deposition of different microorganisms on the surface of the material, followed by growth and spreading of the colonies forming a highly complex structure, culminating in microbial evolution and adaptation towards a stronger resistance to antibiotics and biocides, the appearance of super-biofilm with super-mucous and super-adhesive opportunistic strains, etc. [6–10]. Bacteria foul medical devices and implants, e.g., polymeric materials used as internal or invasive devices such as catheters, components of cardiac pacemakers, artificial heart valves and joints. The formed biofilm can initiate degradation of the material, as well as hospital-acquired infections, for example of small medical devices, because of a high concentration of microorganisms. These implant-associated biofilms are often difficult to remove, even after cleaning the implants pre-operatively with oxidisers and detergents or treating them with antibiotics, and in certain situations replacement surgery may be required [6].

The introduction of antimicrobial agents into the base polymer of these articles is considered the most efficient approach to prevent the growth of biofilms on their surface. A wide variety of organic and inorganic biocides is available, whether synthetic or nature-inspired [11–15]. The choice of appropriate biocides for PA-11 is strongly limited because of the high processing temperatures of the polymer, up to 300 °C. Currently, silver-based compounds are the most widely used antimicrobial additives for PA-11 because of their excellent thermal stability [16,17], as well as their low toxicity to human cells [18]. Silver nanoparticles are regarded as the most promising biocides for polyamide resins since their high surface area ensures an efficient release of Ag^+ species into the medium [19–21]. However, it should be noted that silver nanoparticles are hard to disperse in a polymer matrix because of their strong aggregation ability [16,17,21]. Moreover, silver ions are known to interact with polyamides during melt processing and cause an undesirable discolouration of polymer articles. Therefore, many antimicrobial formulations contain silver-based compounds intercalated into inorganic anion exchangers or encapsulated using soluble ceramics [16,17].

Thus, there is a growing demand for the development of low-cost and low toxic antimicrobial agents that combine good compatibility and processability with polyamide resins, as well as high leaching resistance from polymer matrix.

Copper and its compounds have also emerged as promising antimicrobial additives for polyamides, being much cheaper than silver. Thus, a commercially available ionic copper-based additive, Plasticopper, was incorporated into the PA-11 matrix during the polymer processing stage [22]. The incorporation of 5% and 10% copper was found to have a reinforcing effect on the composites and did not adversely affect their mechanical performance. These composite systems showed long-term antimicrobial activity against Gram-negative bacteria (E. coli) with a reduction of the bacterial population of more than 99.99% [22].

Nowadays, cationic polymers are being considered as a new generation of biocides because of their enhanced antimicrobial activity, as well as their low toxicity to human cells, compared to common low molecular cationic surfactants [23,24]. In particular, polyhexamethylene guanidine (PHMG) salts, comprising guanidinium cations in the main chain, are receiving increasing attention since they display a broad range of antimicrobial activity against bacteria, fungi and viruses [25–31], as well as antifouling activity against macrofoulers in an aquatic environment [32,33]. It should also be noted that PHMG salts showed a much lower acute toxicity than copper-based biocides [33]. The high activity of guanidinium-based polymeric biocides against microorganisms is caused by the presence of multiple positive charges within a single molecule that are able to compensate the negative charges present on the outer cell membranes of microbes. Because of these strong electrostatic interactions,

PHMG is able to attack the cellular envelope, and subsequently associates itself with the head groups of the acidic phospholipids. The presence of hydrophobic aliphatic chains in the PHMG backbone ensures a better partition to the hydrophobic regions of the phospholipid membrane, resulting in a change of membrane permeability and lethal leakage of cytoplasmic materials [27–31].

Poorly water-soluble PHMG salts such as PHMG stearate, PHMG sulfanilate, or PHMG dodecylbenzenesulfonate (PHMG-DBS) have been reported as efficient antimicrobial additives for polycaprolactone [34], polylactide [35], polyamides [36,37] and silicones [38]. PHMG-DBS was found to have sufficient thermal stability to be melt processed with PA-11 and PA-12 resins by conventional methods [36,37]. PA-11 films containing 5–7 wt% of PHMG-DBS showed a high activity against *E. coli*, as well as an excellent resistance against leaching of the polymeric biocide [37].

Another successful approach involves the intercalation of the cationic polymer (partially aminated poly(vinylbenzyl chloride)) into a smectic clay, montmorillonite, to produce a modified organoclay containing 33 wt% of polymeric biocide [39]. Polymerically modified organoclay was found to have sufficient thermal stability for joint processing with PA-6 resin by melt extrusion. The obtained nanocomposites were active against both Gram-negative *E. coli* and Gram-positive *S. aureus* bacteria and demonstrated up to a 2-log reduction in the viable cells adhering to the material surface at an organoclay content of 5 wt%. The mode of antimicrobial action of this material was determined as contact-active because the biocide does not leach out [39].

Despite the evidence for a pronounced antibacterial and antifungal activity of contact-active polyamide composites, their activity against biofilms has not yet been studied. It is worth noting that antibiofilm characteristics do not always parallel antibacterial characteristics. There are several examples of compounds that were added to polymers and possessed antibacterial characteristics, but could not decrease fouling, and vice versa [40–42]. In the present study, a new thermally stable hydrophobic cationic polymer, polyhexamethylene guanidine 2-naphtalene sulfonate (PHMG-NS), was synthesised. In contrast to the previously reported polymeric biocide PHMG-DBS, which sticks together during storage, PHMG-NS forms a fine powder that makes it a good candidate to be applied in PA-11 based powder coating formulations. The aim of our research was to investigate the antibiofilm activity of PA-11 films modified with PHMG-NS biocide against the biofilm-forming model bacterial strains, opportunistically pathogenic *E. coli* K12 and *S. aureus* ATCC 25923.

2. Results and Discussion

2.1. FTIR Analysis of PA-11/PHMG-NS Films

Infrared spectroscopy was employed both to identify the presence of PHMG-NS inside the polymer films and reveal potential interactions between PA-11 and the biocide. Figure 1a shows infrared spectra of PHMG-Cl and PHMG-NS in the 400–4000 cm^{-1} region and Figure 1b shows infrared spectra in the 960–1830 cm^{-1} region of PA-11 and PA-11/PHMG-NS films containing 5%, 7% and 10% of PHMG-NS. As previously described for PHMG-Cl, which was the precursor compound for making PHMG-NS, the very broad bands in the region of 2600–3700 cm^{-1} are attributed to the CH_2, NH_2, and OH stretching vibrations [33]. The modification of PHMG-Cl to PHMG-NS does not change the position of vibrational modes, whose maxima are found at approximately 2856 and 2932 cm^{-1}, respectively, and attributed to the symmetric $\nu_s(CH_2)$ and asymmetric $\nu_{as}(CH_2)$ stretching vibrations of the methylene groups. However, the bands attributed to the symmetric $\nu_s(NH_2)$ and asymmetric $\nu_{as}(NH_2)$ stretching vibrations of amine groups shift to higher wavenumbers at about 3194 and 3313 cm^{-1}. The IR spectra show also strong absorption bands between 1500 and 1800 cm^{-1}, characteristic of both the C=N stretching and the NH_2 scissoring modes. The central position of these broad bands does not shift between PHMG-Cl and PHMG-NS. The strong absorption bands observed at 1177, 1090, 1030 and 673 cm^{-1} can be assigned to the sulphonic group of the 2-naphthalenesulfonate. Two of these later vibrational modes can easily be observed at 1092 cm^{-1} and 1032 cm^{-1} in Figure 1b (dashed lines) with PA-11/PHMG-NS films containing 5%, 7% and 10% of PHMG-NS, thus confirming the presence of the biocide in the films. Overall, the IR spectra of the modified films are similar to each other revealing that the introduction of PHMG-NS does not significantly influence the vibrational bands of PA-11. However, a noticeable change can be observed in Figure 1b: the small intensity band assigned to the carbonyl (C=O) stretching vibrations for PA-11 (at 1727 cm^{-1}) shifts toward higher wavenumbers as a function of the PHMG-NS content and reaches 1734 cm^{-1} for films containing 10% of PHMG-NS (Figure 1b, black arrow). This feature suggests a modification of the specific environment of the C=O group. The guanidinium cation is known to participate in direct hydrogen bonding with backbone carbonyl groups of proteins [43], which suggests a similar interaction between the guanidinium cations of PHMG-NS and the amide carbonyl groups of PA-11.

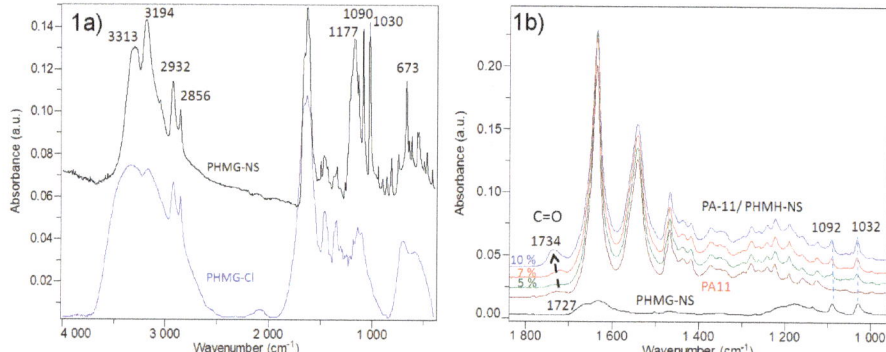

Figure 1. IR spectra: (**a**) PHMG-Cl and PHMG-NS; and (**b**) PHMG-NS, PA-11 and PA-11/PHMG-NS film with 5%, 7% and 10% of PHMG-NS.

2.2. Surface Properties of PA-11/PHMG-NS Films

According to the contact angle measurements data, an introduction of 5 wt% of PHMG-NS into a PA-11 film led to an enhanced hydrophilicity of the surface, which can be attributed to the increase of the polar functional groups on the polyamide surface. However, further increase of PHMG-NS content had little impact on the contact angle value (Table 1). The results of the electrophysical study of the PA-11/PHMG-NS films indicate a sharp increase of the positive surface charge density at a PHMG-NS content of 7 wt% and more (Table 1). Probably, it can be explained by the formation of an uncompensated positive charge of the guanidinium cations at the polymer surface because of specific interactions between the hydrophobic fragments of the PHMG-NS and the PA-11 matrix. It should be noted that both the improved hydrophilicity and the positive charge of the polymer surface are considered to be important factors that determine the antimicrobial efficacy [44–46].

Table 1. Surface properties of PA-11/PHMG-NS films.

Sample	Contact Angle (Degree)	Surface Charge Density (C/cm^2)
PA-11	80 ± 2	(0.47 ± 0.02) × 10^{-10}
PA-11/PHMH-NS (5%)	70 ± 2	(1.2 ± 0.1) × 10^{-10}
PA-11/PHMH-NS (7%)	68 ± 2	(6.5 ± 0.3) × 10^{-10}
PA-11/PHMH-NS (10%)	68 ± 2	(27 ± 1) × 10^{-10}

2.3. Mechanical and Thermal Properties of PA-11/PHMG-NS Composites

It has been established that inorganic biocides have a reinforcing effect on the polyamide matrix caused by the formation of strong interfacial interactions, leading to a reduction in the mobility of polymer chains [22,39]. For example, heterogeneous PA-11/Cu antimicrobial nanocomposites showed an increase of the yield strength from 45 to 54 MPa when 2–10% of a copper additive was introduced [22]. The introduction of 5% of cationic biocide intercalated organoclay into PA-6 improved the yield strength by 44.6% [39].

The polymeric biocide PHMG-NS forms homogeneous composites with PA-11 because of its low melting temperature, as well as its good compatibility with the polymer matrix. Tensile testing of PA-11/PHMG-NS samples was performed to evaluate the effect of the antimicrobial additive on the mechanical properties of polyamide. PA-11 films containing 5% and 7% of PHMG-NS have tensile strength values similar to pure polyamide. A further increase of the polymeric biocide content to 10% led to a deterioration of the mechanical properties of the material (Table 2).

Table 2. Mechanical properties of PA-11/PHMG-NS composites.

Sample	Tensile Strength, MPa	Elongation at Break, %
PA-11	45 ± 2	24 ± 4
PA-11/PHMG-NS (5%)	45 ± 1	25 ± 5
PA-11/PHMG-NS (7%)	43 ± 2	15 ± 3
PA-11/PHMG-NS (10%)	27 ± 2	6 ± 2

The results of the thermal characterisation of the polymeric biocide PHMG-NS, PA-11 and PA-11/PHMG-NS containing 10 wt% of polymeric biocide are summarised in Figure 2 and Table 3. According to the TGA data, PHMG-NS has a thermal decomposition point (which was defined as the temperature of 5% weight loss ($T_{\Delta m} = 5\%$) at 357 °C. The peak mass loss temperature of PHMG-NS is 392 °C (Figure 2a). Pure PA-11 begins to decompose at 425 °C and the maximum rate of thermal degradation was observed at 431 °C (Figure 2b). The PA-11/PHMG-NS composite containing 10 wt% of PHMG-NS is thermally stable to at least 391 °C, and the peak mass loss was found at 465 °C (Figure 2c). At a lower PHMG-NS content, the thermal stability of a composite becomes closer to pure PA-11 (Table 3). Hence, PHMG-NS has excellent thermal stability and can be used for joint melt processing with polyamide resins by conventional methods, as previously reported for the polymeric biocide PHMG-DBS [36,37]. However, PHMG-NS seems to have a broader application range, due to its hydrophobic powder state, whereas PHMG-DBS has a tendency for aggregation during storage. These properties of PHMG-NS allow for its introduction into PA-11-based powder coatings for covering metal articles, by conventional methods using a fluidised bed method of air suspension of a composite material or an electrostatic spraying process.

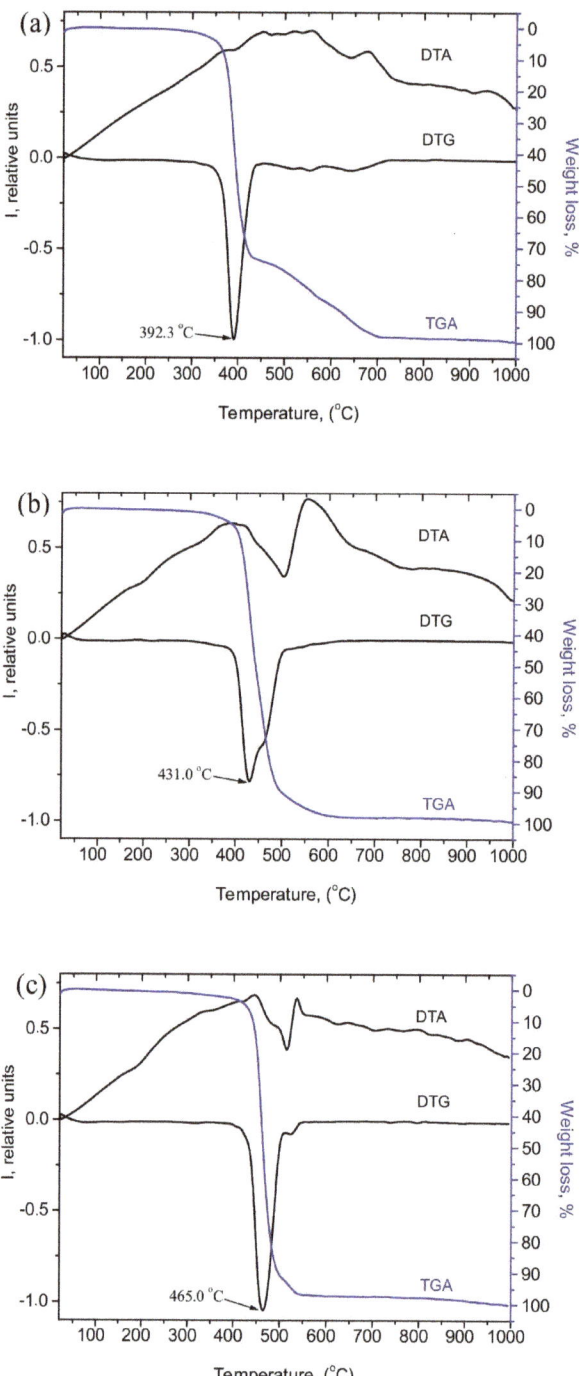

Figure 2. TGA curves in air of: PHMG-NS (**a**); PA-11 (**b**); and PA-11/PHMH-NS (10%) (**c**).

Table 3. TGA data for PHMG-NS and PA-11/PHMG-NS composite*.

Sample	$T_{\Delta m} = 5\%$, °C	$T_{\Delta m} = 10\%$, °C	$T_{\Delta m} = 20\%$, °C	$T_{\Delta m} = 50\%$, °C
PHMG-NS	357	372	381	398
PA-11	425	441	450	463
PA-11/PHMG-NS (5%)	413	434	445	456
PA-11/PHMG-NS (7%)	405	430	442	449
PA-11/PHMG-NS (10%)	391	408	420	443

* Standard error $n \pm 1$.

2.4. Antibiofilm Efficacy of PA-11/PHMG-NS Films

The antibiofilm/antifouling properties of PA-11 modified with the polymeric biocide PHMG-NS were evaluated using two opportunistic biofilm-forming model strains: the Gram-negative *E. coli* K12 belonging to the Enterobacteriaceae family [47] and the Gram-positive *S. aureus* ATCC 25923 [48]. Overall, *E. coli* has been shown to be more resistant to PHMG-containing biocides than the Gram-positive opportunists, such as methicillin-resistant *Staphylococcus aureus* [34,35,38,49]. In addition, its enzymes are more stable when in contact with PHMG derivatives [35]. Principally, both strains were able to form solid–liquid biofilms to the PA-11 films within three days of cultivation. The level of biofilm biomass attached to a PA-11 film containing 5%, 7% or 10% of PHMG-NS was found to be significantly different from those on the control PA-11 films in the Crystal Violet assay (Figure 3) [50]. The biofilm formation decreased approximately three times for the samples containing 7% and 10% of PHMG-NS.

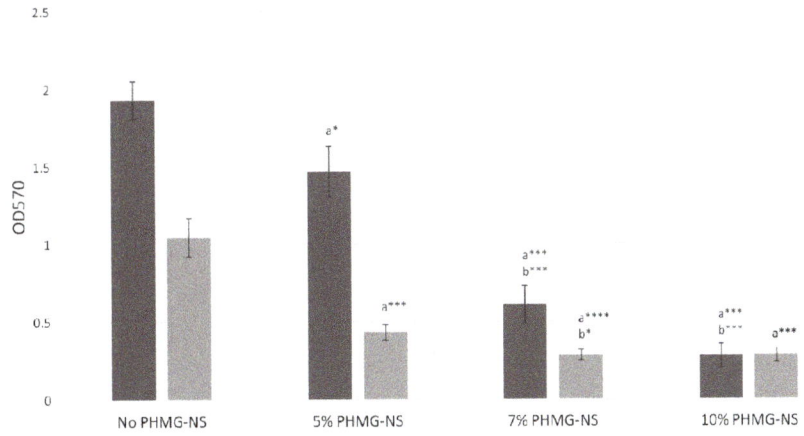

Figure 3. The level of biomass of *E. coli* K12 (dark grey) and *S. aureus* ATCC 25923 (light grey) biofilms formed onto PA-11 films containing 5%, 7% and 10% of PHMG-NS following 72 h of incubation determined by Crystal Violet staining and measured as the optical density at 570 nm (OD570). a: statistical significance compared to control (No PHMG-NS); b: statistical significance compared to 5% PHMG-NS. * $p < 0.05$, *** $p < 0.005$, **** $p < 0.001$.

The Crystal Violet assay measures the overall level of organic layers formed on a plastic surface, containing bacterial cells and numerous organic molecules integrated into the biofilm matrix. Of course, contact-active antimicrobial surfaces are often coated with a layer of dead microbes, to which newly approaching microbes can also adhere and proliferate [51]. Hence, a higher level of Crystal Violet staining does not always correspond to a higher metabolic activity of a biofilm. To assess whether the metabolic activity of the biofilm could be related to the overall number of living bacterial cells in the biofilms, an MTT test was performed in parallel [52]. In this assay, a similar tendency was revealed. All PHMG-NS-containing PA-11 films showed a significant reduction in biofilm metabolic activity (Figure 4). The level of biofilm metabolic activity was 2.5 times lower on the PA-11/PHMG-NS (5%) than on the control PA-11 films. There was a significant difference between the growth under control conditions and the growth on PA-11 containing 5%, 7% and 10% of the polymeric biocide. There was no significant difference between samples containing 5% and 7% PHMG-NS, and between PA-11/PHMG-NS (7%) and PA-11/PHMG-NS (10%). Generally, there was a fivefold decrease in the biofilm metabolic activity for polymer films containing 7% PHMG-NS compared to the control PA-11 films for both bacterial strains ($p < 0.001$ for *E. coli* and $p < 0.01$ for *S. aureus*), and there was almost no metabolic activity on films with 10% PHMG-NS inoculated with *E. coli*.

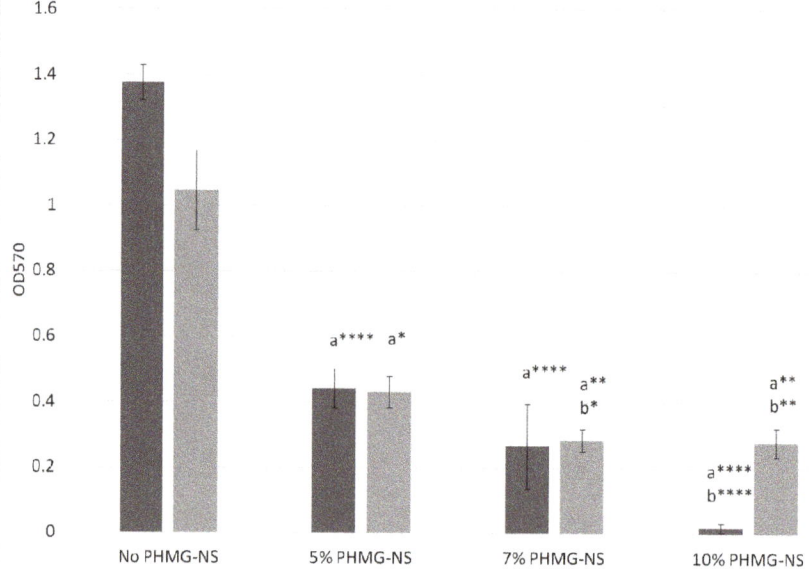

Figure 4. The level of metabolic activity of *E. coli* K12 (dark grey) and *S. aureus* ATCC 25923 (light grey) biofilms formed onto PA-11 films containing 5%, 7% and 10% of PHMG-NS following 72 h of incubation determined by MTT staining and measured as the optical density at 570 nm (OD570). a: statistical significance compared to control (No PHMG-NS); b: statistical significance compared to 5% PHMG-NS. * $p < 0.05$, ** $p < 0.01$, **** $p < 0.001$.

The bacterial toxicity of the PA-11/PHMG-NS films for the planktonic part of the bacterial culture was evaluated by measuring both the optical density and the colony forming units (CFU) count in the overbiofilm layer in 72-h stationary biofilm-forming K12 and ATCC 25923 cultures. There was no significant difference in optical density between any of the four samples (Figure 5) except a minor and possible negligible decrease of ATCC 25923 in the presence of PA-11/PHMG-NS (10%) ($p < 0.05$). The planktonic CFU numbers in the media in contact with the control and 5% PHMG-NS films were, respectively, tenfold and fivefold higher than the CFU of the plankton in contact with the PA-11/PHMG-NS (10%) and the PA-11/PHMG-NS (7%) films for K12. There was also a tenfold decrease in plankton density in PA-11 films doped with 5% and 7% of PHMG-NS and a fivefold decrease for PA-11/PHMG-NS (10%) compared to control PA-11 for ATCC 25923. However, there was no significant difference in effect between the different polyamide films on the planktonic bacteria in a biofilm-forming culture, suggesting a low release rate of the biocide into the medium in the experimental conditions presented here.

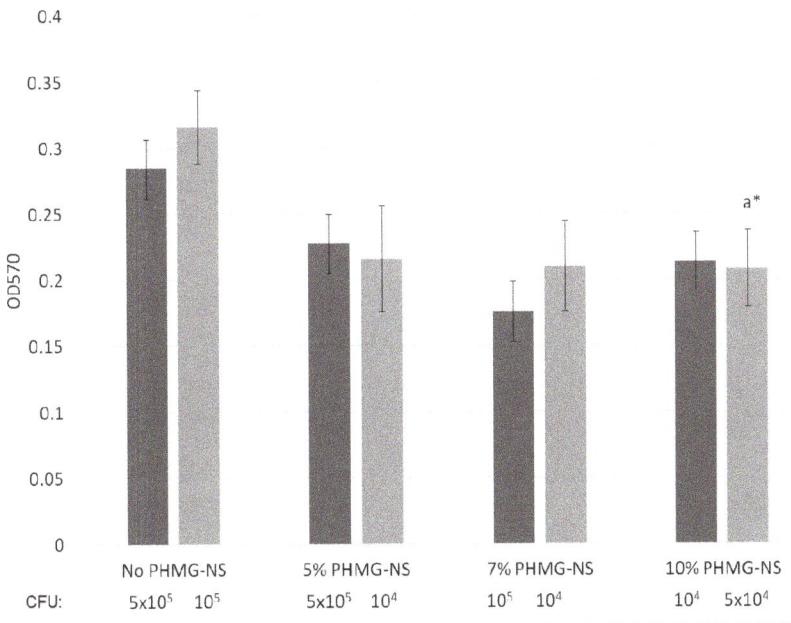

Figure 5. The level of planktonic cell biomass (overbiofilm layer indicated by the optical density at 570 nm (OD570)) of K12 (dark grey) and ATCC 25923 (light grey) in the presence of PA-11 films containing 5%, 7% and 10% of PHMG-NS following 72 h of incubation, correlated with the corresponding CFU counts. a: statistical significance compared to control (No PHMG-NS); * $p < 0.05$.

The behaviour of the planktonic part of the culture raised a question about the antibiofilm properties of the PA-11 films after water exposure. To investigate this, pieces of polymer containing 7% and 10% of PHMG-NS were exposed to water for seven days. The biofilm assay did not show any significantly different antibiofilm properties between the exposed and the non-exposed films.

Despite the absence of any significant effect of the presence of PHMG-NS in the PA-11 on the growth of planktonic cells, visual observation of the 72-h cultures revealed that the biofilm formation on the solid–liquid interface of the microcosms was unexpectedly reduced by the presence of at least 7% of PHMG-NS in the PA-11 films (direct observations). This raises a question: is there any distant effect of non-leaching PHMG-NS onto biofilm formation in a microcosm? Biofilms consist of bacterial cells embedded into a matrix of extracellular polymers composed of polysaccharides, proteins and nucleic acids (mostly DNA) [53]. Extracellular DNA (eDNA) has been known to play quite an important role in the initiation and the development of biofilms of many bacteria [54–57], among which those made by *E. coli* and *S. aureus* [58,59]. eDNA is a negatively charged molecule which might interact with the positively-charged PHMG-NS-containing PA-11. To check this hypothesis, the total eDNA content in the culture was precipitated from the solid–liquid interface biofilms formed after 72 h in the microcosms (Figure 6). There was a significant decrease in eDNA content in the biofilms formed in the presence of PA-11/PHMG-NS (7%) and PA-11/PHMG-NS (10%) for K12 ($p < 0.001$) and in the presence of only PA-11/PHMG-NS (10%) for ATCC 25923 ($p < 0.05$ compared to the control culture and $p < 0.001$ compared to the 5% PHMG-NS treatment), each time compared to the eDNA amount found in microcosms exposed to control PA-11 and PA-11/PHMG-NS (5%), while there were no such differences in the overbiofilm layer in any of the microcosms (Figure 7). Such a decrease in eDNA in the solid–liquid interface biofilms, in contrast with the constant level in the overbiofilm culture, might suggest that at least one of the antibiofilm mechanisms of PHMG-NS-containing PA-11 is associated with eDNA reduction, which in turn may have an influence on the initial stages of bacterial biofilm formation. Moreover, decreasing the level of eDNA would hypothetically reduce an abundance of resistance genes spread horizontally in a hospital-related environment, as eDNA associated with biofilms has been considered a hotspot for deposition and recombination of antibiotic resistance genes [60,61].

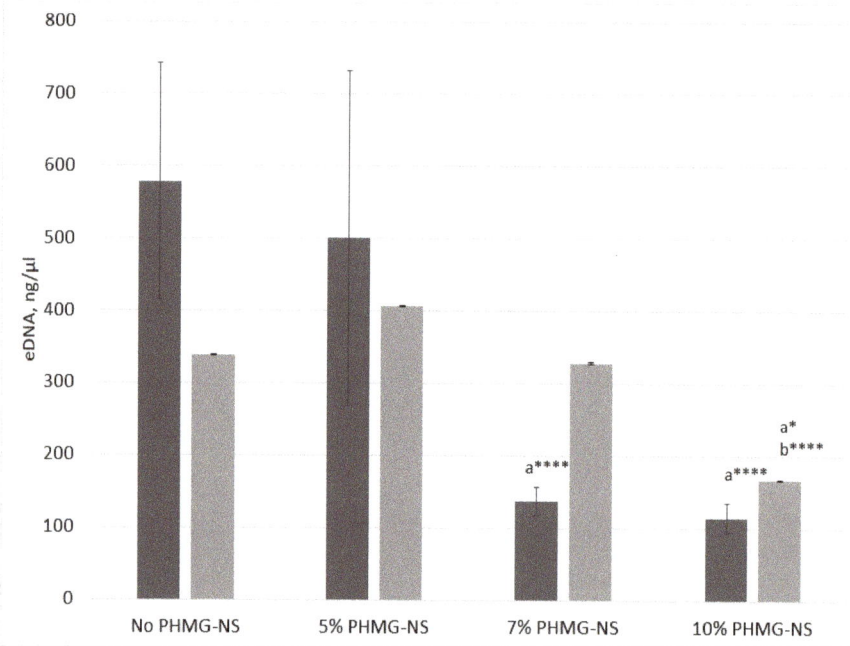

Figure 6. Amount of eDNA precipitated from a biofilm layer (solid-bottom phase) of 72-h-old biofilm-formed K12 (dark grey) and ATCC 25923 (light grey) cultures with PA-11 films containing 5%, 7% and 10% of PHMG-NS. a, statistical significance compared to control (No PHMG-NS); b: statistical significance compared to 5% PHMG-NS. * $p < 0.05$ **** $p < 0.001$.

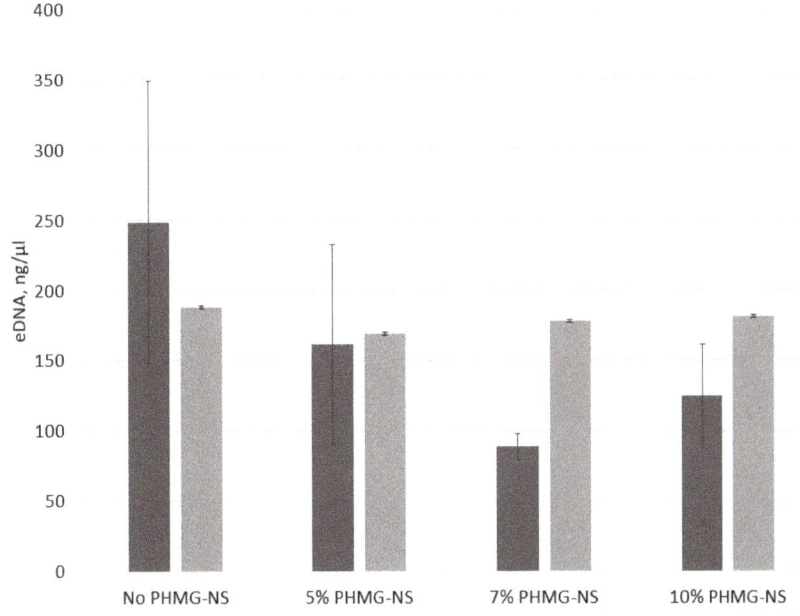

Figure 7. Amount of eDNA precipitated from overbiofilm layer (liquid plankton phase) of 72-h-old biofilms-formed K12 (dark grey) and ATCC 25923 (light grey) cultures with PA-11 films containing 5%, 7% and 10% of PHMG-NS.

It is worth noting that the reported antimicrobial polyamide composites have never before been studied for their activity against biofilms. However, polylactide films containing hydrophobic PHMG salts were found to strongly inhibit the activity of bacterial intracellular dehydrogenases, which prevented the formation of microbial biofilms on the polymer surface [35].

2.5. Leaching Resistance of PHMG-NS from PA-11 Films

The water solubility of PHMG-NS was found to be 0.24 g/L. Thus, given the possibility of a non-covalent association between the PA-11 matrix and PHMG-NS, a gradual release of polymeric biocide into the aqueous medium could be expected. Figure 8 contains UV-visible spectra of PHMG-NS (Curve 1), as well as its precursor PHMG-Cl (Curve 3), which is highly soluble in water. As one can see from these spectra, the characteristic ultraviolet absorption of the guanidyl carbon-to-nitrogen double bond of PHMG allows for a spectrophotometric analysis of either compound in aqueous solutions [62]. However, the adsorption peak of the 2-naphthalene sulfonate anion at 227 nm is the most expressive (Figure 8, Curve 2) and therefore was used for PGMG-NS detection.

After three days of contact with warm water, the PA-11/PHMG-NS (7%) film had lost less than 1% of its biocide contents (Figure 8, Curve 4). No further release of biocide was detected after 7, 14 and 21 days of exposure, which indicates that the biocide-doped polymer is highly resistant to leaching, which in turn is important for the potential durability of the antimicrobial activity of the material. It is worth noting that PA-11 has a much lower water absorption than other commercial polyamides [1], which may be a crucial factor in the determination of low biocide release rate [19]. Moreover, the cooperative hydrogen bonding of both guanidinium cations and 2-naphthalenesulfonate anions with the polar amide groups may also ensure the high retention of PHMG-NS in PA-11.

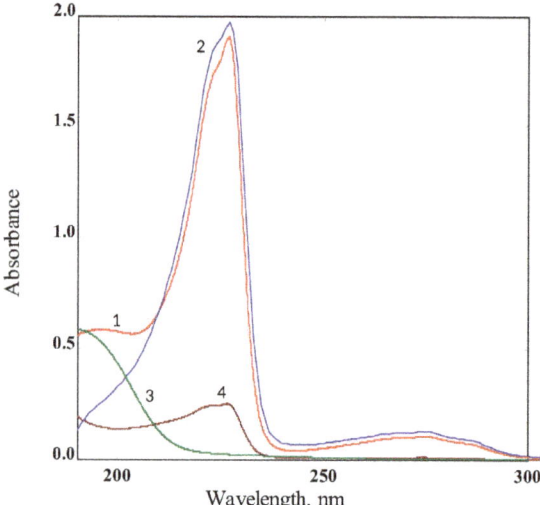

Figure 8. UV-visible spectra of: PHMG-NS (1); sodium 2-naphthalene sulfonate (2); PHMG hydrochloride (3) (C = 4.5 × 10^{-5} mol/L), and water solution after seven-day contact with PA-11/PHMG-NS (7%) film (4).

Even though the non-covalent association between the bioactive compounds and the polymer matrix has been a major advantage to optimise the antimicrobial performance [24,51], the question always remains: is the system contact-active or biocide-releasing? It was shown for antimicrobial polyamide nanocomposites containing silver- or copper-based inorganic biocides that they release Ag or Cu ions into the surrounding aqueous medium in a steady and prolonged manner [19–22]. At the same time, biocide release was detected neither for polylactides, polyamides or silicones containing hydrophobic PHMG salts [35–38] nor for PA-6 containing cationic biocide-modified organoclays [39]. Thus, the mode of antimicrobial action of these materials can be determined as contact-active because of the non-leachable form of the biocide. Bacterial membranes are known to carry a large number of negative charges and therefore can adsorb on positively charged polymer surfaces [24,46,63]. Upon adsorption on a cationic solid substrate, the electrostatic compensation of the negative charges of the bacterial envelope is provided by the cationic charges of the substrate, and the bacteria lose their natural counterions. It has been suggested that this counterion release initiates bacterial death. In the case of Gram-negative bacteria such as *E. coli*, Mg^{2+} and Ca^{2+} ions, which stabilise the outer membrane of the bacterial cell, are expelled during the adsorption of the bacteria on the charged substrate. Thus, the outer membrane is destabilised, leading to non-viable cells [24].

In our study, the low antimicrobial activity of PA-11/PHMG-NS films against planktonic bacteria may indicate that its antimicrobial action is based on contact-killing. The negligible release of polymeric biocide from polyamide matrix may also testify in favour of this assumption. As mentioned above, the antibiofilm properties of both PA-11/PHMG-NS (7%) and (10%) films were not altered after a seven-day water exposure, suggesting that the contact-killing mode of action as well as the anti-eDNA effect were the main elements in the antibiofilm/antifouling mechanism.

3. Materials and Methods

3.1. Materials

The following chemicals were used without further purification for the synthesis of the polymeric biocide: guanidine hydrochloride, 98% (Applichem, Darmstadt, Germany), hexamethylenediamine

(98%), 2-naphtalenesulphonic acid, sodium salt (technical grade, Sigma-Aldrich, Taufkirchen, Germany), and ethanol (95%). Rilsan®PA11 (granules) was supplied by Arkema (King of Prussia, PA, USA).

3.2. Synthesis of Polymeric Biocide PHMG-NS

PHMG-NS was synthesised according to the following procedure (Scheme 1).

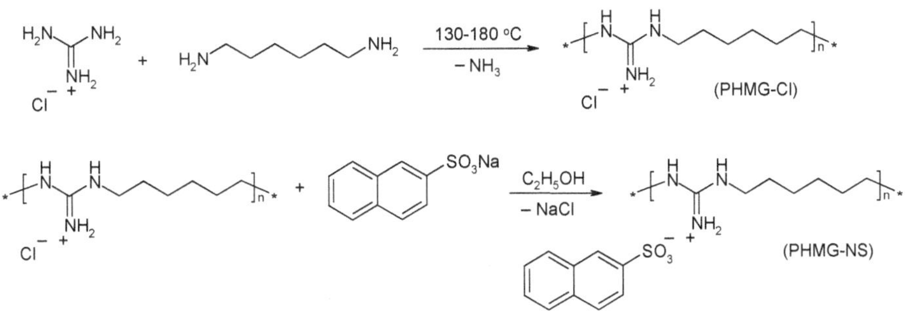

Scheme 1. Synthesis of polymeric biocide PHMG-NS.

A mixture of guanidine hydrochloride (10 g, 0.104 mol) and hexamethylenediamine (12 g, 0.103 mol) was placed into a round-bottomed flask (250 mL) and heated at 80 °C for 4 h under constant stirring. Subsequently, the reaction was carried out for 5 h at 130–140 °C and 5 h at 180 °C to obtain a highly viscous melt. After cooling the reaction mixture to room temperature, a vitreous solid PHMG-Cl was obtained. It was dissolved in water (200 mL) and precipitated by adding 100 mL of a saturated sodium chloride solution. The polymer was isolated by decantation and dried at 140 °C for 24 h. The product yield was 13 g (72%). The intrinsic viscosity was 0.09 dL/g for a PHMG-Cl solution in 0.1 N NaCl at 25 °C.

Sodium 2-naphtalenesulfonate (13.6 g, 0.06 mol) was added to the solution of PHMG-Cl (10 g, 0.055 mol) in 200 mL of ethanol and the mixture was stirred for 12 h at 60 °C (Scheme 1). The formed sodium chloride precipitate was filtered off and the solution was poured into water (500 mL). The white slurry of PHMG-NS was separated by the decantation and washed with water. The wet product was dried at 130 °C for 24 h and then powdered in an agate mortar. The product yield was 16 g (87%). The PHMG-NS salt has a melting point of 105–110 °C. Its water solubility was found to be 0.24 g/L.

The ^{1}H NMR and elemental analysis data for PHMG-Cl and PHMG-DBS are shown in the Supplementary Materials.

3.3. Preparation of PA-11/PHMG-NS Composite Films

PA-11 granules were dissolved in formic acid (98%) at 50 °C to obtain a 10 wt%. solution. An equal volume of isopropanol was added dropwise to the stirred solution to precipitate the polyamide powder. It was filtered off and then washed successively with sodium hydroxide (5%) and water. The obtained fine powder was dried in vacuum (1 mbar) at 70 °C for 12 h.

The mixture of PA-11 and PHMG-NS powders was ground for 3 min in an agate mortar followed by compression moulding at 240 °C. Composite polyamide films (45 mm × 45 mm) were obtained containing 5, 7 and 10 wt% of polymeric biocide.

3.4. Characterisation of PA-11/PHMG-NS Composite

To characterise the chemical properties of the modified PA-11 films, the samples were first placed on the Platinum diamond ATR module and IR spectra were recorded using a Bruker Vertex-70V FTIR spectrometer (all Bruker Optics Inc., Ettlingen, Germany) equipped with a L-alanine-doped deuterated triglycine sulphate (DLaDTGS) detector. Spectra were acquired with a resolution of 2 cm^{-1} in the spectral region from 400 to 5000 cm^{-1} as the co-addition of 100 scans. Acquisition of these spectra was done with Bruker OPUS software (version 6.5, Ettlingen, Germany).

Mechanical testing of the polyamide samples was performed using a P-50 universal tensile testing machine (Milaform, Moscow, Russia) at a deformation rate of 10 mm/min. The obtained films were cut into specimens with the size of 40 mm × 10 mm × 0.15 mm. An average value (with standard deviation) for the tensile strength was obtained from three samples of each film.

Contact angle measurements were performed using a Drop Shape Analyzer DSA25E (Krüss, Hamburg, Germany) by the sessile drop method. The contact angle was estimated, using ImageJ software (version 1.50i, Bethesda, MD, USA), as the tangent normal to the water drop (3 mL) at the intersection between the sessile drop and the polymer surface. All reported contact angles are the average of at least five measurements taken at different locations on the polymer surface.

The surface charge density of the PA-11/PHMG-NS films was determined with the contactless inductive method [37]. The surface charge of the samples was determined by comparing the voltage amplitudes of the capacitor with PA-11 films and of the capacitor with a known calibrated electret. The measurements were carried out immediately after the samples were positioned into the measuring assembly, as well as 5 min later to estimate the changes of the surface charge with time.

Thermal gravimetric analysis (TGA) data for the polymeric biocide and modified PA-11 samples were obtained using a TGA Q500 (TA Instruments, Eschborn, Germany). About 10 mg of each sample were heated from 30 °C to 700 °C with a heating rate of 10 °C/min under an air atmosphere.

3.5. Biocide Release

The solubility of pure PHMG-NS in water was determined by stirring 1 g of the polymeric biocide powder in 100 mL of water for 24 h at room temperature. Then, the solution was filtered and evaporated. The weight of the solid residue was determined.

The release of PHMG-NS from the PA-11 film was investigated by UV-visible spectrophotometric analysis using a Jenway 6850 spectrometer (Stone, United Kingdom). The calibrating graph was obtained by measuring the absorbance of PHMG-NS aqueous solutions in a concentration range of 1×10^{-5}–5×10^{-5} mol/L at 227 nm, which is the characteristic peak of the naphthalene ring. For the evaluation of the leaching rate of polymeric biocide, 2 g of PA-11/PHMG-NS (7%) film was placed into a closed 1 L conical flask containing 750 mL of deionised water. The sample was kept at 37 °C at constant stirring. Three millilitres of each solution were taken periodically and analysed by measuring the absorbance at said wavelength to determine the concentration of the released biocide. The biocide release ratio was determined as the percentage of PHMG-NS released into the solution from its total quantity in the film. Each measurement has been repeated three times.

3.6. Biofilm Assay

The resistance to biofouling, i.e., the antibiofilm characteristics of the PA-11/PHMG-NS films, was evaluated by assessing the capability of two biofilm-forming model strains, *E. coli* K12 and *Staphylococcus aureus* ATCC 25923, to form attached biofilms on the surface of polymer samples following three days of stationary incubation. Each PA-11/PHMG-NS film was cut into pieces of 1 cm^2 each. The pieces were sterilised by autoclaving at 105 °C for 30 min. Water-treated pieces of plastics were prepared by exposition of 1 g of plastic films in 500 mL of deionised water for 7 days.

Each piece was then placed in a well of a sterile polystyrene 24-well plate in which 2 mL of Luria Broth (LB) medium were added, inoculated with 10 µL of an overnight inoculum culture containing 10^9 CFU/mL; there were eight replicas per variant. The plate was incubated at 37 °C for 72 h. The control for incubation was performed by incubating the films in sterile LB with four replicas. After incubation, each film piece was removed and washed three times to remove planktonic and poorly attached biofilm mass.

To measure the level of biofilm biomass attached to the plastics, a Crystal Violet assay was performed. To this end, eight pieces with attached biofilms were placed in a glass vial, stained with

1 mL of a 0.05% Crystal Violet stain solution for 30 min, and washed three times in water, after which the stain was eluted by incubating the piece in 500 µL of 96% ethanol for an hour. The eluted stain in each 200 µL aliquot was quantified by absorbance measurements at 570 nm in a BioTek ELx800 microplate spectrophotometer. Net biofilm attachment was calculated by subtracting the control values, corresponding to an incubation in LB.

A biofilm metabolic assay was performed for eight pieces as well. For this, each piece was placed in a glass vial with 500 µL of a 0.05% methylthiazolyldiphenyltetrazolium bromide (MTT) solution (Sigma-Aldrich, Taufkirchen, Germany) and incubated at 37 °C for 20 h. Then, the film and the MTT solution were removed from each vial and placed in a 1.5 mL plastic tube, which was spun down at 13,000× g for 15 min (Eppendorf 5424 Microcentrifuge (Fisher Scientific, Pittsburg, PA, USA). The supernatant was discarded and the sediment was dissolved again in 500 µL of DMSO. Again, staining intensities of 200 µL were evaluated using absorbance measurements at 570 nm. Net biofilm metabolic activity was calculated by subtracting the control values, corresponding to an incubation in LB.

3.7. Bacteria Toxicity Assay

The toxicity of the PA-11/PHMG-NS films was assessed on the basis of the optical density as well as the colony forming units number of the overbiofilm planktonic culture. For this, 200 µL of the overbiofilm planktonic culture of each treatment were transferred into a sterile polystyrene 96-well plate. The optical density was measured spectrophotometrically at 570 nm [64]. One hundred microlitres of each overbiofilm planktonic culture were used for preparing dilution series which were subsequently plated on LB agar plates for a colony forming units determination.

3.8. eDNA Assay

The amount of extracellular DNA (eDNA) was measured after its precipitation from cell-free supernatants. For this, 500 µL of the aforementioned biofilm culture and 550 µL of the bottom culture containing solid–liquid interface biofilms of the same microcosm, in which the PA-11/PHMG-NS films had been incubated for 72 h, were vortexed for 1 min and spun down at 13,000× g for 15 min (Eppendorf 5424 Microcentrifuge). Five hundred microlitres of each supernatant were removed and transferred into new 1.5 mL plastic tubes. One millilitre of chilled 96% ethanol and 50 µL of a 3 M sodium acetate solution (pH 5.2) were added to the supernatants, which were then incubated overnight at −20 °C. Then, the samples were spun down at 13,000× g for 15 min and the supernatants were removed. One millilitre of 70% ethanol was added into each of the tubes, which were then spun down again at 13,000× g for 15 min to wash the pellet. The supernatants were removed and the sediments were dried to full ethanol evaporation. Two hundred microlitres of Tris-EDTA (TE) buffer were added to dissolve each sample. eDNA concentration was measured using a NanoDrop 2000 spectrometer (Thermo Fisher Scientific, Waltham, MA, USA).

3.9. Statistical Analysis

The obtained data were processed statistically using the software package Statistica 7 or MS Excel for Windows. All results are presented as mean ± standard deviation. A value of $p < 0.05$ was considered statistically significant.

4. Conclusions

A new, thermally stable polymeric biocide polyhexamethylene guanidine 2-naphtalenesulfonate (PHMG-NS) was synthesised by anion metathesis between polyhexamethylene guanidine hydrochloride and sodium 2-naphtalenesulfonate. In dried conditions, PHMG-NS can be prepared as fine powder, which makes it suitable as an antimicrobial additive for polymer articles and protective coatings. It has a melting point of 105–110 °C and a limited water solubility of 0.024 g/L. According to thermogravimetric analysis, PHMG-NS is thermally stable to at least 357 °C, which indicates its availability for joint melt processing with polyamide resins by common methods. Polyamide 11 (PA-11) films containing 5, 7 and 10 wt% of PHMG-NS have been obtained by compression moulding at 240 °C. The introduction of PHMG-NS into PA-11 films was found to significantly increase its surface hydrophilicity, as well as positive surface charge density. PA-11/PHMG-NS composites showed no changes of tensile strength at PHMG-NS content up to 7%, as well as high thermal decomposition point about 400 °C.

The antibiofilm properties of PA-11 modified with the polymeric biocide PHMG-NS were evaluated using the opportunistic biofilm-forming model bacterial strains *E. coli* K12 and *S. aureus* ATCC 25923. There was a substantial decrease in biofilm metabolic activity as well as in biofilm biomass for PA-11 films containing 7% and 10% of PHMG-NS for both strains. At the same time, there was no significant difference between the different PA-11/PHMG-NS films with regard to their effect on the planktonic bacteria in a biofilm-forming culture. The last fact may be due to the negligible biocide release into the medium. Indeed, the study of PHMG-NS release behaviour from the PA-11 films showed a low leaching ratio of less than 1% after 21 days, confirming its high retention in polymer matrix and maintenance its antibiofilm characteristics. Thus, it has been suggested that at least one mechanism of antibiofilm activity of PHMG-NS-containing PA-11 is associated with a reduction of eDNA, which affects the initial stages of bacterial biofilm formation and, thus, may decrease the spread of antibiotic resistance genes in a hospital-related environment.

Supplementary Materials: Supplementary materials can be found at http://www.mdpi.com/1422-0067/20/2/348/s1.

Author Contributions: O.M. designed and performed antibiofilm experiments, as well as spectrophotometric control of biocide release; J.-F.B. performed infrared analysis; O.T. synthesised polymeric biocide and prepared polymer composites; S.M. performed electrophysical investigations; T.C. performed thermal investigations; O.D. performed surface analysis; G.P. analysed the data; S.R. conceived and designed the experiments; and O.M. and S.R. wrote the paper.

Acknowledgments: The authors would like to thank NATO Science for Peace and Security multi-year project SPS 984834 "Fighting maritime corrosion and biofouling with task-specific ionic compounds" for its financial support of the project.

Conflicts of Interest: The authors declare no conflict of interest.

Abbreviations

PA-11	Polyamide 11
PHMG-Cl	Polyhexamethylene guanidine hydrochloride
PHMG-NS	Polyhexamethylene guanidine 2-naphtalenesulfonate
LB	Luria Broth
MTT	Methylthiazolyldiphenyltetrazolium bromide
eDNA	Extracellular DNA
TE buffer	Tris-EDTA buffer
CFU	colony forming units

References

1. *RILSAN®PA11: Created from a Renewable Source (Product Data Sheet)*; Arkema: Puteaux, France, 2005.
2. *Fine Powders: A Durable Coating for Durable Products (Product Data Sheet)*; Arkema: Colombes, France, 2010.
3. Klun, U.; Friedrich, Z.; Kržan, A. Polyamide 6 fibre degradation by a lignolytic fungus. *Polym. Degrad. Stab.* **2003**, *79*, 99–104. [CrossRef]
4. Tomita, K.; Ikeda, N.; Ueno, A. Isolation and characterization of a thermophilic bacterium, Geobacillus thermocatenulatus, degrading nylon 12 and nylon 66. *Biotechnol. Lett.* **2003**, *25*, 1743–1746. [CrossRef] [PubMed]
5. Chonde Sonal, G.; Chonde Sachin, G.; Raut, P.D. Studies on Degradation of synthetic polymer Nylon 6 and Nylon 6, 6 by Pseudomonas aeruginosa NCIM 2242. *IJETCAS* **2013**, *4*, 362–369. [CrossRef]

6. Kaali, P.; Strömberg, E.; Karlsson, S. Prevention of biofilm assotiated infections and degradation of polymeric materials used in biomedical applications. In *Biomedical Engineering, Trends in Material Science*; Laskovski, A.N., Ed.; In Tech: Rijeka, Slovenia, 2011; Chapter 22, pp. 513–541.
7. Moshynets, O.V.; Spiers, A.J. Viewing biofilms within the larger context of bacterial aggregations. In *Microbial Biofilms—Importance and Applications*; Dhanasekaran, D., Thajuddin, N., Eds.; InTech: Rijeka, Croatia, 2016; pp. 3–22, ISBN 978-953-2436-8.
8. Koza, A.; Kusmierska, A.; McLauglin, K.; Moshynets, O.; Spiers, A.J. Adaptive radiation of P. fluorescens SBW25 in experimental microcosms provides an understanding of the evolutionary ecology and molecular biology of A-L interface biofilm-formation. *FEMS Microbiol. Lett.* **2017**, *364*. [CrossRef]
9. McLaughlin, K.; Folorunso, A.O.; Deeni, Y.Y.; Foster, D.; Gorbatiuk, O.; Hapca, S.M.; Immoor, C.; Koza, A.; Mohammed, I.U.; Moshynets, O.; et al. Biofilm formation and cellulose expression by Bordetella avium 197N, the causative agent of bordetellosis in birds and an opportunistic respiratory pathogen in humans. *Res. Microbiol.* **2017**, *168*, 419–430. [CrossRef] [PubMed]
10. Donlan, R.M.; Costerton, J.W. Biofilms: Survival mechanisms of clinically relevant microorganisms. *Clin. Microbiol. Rev.* **2002**, *15*, 167–193. [CrossRef] [PubMed]
11. Nichols, D. *Biocides in Plastics. Rapra Review Reports*; Rapra Technology: Shrewsbury, UK, 2005; Volume 15, Report 180.
12. Rabin, N.; Zheng, Y.; Opoku-Temeng, C.; Du, Y.; Bonsu, E.; Sintim, H.O. Agents that inhibits bacterial biofilm formation. *Future Med. Chem.* **2015**, *7*, 647–671. [CrossRef] [PubMed]
13. Vitiello, G.; Pezzella, A.; Zanfardino, A.; Varcamonti, M.; Silvestri, B.; Costantini, A.; Branda, F.; Luciani, G. Titania as driving agent for DHICA polymerization: A novel strategy for the design of bioinspired antimicrobial nanomaterials. *J. Mater. Chem. B* **2015**, *3*, 2808–2815. [CrossRef]
14. Vitiello, G.; Pezzella, A.; Zanfardino, A.; Varcamonti, M.; Silvestri, B.; Giudicianni, P.; Costantini, A.; Varcamonti, M.; Branda, F.; Luciani, G. Antimicrobial activity of eumelanin-based hybrids: The role of TiO_2 in modulating the structure and biological performance. *Mater. Sci. Eng. C* **2017**, *75*, 454–462. [CrossRef]
15. Vitiello, G.; Silvestri, B.; Luciani, G. Learning from nature: Bioinspired strategies towards antimicrobial nanostructured systems. *Curr. Top. Med. Chem.* **2018**, *18*, 22–41. [CrossRef] [PubMed]
16. Kuratsuji, T.; Shimizu, H. Polyamide Based Antibacterial Powder Paint Composition. U.S. Patent 20030171452, 11 September 2003.
17. Lapeyre, A.; Ganset, C. Polyamide-Based Powder and Its Use for Obtaining an Antibacterial Coating. U.S. Patent 8303970, 4 August 2005.
18. Williams, R.L.; Doherty, P.J.; Vince, D.J.; Grashoff, G.J.; Williams, D.F. The biocompatibility of silver. *Crit. Rev. Biocompat.* **1989**, *5*, 221–223.
19. Kumar, R.; Münstedt, H. Silver ion release from antimicrobial polyamide/silver composites. *Biomaterials* **2005**, *26*, 2081–2088. [CrossRef] [PubMed]
20. Damm, C.; Münstedt, H.; Rösch, A. Long-term antimicrobial polyamide 6/silver-nanocomposites. *J. Mater. Sci.* **2007**, *42*, 6067–6073. [CrossRef]
21. Damm, C.; Münstedt, H.; Rösch, A. The antimicrobial efficacy of polyamide 6/silver-nano- and microcomposites. *Mater. Chem. Phys.* **2008**, *108*, 61–66. [CrossRef]
22. Thokala, N.; Kealey, C.; Kennedy, J.; Brady, D.B.; Farrell, J.B. Characterization of polyamide 11/copper antimicrobial composites for medical device applications. *Mater. Sci. Eng. C* **2017**, *78*, 1179–1186. [CrossRef] [PubMed]
23. Gilbert, P.; Moore, L.E. Cationic antiseptics: Diversity of action under a common epithet. *J. Appl. Microbiol.* **2005**, *99*, 703–715. [CrossRef] [PubMed]
24. Carmona-Ribeiro, A.M.; de Melo Carrasco, L.D. Cationic antimicrobial polymers and their assemblies. *Int. J. Mol. Sci.* **2013**, *14*, 9906–9946. [CrossRef]
25. Zhang, Y.M.; Jiang, J.M.; Chen, Y.M. Synthesis and antimicrobial activity of polymeric guanidine and biguanidine salts. *Polymer* **1999**, *40*, 6189–6198. [CrossRef]
26. Oulè, M.K.; Azinwi, R.; Bernier, A.M.; Kablan, T.; Maupertuis, A.M.; Mauler, S.; Koffi- Nevry, R.; Dembèlè, K.; Forbes, L.; Diop, L. Polyhexamethylene guanidine hydrochloride-based disinfectant: A novel tool to fight meticillin-resistant Staphylococcus aureus and nosocomial infections. *J. Med. Microbiol.* **2008**, *57*, 1523–1528. [CrossRef]

27. Qian, L.; Guan, Y.; He, B.; Xiao, H. Modified guanidine polymers: Synthesis and antimicrobial mechanism revealed by AFM. *Polymer* **2008**, *49*, 2471–2475. [CrossRef]
28. Zhou, Z.; Wei, D.; Guan, Y.; Zheng, A.; Zhong, J.-J. Damage of Escherichia coli membrane by bactericidal agent polyhexamethylene guanidine hydrochloride: Micrographic evidences. *J. Appl. Microbiol.* **2010**, *108*, 898–907. [CrossRef]
29. Zhou, Z.; Wei, D.; Guan, Y.; Zheng, A.; Zhong, J.-J. Extensive in vitro activity of guanidine hydrochloride polymer analogs against antibiotics-resistant clinically isolated strains. *Mater. Sci. Eng.* **2011**, *31*, 1836–1843. [CrossRef]
30. Zhou, Z.; Zheng, A.; Zhong, J. Interactions of biocidal guanidine hydrochloride polymer analogs with model membranes: A comparative biophysical study. *Acta Biochim. Biophys. Sin.* **2011**, *43*, 729–737. [CrossRef]
31. Choi, H.; Kim, K.-J.; Lee, D.J. Antifungal activity of the cationic antimicrobial polymer-polyhexamethylene guanidine hydrochloride and its mode of action. *Fungal Biol.* **2017**, *121*, 53–60. [CrossRef]
32. Han, J.-S.; Lim, K.-M.; Park, S.-J.; Song, W.-S. Polyhexamethyleneguanidine Phosphate Powder, Method of Making the Same and Antimicrobial Resin Containing the Same. Eur. Patent 1 110 948, 17 May 2001.
33. Protasov, A.; Bardeau, J.-F.; Morozovskaya, I.; Boretska, M.; Cherniavska, T.; Petrus, L.; Tarasyuk, O.; Metelytsia, L.; Kopernyk, I.; Kalashnikova, L.; et al. New promising antifouling agent based on polymeric biocide polyhexamethylene guanidine molybdate. *J. Environ. Toxicol.* **2016**, *36*, 2543–2551. [CrossRef]
34. Swiontek Brzezinska, M.; Walczak, M.; Jankiewizs, U.; Pejchalová, M. Antimicrobial activity of polyhexamethylene guanidine derivatives introduced into polycaprolactone. *J. Polym. Environ.* **2018**, *26*, 589–595. [CrossRef]
35. Walczak, M.; Richert, A.; Burkowska-But, A. The effect of polyhexamethylene guanidine hydrochloride (PHMG) derivatives introduced into polylactide (PLA) on the activity of bacterial enzymes. *J. Ind. Microbiol. Biotechnol.* **2014**, *41*, 1719–1724. [CrossRef]
36. Rogalskyy, S.; Bardeau, J.-F.; Tarasyuk, O.; Fatyeyeva, K. Fabrication of new antifungal polyamide-12 material. *Polym. Int.* **2012**, *61*, 686–691. [CrossRef]
37. Rogalsky, S.; Bardeau, J.-F.; Wu, H.; Lyoshina, L.; Bulko, O.; Tarasyuk, O.; Makhno, S.; Cherniavska, T.; Kyselov, Y.; Koo, J.H. Structural, thermal and antibacterial properties of polyamide 11/polymeric biocide polyhexamethylene guanidine dodecylbenzenesulfonate composites. *J. Mater. Sci.* **2016**, *51*, 7716–7730. [CrossRef]
38. Ghamrawi, S.; Bouchara, J.-P.; Tarasyuk, O.; Rogalsky, S.; Lyoshina, L.; Bulko, O.; Bardeau, J.-F. Promising silicones modified with cationic biocides for the development of antimicrobial medical devices. *Mater. Sci. Eng. C* **2017**, *75*, 969–979. [CrossRef]
39. Nigmatullin, R.; Gao, F.; Konovalova, V. Permanent, non-leaching antimicrobial polyamide nanocomposites based on organoclays modified with a cationic polymer. *Macromol. Mater. Eng.* **2009**, *294*, 795–805. [CrossRef]
40. Li, G.; Shen, J. A study of pyridinium-type functional polymers. IV. Behavioral features of the antibacterial activity of insoluble pyridinium-type polymers. *J. Appl. Polym. Sci.* **2000**, *78*, 676–684. [CrossRef]
41. Desai, D.G.; Liao, K.S.; Cevallos, M.E.; Trautner, B.W. Silver or nitrofurazone impregnation of urinary catheters has a minimal effect on uropathogen adherence. *J. Urol.* **2010**, *184*, 2565–2571. [CrossRef]
42. Ghatak, P.D.; Mathew-Steiner, S.S.; Pandey, P.; Roy, S.; Se, C.K. A surfactant polymer dressing potentiates antimicrobial efficacy in biofilm disruption. *Sci. Rep.* **2018**, *8*, 873. [CrossRef]
43. Shao, Q.; Fan, Y.; Yang, L.; Gao, Y.Q. Counterion effects on the denaturing activity of guanidinium cation to protein. *J. Chem. Theory Comput.* **2012**, *8*, 4364–4373. [CrossRef]
44. Jansen, B.; Peters, G. Modern strategies in the prevention of polymer-associated infections. *J. Hosp. Infect.* **1991**, *19*, 83–88. [CrossRef]
45. An, Y.H.; Friedman, R.J. Concise review of mechanisms of bacterial adhesion to biomaterial surfaces. *J. Biomed. Mater. Res.* **1998**, *43*, 338–348. [CrossRef]
46. Kügler, R.; Bouloussa, O.; Rondelez, F. Evidence of a charge-density threshold for optimum efficiency of biocidal cationic surfaces. *Microbiology* **2005**, *151*, 1341–1348. [CrossRef]
47. Reisner, A.; Haagensen, J.A.J.; Schembri, M.A.; Zechner, E.L.; Molin, S. Development and maturation of Escherichia coli K-12 biofilms. *Mol. Microbiol.* **2003**, *48*, 933–946. [CrossRef]
48. Avila-Novoa, M.G.; Iniguez-Moreno, M.; Solis-Velazquez, O.A.; Gonzalez-Gomez, J.P.; Guerrero-Medina, P.J.; Gutierrez-Lomeli, M. Biofilm formation by Staphyloccus aureus isolated from food contact surface in the dairy industry of Jalisco, Mexico. *J. Food Qual.* **2018**. [CrossRef]

49. Zhou, Z.; Wei, D.; Lu, Y. Polyhexamethylene guanidine hydrochloride bactericidal advantages over chlorhexidine bigluconate against ESKAPE bacteria. *Biotechnol. Appl. Biochem.* **2014**. [CrossRef]
50. Moshynets, O.; Koza, A.; Dello Sterpaio, P.; Kordium, V.; Spiers, A.J. Up-dating the Cholodny method using PET films to sample microbial communities in soil. *Biopolym. Cell* **2011**, *27*, 199–205. [CrossRef]
51. Siedenbiedel, F.; Tiller, J.C. Antimicrobial polymers in solution and on surfaces: Overview and functional principles. *Polymers* **2012**, *4*, 46–71. [CrossRef]
52. Wang, H.; Chen, H.; Wang, F.; Wei, D.; Wang, X. An improved 3-(4,5-dimethylthiazol-2-yl)-2,5-diphenyl tetrazolium bromide (MTT) reduction assay for evaluating the viability of *Escherichia coli* cells. *J. Microbiol. Methods* **2010**, *82*, 330–333. [CrossRef]
53. Flemming, H.C.; Wingender, J. The biofilm matrix. *Nat. Rev. Microbiol.* **2010**, *8*, 623–633. [CrossRef]
54. Allesen-Holm, M.; Barken, K.B.; Yang, L.; Klausen, M.; Webb, J.S.; Kjelleberg, S.; Molin, S.; Givskov, M.; Tolker-Neilsen, T. A characterization of DNA release in *Pseudomonas aeruginosa* cultures and biofilms. *Mol. Microbiol.* **2006**, *59*, 1114–1128. [CrossRef]
55. Thomas, V.C.; Hiromasa, Y.; Harma, N.; Thurlow, L.; Tomich, J.; Hancock, L.E. A fratricidal mechanism is responsible for eDNA release and contributes to biofilm development of *Enterococcus faecalis*. *Mol. Micriol.* **2009**, *72*, 1022–1036. [CrossRef]
56. Montanaro, L.; Poggi, A.; Visai, L.; Ravaioli, S.; Campoccia, D.; Speziale, P.; Arciola, C.R. Extracellular DNA in biofilms. *Int. J. Artif. Organs* **2011**, *34*, 824–831. [CrossRef]
57. Christner, M.; Heinze, C.; Busch, M.; Franke, G.; Hentschke, M.; Duhring, S.B.; Buttner, H.; Kotasinska, M.; Wischnewski, V.; Kroll, G.; et al. sarA negatively regulats staphylococcus epidermidis biofilm formation by modulation expression of 1 MDa extracellular matrix binding protein and autolysis-dependent release of eDNA. *Mol. Microbiol.* **2012**, *86*, 394–410. [CrossRef]
58. Wu, J.; Xi, C. Evaluation of different methods for extracting extracellular DNA from the biofilm matrix. *Appl. Environ. Microbiol.* **2009**, 5390–5395. [CrossRef]
59. Schwartz, K.; Ganesan, M.; Payne, D.E.; Solomon, M.J.; Boles, B.R. Extracellular DNA facilitates the formation of functional amyloids in Staphylococcus aureus biofilms. *Mol. Microbiol.* **2016**, *99*, 123–134. [CrossRef]
60. Hannan, S.; Ready, D.; Jasni, A.S.; Rogers, M.; Pratten, J.; Roberts, A.P. Transfer of antibiotic resistance by transformation with eDNA within oral biofilms. *FEMS Immunol. Med. Microbiol.* **2010**, *59*, 345–349. [CrossRef]
61. Itzek, A.; Zheng, L.; Chen, Z.; Merritt, J.; Kreth, J. Hydrogen peroxide-dependent DNA release and transfer of antibiotic resistance genes in *Streptococcus gordonii*. *J. Bacteriol.* **2011**, *193*, 6912–6922. [CrossRef]
62. Wei, D.; Zhou, R.; Guan, Y.; Zheng, A.; Zhang, Y. Investigation on the reaction between polyhexamethylene guanidine hydrochloride oligomer and glycidyl methacrylate. *J. Appl. Polym. Sci.* **2013**, *127*, 666–674. [CrossRef]
63. Lewis, K.; Klibanov, A.M. Surpassing nature: Rational design of sterile-surface materials. *Trends Biotechnol.* **2005**, *23*, 343–348. [CrossRef]
64. Sambrook, J.; Fritsch, E.F.; Maniatis, T. *Molecular Cloning: A Laboratory Manual*, 2nd ed.; Cold Spring Harbor Laboratory Press, Cold Spring Harbor: New York, NY, USA, 1989; Volume 3, ap. B.11 and B.23.

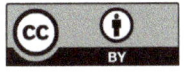

© 2019 by the authors. Licensee MDPI, Basel, Switzerland. This article is an open access article distributed under the terms and conditions of the Creative Commons Attribution (CC BY) license (http://creativecommons.org/licenses/by/4.0/).

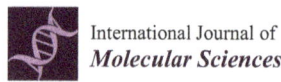

Article

Synthesis, Characterization, and Antimicrobial Properties of Peptides Mimicking Copolymers of Maleic Anhydride and 4-Methyl-1-pentene

Marian Szkudlarek [1], Elisabeth Heine [1,*], Helmut Keul [1], Uwe Beginn [2,*] and Martin Möller [1,*]

[1] DWI Leibniz Institute for Interactive Materials and Institute of Technical and Macromolecular Chemistry, RWTH Aachen University, Forckenbeckstraße 50, D-52056 Aachen, Germany; szkudlarekmh@gmail.com (M.S.); keul@dwi.rwth-aachen.de (H.K.)
[2] Institut für Chemie, Universität Osnabrück, OMC, Barbarastraße 7, D-49076 Osnabrück, Germany
* Correspondence: heine@dwi.rwth-aachen.de (E.H.); ubeginn@uni-osnabrueck.de (U.B.); moeller@dwi.rwth-aachen.de (M.M.); Tel.: +49-541-9692790 (U.B.); +49-241-8023302 (M.M.)

Received: 9 August 2018; Accepted: 29 August 2018; Published: 4 September 2018

Abstract: Synthetic amphiphilic copolymers with strong antimicrobial properties mimicking natural antimicrobial peptides were obtained via synthesis of an alternating copolymer of maleic anhydride and 4-methyl-1-pentene. The obtained copolymer was modified by grafting with 3-(dimethylamino)-1-propylamine (DMAPA) and imidized in a one-pot synthesis. The obtained copolymer was modified further to yield polycationic copolymers by means of quaternization with methyl iodide and dodecyl iodide, as well as by being sequentially quaternized with both of them. The antimicrobial properties of obtained copolymers were tested against *Escherichia coli*, *Pseudomonas aeruginosa*, *Staphylococcus epidermidis*, and *Staphylococcus aureus*. Both tested quaternized copolymers were more active against the Gram-negative *E. coli* than against the Gram-positive *S. aureus*. The copolymer modified with both iodides was best when tested against *E. coli* and, comparing all three copolymers, also exhibited the best effect against *S. aureus*. Moreover, it shows (limited) selectivity to differentiate between mammalian cells and bacterial cell walls. Comparing the minimum inhibitory concentration (MIC) of Nisin against the Gram-positive bacteria on the molar basis instead on the weight basis, the difference between the effect of Nisin and the copolymer is significantly lower.

Keywords: cationic polymers; imidization; quaternization; antimicrobial properties; hemolytic activity

1. Introduction

Since in 1960s, Cornell and Donaruma [1] have described 2-methacryloxytropones-based polymers that exhibited antibacterial activity, and antimicrobial copolymers have since gained significant interest. Over the last decades, a large number of publications and multiple reviews exploring antimicrobial polymers have been published. In the 1990s and at the beginning of 21st century, the main focus was on the synthesis and chemical nature of the polymers [2]. For example, Kenawy et al. [3] classified antimicrobial copolymers regarding their structure as quaternary ammonium salts (QAS) [4–20], phosphonium salts [20–27], sulfonic acid derivatives (salts, sulfonamides), and N-halamines. In most recent reviews, the main focus has been on the bactericidal mechanism and influence of relevant parameters such as molecular weight and charge distribution [28]. The antimicrobial properties of maleic anhydride copolymers with olefins [29] and styrene [30–32] have been investigated since the 1960s. In all cases, succinic anhydride functionality was used as a base for further modification in order to introduce an antibacterial moiety (diamine, aminophenol, etc.). From this perspective, the modified maleic anhydride copolymers belong to one of the groups mentioned above. These polymers are usually amphiphilic and act as surfactants.

At the same time, antimicrobial peptides represent a large group of natural compounds with a broad spectrum of antimicrobial activity [33–36]. The antimicrobial activity of these molecules also comes from their amphiphilic structure [34].

In the past, much effort has been made to understand the mechanism of cytotoxicity of amphiphilic peptides. One of the examples is Melittin from bee venom, which has the highest hemolytic activity. Compared to Magainin from *Xenopus* frog skin, it has a high content of hydrophobic residues. It has a 26-amino-acid-residue-long sequence with a characteristic cluster of lysine and arginine residues. Magainins, 23-residue-long peptides, are essentially toxic for bacterial strains while being poorly hemolytic [37]. Synthetic peptides of different composition and structure have been widely investigated for their antimicrobial properties. Particular attention has been paid to peptides, which are only constituted by nonpolar leucine and charged lysine, so-called LK-peptides [37,38]. These molecules are ideally amphiphilic and proper choice of the Lys:Leu ratio as well as the chain length enables designing structures most similar to natural toxins.

With the aim to design an optimum antimicrobial polymer and to set up a structure–function relationship, many groups, including ours, have constructed amphiphilic polymers with different backbones and specific cationic and hydrophobic residues in defined ratios mimicking antimicrobial peptides. An overview on the peptide mimetic design of antimicrobial polymers can be found, e.g., in [39]. Specific design can lead to broad-spectrum antibacterials or polymers with Gram-selectivity [40].

The aim of creating a new synthetic, amphiphilic structure with strong antimicrobial properties comparable to natural antimicrobial peptides led to the choice of an alkene and maleic anhydride copolymer. Lower alkenes and maleic anhydride yield alternating copolymers. This ensures a constant 1:1 ratio of the hydrophobic and cationic part similar to those in Leu:Lys 1:1 LK-peptides. The choice of 4-methyl-1-pentene as a hydrophobic comonomer is based on the similarity of its structure with leucine (cf. Scheme 1), while the choice of maleic anhydride leaves ample space for further design of the hydrophilic part by means of chemical modification.

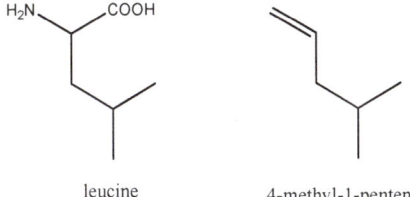

Scheme 1. Comparison of the structure of leucine with 4-methyl-1-pentene.

This work covers polymeric quaternary ammonium salts obtained by chemical modification of maleic anhydride 4-methyl-1-pentene copolymers. The free radical copolymerization of maleic anhydride with 4-methyl-1-pentene leads to alternating copolymers, which were grafted using N,N-substituted diamines. Although the antimicrobial activity of nonquaternized N,N-substituted derivatives has been reported [1], biocidal activity should be enhanced by quaternization of the tertiary amine groups with different alkyl halides. The higher biological activity of positively charged moieties can be explained by electrostatic interaction with negatively charged cell surfaces. The advantage of polycations is based on the higher charge density that allows highly extended adsorption on the bacterial cell. The expected penetration of the cell wall and disruption of the membrane by the lipophilic alkane chain releases cytoplasmic constituents and leads to the death of the cell.

2. Results and Discussion

2.1. Copolymerization of Maleic Anhydride with 4-Methyl-1-pentene

Alternating copolymers of maleic anhydride with alkenes were obtained by free-radical copolymerization in solution in the presence of radical initiators [41–45]. However, copolymers which contain an excess of olefin have also been described in the literature [46,47], but as a general rule, alternating copolymers are formed, in particular, when an excess of anhydride was used.

The alternating copolymer of 4-methyl-1-pentene with maleic anhydride (MSA) was synthesized accordingly via free-radical polymerization. The copolymerization was carried out under homogenous conditions in anhydrous 2-butanone (MEK) at 80 °C in the presence of benzoyl peroxide (BPO) as an initiator. Scheme 2 depicts the copolymerization reaction of 4-methyl-1-pentene with maleic anhydride.

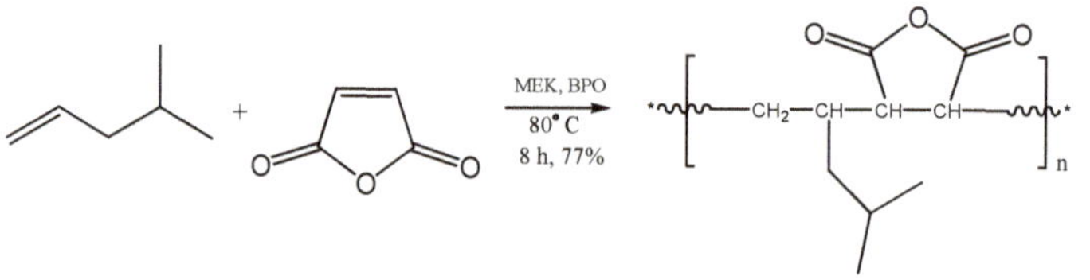

Scheme 2. Copolymerization of maleic anhydride (MSA) with 4-methyl-1-pentene.

An excess of maleic anhydride was used to ensure the equimolar composition of the resulting copolymer. The product was separated from the reaction mixture by precipitation in a Et$_2$O:MeOH (4:1, vol:vol) mixture. For its molecular weight determination by gel permeation chromatography (GPC), the succinic anhydride units of the copolymer were methanolized at room temperature. The methanolysis was necessary because maleic anhydride copolymer adsorbed on the inline filter, impeding any measurement. GPC measurement of the methanolyzed copolymer was performed in THF with PMMA standards and the determined values were: M_n = 5800 and M_w/M_n = 1.67.

The composition of the obtained polymer could not be determined by ^{1}H-NMR because of overlapping signals of both monomers. Figure 1a depicts a typical ^{1}H-NMR-spectrum of a P[MP-alt-MSA] copolymer. The range of overlapping signals between 1 and 4 ppm precludes the calculation of the polymer composition for the non-methanolyzed copolymers (MSA protons 3.25 ppm) as well as methanolyzed products (MSA protons 2.8 ppm) [47].

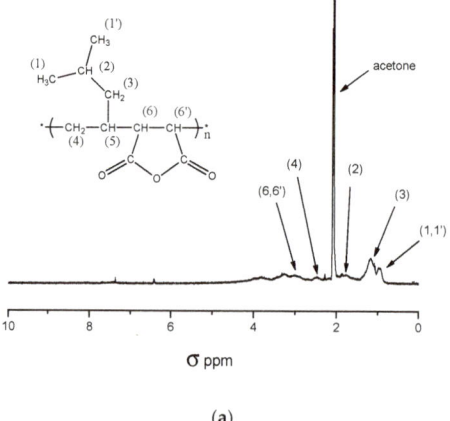

(a)

Figure 1. Cont.

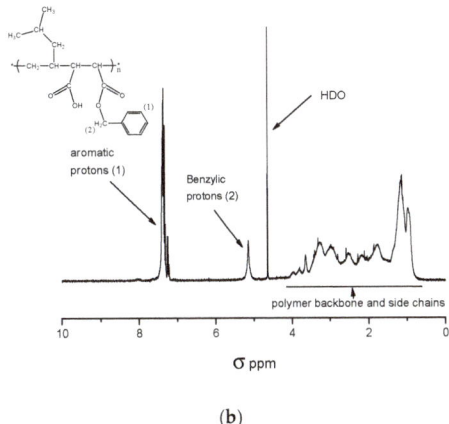

(b)

Figure 1. (a) ^{1}H-NMR spectrum of P[MP-alt-MSA] measured in acetone d$_6$; (b) ^{1}H-NMR spectrum of P[MP-alt-MSA] esterified with benzyl alcohol measured in D$_2$O.

Treatment of the copolymer with benzyl alcohol in MEK results in the formation of monobenzyl esters. This method allows determining the content of protons of succinic acid benzyl ester since the benzyl group's NMR signals were well separated from the other polymer peaks. Figure 1b depicts the ^{1}H-NMR spectrum of a P[MP-alt-MSA] copolymer after reaction with benzyl alcohol. The aromatic protons as well as the benzylic protons are well separated from the signals of the polymer backbone and the alkyl side groups. The monomer composition was calculated from the integrated signal intensity of the benzylic protons and that of the alkyl signals between 0.8 and 5.2 ppm according to Equation (1):

$$F_{MSA} = \frac{\frac{A}{m}}{\frac{A}{m} + \frac{B}{n}} \quad (1)$$

A—integration value of benzylic proton signal (σ = 4.90–5.30 ppm),
m—number of benzylic protons = 2,
B—integration value of polymer backbone and side chains proton signal (σ = 0.70–4.2),
n—number of protons in signal mentioned in B = 14.

This method was developed for determination of the MSA content in terpolymers, and it was proved that, without a catalyst, only one carboxyl group was esterified [48]. It is very useful and precise in the range of error of the used spectroscopic method. The 46 ± 5% of calculated content of succinic anhydride in the copolymer is reasonable and allowed us to assume that an alternating copolymer was obtained. The composition of the copolymer was also determined by elemental analysis. The obtained results correspond well to the composition calculated for alternating copolymer (see Table 1).

Table 1. Comparison of the experimental and calculated elemental composition of an alternating copolymer poly[(4-methyl-1-pentene)-alt-maleic anhydride] (C$_{10}$H$_{14}$O$_3$).

Composition	Carbon	Hydrogen	Oxygen
Calculated for C,H,O	65.90	7.70	26.40
Found	65.54	7.85	26.61

2.2. Grafting of DMAPA onto P[MP-alt-MSA] Copolymer

2.2.1. Model Reaction of Amidoacidification

Maleic anhydride can easily react with 3-(dimethylamino)-1-propylamine (DMAPA) to yield 3-(N,N-dimethylamino)propyl maleamic acid (M1). The reaction was carried out in chloroform by addition of the amine to MSA at room temperature and subsequent heating to 60 °C. The reaction is exothermic and proceeds easily, hence, the heating step was performed to ensure complete reaction. The product was precipitated in a fivefold excess of acetone and dried. The desired compound has been obtained as a white powder. Scheme 3 depicts the reaction of maleic anhydride with DMAPA.

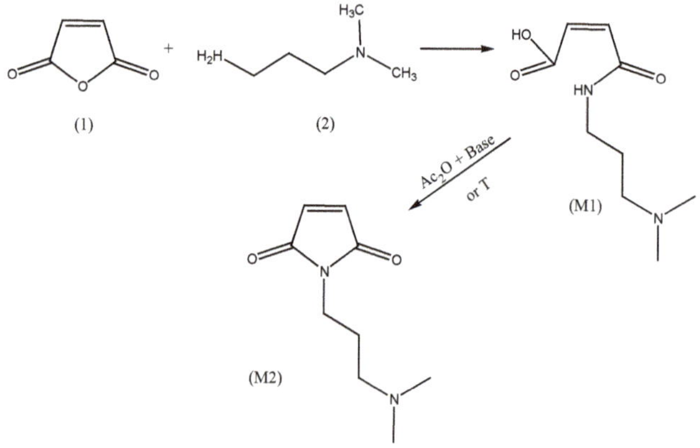

Scheme 3. Model reaction of amidoacidification and imidization of maleic anhydride with -(dimethylamino)-1-propylamine (DMAPA).

Because of its molecular asymmetry, the product can be easily identified and distinguished from nonreacted MSA by means of ^{1}H-NMR. In the course of the reaction, the single peak of MSA around 7 ppm (double bond protons) disappeared and two doublets appeared at 6.33 and 5.96 ppm, respectively (see Figure 2).

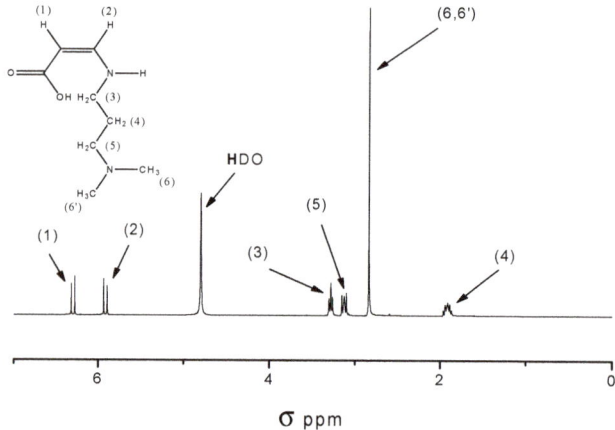

Figure 2. ^{1}H-NMR spectra of cis-3-(N,N-dimethylamino)propyl maleamic acid.

2.2.2. Amidoacidification and Imidization of Poly[(4-methyl-1-pentene)-alt-maleic Anhydride

Scheme 4 depicts the reaction of the anhydride moiety in the polymeric chain (C1) with DMAPA, yielding amidacid (C2), and followed by thermal imidization, which yields the cyclic N-substituted imide (C3).

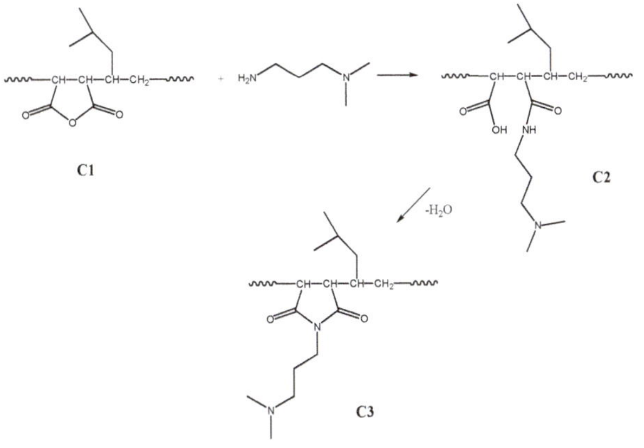

Scheme 4. Amidoacidification and imidization of MSA copolymer.

The amidoacidification of maleic anhydride copolymer with N,N-dimethylamino-1-propyl amine (DMAPA) was performed analogously to the model reaction [18,44,49–60]. The amine was added dropwise to a dimethylformamide DMF solution of the copolymer. The product precipitated from the reaction mixture and could be easily obtained in its pure form. Because of the heterogeneity of the reaction mixture, an excess of amine was used and the mixture was stirred for about 20 h to obtain an almost quantitative conversion. This intermediate product was separated by filtration and analysed.

The prepared macromolecular amic acid could not be characterized well by means of NMR spectroscopy because of the occurrence of broad overlapping signals. The IR spectra of the amidoacidified copolymer C2 shown in Figure 3 corresponded to the comparative spectrum of the model product (Figure 3 M1) from the reaction of maleic anhydride with DMAPA.

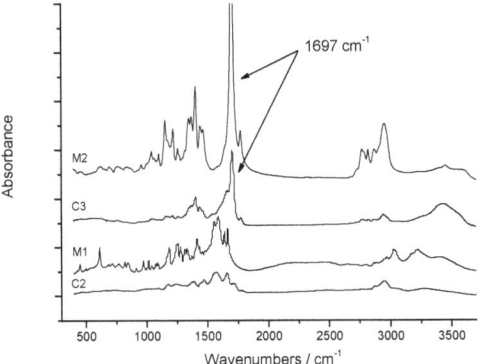

Figure 3. IR spectra of amidoacidified C2, thermally imidized C3, and model compounds M1 and M2 (3-(N,N-dimethylamino)propyl maleamic acid and 3-(N,N-dimethylaminopropyl)maleimide). The characteristic absorption band of cyclic imides in C3 and M2 at 1697 cm^{-1} are shown.

To determine the content of modified succinic anhydride moieties, elemental analysis was employed. The standard measurement for carbon, hydrogen, and nitrogen determination showed a strong correlation to the calculated values for the hydrogen and nitrogen content while measured content of carbon strongly differed from the calculated value (Table 2). However, the product was found to be hygroscopic [50] and the standard analytical treatment did not include a drying step. When one recalculates the elemental composition of the copolymer assuming that each amic acid unit additionally binds two molecules of water, the determined elemental composition becomes reasonable (see Table 2, #3).

Table 2. Comparison of the CHN elemental analysis results of the amidoacidified copolymer with calculated values.

#	Composition	Carbon	Hydrogen	Nitrogen
#1	Calculated for $C_{15}H_{28}N_2O_3$	64.30	9.80	9.80
#2	Calculated for $C_{15}H_{28}N_2O_3 \cdot 2H_2O$	56.23	10.07	8.74
#3	Found	56.18	9.73	9.78

The abovementioned hypothesis was verified in a simple experiment. A small sample of the C2 was dried in vacuo to a constant weight and placed in an open vessel on a very precise balance to absorb the humidity from air. A rapid increase in weight of the sample was observed. The calculated difference between initial mass of the sample and the mass after 12 h of exposure to humid air showed that the composition of the copolymer was $C_{15}H_{28}N_2O_3 \cdot 1.86H_2O$. The difference between the expected and obtained values can be explained as a result of insufficient drying, absorption of water during transfer from the drying oven to balance (the initial period of the experiment showed a rapid increase of the weight), degree of modification lower than assumed 100%, or impurities. Most probably it should be treated as the combination of several reasons, although the measured value of ~1.9 moles H_2O per amic acid unit is very close to the postulated stoichiometric 1:2 composition.

2.2.3. Chemical Imidization

The imidization reaction of amic acid in the presence of a dehydration agent and a base has been described in many publications [51,52,58–60]. The most common reagents are acetic anhydride in the presence of triethylamine or sodium acetate. This reaction is usually carried out under mild conditions (temperature 80–90 °C) and is useful for the synthesis of a wide range of N-substituted imides.

The reaction was first tested by means of a model reaction between cis-3-(3-dimethylaminopropyl carbamoyl) acrylic acid and acetic anhydride. As depicted in Scheme 3, the substrate (M1) was heated at 90 °C for 4 h in the presence of acetic anhydride (dehydrating agent) and sodium acetate (catalyst).

At the end of the reaction time, the mixture was cooled down and sodium acetate was separated by filtration. Acetic anhydride, as well as acetic acid formed during the reaction, were distilled off under reduced pressure. The product was obtained as a brown oily liquid.

^{1}H-NMR analysis of the crude 3-(3-dimethylaminopropyl)maleimide (see Figure 4) shows trace signals of double-bond protons (between 6 and 6.5 ppm) from unreacted maleic acid amide, which is about 2% in respect to maleimide.

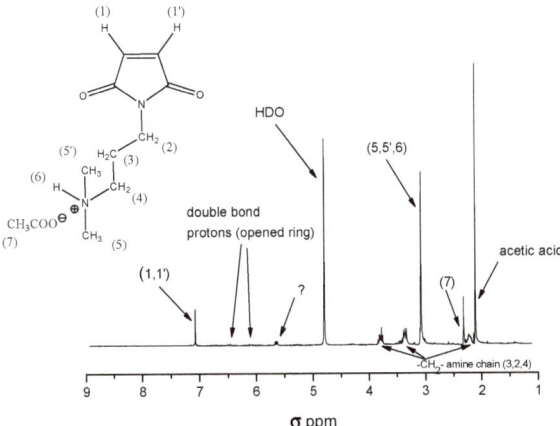

Figure 4. ^{1}H-NMR spectra of crude 3-(3-dimethylaminopropyl)maleimide. Characteristic peak at ~7 ppm confirms the ring formation.

However, the singlet at ~7 ppm shows that the five-membered ring has been successfully formed. The comparison between the signals at σ = 7 ppm and aliphatic protons (σ = 2–4 ppm), which belong to the amine chain, shows that less than 50% of the material that has been obtained was converted to the required compound. The excess of aliphatic amine protons cannot be explained by incomplete conversion of the amic acid because of the very low signal intensity of its double-bond protons. Also, a very strong signal of acetic acid has been registered, although the sample was kept under vacuum for long time.

The IR spectrum (Figure 3) shows the characteristic absorption bands of cyclic imides at 1697 and 1714 cm^{-1} that confirm the imide formation.

The reaction of amidoacidified C2 in the presence of Ac$_2$O and both mentioned bases always yielded dark brown products of sometimes even tarry consistency. Although characteristic absorption bands of imides were observed, no way was found to purify the macromolecular product or at least to remove the dark color.

2.2.4. Thermal Imidization

Because of the poor quality of obtained products, other possibilities of imidization were explored. Thermal imidization of amic acids as a main synthesis method has been described in many organic chemistry handbooks and publications [18,53–58].

TGA analysis of copolymer 2 was performed in order to determine suitable conditions for the reaction. The calculated mass difference between amic acid form of the copolymer and its imidized form was 6.5%. The thermogravimetric analysis showed a weight loss of approximately 7% in the temperature range between 80 and 130 °C, which was attributed to the formation of the cyclic imide by elimination of water (see Figure 5).

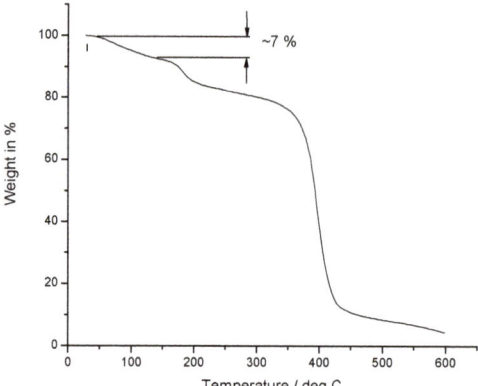

Figure 5. Thermogravimetric analysis (TGA) measurement of amic acid form C2.

The imidization of C2 was carried out in DMF at 120 °C. The imidized copolymer C3 was obtained in form of a pale cream-colored powder which was soluble in acetone. For comparison, the amidoacidified C2 was insoluble in acetone. The infrared spectroscopy (see Figure 3) showed a characteristic absorption band of imides at 1567 cm^{-1}.

The advantage of thermal imidization is its simplicity and the improved product quality as well as the absence of other reagents. It is of paramount importance for an antibacterial test to avoid the presence of low-molecular-weight toxic agents, which can cause false positive results.

The molecular weight of the imidized copolymer was measured by THF-GPC. The measurement showed an increase of the molecular weight of the copolymer after modification from M_n = 5800 to M_n = 8800. This increase in M_n is partially caused by the modification as well as by removal of the low molecular weight fraction during purification. This is indicated also by a change of the polydisperisity of the sample from M_w/M_n = 1.67 to M_w/M_n = 1.47.

2.3. Quaternization of C3

The quaternization reaction was carried out in solution according to the method described in the literature [18,50,53–55,61–63]. The C3 copolymer was dissolved in DMSO and reacted with methyl iodide to give copolymer C4. With a mixture of methyl iodide and dodecyl iodide (1:1, mol:mol), copolymer C5 was obtained and applying dodecyl iodide alone yielded copolymer C6. The reaction was performed at room temperature in the presence of an excess of alkyl iodide (with respect to amine groups), yielding quantitative conversion of the tertiary amine.

According to the literature, a long alkyl chain within the ammonium group shows better biocidal properties [2,64,65]. For this reason, three different quaternized polymers have been prepared bearing trimethyl ammonium, dimethyl-dodecyl ammonium groups, as well as a 1:1 (mol:mol) mixture of both ammonium moieties as the quaternary ammonium side groups.

The IR spectra of quaternized copolymers showed no significant changes because the absorption bands characteristic for ammonium salts overlap with absorption bands of the nonquaternized copolymer (~1500 and 3000 cm^{-1}).

2.4. Solubility in Selected Solvents

The different polarity of the copolymers C3, C4, C5, and C6 is also reflected in the different solubility (see Table 3).

Table 3. Solubility of imidized C3 and quaternized C4, C5, and C6 in chosen solvents (10 mg of copolymer/mL). (+) well soluble (>10 wt %); (−) nonsoluble (<1 wt %).

Solvent	C3	C4	C5	C6
Water	+	+	+	−
Methanol	+	−	+	−
Ethanol	+	−	+	−
Acetone	+	−	+	+
2-Butanone	+	−	+	+
Ethyl acetate	+	−	−	−
THF	+	−	+	+
DMSO	+	+	+	−
DMF	+	+	+	−
Chloroform	+	−	−	+

THF = tetrahydro furane, DMSO = dimethyl sulfoxide, DMF = dimethylformamide.

The introduction of cationic moieties into the polymeric chains strongly increases the polarity of the copolymer and has a huge influence on the solubility. While nonquaternized copolymer C3 was well soluble in all of the chosen solvents, the methyl-iodide-quaternized copolymer C4 was soluble only in very polar solvents such as water and DMSO but insoluble even in lower alcohols such as methanol and ethanol. The introduction of long alkyl chains by quaternization with dodecyl iodide makes copolymer C6 insoluble in water, DMSO, DMF, and alcohols but well soluble in ketones, THF, and chloroform. The simultaneous quaternization with both methyl iodide and dodecyl iodide (C5) ensures good solubility in very polar solvents (water, DMSO) as well as less polar as 2-butanone. The solubility of the quaternized copolymers in water is of utmost importance for antimicrobial investigations.

2.5. Thermal Properties

Figure 6 depicts the TGA thermograms of copolymer C3 and its quaternized derivatives C4, C5, and C6. The nonquaternized copolymer C3 (curve 1) is the thermally most stable polymer and shows only slight weight loss below 200 °C. The highest weight loss is observed above 300 °C. Any modification of C3 by quaternization causes a decrease in thermal stability of the polymer due to Hofmann elimination of the ammonium groups [61]. The Hofmann elimination occurs when quaternary ammonium salts are exposed to high temperatures and the reaction yields an alkene and a tertiary amine and a low-molecular-weight compound specific for the counterion (e.g., water, HCl, HI, etc.).

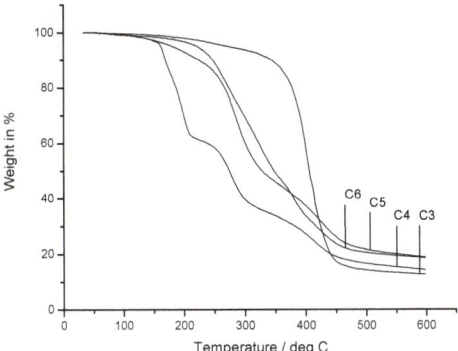

Figure 6. TGA measurement of nonquaternized C3 and quaternized copolymers: C4 (-N(CH$_3$)$_3^+$), C5 ((-N(CH$_3$)$_3^+$ + -N(CH$_3$)$_2$ C$_{12}$H$_{25}^+$), and C6 (-N(CH$_3$)$_2$ C$_{12}$H$_{25}^+$).

The quaternization with methyl iodide causes the C4 (curve 2) to decompose above 150 °C via a three-stage thermal degradation. The first stage starts at 150 °C and ends at 200 °C with a weight loss of 32% corresponding to the loss of HI (31 wt %). Even partial quaternization with long alkyl-chain iodide versus methyl iodide increased the thermal stability, as observed in curves 3 and 4 (C5 and C6) in Figure 6.

However, such derivatives also show faster thermal degradation than nonquaternized C3. In all cases, the investigated copolymers showed a certain weight loss at relatively low temperatures around 100 °C, most probably caused by a loss of adsorbed water because of the hygroscopic nature of salts.

DSC measurement of dodecyl-iodide-quaternized copolymer is typical for all ammonium copolymers based on the C3 copolymer in the temperature range of −50 to 200 °C. Each copolymer showed two thermal transitions: one at 17 °C and a second one in the region of 80–105 °C (see Table 4). The temperature of the second transition seems to depend on the type of quaternizing agent and is about 20 °C higher for copolymers quaternized with dodecyl iodide. There is a correlation with the TGA data where the presence of dodecyl iodide increased the thermal stability. Since the copolymers undergo decomposition in this range of temperatures, reverse heating does not reproduce the curves. Only the first transition is fully reproducible. The fact that the presence of longer alkyl chain gives a higher T_g value is not in line with the expectations. It is known that polymers which contain longer alkyl side chains exhibit lower glass transition temperatures than the shorter ones due to the plastifying effect. Although there has been no melting temperature observed, this phenomenon can be assigned to the formation of ordered structures on the micro or even nano scale. These types of crystalline structures usually do not give any measurable thermal response and further investigation is required. Detailed values of the thermal transition of the investigated copolymers are summarized in Table 4.

Table 4. Transition temperatures for nonquaternized C3 and its cationic modifications.

#	Transition 1 (°C)	Transition 2 (°C)	Functional Group
C3	18	88	$-N(CH_3)_2$
C4	17	85	$-N(CH_3)_3^+$
C5	17	104	$-N(CH_3)_3^+ + -N(CH_3)_2 \, C_{12}H_{25}^+$
C6	18	101	$-N(CH_3)_2 \, C_{12}H_{25}^+$

2.6. Investigation of Antimicrobial Properties of the Cationic Copolymer

In the World Health Organization's (WHO) "global priority list of antibiotic-resistant bacteria to guide research, discovery, and development of new antibiotics" of February 2017, experts agreed on grouping pathogens according to the species and the type of antibiotic resistance and classified the results in three priority tiers: critical, high, and medium.

Our selected bacteria belong to genera that were grouped into the priorities critical and high, i.e., here, the prevalence of resistance against antibiotic treatments is extremely high. With our research field, to prepare antimicrobially functional polymers, we would like to contribute to the reduction of the spread of these bacteria.

Amphiphilic polymers with quaternary ammonium groups are known to have antimicrobial properties [20]. Thus, the water soluble C3, C4, and C5 were tested for their antimicrobial efficacy.

In order to find the MIC of the copolymers, bacterial growth of strains belonging to clinically relevant genera was monitored in the presence of all the copolymers. The tests were performed in microwell plates and the proliferation potential of the bacteria was monitored at 37 °C by measuring the optical density at 612 nm for 20 h using a microwell plate incubator/reader in comparison to a reference without the respective polymer. The MIC values are summarized in Table 5.

Table 5. Minimum inhibitory concentration (MIC) of the polymeric materials in bidistilled water and Mueller-Hinton broth (MHB) against bacteria (1–2 × 10⁶ cfu/mL) (MIC$_{100}$: complete growth inhibition during the monitoring time of 20 h) compared to reference Nisin, and hemolytic effect (HC$_{50}$).

Polymer	MIC$_{100}$ in µg/mL				HC$_{50}$ in µg/mL
	E. coli ATCC 23716	P. aeruginosa ATCC27853	S. aureus ATCC 6538	S. epidermidis ATCC 12228	
C3	20	100	>1000	20	100 *
C4	200	>>1000	1000	20	>>1000 **
C5	10	200	100	20	60 #
NISIN	100	>200	3	3	>>340 +

* Agglutination of red blood cells (RBC) at all concentrations tested 10–1000 µg/mL; ** agglutination of RBC at 20–1000 µg/mL; # no agglutination of RBC, + at 340 µg/mL = 100 mM Nisin only 10.8% of the RBC are lysed. Nisin (Handary 97.9%).

The novelty of this paper is (i) the polymer backbone based on maleic anhydride and 4-methyl-1-pentene and (ii) the fact that the results obtained for *E. coli* and *S. aureus* were not as expected based on a great amount of papers showing that amphiphilic polymers with different backbones and manifold kinds of cationic and hydrophobic residues are more active against Gram-positive bacteria (lower MIC values) than against Gram-negative bacteria.

The polymers are more effective by a factor of 5–10 against the Gram-negative *E. coli* than against the Gram-positive *S. aureus*. This selectivity, although with a lower factor, was also found in [66], who prepared lysine and arginine mimicking amino and guanidine propyl methacrylamide copolymers; in the latter, the amine-containing copolymers were best.

Compared to polymer C4 (modified with methyl iodide), polymers C3 (nonquaternized) and C5 (modified with both iodides, methyl and dodecyl iodide) are more active against the Gram-negative bacteria *E. coli* and *P. aeruginosa*, whereas, in the case of *S. aureus*, C5 was the most active polymer compared to C3 and C4, with the nonquaternized C3 being the least active in the latter case. Previous studies in our group, although with a different polymer backbone, have shown that the best results against *S. aureus* were obtained with the cationic residue directly linked to the aliphatic residue without a spacer in between [67], and that longer alkyl chains showed best efficacy [68] and, thus, confirm these results. Regarding the solubility properties (Table 3), C3 and C5 show similar solubilities in the different solvents compared to C4. The limited solubility of the latter seems to restrict the effect against *E. coli*, *P. aeruginosa*, and *S. aureus* since the hydrophilic–lipophilic balance is decisive for the efficacy of the respective polymer.

Against *S. epidermidis*, all three polymers are equally active in a comparable range, such as C3 and C5 against *E. coli*.

Comparing the MIC for the Gram-negative bacteria gave 5- (C3) to 20-fold (C5) higher values for *P. aeruginosa* than for *E. coli*, meaning that *E. coli* is 5–20 times better inhibited compared to *P. aeruginosa*. Gram-negative bacteria are known to actively secrete outer membrane vesicles (OMVs) from the outer membrane (OM) [69]. OMV production is correlated with an increased rate of survival upon antimicrobial peptide treatment [70] In *Pseudomonas putida*, OMVs are generated, e.g., as a response to stress caused by cationic surfactants which can contribute to OMV biogenesis, through a physical mechanism by induction of the curvature of the membrane [71]. Although OMV production is common in many bacteria, the extent and mechanism of OMV production is species specific, and thus, the higher MIC values for *P. aeruginosa* might be due to the level of OMV production, since environmental stresses result in increased OMV formation by *P. aeruginosa* [72].

For the Gram-negative bacteria *E. coli* and *P. aeruginosa* and for the Gram-positive *S. aureus*, C5 quaternized with the long alkyl chain, i.e., the repeat unit structure with the hydrophobic moiety being directly accompanied by the charged moiety, exhibits a higher efficacy compared to C4 quaternized with methyl iodide (this was also confirmed for functionalized polymers with polglycidol backbone [73]).

C5 exhibits a more ordered structure due to phase separation and orientation of the hydrophobic $C_{12}H_{25}$ chains to hydrophobic domains (see also the discussion on the thermal properties in Section 2.5).

Whereas polymers C3 and C4 led to an agglutination of human RBC at all concentrations tested (10–1000 µg/mL), C5 did not agglutinate RBC but showed lysis of 50% of the RBC relative to the positive control (HC_{50}) at a concentration of 60 µg/mL. The higher value of HC_{50} compared to the MIC_{100} against *E. coli* (10 µg/mL) proved that polymer C5 has a selectivity to differentiate between mammalian cells and bacterial cell walls. However, since the values are overall in the same order of magnitude, the selectivity is low.

Since the investigated antimicrobial copolymers were designed to mimic peptides, a comparison with a reference compound is needed. The type A lantibiotics, e.g., Pep5 or Nisin, are in general of linear conformation and all the Nisin type peptides are positively charged [33]. Combination of the cationic nature and the presence of leucine makes Nisin a good reference.

Nisin is a 34-residue-long peptide which is predominantly active against Gram-positive bacteria (Nisin is also active against Gram-negative bacteria but only after a pretreatment) [74]. It is generally accepted that the bacterial plasma membrane is the target for Nisin, and that Nisin kills the cells by pore formation and inhibition of peptidoglycan synthesis. The pore formation causes collapse of vital ion gradients, resulting in cell death [75]. In this study, it was shown that Nisin, compared to the copolymer modified with both iodides, is highly active against Gram-positive bacteria, and, as expected, 30 to more than 60 times less active against Gram-negative bacteria. Moreover, comparing the MIC of Nisin against the Gram-positive bacteria on the molar basis instead on the weight basis, the difference between the effect of Nisin and the copolymer is significantly lower.

This gap indicates that the activity of the peptides is determined not only by the amphiphilic nature but most probably the secondary peptide structure plays also a substantial role.

3. Materials and Methods

3.1. Materials

Maleic anhydride (MSA, Merck, Darmstadt, Germany, for synthesis) was sublimed under reduced pressure (50 °C, 2.4×10^{-2} bar), benzoyl peroxide (BPO, Merck, for synthesis) was recrystallized from a chloroform:methanol mixture (1:5 vol:vol), 2-butanone (MEK, Merck, p.a.), and other solvents (technical grade) were dried over calcium hydride (Fluka, Seelze, Germany) and distilled before use. 4-methyl-1-pentene (Aldrich, Darmstadt, Germany, for synthesis), methyl iodide (ABCR, Karlsruhe, Germany), benzyl alcohol (Merck, for synthesis), dimethyl sulfoxide (Fluka, p.a.), acetic anhydride (Merck, for synthesis), 3-dimethylaminopropylamine (Aldrich), succinic anhydride (Merck, p.a.), triethylamine (Fluka, p.a.), and anhydrous sodium acetate (Merck, p.a.) were used without additional purification. The inorganic salts sodium chloride, sodium dihydrogen phosphate monohydrate, and disodium hydrogen phosphate dehydrate (all Merck) were used as received.

Bacteria have been provided by the German Resource Centre for Biological Material.

(Leibniz-Institut DSMZ-Deutsche Sammlung von Mikroorganismen und Zellkulturen GmbH, Braunschweig, Germany) and (LGC Standards GmbH, Wesel, Germany). Gram-negative bacteria: *Escherichia coli* (DSM 498, ATCC 23716) and *Pseudomonas aeruginosa* (DSM 1117, ATCC 27853).

Gram-positive bacteria: *Staphylococcus aureus* (ATCC 6538) and *Staphylococcus epidermidis* (DSM 1798, ATCC 12228).

Nutrient solutions: (1) NL1: 0.5 g of meat extract (Merck) and 0.3 g of peptone obtained from casein (Merck) were dissolved in 99.2 g of sterile water; (2) Mueller-Hinton Broth (Carl Roth GmbH, Karlsruhe, Germany) per L: 2.0 g Beef Extract Powder, 17.5 g Acid Digest of Casein, 1.5 g Starch pH 7.4 ± 0.2.

Phosphate buffered saline (PBS): 100 mL of phosphate buffer and 1.8 g of sodium chloride were placed in a 200-mL measuring flask and filled with distilled water *ad* 200 mL.

3.2. Measurements/Apparatus

Size exclusion chromatography was performed using a system consisting of an LC 1120 pump (Polymer Laboratories, Church Stretton, UK), a UV detector ERC-7215, an RI detector ERC-7515A (ERMA CR INC., Kawaguchi, Japan),), a precolumn (50 × 8 mm) of nominal pore size 50 Å, and four columns (300 × 8 mm) filled with MZ-Gel SDplus of nominal pore size 50, 100, 1000, and 10,000 Å (MZ-Analysentechnik, Mainz, Germany). The set was calibrated with PMMA and PS standards from Polymer Laboratories. The sample concentration was 7 mg of polymer in 1 mL of tetrahydrofuran, and the injected volume of the sample was 100 µL. The tetrahydrofuran was stabilized with 2,6-di-tert-butyl-4-methylphenol (250 mg/L).

^{1}H-NMR spectra were obtained on a Bruker DPX-300 spectrometer in acetone-d_6 and D_2O at 300 MHz. MestRe-C 4.9.0.0 was used as evaluation software. The solvent peak as the reference signal was used.

IR spectra were measured with on an FTIR Thermo Nicolet Nexus spectrometer in KBr-pellets with a resolution of 4 cm^{-1}.

Thermogravimetric analysis (TGA) was performed by means of NETZSCH TG 209c thermo balance under nitrogen atmosphere at a nitrogen flow of 15 mL/min. Samples of 9–11 mg were placed in a standard NETZSCH alumina 85-µL crucible. The heating rate was 10 K min^{-1}.

Differential scanning calorimetry (DSC) measurements were performed by means of a Netzsch DSC 204 unit. Samples (typical weight: ~9 mg) were enclosed in standard Netzsch 25-µL aluminium crucibles. Indium and palmitic acid were used as calibration standards. Heating and cooling rates were 10 °C min^{-1}.

CHN elemental analysis was performed by means of a Carlo Erba MOD-1106 elemental analysis apparatus at the Institute of Organic Chemistry of the RWTH Aachen. Each measurement was performed twice.

The optical density measurements were performed by means of an Infinite 200 Pro (Tecan, Männedorf, Switzerland) Multiwell plate Reader/Incubator at a wavelength of 612 nm in cycles of 30 min for 20 h.

3.3. Syntheses

3.3.1. Poly[(4-methyl-1-pentene)-alt-maleic anhydride] (Copolymer 1, C1)

In a 100-mL round-bottomed flask equipped with a reflux condenser and a valve, maleic anhydride (7 g, 71 mmol, 55 mol %) and 4-methyl-1-pentene (5.04 g 60 mmol) were dissolved in dry MEK (35 mL). To this mixture, BPO (0.3 g, 1.23 mmol, 0.93 mol %) was added and the mixture was degassed three times by freeze–pump–thaw cycles and filled with nitrogen. The reaction mixture was placed in an oil bath at 80 °C for 8 h. After the given time, the reaction mixture was cooled to ambient temperature and the polymer was precipitated in a mixture of diethylether:methanol (4:1 vol:vol), separated by filtration, and dried under vacuum at 40 °C for 8 h. The copolymer (9.3 g, 77% yield) was obtained as a white solid. The molecular weight of the obtained copolymer was determined by gel permeation chromatography in tetrahydrofuran THF-GPC using PMMA standard: M_n = 5800, Đ = M_w/M_n = 1.67. The characteristic absorption peaks of IR spectra were: 1852, 1777 (C=O); 927 (C-O-C) cm^{-1}. Elemental analysis for $C_{10}H_{14}O_3$; calculated: C 65.9; H 7.7; O 26.4 wt %, found: C 65.54; H 7.85; O 26.61 wt %. ^{1}H-NMR (acetone-d_6, δ in ppm): 0.71–4.03; (m, backbone, and side chains)

3.3.2. Determination of the Maleic Anhydride Content of C1 by ^{1}H-NMR

C1 (100 mg) was dissolved in 2-butanone (5 mL) and benzyl alcohol (0.5 g) was added. The mixture was heated at 50 °C under reflux for 18 h. The product was precipitated in a diethylether/methanol (1:1) mixture and dried under vacuum at 40 °C for 8 h. ^{1}H-NMR (CDCl$_3$, δ in ppm): 7.16–7.49 (m, 5H, aromatic); 5.11 (2H, -O-CH$_2$-); 0.71–4.03 (m, 14H, backbone, and side chains)

3.3.3. Amidoacidification of C1 to Poly[(4-methyl-1-pentene)-alt-(1-(3-N,N-dimethylaminopropyl)malemic acid)] (Copolymer 2, C2)

C1 (2.0 g) was dissolved in dry dimethylformamid (DMF) (45 mL) and -(dimethylamino)-1-propylamine (DMAPA) (1.19 g, 11.7 mmol) was added dropwise for 2 h to the stirred solution using a syringe pump at room temperature (RT). During the addition phase, precipitation of the product occurred. The mixture was stirred for an additional 24 h, and the precipitated product, a cream-colored solid, was filtered off and dried at 40 °C under reduced pressure for 8 h. The characteristic absorption peaks of IR spectra were: 1714; 1657; 1567 cm^{-1}.

3.3.4. Thermal Imidization of C2 to Poly[(4-methyl-1-pentene)-alt-(1-(3-N,N-dimethylaminopropyl)maleimide)] (Copolymer 3a, C3a)

Amidoacidified C2 (1.0 g) was dissolved in DMF (20 mL) and heated under reflux at 120 °C for 24 h. The product was precipitated from diethylether and dried under vacuum at 40 °C for 5 h. The molecular weight of the obtained copolymer was determined by THF-GPC using PMMA standard: M_n = 8600, Đ = 1.46. The characteristic absorption peaks of IR spectra were: 1772; 1697 cm^{-1}. Elemental analysis for $C_{15}H_{26}O_2N_2$; calculated: C 67.7; H 9.8; N 10.5; O 12.0 wt %; found: C 67.09; H 9.70; N 10.11; O 11.10 wt %.

3.3.5. Chemical Imidization of Amidoacidified C2 (Copolymer 3b, C3b)

The amidoacidified C2 (0.5 g) was dissolved in a mixture of DMF, acetic anhydride, 2-butanone triethylamine, or sodium acetate (see Table 6 for detailed composition). The reaction mixture was either heated under reflux or stirred at RT under a protective atmosphere of nitrogen for 12–18 h. The product was precipitated in diethylether as a dark-brown solid and dried under vacuum at 40° for 24 h. The repeated precipitation had no influence on the appearance. The characteristic absorption peaks of IR spectra were: 1770; 1697 cm^{-1}.

Table 6. Composition of the reaction mixtures, reaction conditions for the chemical imidization of C2, yield, and appearance of the product.

#	DMF (g)	Ac$_2$O (g)	MEK (g)	Et$_3$N (g)	CH$_3$COONa (g)	T (°C)	t (h)	Yield %	Appearance
1	15	15	-	0.1	-	RT	12	88	brown powder
2	15	15	-	0.1	-	80	18	70	brown powder
3	20	1.07	-	1.41	-	80	24	62	brown, tarry
4	-	1.0	15	0.8	-	90	18	87	grey powder
5	-	0.55	15	0.73	-	90	12	90	grey powder
6	-	7	-	1	-	80	20	78	grey powder
7	-	10	-	-	0.1	80	18	69	brown powder

DMF = dimethylformamid, Ac$_2$O = acetic anhydride, MEK = 2-butanone, Et$_3$N = triethylamine, CH$_3$COONa = sodium acetate, RT = room temperature.

3.3.6. Preparation of Imide C3 in a One-Pot Reaction (Copolymer 3c, C3c)

C1 (3.5 g) was dissolved in dry DMF (20 mL) and placed in a 250-mL round-bottomed flask. Within 2 h, DMAPA (2.5 g) dissolved in dry DMF (40 mL) was added by means of a syringe pump at room temperature. The dispersion of the precipitated product was stirred additionally for 12 h and the mixture was placed in an oil bath heated to 120 °C for another 24 h. The product was purified by precipitation in 400 mL of diethylether. After drying the precipitate under vacuum at 40 °C for 8 h, a cream-colored powder was obtained (3.2 g, 97.5%). The molecular weight of the obtained copolymer was determined by THF-GPC using PMMA standard: M_n = 9350, Đ = 1.40. The characteristic absorption peaks of IR spectra were: 1772; 1697 cm^{-1}. Elemental analysis for $C_{15}H_{26}O_2N_2$; calculated: C 67.7; H 9.8; N 10.5; O 12.0 wt %; found: C 67.16; H 9.76; N 10.21; O 12.87 wt %.

3.3.7. Synthesis of Poly[(4-methyl-1-pentene)-alt-(1-(3-N,N,N-trimethylammonium-propyl)-maleimidoiodide)] by Quaternization of Imidized C3 with Methyl Iodide (Copolymer 4, C4)

Thermally imidized C3a (0.1 g) was dissolved in dimethyl sulfoxide DMSO (4 mL) and placed in a 25-mL round-bottomed flask. Methyl iodide (0.1 mL) was added and the mixture was stirred at room temperature for 18 h. The product was precipitated in THF and dried under vacuum at 40 °C for 12 h. The product (0.147 g, 96%) was obtained as a lemon-yellowish powder. Elemental analysis for $C_{16}H_{29}O_2N_2I$; calculated: C 47.1; H 7.2; N 6.9; O 7.6; I 31.2 wt %; found: C 46.63; H 7.0; N 6.97; O 7.87 wt %.

3.3.8. Sequential Quaternization of Imidized C3 with Methyl and Dodecyl Iodide (Copolymer 5, C5)

Thermally imidized C3a (0.3 g) was placed in a 25-mL round-bottomed flask and dissolved in a mixture of acetone (10 mL) and DMSO (5 mL). Dodecyl iodide (0.164 g, 0.564 mmol, 50% with respect to the N,N-dimethylammonium groups) of) was added and the mixture was stirred for 48 h. In a subsequent step, methyl iodide (0.2 g, 1.4 mmol) dissolved in DMSO (5 mL) was added and the reaction mixture was stirred for another 24 h. The product was precipitated in a THF/hexane (4:1) mixture, separated, and dried under vacuum at 40 °C for 8 h. Elemental analysis for $C_{43}H_{80}O_4N_4I_2$; calculated: C 53.2; H8.2; N5.8; O 6.6; I 26.2 wt %; found: C 53.0; H 8.17; N 5.84; O 6.9 wt %.

3.3.9. Synthesis of Poly[(4-methyl-1-pentene)-alt-(1-(3-N,N-dimethyl-N-dodecylammoniumpropyl)-maleimidoiodide)] (Copolymer 6, C6)

Thermally imidized C3a (0.1g) was dissolved in acetone (4 mL) and placed in a 25-mL round-bottomed flask and dodecyl iodide (0.1 mL) was added. The flask was closed with a glass stopper and the mixture was stirred for 48 h. The product was precipitated in hexane, filtered, and dried under vacuum at 40 °C for 8 h. Elemental analysis for $C_{27}H_{51}O_2N_2I$; calculated: C 57.6; H 9.0; N 5.0; O 5.7; I 22.7 wt %; found: C 57.56; H 9.06; N 5.01; O 5.88 wt %.

3.3.10. Synthesis of 3-(N,N-dimethylamino)propyl Maleic Acid Amide (M1)

Maleic anhydride (7.0 g, 71 mmol) was dissolved in dry chloroform (100 mL) and placed in a 250-mL flask. A solution of DMAPA (6.8 g, 67 mmol) in chloroform (20 mL) was added dropwise and stirred for 1 h at 60 °C. After the addition period, the reaction mixture was heated at 60 °C for 1 h. The product was precipitated in a fivefold excess of acetone (with respect to the volume of the reaction mixture), separated, and dried under vacuum at 40 °C for 8 h. The product (12.2 g, 88%) was obtained as a white powder. The characteristic absorption peaks of IR spectra were: 1710, 1650, 1588 cm^{-1}. ^{1}H-NMR (D$_2$O, δ in ppm): 6.33 (dd, 1H, C = CH-CON-, ^3J = 12 Hz); 5.96 (dd, 1H, C = CH-COOH, ^3J = 12 Hz); 3.33 (t, 2H, -NH-CH$_2$-CH$_2$-CH$_2$-N(CH$_3$)$_2$, ^3J = 6 Hz); 3,17 (t, 2H, -NH-CH$_2$-CH$_2$-CH$_2$-N(CH$_3$)$_2$, ^3J = 9 Hz); 2,88 (s, 6H, -NH-CH$_2$-CH$_2$-CH$_2$N-(CH$_3$)$_2$); 1,95 (q, 2H, -NH-CH$_2$-CH$_2$-CH$_2$N-(CH$_3$)$_2$) ^3J = 6 Hz).

3.3.11. Chemical Imidization (Z)-4-(N,N-dimethylamino)propylamino-4-oxobut-2-enoic Acid (M2)

with a reflux condenser for 4 h at 90 °C. After cooling to ambient temperature, the reaction mixture Maleamic acid (1.0 g, 5 mmol) and sodium acetate (0.2 g, 2 mmol) were dissolved in acetic anhydride (30 mL) and heated in a 50-mL round-bottomed flask equipped was filtered to remove sodium acetate, and acetic anhydride was distilled off under reduced pressure. A brown oily product (0.8 g, 72%) was obtained. The characteristic absorption peaks of the IR spectra were: 1773; 1697 cm^{-1}. ^{1}H-NMR (D$_2$O, δ in ppm): 6.86 (s, 2H, -OC-CH = CH-CO-); 3.62 (t, 2H, -NH-CH$_2$-CH$_2$-CH$_2$-N(CH$_3$)$_2$, ^3J = 6 Hz); 3.14 (t, 2H, -NH-CH$_2$-CH$_2$-CH$_2$-N(CH$_3$)$_2$, ^3J = 9 Hz); 2.86 (s, 6H, -NH-CH$_2$-CH$_2$-CH$_2$N-(CH$_3$)$_2$); 1.98 (q, 2H, -NH-CH$_2$-CH$_2$-CH$_2$N-(CH$_3$)$_2$) ^3J = 6 Hz).

3.3.12. Synthesis of 3-(N,N-dimethylamino)propyl Succinamic Acid (M3)

DMAPA (3.6 g, 35 mmol) was added slowly to a solution of succinic anhydride 3.5 g (35 mmol) in dry acetone (20 mL). The mixture was stirred for 2 h at room temperature. The precipitated product was filtered and immediately used for the thermal imidization reaction without further characterization.

3.3.13. Thermal Imidization of (Z)-4-(N,N-dimethylamino)propylamino-4-oxobutanoic Acid (M4)

3-(N,N-dimethylamino)propyl succinamic acid obtained from the reaction of succinic anhydride and DMAPA was heated under flowing nitrogen at 170 °C for 2 h. A brownish oily liquid (6.3 g, 98%) was obtained. The characteristic absorption peaks of IR spectra were: 1770; 1697 cm^{-1}. ^{1}H-NMR (D$_2$O, δ in ppm): 3.23 (t, 2H, -NH-$\underline{CH_2}$-CH$_2$-CH$_2$-N(CH$_3$)$_2$, ^3J = 6 Hz); 2.97 (t, 2H, -NH-CH$_2$-CH$_2$-$\underline{CH_2}$-N(CH$_3$)$_2$, ^3J = 6 Hz); 2.73 (s, 6H, -NH-CH$_2$-CH$_2$-CH$_2$N-$\underline{(CH_3)_2}$); 2.41 (s, 4H, -OC-$\underline{CH_2}$-$\underline{CH_2}$-CO-); 1.85 (q, 2H, -NH-CH$_2$-$\underline{CH_2}$-CH$_2$N-(CH$_3$)$_2$.

3.4. Antimicrobial Tests

The antibacterial activity of the amphiphilic polymers in solution was determined by measuring the minimum inhibitory concentration (MIC) using the test bacteria mentioned above. Suspensions of strains with known colony forming units (CFU; 2 × 10^6 CFU/mL) were incubated at 37 °C in nutrient solution (Mueller-Hinton Broth, MHB) with different concentrations of the polymer samples. The polymer samples were solubilized in bidistilled water and added to the nutrient solution at a constant ratio of 1:10. The growth of the bacteria was followed during the incubation over 20 h by measuring the optical density at 612 nm every 30 min (with 1000 s of shaking at 100 rpm per 30 min cycle by using a microwell plate reader/incubator (TECAN Infinite 200 Pro, Tecan Trading AG, Männedorf, Switzerland). The testing was performed with defined concentrations specifically for each polymer until, within the monitoring time of 20 h, no bacterial growth curve was recorded. All experiments were performed in triplicate duplicates and MIC determination was repeated on three different days. The polymers were not sterilized. Sterile controls (defined polymer concentrations in nutrient solution without bacteria) were assessed in every growth curve monitoring testing series. MICs were determined according to broth microdilution in 96-well microtitre plates [76]. The MIC corresponds to the concentration of the test substance at which a complete inhibition of the growth of the inoculated bacteria was observed by comparison with control samples without test substance.

3.5. Hemolytic Activity

Hemolytic activity was assessed according to the literature [77]. Human erythrocytes (from healthy donors, red blood cells (RBC), 0, Rh positive, citrate-phosphate-dextrose-adenine-stabilized; CPDA1 Sarstedt Germany) were obtained by centrifugation (3500 rpm, 12 min) to remove plasma, washed three times in PBS (0.01 M phosphate buffered saline, Sigma Aldrich Chemie GmbH, Steinheim, Germany), and diluted in PBS to obtain a stock solution of 2.5 × 10^8–3.0 × 10^8/mL RBC. Solutions of defined polymer concentration (250 µL) were pipetted into 250 µL of the stock solution, the final amount of RBC being 1.2 × 10^8–1.5 × 10^8 RBC/mL. The RBC were exposed for 60 min at 37 °C under 3D-shaking, centrifuged thereafter (4000 rpm, 12 min), and the absorption of the supernatant (diluted 10-fold in PBS) was determined at 414 nm in a microplate reader. As reference solutions, (i) PBS for determining spontaneous hemolysis and (ii) 1% Triton X-100 for 100% hemolysis (positive control) were used. Hemolysis was plotted as a function of polymer concentration and the hemolytic activity was defined as the polymer concentration that causes 50% hemolysis of human RBC relative to the positive control (HC$_{50}$).

4. Conclusions

Maleic anhydride copolymers are versatile, easy-for-modification materials which can be used as a base for a wide range of antimicrobial copolymers.

The modification of P[MP-alt-MSA] copolymer with diamine to poly[(4-methyl-1-pentene)-alt-(1-(3-*N*,*N*-dimethylaminopropyl)maleimide)] can be performed as a one-pot synthesis without using any additives in relatively mild conditions. Poly[(4-methyl-1-pentene)-alt-(1-(3-*N*,*N*-dimethylaminopropyl)maleimide)] can be easily converted into a polycationic material by means of any alkyl iodide. Sequential quaternization with methyl iodide and dodecyl iodide—which introduce a hydrophobic long-alkyl-chain moiety, but thanks to methyl iodide, ensure solubility in polar solvents—shows the best properties in the sense of antimicrobial activity.

The antimicrobial properties of poly[(4-methyl-1-pentene)-alt-(1-(3-*N*,*N*,*N*-trimethylammoniumpropyl)-maleimidoiodide)] are even lower than the properties of the nonquaternized copolymer.

The polymers are more effective by a factor of 5–10 against the Gram-negative *E. coli* than against the Gram-positive *S. aureus*. Compared to poly[(4-methyl-1-pentene)-alt-(1-(3-*N*,*N*,*N*-trimethylammoniumpropyl)-maleimidoiodide)], polymers poly[(4-methyl-1-pentene)-alt-(1-(3-*N*,*N*-dimethylaminopropyl)maleimide)] and poly[(1-(3-*N*,*N*,*N*-trimethylammonium-propyl)-maleimidoiodide)-co-(1-(3-*N*,*N*-dimethyl-*N*-dodecylammoniumpropyl) maleimidoiodide)-alt-(4-methyl-1-penten)] are more active against the Gram-negative bacteria *E. coli* and *P. aeruginosa*, whereas, in the case of *S. aureus*, only poly[(1-(3-*N*,*N*,*N*-trimethylammonium-propyl)-maleimidoiodide)-co-(1-(3-*N*,*N*-dimethyl-*N*-dodecylammoniumpropyl) maleimidoiodide)-alt-(4-methyl-1-penten)] was the most active polymer compared to the nonquaternized polymer and the polymer quaternized with methyl iodide. The nonquaternized copolymer was the least active in the latter case.

The MIC of the synthetic copolymers is higher than of the natural peptide Nisin. However, the freedom in designing the basic polymer, molecular weight, as well as the way of modification and, in particular, the much lower price of the synthetic compounds show the potential of the presented strategy to develop new "surface protection".

Author Contributions: Supervision, U.B. and M.M.; Writing—original draft, M.S., E.H., and H.K.

Acknowledgments: The authors gratefully acknowledge the excellent technical assistance of Rita Gartzen who performed the antimicrobial tests.

Conflicts of Interest: The authors declare no conflict of interest.

References

1. Cornell, R.J.; Donaruma, L.G. 2-Methacryloxytropones. Intermediates for synthesis of biologically active polymers. *J. Med. Chem.* **1965**, *8*, 388–390. [PubMed]
2. Tashiro, T. Antibacterial and bacterium adsorbing macromolecules. *Macromol. Mater. Eng.* **2001**, *286*, 63–87. [CrossRef]
3. Kenawy, E.R.; Mahmoud, Y.A.G. Biologically active polymers, 6-synthesis and antimicrobial activity of some linear copolymers with quaternary ammonium and phosphonium groups. *Macromol. Biosc.* **2003**, *3*, 107–116. [CrossRef]
4. Sanda, F.; Endo, T. Syntheses and functions of polymers based on amino acids. *Macromol. Chem. Phys.* **1999**, *200*, 2651–2661. [CrossRef]
5. Ilker, M.F.; Nusslein, K.; Tew, G.N.; Coughlin, E.B. Tuning the hemolytic and antibacterial activities of amphiphilic polynorbornene derivatives. *J. Am. Chem. Soc.* **2004**, *126*, 15870–15875. [CrossRef] [PubMed]
6. Rivas, B.L.; Pereira, E.D.; Mondaca, M.A. Biostatic behavior of side chain charged-polycations and polymer-ag complexes. *Polym. Bull.* **2003**, *50*, 327–333. [CrossRef]
7. Tashiro, T. Removal of bacteria from water by systems based on insoluble polystyrene-polyethyleneimine. *J. Appl. Polym. Sci.* **1992**, *46*, 899–907. [CrossRef]
8. Hazzizalaskar, J.; Nurdin, N.; Helary, G.; Sauvet, G. Biocidal polymers active by contact.1. Synthesis of polybutadiene with pendant quaternary ammonium groups. *J. Appl. Polym. Sci.* **1993**, *50*, 651–662. [CrossRef]
9. Nurdin, N.; Helary, G.; Sauvet, G. Biocidal polymers active by contact. II. Biological evaluation of polyurethane coatings with pendant quaternary ammonium-salts. *J. Appl. Polym. Sci.* **1993**, *50*, 663–670. [CrossRef]

10. Nurdin, N.; Helary, G.; Sauvet, G. Biocidal polymers active by contact. III. Aging of biocidal polyurethane coatings in water. *J. Appl. Polym. Sci.* **1993**, *50*, 671–678. [CrossRef]
11. Hazzizalaskar, J.; Helary, G.; Sauvet, G. Biocidal polymers active by contact. IV. Polyurethanes based on polysiloxanes with pendant primary alcohols and quaternary ammonium groups. *J. Appl. Polym. Sci.* **1995**, *58*, 77–84. [CrossRef]
12. Sauvet, G.; Fortuniak, W.; Kazmierski, K.; Chojnowski, J. Amphiphilic block and statistical siloxane copolymers with antimicrobial activity. *J. Appl. Polym. Sci.* **2003**, *41*, 2939–2948. [CrossRef]
13. Ikeda, T.; Hirayama, H.; Suzuki, K.; Yamaguchi, H.; Tazuke, S. Biologically-active polycations. 6. Polymeric pyridinium salts with well-defined main chain structure. *Macromol. Chem.* **1986**, *187*, 333–340. [CrossRef]
14. Li, G.J.; Shen, J.R.; Zhu, Y.L. Study of pyridinium-type functional polymers. II. Antibacterial activity of soluble pyridinium-type polymers. *J. Appl. Polym. Sci.* **1998**, *67*, 1761–1768. [CrossRef]
15. Sauvet, G.; Dupond, S.; Kazmierski, K.; Chojnowski, J. Biocidal polymers active by contact. V. Synthesis of polysiloxanes with biocidal activity. *J. Appl. Polym. Sci.* **2000**, *75*, 1005–1012. [CrossRef]
16. Tashiro, T. Removal of *Escherichia-coli* from water by systems based on insoluble polystyrene-poly(ethylene glycol)s, polystyrene-polyethylenimines, and polystyrene-polyethylenepolyamines quaternized. *J. Appl. Polym. Sci.* **1991**, *43*, 1369–1377. [CrossRef]
17. Augusta, S.; Gruber, H.F.; Streichsbier, F. Synthesis and antibacterial activity of immobilized quaternary ammonium-salts. *J. Appl. Polym. Sci.* **1994**, *53*, 1149–1163. [CrossRef]
18. Fields, J.E.; Johnson, J.H. Air Purification Process. U.S. Patent 3,340,680, 1 February 1967.
19. Destais, N.; Ades, D.; Sauvet, G. Synthesis, characterization and biocidal properties of epoxy resins containing quaternary ammonium salts. *Polym. Bull.* **2000**, *44*, 401–408. [CrossRef]
20. Kenawy, E.R.; Abdel-Hay, F.I.; El-Raheem, A.; El-Shanshoury, R.; El-Newehy, M.H. Biologically active polymers: Synthesis and antimicrobial activity of modified glycidyl methacrylate polymers having a quaternary ammonium and phosphonium groups. *J. Control. Release* **1998**, *50*, 145–152. [CrossRef]
21. Kenawy, E.R.; Abdel-Hay, F.I.; El-Shanshoury, A.E.R.R.; El-Newehy, M.H. Biologically active polymers. V. Synthesis and antimicrobial activity of modified poly(glycidyl methacrylate-co-2-hydroxyethyl methacrylate) derivatives with quaternary ammonium and phosphonium salts. *J. Polym. Sci. Part A Polym. Chem.* **2002**, *40*, 2384–2393. [CrossRef]
22. Kanazawa, A.; Ikeda, T.; Endo, T. Polymeric phosphonium salts as a novel class of cationic biocides. 8. Synergistic effect on antibacterial activity of polymeric phosphonium and ammonium-salts. *J. Appl. Polym. Sci.* **1994**, *53*, 1245–1249. [CrossRef]
23. Kanazawa, A.; Ikeda, T.; Endo, T. Novel polycationic biocides-synthesis and antibacterial activity of polymeric phosphonium salts. *J. Polym. Sci. Part A Polym. Chem.* **1993**, *31*, 335–343. [CrossRef]
24. Kanazawa, A.; Ikeda, T.; Endo, T. Polymeric phosphonium salts as a novel class of cationic biocides. 2. Effects of couter anion and molecular-weight on antibacterial activity of polymeric phosphonium salts. *J. Polym. Sci. Part A Polym. Chem.* **1993**, *31*, 1441–1447. [CrossRef]
25. Kanazawa, A.; Ikeda, T.; Endo, T. Polymeric phosphonium salts as a novel class of cationic biocides. 9. Effect of side-chain length between main-chain and active group on antibacterial activity. *J. Polym. Sci. Part A Polym. Chem.* **1994**, *32*, 1997–2001. [CrossRef]
26. Kanazawa, A.; Ikeda, T.; Endo, T. Polymeric phosphonium salts as a novel class of cationic biocides. 10. Antibacterial activity of filters incorporating phosphonium biocides. *J. Appl. Polym. Sci.* **1994**, *54*, 1305–1310. [CrossRef]
27. Kanazawa, A.; Ikeda, T.; Endo, T. Polymeric phosphonium salts as a novel class of cationic biocides. 7. Synthesis and antibacterial activity of polymeric phosphonium salts and their model compounds containing long alkyl chains. *J. Appl. Polym. Sci.* **1994**, *53*, 1237–1244. [CrossRef]
28. Timofeeva, L.; Kleshcheva, N. Antimicrobial polymers: Mechanism of action, factors of activity, and applications. *Appl. Microbiol. Biotechnol.* **2011**, *89*, 475–492. [CrossRef] [PubMed]
29. Monsanto Company. Pharmaceutical Compositions. GB Patent 1,260,451, 19 January 1972.
30. Patel, H.; Raval, D.A.; Madamwar, D.; Patel, S.R. Polymeric prodrug: Synthesis, release study and antimicrobial property of poly(styrene-co-maleic anhydride)-bound acriflavine. *Angew. Macrom. Chem.* **1998**, *263*, 25–30. [CrossRef]
31. Jeong, J.H.; Byoun, Y.S.; Ko, S.B.; Lee, Y.S. Chemical modification of poly(styrene-alt-maleic anhydride) with antimicrobial 4-aminobenzoic acid and 4-hydroxybenzoic acid. *J. Ind. Eng. Chem.* **2001**, *7*, 310–315.

32. Jeong, J.H.; Byoun, Y.S.; Lee, Y.S. Poly(styrene-alt-maleic anhydride)-4-aminophenol conjugate: Synthesis and antibacterial activity. *React. Funcct. Polym.* **2002**, *50*, 257–263. [CrossRef]
33. Bierbaum, G. Antibiotische Peptide-Lantibiotika. *Chemother. J.* **1999**, *8*, 204–209.
34. Zasloff, M. Antimicrobial peptides of multicellular organisms. *Nature* **2002**, *415*, 389–395. [CrossRef] [PubMed]
35. Zasloff, M. Magainins, a class of antimicrobial peptides from xenopus skin-isolation, characterization of 2 active forms, and partial cdna sequence of a precursor. *Proc. Natl. Acad. Sci. USA* **1987**, *84*, 5449–5453. [CrossRef] [PubMed]
36. Broekaert, W.F.; Terras, F.R.; Cammue, B.P.; Osborn, R.W. Plant Defensins: Novel Antimicrobial Peptides as Components of the Host Defense System. *Plant Physiol.* **1995**, *108*, 1353–1358. [CrossRef] [PubMed]
37. Cornut, I.; Büttner, K.; Dasseux, J.L.; Dufourcq, J. The amphipathic α-helix concept: Application to the de novo design of ideally amphipathic Leu, Lys peptides with hemolytic activity higher than that of melittin. *FEBS Lett.* **1994**, *349*, 29–33. [CrossRef]
38. Beven, L.; Castano, S.; Dufourcq, J.; Wieslander, A.; Wroblewski, H. The antibiotic activity of cationic linear amphipathic peptides: Lessons from the action of leucine/lysine copolymers on bacteria of the class Mollicutes. *Eur. J. Biochem.* **2003**, *270*, 2207–2217. [CrossRef] [PubMed]
39. Kuroda, K.; Caputo, G.A. Antimicrobial polymers as synthetic mimics of host-defense peptides. *WIRE Nanomed. Nanobiotechnol.* **2013**, *5*, 49–66. [CrossRef] [PubMed]
40. Lienkamp, K.; Tew, G.N. Synthetic mimics of antimicrobial peptides (SMAMPs). *Chem. Eur. J.* **2009**, *15*, 11784–11800. [CrossRef] [PubMed]
41. Arnold, M.; Rätzsch, M. The copolymerization of maleic anhydride with propene and isobutene. *Macromol. Chem.* **1986**, *187*, 1593–1596. [CrossRef]
42. Nash, J.F.; Lin, T.-M. Resin Compositions and Method for Controlling Diarrhea. U.S. Patent 3,224,941, 21 December 1965.
43. Komber, H. The 1H and 13C NMR spectra of alternating isobutene/maleic anhydride copolymer and the corresponding acid and sodium salt—A stereochemical analysis. *Macromol. Chem. Phys.* **1996**, *197*, 343–353. [CrossRef]
44. Bortel, E.; Styslo, M. On the chemical communications of poly(maleic anhydride-co-isobutene) by means of hydrolysis, ammoniation or aminations. *Macromol. Chem. Phys.* **1990**, *191*, 2653–2662. [CrossRef]
45. Bortel, E.; Styslo, M. On the structure of radically obtained maleic anhydride/C4-alkene copolymers. *Macromol. Chem. Phys.* **1988**, *189*, 1155–1165. [CrossRef]
46. Kenawy, E.R. Biologically active polymers. Iv. Synthesis and antimicrobial activity of polymers containing 8-hydroxyquinoline moiety. *J. Appl. Polym. Sci.* **2001**, *82*, 1364–1374. [CrossRef]
47. Iwabuchi, S.; Watanabe, Y.; Nakahira, T.; Kojima, K. Vinylhydroquinone. V. Tri-n-butylborane-initiated copolymerization of maleic anhydride and redox property of copolymers. *J. Polym. Sci. Polym. Chem. Ed.* **1979**, *17*, 1721–1726. [CrossRef]
48. Szkudlarek, M.; Beginn, U.; Keul, H.; Möller, M. Synthesis of Terpolymers with Homogeneous Composition by Free Radical Copolymerization of Maleic Anhydride, Perfluorooctyl and Butyl or Dodecyl Methacrylates: Application of the Continuous Flow Monomer Addition Technique. *Polymers* **2017**, *11*, 610. [CrossRef]
49. Kenawy, E.-R.; Sakran, M.A. Controlled release of polymer conjugated agrochemicals. System based on poly(methyl vinyl ether-alt-maleic anhydride). *J. Appl. Polym. Sci.* **2001**, *80*, 415–421. [CrossRef]
50. Lee, W.-F.; Chen, Y.-M. Poly(sulfobetaine)s and corresponding cationic polymers. VIII. Synthesis and aqueous solution properties of a cationic poly(methyl iodide quaternized styrene-N,N-dimethylaminopropyl maleamidic acid)copolymer. *J. Appl. Polym. Sci.* **2000**, *80*, 1619–1626. [CrossRef]
51. Kang, Y.; Seo, Y.-H.; Lee, C. Synthesis and Conductivity of PEGME Braneded Poly(ethylene-alt-maleimide) Based Solid Polymer Electrolyte. *Bull. Korean Chem. Soc.* **2000**, *21*, 241–244.
52. Lee, S.S.; Ahn, T.O. Direct Polymer reaction of poly(styrene-co-maleic anhydride): Polymeric imidization. *J. Appl. Polym. Sci.* **1998**, *71*, 1187–1196. [CrossRef]
53. Lee, W.-F.; Hwong, G.-Y. Polysulfobetaines and corresponding cationic polymers. IV. Synthesis and aqueous solution properties of cationic poly(MIQSDMAPM). *J. Appl. Polym. Sci.* **1996**, *59*, 599–608. [CrossRef]

54. Lee, W.-F.; Huang, G.-Y. Polysulfobetaines and corresponding cationic polymers. VI. Synthesis and aqueous solution properties of cationic poly(methyl iodide quaternized acrylamide-N,N-dimethylaminopropylmaleimide copolymer) [poly(MIQADMAPM)]. *J. Appl. Polym. Sci.* **1996**, *60*, 187–199. [CrossRef]
55. Lee, W.-F.; Chen, C.-F. Poly(sulfobetaine)s and corresponding cationic polymers. VII. Thermal degradation of copolymers derived from poly(acrylamide co-N,N-dimethylaminopropylmaleimide). *J. Appl. Polym. Sci.* **1997**, *66*, 95–103. [CrossRef]
56. Rice, L.M.; Grogan, C.H.; Reid, E.E. Hypotensive Agents. III. Dialkylaminoalkyl Pyrrolydine Derivatives. *J. Am. Chem. Soc.* **1953**, *75*, 2261–2262. [CrossRef]
57. Meng, Y.Z.; Tjong, S.C.; Hay, A.S.; Wang, S.J. Synthesis and proton conductivities of phosphonic acid containing poly-(arylene ether)s. *J. Polym. Sci. Part A Polym. Chem.* **2001**, *39*, 3218–3226. [CrossRef]
58. Sung, P.-H.; Chen, C.-Y.; Wu, S.-Y.; Huang, J.Y. Styrene/maleimide copolymer with stable second-order optical nonlinearity. *J. Polym. Sci. Part A Polym. Chem.* **1996**, *34*, 2189–2194. [CrossRef]
59. Liu, Y.L.; Liu, Y.L.; Jeng, R.J.; Chiu, Y.-S. Triphenylphosphine oxide-based bismaleimide and poly(bismaleimide): Synthesis, characterization, and properties. *J. Polym. Sci. Part A Polym. Chem.* **2001**, *39*, 1716–1725. [CrossRef]
60. Wang, C.-S.; Hwang, H.-J. Investigation of bismaleimide containing naphthalene unit. II. Thermal behavior and properties of polymer. *J. Polym. Sci. Part A Polym. Chem.* **1996**, *34*, 1493–1500. [CrossRef]
61. Alfaia, A.J.I.; Calado, A.R.T.; Reis, J.C.R. Quaternization reaction of aromatic heterocyclic imines in methanol—A case of strong anti-reactivity selectivity principle with isoselective temperature. *Eur. J. Org. Chem.* **2000**, *2000*, 3627–3631. [CrossRef]
62. Johnson, T.W.; Klotz, I.M. Preparation and characterization of some derivatives of poly(ethyleneimine). *Macromolecules* **1974**, *7*, 149–153. [CrossRef]
63. Bütün, V.; Armes, S.P.; Billingham, N.C. Selective quaternization of 2-(dimethylamino)ethyl methacrylate residues in tertiary amine methacrylate diblock copolymers. *Macromolecules* **2001**, *34*, 1148–1159. [CrossRef]
64. Vogl, O.; Tirrell, D. Functional polymers with biologically active groups. *J. Macromol. Sci. Chem.* **1979**, *A13*, 415–439. [CrossRef]
65. Worley, S.D.; Sun, G. Biocidal Polymers. *Trends Polym. Sci.* **1996**, *4*, 364–370.
66. Exley, E.E.; Pasley, L.C.; Sahukhal, G.S.; Abel, B.A.; Brown, T.D.; McCormick, C.L.; Heinhorst, S.; Koul, V.; Choudhary, V.; Elasri, M.O.; et al. Antimicrobial Peptide Mimicking Primary Amine and Guanidine Containing Methacrylamide Copolymers Prepared by Raft Polymerization. *Biomacromolecules* **2015**, *16*, 3845–3852. [CrossRef] [PubMed]
67. He, Y.; Heine, E.; Keusgen, N.; Keul, H.; Moeller, M. Synthesis and Characterization of Amphiphilic Monodisperse Compounds and Poly(ethylene imine)s: Influence of Their Microstructures on the Antimicrobial Properties. *Biomacromolecules* **2012**, *13*, 612–623. [CrossRef] [PubMed]
68. Kiss, E.; Heine, E.T.; Hill, K.; He, Y.C.; Keusgen, N.; Penzes, C.B.; Schnoller, D.; Gyulai, G.; Mendrek, A.; Keul, H.; et al. Membrane Affinity and Antibacterial Properties of Cationic Polyelectrolytes with Different Hydrophobicity. *Macromol. Biosci.* **2012**, *12*, 1181–1189. [CrossRef] [PubMed]
69. Roier, S.; Zingl, F.G.; Cakar, F.; Schild, S. Bacterial outer membrane vesicle biogenesis: A new mechanism and its implications. *Microb. Cell* **2016**, *3*, 257–259. [CrossRef] [PubMed]
70. Manning, A.J.; Kuehn, M.J. Contribution of bacterial outer membrane vesicles to innate bacterial defense. *BMC Microbiol.* **2011**, *11*, 258–272. [CrossRef] [PubMed]
71. Heredia, R.M.; Boeris, P.S.; Liffourrena, A.S.; Bergero, M.F.; López, G.A.; Lucchesi, G.I. Release of outer membrane vesicles in *Pseudomonas putida* as a response to stress caused by cationic surfactants. *Microbiology* **2016**, *162*, 813–822. [CrossRef] [PubMed]
72. MacDonald, I.A.; Kuehn, M.J. Stress-induced outer membrane vesicle production by *Pseudomonas aeruginosa*. *J. Bacteriol.* **2013**, *195*, 2971–2981. [CrossRef] [PubMed]
73. Marquardt, F.; Stöcker, C.; Gartzen, R.; Heine, E.; Keul, H.; Möller, M. Novel Antibacterial Polyglycidols: Relationship between Structure and Properties. *Polymers* **2018**, *10*, 96. [CrossRef]
74. Sahl, H.-G.; Jack, R.W.; Bierbaum, G. Biosynthesis and biological activities of lantibiotics with unique post-translational modifications. *Eur. J. Biochem.* **1995**, *230*, 827–853. [CrossRef] [PubMed]
75. Breukink, E.; de Kruijff, B. The lantibiotic Nisin, a special case or not? *Biochim. Biophys. Acta* **1999**, *1462*, 223–234. [CrossRef]

76. Deutsches Institut für Normung. *Medical Microbiology—Susceptibility Testing of Microbial Pathogens to Antimicrobial Agents—Part 7: Determination of the Minimum Bactericidal Concentration (MBC) with the Method of Microbouillondilution*; Deutsches Institut für Normung: Berlin, Germany, 2009.
77. Wang, Y.; Xu, J.; Zhang, Y.; Yan, H.; Liu, K. Antimicrobial and hemolytic activities of copolymers with cationic and hydrophobic groups: A comparison of block and random copolymers. *Macromol. Biosci.* **2011**, *11*, 1499–1504. [CrossRef] [PubMed]

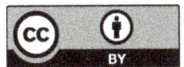

© 2018 by the authors. Licensee MDPI, Basel, Switzerland. This article is an open access article distributed under the terms and conditions of the Creative Commons Attribution (CC BY) license (http://creativecommons.org/licenses/by/4.0/).

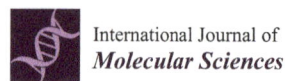

Article

Providing Antibacterial Activity to Poly(2-Hydroxy Ethyl Methacrylate) by Copolymerization with a Methacrylic Thiazolium Derivative

Alexandra Muñoz-Bonilla *, Daniel López and Marta Fernández-García *

Instituto de Ciencia y Tecnología de Polímeros (ICTP-CSIC), C/ Juan de la Cierva 3, 28006 Madrid, Spain; daniel@ictp.csic.es
* Correspondence: sbonilla@ictp.csic.es (A.M.-B.); martafg@ictp.csic.es (M.F.-G.); Tel.: +34-91-258-7530 (M.F.-G.)

Received: 28 November 2018; Accepted: 16 December 2018; Published: 19 December 2018

Abstract: Antimicrobial polymers and coatings are potent types of materials for fighting microbial infections, and as such, they have attracted increased attention in many fields. Here, a series of antimicrobial copolymers were prepared by radical copolymerization of 2-hydroxyethyl methacrylate (HEMA), which is widely employed in the manufacturing of biomedical devices, and the monomer 2-(4-methylthiazol-5-yl)ethyl methacrylate (MTA), which bears thiazole side groups susceptible to quaternization, to provide a positive charge. The copolymers were further quantitatively quaternized with either methyl or butyl iodide, as demonstrated by nuclear magnetic resonance (NMR) and attenuated total reflection Fourier-transform infrared spectroscopy (ATR-FTIR). Then, the polycations were characterized by zeta potential measurements to evaluate their effective charge and by differential scanning calorimetry (DSC) and thermogravimetric analysis (TGA) to evaluate their thermal properties. The ζ-potential study revealed that the quaternized copolymers with intermediate compositions present higher charges than the corresponding homopolymers. The cationic copolymers showed greater glass transition temperatures than poly(2-hydroxyethyl methacrylate) (PHEMA), with values higher than 100 °C, in particular those quaternized with methyl iodide. The TGA studies showed that the thermal stability of polycations varies with the composition, improving as the content of HEMA in the copolymer increases. Microbial assays targeting Gram-positive and Gram-negative bacteria confirmed that the incorporation of a low number of cationic units into PHEMA provides antimicrobial character with a minimum inhibitory concentration (MIC) of 128 µg mL^{-1}. Remarkably, copolymers with MTA molar fractions higher than 0.50 exhibited MIC values as low as 8 µg mL^{-1}.

Keywords: antimicrobial polymers; quaternary ammonium; 2-hydroxyethyl methacrylate; thermal stability

1. Introduction

In the last few years, antimicrobial polymers have attracted substantial scientific and industrial attention because of their unique properties and applications in the design and production of many materials, including medical devices, textiles, packaging, and purification systems [1–3]. Of special concern is bacterial contamination on the surfaces of medical devices, such as catheters or implants, which are responsible for many hospital-acquired infections (HAI), also known as nosocomial infections. The most common and serious HAIs are catheter-associated urinary tract infections, central line-associated bloodstream infections, ventilator-associated pneumonia, and surgical site infections, among others [4,5]. Coatings able to eliminate bacterial contamination on these material surfaces and, thus, prevent such infections have emerged as very efficient prophylactic strategies. These coatings can either repel microbes, avoiding microbial attachment, or kill microorganisms upon contact or in the surrounding by biocidal release [6]. In particular, self-disinfecting coatings with killing or bactericidal activity have demonstrated high efficiency and are typically obtained by incorporating antimicrobial agents, including antibiotics [7,8], antimicrobial peptides [9,10], silver and copper compounds [11,12], zinc oxide [13], titanium dioxide particles [14,15], etc., onto the surface. Alternatively, the use of antimicrobial polymers as contact-active coatings with inherent biocidal activity has gained importance, because antimicrobial polymers offer some advantages, such as chemical stability, high and long-term activity, low toxicity, and reduced potential to generate resistance [16,17]. Most of these antimicrobial polymers are polycations, in particular polymers with quaternary ammonium groups [18,19], which are able to interact with the negatively charged bacterial wall, disrupting the integrity of the membrane and leading to the death of the bacteria. Recently, we developed a series of polycations based on polymethacrylates bearing pendant 1,3-thiazolium groups, which have demonstrated high activity against a broad spectrum of bacteria [20–22]. In addition, antimicrobial polymeric coatings have been prepared from these polycations by blending with hydrophobic polymers typically used in medical devices, such as polyacrylonitrile or polystyrene [23–25].

Concerning hydrophilic polymer materials, poly(2-hydroxyethyl methacrylate) (PHEMA) is one of the most widely used in the manufacture of medical devices, such as contact and intraocular lenses, and medical device coatings [26,27], because it exhibits blood and cell biocompatibility, low cytotoxicity, and thrombogenicity [28,29]. In addition, a variety of antimicrobial agents has been included into hydrogels and materials based on PHEMA to provide biocidal character as an additional property [26,30–32]. Herein, we prepared copolymers systems composed of 2-hydroxyethyl methacrylate (HEMA) and a methacrylic monomer bearing thiazolium moieties (MTARI) with the purpose of incorporating antimicrobial properties into PHEMA. Several copolymer compositions were prepared and evaluated for an adequate balance of structural, thermal, and antimicrobial properties.

2. Results and Discussion

2.1. Synthesis of Cationic Polyelectrolytes: P(MTARI-co-HEMA) Copolymers

First, the synthesis of P(MTA-co-HEMA) copolymers was performed by free radical polymerization of HEMA and 2-(4-methylthiazol-5-yl)ethyl methacrylate (MTA) comonomers, using different feed molar ratios, i.e., feed molar fraction of MTA, f_{MTA} = 0.0, 0.2, 0.4, 0.6, 0.8, and 1.0 (Scheme 1).

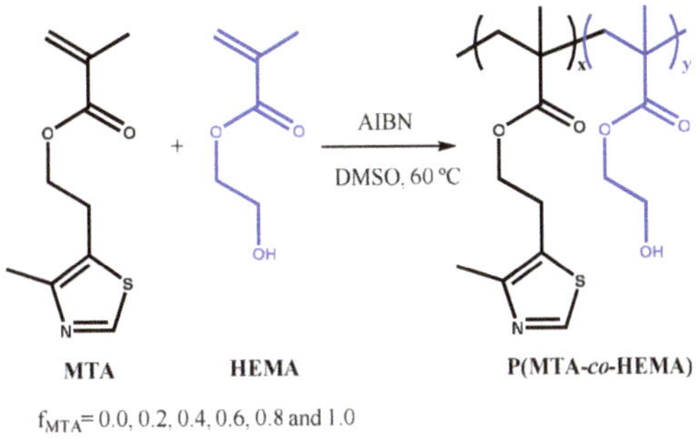

Scheme 1. Schematic representation of the synthesis of the P(MTA-co-HEMA) copolymers with different molar compositions. AIBN: 2,2′-azobisisobutyronitrile.

The copolymerizations almost reached full conversion after 24 h for all the initial f_{MTA}, which was confirmed gravimetrically and by ^{1}H-NMR (the double bonds completely disappeared from the bulk of the reactions). Similarly, the molar fractions of MTA in the obtained copolymers (F_{MTA}) were determined by ^{1}H-NMR, and as expected, these values were found to be very close to the f_{MTA} values (Table 1) as the conversion was nearly complete ($f_{MTA} \cong F_{MTA}$). Table 1 summarizes the average molecular weight (M_n) and the polydispersity indexes (PDI) of the P(MTA-co-HEMA) copolymers determined by gel permeation chromatography (GPC). The molecular weights ranged from 35 to 87 kDa, while the PDI values were around 1.9–2.4, similar to those typically obtained in radical polymerization.

Table 1. Characterization of the P(MTA-co-HEMA) copolymers.

f_{MTA}	F_{MTA}	M_n (kDa)	PDI
0.00	0.00	86.8	2.1
0.20	0.18	60.8	2.0
0.40	0.37	59.2	2.4
0.60	0.56	42.6	2.2
0.80	0.76	34.5	2.2
1.00	1.00	36.6	1.9

Subsequently, the corresponding polycations with different charge balances were prepared by N-alkylation of the P(MTA-co-HEMA) copolymers with either butyl or methyl iodide, as shown in Scheme 2.

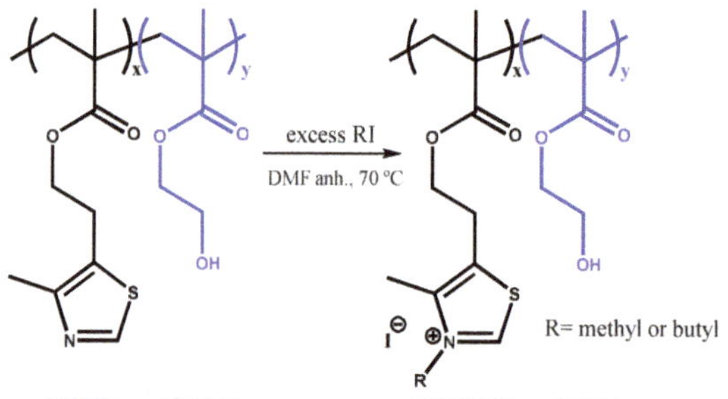

Scheme 2. Schematic representation of the quaternization of the P(MTARI-co-HEMA) polycations with alkyl iodide (RI). DMF: N,N-dimethylformamide.

To ensure the complete quaternization of all the thiazole groups present in the copolymers, the reaction was carried out with an excess of the alkylating agent at 70 °C. After one week, complete quaternization was reached for all the cases as revealed by ^{1}H-NMR spectra. As an example, Figure 1 depicts the spectra of the quaternized copolymers with butyl iodide, P(MTABuI-co-HEMA), and their corresponding homopolymers, PHEMA and PMTABuI. The MTA homopolymer (PMTA) spectrum is also depicted for comparative purposes to visualize the shift alteration produced by the protonation. It can be clearly seen that the signals corresponding to the aromatic protons of 1,3-thiazole, –N=CH–S, at ~8.8 ppm shifted to ~10.1–10.2 ppm after the N-alkylation to obtain 1,3-thiazolium group, –N$^+$=CH–S, which confirmed that all the modifications were achieved quantitatively [33,34]. In addition, new signals appeared at ~4.4 ppm due to the alkylating agent (i.e., –N$^+$–CH$_2$– in the case of butyl iodide). The intensity of this signal increased as the content of MTA increased in the copolymer, that is, with increasing values of F_{MTA}. This event was concomitant with a decrease in the intensity of the signals attributed to the HEMA units, such as the peak at 4.8 ppm that corresponded to the proton of the hydroxyl group. The copolymers were also characterized by ATR-FTIR spectroscopy. As an example, Figure 2 shows the spectra of the unquaternized and quaternized copolymers with both alkylating agents with an active comonomer composition of 0.8, viz. P(MTA$_{0.8}$-co-HEMA$_{0.2}$), P(MTAMeI$_{0.8}$-co-HEMA$_{0.2}$), and P(MTABuI$_{0.8}$-co-HEMA$_{0.2}$), respectively. The carbonyl stretching vibration (C=O) at around 1720 cm^{-1}, characteristic of methacrylic monomers, the O–H stretching region around 3700–3100 cm^{-1}, and the C–O band at ca. 1250 cm^{-1}, typical of HEMA polymers, can be observed clearly in the spectra. The band corresponding to the C=N– stretching vibration of MTA appeared at 1550 cm^{-1}. This band vanished when the copolymers were modified with the alkyl iodine agents, and a new band emerged at ca. 1590 cm^{-1}, characteristic of the C=N$^+$– stretching vibration.

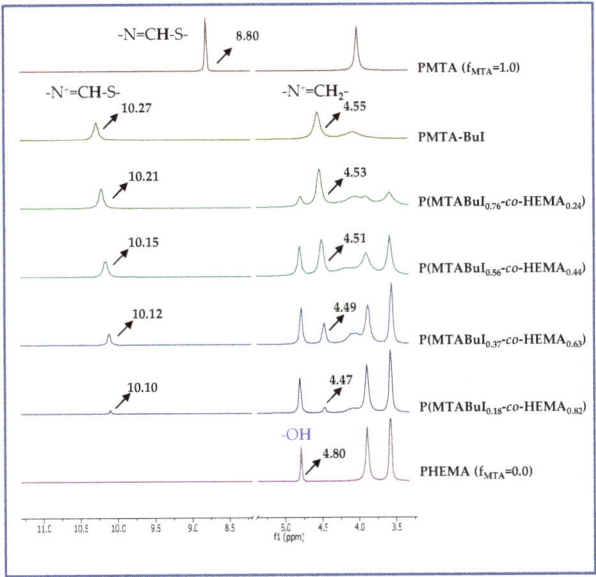

Figure 1. Schematic representation of the preparation of the P(MTARI-co-HEMA) polycations by quaternization with alkyl iodide (RI). Representative region of ^{1}H-NMR spectra in DMSO-d6 of P(MTABuI-co-HEMA), PMTA, PMTABuI, and PHEMA.

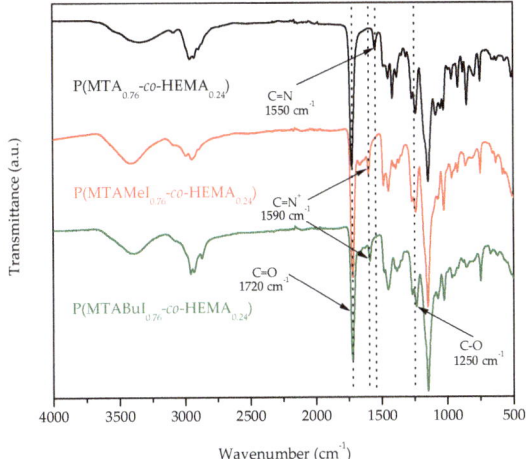

Figure 2. Attenuated total reflection Fourier-transform infrared spectroscopy (ATR-FTIR) spectra of P(MTA$_{0.8}$-co-HEMA$_{0.2}$), P(MTAMeI$_{0.8}$-co-HEMA$_{0.2}$), and P(MTABuI$_{0.8}$-co-HEMA$_{0.2}$).

2.2. Characterization of the Synthetized Copolymers: P(MTA-co-HEMA), and P(MTARI-co-HEMA)

Once the copolymer precursors, P(MTA-co-HEMA), and the polycations P(MTARI-co-HEMA) were successfully prepared, they were characterized to estimate their antimicrobial potential. It is well known that such activity is dependent on different parameters, such as the nature of the charge; the hydrophobic groups; the balance of cationic to hydrophobic moieties; the polymer composition;

and the molecular weight [1,35,36]. Then, the ζ-potential of the polycations was determined, and the obtained values are represented in Figure 3.

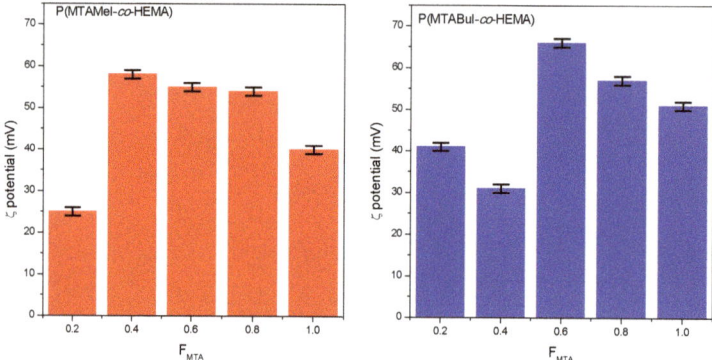

Figure 3. Variation of the ζ-potential of the quaternized copolymer series as a function of the composition.

Interestingly, the compositions with higher contents of MTA presented greater zeta potential values than their corresponding quaternized homopolymers. They presented values near to +60 or higher, which indicated the good stability of the aggregation in comparison with the homopolymers, especially with respect to the PMTAMeI, which has moderate stability with a ζ-potential of +40. In fact, the PMTABuI homopolymer was more stable and positively charged than the PMTAMeI: therefore, higher antimicrobial activity was to be expected.

Subsequently, the thermal properties of the obtained copolymers were analyzed given that they were of great importance for the applicability of these antimicrobial polymers. The copolymers were first analyzed by differential scanning calorimetry (DSC), and the glass transition temperatures, T_g, are given in Table 2. Figure 4a displays the DSC curves of the unquaternized copolymers, while Figure 4b represents the T_g variation of all the series as a function of the copolymer composition, F_{MTA}.

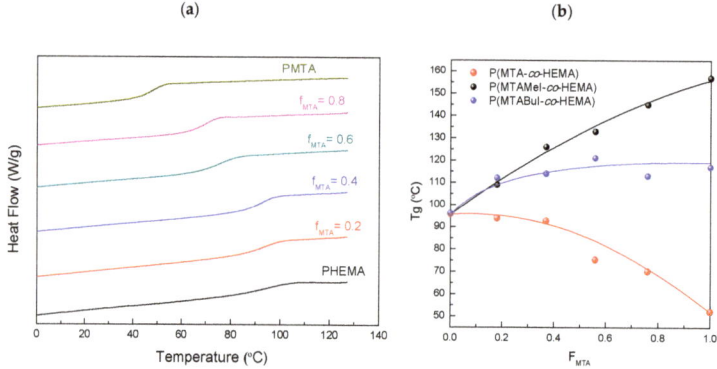

Figure 4. (a) Differential scanning calorimetry (DSC) curves of the pristine (PMTA-*co*-HEMA) copolymers; and (b) The glass transition temperatures of the P(MTA-*co*-HEMA), P(MTAMeI-*co*-HEMA), and P(MTABuI-*co*-HEMA) copolymers as a function of the MTA or MTARI content in the copolymer, F_{MTA}.

From these data, it was observed that the T_g values of the copolymers shifted to lower temperatures as the content of MTA, F_{MTA}, increased up to 49 °C for the PMTA homopolymer. In contrast, the polycations obtained after quaternization followed the contrary trend; their T_g increased with the amount of the MTARI cationic units for both series of copolymers—those quaternized with methyl iodide (P(MTAMeI-co-HEMA)) and those quaternized with butyl iodide (P(MTABuI-co-HEMA)). Also, both series of cationic copolymers exhibited greater T_g than the PHEMA homopolymer. It was noticeable that the P(MTAMeI-co-HEMA) copolymers achieved higher T_g values in comparison with the P(MTABuI-co-HEMA) series due to the effect of the length of the alkylating agent. The incorporation of a long and flexible alkyl chain, such as a butyl group, improved the mobility of the copolymers and reduced their T_g.

Table 2. Thermal characteristic parameters determined by DSC and TGA of the synthesized copolymers. Glass transition temperature, T_g; initial degradation temperature, T_d^{onset}; temperature of the maximum rate of weight loss for each step, T_d^{max}; and the rate of weight loss for each step, $-dw/dT$.

F_{MTA}	T_g (°C)	T_d^{onset} (°C)	T_d^{max1} (°C)	$-dw_1/dT$ (%/°C)	T_d^{max2} (°C)	$-dw_2/dT$ (%/°C)	T_d^{max3} (°C)	$-dw_3/dT$ (%/°C)
				P(MTA-co-HEMA)				
0.00	96	259.0	178.5	0.03	-	-	400.0	0.99
0.18	94	288.0	175.0	0.03	328.5	0.45	441.5	1.26
0.37	92	300.5	100.0	0.02	327.5	0.62	432.5	1.17
0.56	75	301.0	-	-	341.0	0.74	435.0	0.91
0.76	70	294.0	-	-	350.0	0.98	426.0	0.65
1.00	49	300.0	-	-	366.5	1.08	413.5	0.34
				P(MTAMeI-co-HEMA)				
0.00	96	259.0	178.5	0.03	-	-	400.0	0.99
0.18	109	185.0	237.5	0.18	-	-	420.5	1.05
0.37	126	186.5	228.5	0.39	-	-	404.0	0.71
0.56	133	196.5	220.5	0.75	320.0	0.38	429.5	0.71
0.76	145	205.5	228.5	0.89	329.5	0.37	422.0	0.52
1.00	157	209.5	235.5	1.12	341.5	0.41	421.5	0.36
				P(MTABuI-co-HEMA)				
0.00	96	259.0	178.5	0.03	-	-	400.0	0.99
0.18	112	220.0	250.5	0.37	-	-	433.5	1.32
0.37	114	225.0	247.5	0.96	-	-	432.0	0.89
0.56	121	222.0	242.5	1.20	-	-	426.0	0.73
0.76	113	221.0	244.5	1.43	-	-	419.0	0.55
1.00	117	229.0	251.0	1.80	-	-	418.0	0.36

Then, the thermal stability of the different series was analyzed by TGA under an inert atmosphere. Figure 5 displays the TGA curves of the unquaternized and quaternized copolymer, and the thermal degradation parameters are collected in Table 2. The degradation of PHEMA took place in one single stage, considering that a previous step of water elimination occurred because of the hygroscopic character of the polymer (ca. 2–3%). The literature has explained that the resulting product of this breakdown is mainly the HEMA monomer [37–39]. PMTA presented two main stages, and contrary to HEMA, in which depolymerization was the main process, the degradation seemed to be by random chain scission as with poly(methyl methacrylate). In the case of the unmodified copolymers, the behavior was dependent on the HEMA/MTA content. Those copolymers with HEMA predominance presented hygroscopic tendencies and intermediate behaviors between both homopolymer parents. The first main stage, at temperatures higher than 300 °C, is shifted to higher temperatures as the MTA increased, while in the second step, the temperatures decreased. Nevertheless, the stability was improved by the presence of HEMA in the copolymer.

This behavior was more evident in both the quaternized copolymer series. Figure 5b,c show that the incorporation of the HEMA units into the copolymers expanded the thermal stability, which could extend the applicability of these antimicrobial materials. In the case of methyl iodide incorporation, the degradation occurred in three stages instead of the two appearing in the case of butyl iodide. Therefore, the quaternization with a longer alkyl agent stabilized the macromolecular structure of the cationic copolymers. In contrast, the polycations obtained after the quaternization followed the contrary trend; their T_g increased with the amount of the MTARI cationic units for both series of copolymers—those quaternized with methyl iodide (P(MTAMeI-co-HEMA)) and those quaternized with butyl iodide (P(MTABuI-co-HEMA)). Also, both series of cationic copolymers exhibited greater T_g than the PHEMA homopolymer, whose value was almost 100 °C due to the strong inter- and intramolecular interactions [37,40]. It is noticeable that the P(MTAMeI-co-HEMA) copolymers achieved higher T_g values in comparison with the copolymers quaternized with butyl iodide because of the effect of the length of the alkylating agent. The incorporation of a long and flexible alkyl chain, such as a butyl group, improved the mobility of the copolymers and reduced their T_g.

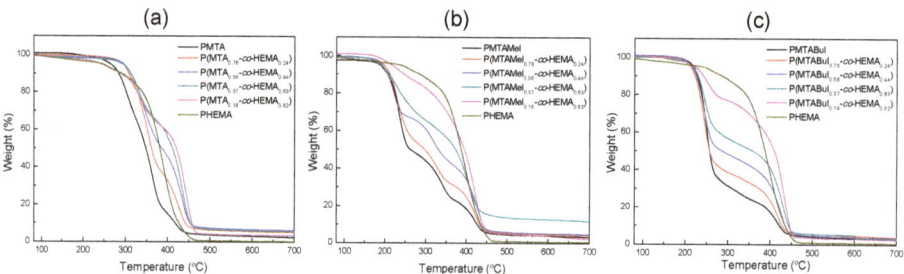

Figure 5. Thermogravimetric analysis of the (**a**) P(MTA-co-HEMA), (**b**) P(MTAMeI-co-HEMA), and (**c**) P(MTABuI-co-HEMA) copolymers.

2.3. Antibacterial Activity Studies

The antimicrobial activity of the prepared polycations, the P(MTAMeI-co-HEMA) and P(MTABuI-co-HEMA) copolymers, was evaluated against the model bacterial strains, Gram-positive *Staphylococcus aureus* and Gram-negative *Pseudomonas aeruginosa*. These polymers were also tested against fungi *Candida parapsilosis*, but they were not effective in the opposite behavior when MTA was copolymerized with acrylonitrile, a hydrophobic monomer [21]. Concretely, the microbroth dilution reference method [41–43] was used, obtaining the minimum inhibitory concentration (MIC) values collected in Table 3. As expected, the homopolymers, PMTAMeI and PMTABuI, exhibited significant antimicrobial activity with very low MIC values, as previously reported [20]. The homopolymer quaternized with butyl iodide showed improved activity against the Gram-negative bacteria in comparison with the methylated polymer, because it augments the hydrophobic balance of the copolymers [35]. In effect, several studies have demonstrated that the incorporation of certain contents of hydrophobic moieties, reaching an adequate hydrophobic/hydrophilic balance, improves the antimicrobial activity of the polymer, because the process facilitates the pass through the hydrophobic cytoplasmic membrane [44,45].

On the other hand, when biocompatible HEMA units are incorporated into the copolymer, the activity tends to diminish. This is due to the decrease in the positive charge density of the corresponding polycations as a result of the incorporation of a non-active monomer. Nevertheless, the copolymers mainly based on HEMA, with MTARI contents as low as $F_{MTA} = 0.18$, still exhibited significant activity—MIC values of 128 µg mL^{-1}. Again, the copolymers containing butyl groups showed better activities than the copolymers quaternized with methyl iodide. Remarkably, the copolymers quaternized with butyl iodide maintained their excellent activity up to a relatively high content of HEMA, with MIC = 8 µg mL^{-1} for the F_{MTA} value of 0.56. In this case, the copolymers might have adopted in-solution conformations in which their positive charges were highly accessible to bacterial membrane.

Table 3. Minimum inhibitory concentration (MIC) of the quaternized copolymers, P(MTAMeI-co-HEMA) and P(MTABuI-co-HEMA), against Gram-positive *Staphylococcus aureus* and Gram-negative *Pseudomonas aeruginosa*.

F_{MTA}	MIC (µg mL^{-1})	
	S. aureus	P. aeruginosa
P(MTAMeI-co-HEMA)		
0.18	128	128
0.37	128	128
0.56	128	128
0.76	8	32
1.00	8	16
P(MTABuI-co-HEMA)		
0.18	128	128
0.37	128	128
0.56	8	8
0.76	8	8
1.00	8	8

Therefore, the obtained copolymers were demonstrated to be promising antimicrobial materials, in which the incorporation of even a low number of cationic units into PHEMA provided significant antibacterial activity and maintained good thermal stability. While higher amounts of the cationic monomer, up to ~50%, maintained the excellent antimicrobial activity, reaching MIC values similar to that found in the homopolymers PMTARI, and improved their thermal stability, the monomer could also enhance their biocompatibility, because PHEMA and PMTARI are not toxics [20,22,28,29].

3. Materials and Methods

3.1. Materials

The monomer 2-(4-methylthiazol-5-yl)ethyl methacrylate (MTA) was synthesized as previously reported [20]. The monomer 2-hydroxyethyl methacrylate (HEMA, 99%; Aldrich, Steinheim, Germany) was distilled prior to use. 2,2'-Azobisisobutyronitrile (AIBN, 98%; Acros, Buch, Switzerland) was recrystallized twice from methanol (MeOH, 99.9%; Aldrich) prior to use. Anhydrous dimethyl sulfoxide (DMSO, 99.8%) and N,N-dimethylformamide (DMF, 99.8%) were purchased from Alfa-Aesar (Karlsruhe, Germany) and were used as received. 1-Iodobutane (BuI, 99%, Aldrich), iodomethane (MeI, 99%; Aldrich), and hexane (96%; Scharlau, Sentmenat, Spain) were used as received.

For the microbiological assays, sodium chloride (NaCl, 0.9%, BioXtra, Steinheim, Germany, suitable for cell cultures) and phosphate buffered saline (PBS, pH 7.4) were obtained from Aldrich. BBL^{TM} Mueller Hinton broth used as microbial growth media was purchased from Becton, Dickinson and Company (Madrid, Spain). Sheep blood (5%) and Columbia Agar plates were acquired from BioMérieux (Madrid, Spain). American Type Culture Collection (ATCC) Gram-positive *Staphylococcus aureus* (*S. aureus*, ATCC 29213) and Gram-negative *Pseudomonas aeruginosa* (*P. aeruginosa*, ATCC 27853) bacteria were obtained from Oxoid^{TM} (Wesel, Germany).

3.2. Synthesis of P(MTA-co-HEMA) Copolymers

P(MTA-co-HEMA)s copolymers with different chemical compositions were synthesized via free radical polymerization of HEMA and MTA comonomers, as shown in Scheme 1. Briefly, both monomers, MTA and HEMA (1 M total concentration), and the initiator, AIBN (5×10^{-2} M), were added into a Schlenk tube and dissolved in anhydrous DMSO. The mixture was deoxygenated by purging with argon over 15 min. Then, the reaction was stirred at 60 °C for 20 h under an argon atmosphere. After that, the mixture was cooled down, and the polymers were isolated by precipitation into distilled water, filtered, and washed several times with water. The solid was dried under a vacuum until a constant weight was reached.

P(MTA-co-HEMA): ^{1}H-NMR (300 MHz, DMSO-d6): δ = 8.80–8.85 (br, 1H; =CH thiazole, MTA), 4.80 (br, 1H; OH, HEMA), 4.02 (br, 2H; OCH$_2$, MTA), 3.90 (br, 2H; –**CH$_2$**–OH, HEMA), 3.59 (br, 2H; –CH$_2$–CO–, HEMA), 3.05 (br, 2H; CH$_2$, MTA), 2.30 (br, 3H; CH$_3$ thiazole, MTA), 1.92–1.24 (br, 2H; CH$_2$, MTA), 0.76–0.57 (br, 3H; CH$_3$, MTA).

3.3. Quaternization of Copolymers: Synthesis of Cationic Polyelectrolytes, P(MTARI-co-HEMA)

The P(MTA-co-HEMA) copolymers were modified by N-alkylation of the thiazole groups of the MTA units with 1-iodobutane or iodomethane, as shown in Scheme 2. The copolymers were added into a sealed tube containing a magnetic stirring bar and dissolved in anhydrous DMF (0.1 mmol L^{-1}). Then, a large excess of alkyl iodide, methyl iodide, or butyl iodide was added (ratio copolymer/alkyl iodide ≈ 1:5). The mixture was purged with argon and heated at 70 °C while being stirred for one week to ensure complete quaternization. Then, the solution was poured into hexane, and the copolymers were obtained as brown oils. The quaternized copolymers were further purified by dialysis against the distilled water to remove the residual products and were freeze dried. The methylated and butylated copolymers were labeled as P(MTAMeI-co-HEMA) and P(MTABuI-co-HEMA), respectively. The degree of quaternization was determined by ^{1}H-NMR spectroscopy [22].

P(MTAMeI-co-HEMA): ^{1}H-NMR (300 MHz, DMSO-d6): δ = 10.16–10.06 (br, 1H; =CH thiazolium, MTAMeI), 4.80 (br, 1H; OH, HEMA), 4.20–3.99 (br, 5H; $^+$NCH$_3$ and OCH$_2$, MTAMeI), 3.90 (br, 2H; –**CH$_2$**–OH, HEMA), 3.59 (br, 2H; –CH$_2$–CO–, HEMA), 3.40 (br, 2H; CH$_2$, MTAMeI), ~2.57 (br, 3H; CH$_3$ thiazolium, MTAMeI), 2.14–1.47 (br, 2H; –CH$_2$–, MTAMeI), 1.80 (br, 2H, –CH$_2$–, HEMA), 1.10–0.60 (br, 3H; CH$_3$, HEMA) 1.07–0.41 (br, 3H; CH$_3$, MTAMeI).

P(MTABuI-co-HEMA): ^{1}H-NMR (300 MHz, DMSO-d$_6$): δ = 10.27–10.10 (br, 1H; =CH thiazolium, MTABuI), 4.80 (br, 1H; OH, HEMA), 4.56–4.45 (br, 2H; $^+$NCH$_2$, MTABuI), 4.09–4.02 (br, 2H; OCH$_2$, MTABuI), 3.90 (br, 2H; –**CH$_2$**–OH, HEMA), 3.59 (br, 2H; –CH$_2$–CO–, HEMA), 3.32 (br, 2H; CH$_2$, MTABuI), ~2.57 (br, 3H; CH$_3$ thiazolium, MTABuI), 1.93–1.65 (br, 2H; CH$_2$, MTABuI), 1.80 (br, 2H, –CH$_2$–, HEMA), 1.10–0.60 (br, 3H; CH$_3$, HEMA), 1.48–1.23 (br, 4H; 2CH$_2$, MTABuI), 0.98–0.34 (br, 6H; 2CH$_3$, MTABuI).

3.4. Characterization Methods

The ^{1}H nuclear magnetic resonance (NMR) spectra were recorded on a Varian System-500 at room temperature using deuterated chloroform (CDCl$_3$) and DMSO-d6 purchased from Sigma-Aldrich as solvents. Fourier-transform infrared (FTIR) spectra were recorded on a Perkin Elmer Spectrum Two instrument with a high-performance, room temperature LiTaO$_3$ (lithium tantalate) detector and a universal attenuated total reflectance (ATR) instrument with a diamond/ZnSe crystal. The absorptions were given in wavenumber (cm^{-1}), and the spectrum was performed in scan range from 4000 to 450 cm^{-1} with a 0.5 cm^{-1} resolution and 16 scans. The molecular weights and polydispersity indexes of the synthetized copolymers were determined by gel permeation chromatography (GPC) on a Waters Division Millipore system and a Waters 2414 refractive index detector with a 1 mL/min^{-1} flow rate of DMF (GPC-grade, stabilized with 0.1 M LiBr, Scharlau) as eluent at 50 °C. The calibration was performed with poly(methyl methacrylate) standards (Polymer Laboratories LTD). The zeta potential measurements were conducted using the Zetasizer Nano series ZS (Malvern Instruments Ltd, Malvern, UK). The zeta potential of the polymers in deionized water was an average of 10 measurements. Differential scanning calorimetry (DSC) measurements were conducted on a TA Q2000 instrument under dry nitrogen (50 cm^3 min^{-1}). The samples were equilibrated at −70 °C and heated to 120 °C at 10 °C/min. Then, they were cooled to −70 °C and again heated to 120 °C at similar scanning rates. The thermogravimetric analysis (TGA) of the copolymers was performed on a TA Instrument (TGA Q500, TA Instruments, New Castle, Delaware, US) at a heating rate of 10 °C/min^{-1} from 40 to 800 °C under a nitrogen atmosphere. The instrument was calibrated both for temperature and weight by standard methods.

3.5. Microbial Growth Inhibition Assays

The antimicrobial activity of the quaternized copolymers was tested against the ATCC microbial strains according to the Clinical Laboratory Standards Institute (CLSI) microbroth dilution reference methods [42,43,46]. The microorganisms were incubated on 5% sheep blood and Columbia Agar plates (BioMérieux) for 24 h at 37 °C in a Jouan IQ050 incubator (Winchester, VA, USA). Then, the microorganism concentration was adjusted with a saline solution to a turbidity equivalent to ca. 0.5 of the McFarland turbidity standard, which corresponds to about 10^8 colony-forming units (CFU) mL^{-1}. The optical density of the microorganism suspensions was measured in a DensiCHEK™ Plus (VITEK, BioMérieux). These suspensions were further diluted with Mueller–Hinton broth to obtain 2×10^6 CFU mL^{-1}. The copolymers were dissolved in a mixture of sterile water and a minimum amount of DMSO (up to 6% v/v as a higher DMSO content was demonstrated to be toxic for these bacterial strains [20,47]) to obtain solutions of 256 µg mL^{-1} for each copolymer. Then, the broth microdilution method was carried out as follows: 100 µL of each copolymer solution was placed in the first column of a 96-well round-bottom microplate. Subsequently, 50 µL of broth was added into the rest of the wells (except in the first column). In the first column, 50 µL of the copolymer solution was diluted by 2-fold serial dilutions in the rest of the wells, and finally, all the wells of the microdilution plates were inoculated with 50 µL of each test microorganism sample to yield a total volume of 100 µL, bacterial concentrations of 5×10^5 CFU mL^{-1}, and copolymer concentrations of 128, 64, 32, 16, 8, 4, 2, 1, 0.5, 0.25, and 0.125 µg mL^{-1}. Positive and negative controls were also performed. The plates were incubated at 37 °C for 24 h, and the MIC was visually determined to be the lowest concentration of the antimicrobial copolymer in which no bacterial growth was observed. The tests were performed in triplicate.

Author Contributions: Conceptualization, M.F.-G.; Methodology, M.F.-G., A.M.-B. and D.L.; Validation, M.F.-G., A.M.-B. and D.L.; Formal Analysis, A.M.-B., D.L. and M.F.-G.; Original Draft Preparation, A.M.-B.; Review and Editing, M.F.-G.; and Funding Acquisition, M.F.-G.

Acknowledgments: This work was supported by grants from el Sistema Nacional de Garantía Juvenil: PEJ-2014-A-85575 and CM_MAD_ICTP_040 (Promoción de Empleo Joven e Implantación de la Garantía Juvenil, 2014 MINECO, and 2015 CSIC, respectively) and el Ministerio de Ciencia, Innovación y Universidades (Project MAT2016-78437-R), la Agencia Estatal de Investigación (AEI, Spain), and el Fondo Europeo de Desarrollo Regional (FEDER, EU). The authors would like to acknowledge Móstoles University Hospital for the assistance with the antimicrobial tests and Ms. M. González for the preparation of polymers.

Conflicts of Interest: The authors declare no conflicts of interest.

Abbreviations

AIBN	2,2'-azobisisobutyronitrile
ATCC	American Type Culture Collection
br	broad
BuI	1-iodobutane
$CDCl_3$	deuterated chloroform
CFU	colony-forming units
CLSI	Clinical Laboratory Standards Institute
DMF	N,N-dimethylformamide
DMSO	dimethyl sulfoxide
DMSO-d6	deuterated dimethyl sulfoxide
DSC	differential scanning calorimetry
$-dw/dT$	rate of weight loss
f_{MTA}	feed molar fraction of MTA
F_{MTA}	molar fraction of MTA in the copolymer

GPC	gel permeation chromatography
HAI	hospital-acquired infections
HEMA	2-hydroxyethyl methacrylate
MeOH	methanol
MeI	iodomethane
MIC	minimum inhibitory concentration
M_n	number average molecular weight
MTA	2-(4-methylthiazol-5-yl)ethyl methacrylate
NMR	nuclear magnetic resonance
P. aeruginosa	*Pseudomonas aeruginosa*
PBS	phosphate buffered saline
PDI	polydispersity indexes
PHEMA	poly(2-hydroxyethyl methacrylate)
PMTA	poly(2-(4-methylthiazol-5-yl)ethyl methacrylate)
P(MTA-*co*-HEMA)	copolymers of HEMA with MTA
RI	alkyl iodide
S. aureus	*Staphylococcus aureus*
T_d^{max}	temperature of maximum rate of weight loss
T_d^{onset}	initial degradation temperature
TGA	thermogravimetric analysis
T_g	glass transition temperature

References

1. Muñoz-Bonilla, A.; Fernández-García, M. Polymeric materials with antimicrobial activity. *Prog. Polym. Sci.* **2012**, *37*, 281–339. [CrossRef]
2. Huang, K.-S.; Yang, C.-H.; Huang, S.-L.; Chen, C.-Y.; Lu, Y.-Y.; Lin, Y.-S. Recent advances in antimicrobial polymers: A mini-review. *Int. J. Mol. Sci.* **2016**, *17*, 1578. [CrossRef] [PubMed]
3. Alvarez-Paino, M.; Munoz-Bonilla, A.; Fernandez-Garcia, M. Antimicrobial polymers in the nano-world. *Nanomaterials* **2017**, *7*, 48. [CrossRef] [PubMed]
4. Hong, K.H.; Sun, G. Structures and photoactive properties of poly(styrene-*co*-vinylbenzophenone). *J. Polym. Sci. Part B Polym. Phys.* **2008**, *46*, 2423–2430. [CrossRef]
5. Nishat, N.; Ahamad, T.; Zulfequar, M.; Hasnain, S. New antimicrobial polyurea: Synthesis, characterization, and antibacterial activities of polyurea-containing thiosemicarbazide–metal complexes. *J. Appl. Polym. Sci.* **2008**, *110*, 3305–3312. [CrossRef]
6. Francolini, I.; Vuotto, C.; Piozzi, A.; Donelli, G. Antifouling and antimicrobial biomaterials: An overview. *Apmis* **2017**, *125*, 392–417. [CrossRef] [PubMed]
7. Hickok, N.J.; Shapiro, I.M. Immobilized antibiotics to prevent orthopaedic implant infections. *Adv. Drug Deliv. Rev.* **2012**, *64*, 1165–1176. [CrossRef]
8. Gao, P.; Nie, X.; Zou, M.; Shi, Y.; Cheng, G. Recent advances in materials for extended-release antibiotic delivery system. *J. Antibiot.* **2011**, *64*, 625–634. [CrossRef]
9. Adlhart, C.; Verran, J.; Azevedo, N.F.; Olmez, H.; Keinanen-Toivola, M.M.; Gouveia, I.; Melo, L.F.; Crijns, F. Surface modifications for antimicrobial effects in the healthcare setting: A critical overview. *J. Hosp. Infect.* **2018**, *99*, 239–249. [CrossRef]
10. Kelly, M.; Williams, R.; Aojula, A.; O'Neill, J.; Trzinscka, Z.; Grover, L.; Scott, R.A.; Peacock, A.F.; Logan, A.; Stamboulis, A.; et al. Peptide aptamers: Novel coatings for orthopaedic implants. *Mater. Sci. Eng. C Mater. Biol. Appl.* **2015**, *54*, 84–93. [CrossRef]
11. Jo, Y.K.; Seo, J.H.; Choi, B.H.; Kim, B.J.; Shin, H.H.; Hwang, B.H.; Cha, H.J. Surface-independent antibacterial coating using silver nanoparticle-generating engineered mussel glue. *ACS Appl. Mater. Interfaces* **2014**, *6*, 20242–20253. [CrossRef] [PubMed]
12. Kubacka, A.; Ferrer, M.; Fernández-García, M.; Serrano, C.; Cerrada, M.L.; Fernández-García, M. Tailoring polymer-TiO$_2$ film properties by presence of metal (ag, cu, zn) species: Optimization of antimicrobial properties. *Appl. Catal. B Environ.* **2011**, *104*, 346–352. [CrossRef]

13. De Lucas-Gil, E.; Reinosa, J.J.; Neuhaus, K.; Vera-Londono, L.; Martín-González, M.; Fernández, J.F.; Rubio-Marcos, F. Exploring new mechanisms for effective antimicrobial materials: Electric contact-killing based on multiple schottky barriers. *ACS Appl. Mater. Interfaces* **2017**, *9*, 26219–26225. [CrossRef]
14. Muñoz-Bonilla, A.; Cerrada, M.; Fernández-García, M.; Kubacka, A.; Ferrer, M.; Fernández-García, M. Biodegradable polycaprolactone-titania nanocomposites: Preparation, characterization and antimicrobial properties. *Int. J. Mol. Sci.* **2013**, *14*, 9249. [CrossRef] [PubMed]
15. Kubacka, A.; Cerrada, M.L.; Serrano, C.; Fernández-García, M.; Ferrer, M.; Fernández-García, M. Plasmonic nanoparticle/polymer nanocomposites with enhanced photocatalytic antimicrobial properties. *J. Phys. Chem. C* **2009**, *113*, 9182–9190. [CrossRef]
16. Siedenbiedel, F.; Tiller, J.C. Antimicrobial polymers in solution and on surfaces: Overview and functional principles. *Polymers* **2012**, *4*, 46–71. [CrossRef]
17. Jain, A.; Duvvuri, L.S.; Farah, S.; Beyth, N.; Domb, A.J.; Khan, W. Antimicrobial polymers. *Adv. Healthc. Mater.* **2014**, *3*, 1969–1985. [CrossRef]
18. Xue, Y.; Xiao, H.; Zhang, Y. Antimicrobial polymeric materials with quaternary ammonium and phosphonium salts. *Int. J. Mol. Sci.* **2015**, *16*, 3626–3655. [CrossRef] [PubMed]
19. Jiao, Y.; Niu, L.-N.; Ma, S.; Li, J.; Tay, F.R.; Chen, J.-H. Quaternary ammonium-based biomedical materials: State-of-the-art, toxicological aspects and antimicrobial resistance. *Prog. Polym. Sci.* **2017**, *71*, 53–90. [CrossRef]
20. Tejero, R.; Lopez, D.; Lopez-Fabal, F.; Gomez-Garces, J.L.; Fernandez-Garcia, M. Antimicrobial polymethacrylates based on quaternized 1,3-thiazole and 1,2,3-triazole side-chain groups. *Polym. Chem.* **2015**, *6*, 3449–3459. [CrossRef]
21. Tejero, R.; Gutiérrez, B.; López, D.; López-Fabal, F.; Gómez-Garcés, J.L.; Fernández-García, M. Copolymers of acrylonitrile with quaternizable thiazole and triazole side-chain methacrylates as potent antimicrobial and hemocompatible systems. *Acta Biomater.* **2015**, *25*, 86–96. [CrossRef] [PubMed]
22. Tejero, R.; López, D.; López-Fabal, F.; Gómez-Garcés, J.L.; Fernández-García, M. High efficiency antimicrobial thiazolium and triazolium side-chain polymethacrylates obtained by controlled alkylation of the corresponding azole derivatives. *Biomacromolecules* **2015**, *16*, 1844–1854. [CrossRef] [PubMed]
23. Cuervo-Rodriguez, R.; Lopez-Fabal, F.; Gomez-Garces, J.L.; Munoz-Bonilla, A.; Fernandez-Garcia, M. Contact active antimicrobial coatings prepared by polymer blending. *Macromol. Biosci.* **2017**, *17*, 1700258. [CrossRef]
24. Tejero, R.; Gutiérrez, B.; López, D.; López-Fabal, F.; Gómez-Garcés, J.; Muñoz-Bonilla, A.; Fernández-García, M. Tailoring macromolecular structure of cationic polymers towards efficient contact active antimicrobial surfaces. *Polymers* **2018**, *10*, 241. [CrossRef]
25. Munoz-Bonilla, A.; Cuervo-Rodriguez, R.; Lopez-Fabal, F.; Gomez-Garces, J.L.; Fernandez-Garcia, M. Antimicrobial porous surfaces prepared by breath figures approach. *Materials* **2018**, *11*, 1266. [CrossRef] [PubMed]
26. Jones, D.S.; McCoy, C.P.; Andrews, G.P.; McCrory, R.M.; Gorman, S.P. Hydrogel antimicrobial capture coatings for endotracheal tubes: A pharmaceutical strategy designed to prevent ventilator-associated pneumonia. *Mol. Pharm.* **2015**, *12*, 2928–2936. [CrossRef] [PubMed]
27. Myung, D.; Duhamel, P.-E.; Cochran, J.R.; Noolandi, J.; Ta, C.N.; Frank, C.W. Development of hydrogel-based keratoprostheses: A materials perspective. *Biotechnol. Prog.* **2008**, *24*, 735–741. [CrossRef] [PubMed]
28. Prasitsilp, M.; Siriwittayakorn, T.; Molloy, R.; Suebsanit, N.; Siriwittayakorn, P.; Veeranondha, S. Cytotoxicity study of homopolymers and copolymers of 2-hydroxyethyl methacrylate and some alkyl acrylates for potential use as temporary skin substitutes. *J. Mater. Sci. Mater. Med.* **2003**, *14*, 595–600. [CrossRef]
29. Allison, B.C.; Applegate, B.M.; Youngblood, J.P. Hemocompatibility of hydrophilic antimicrobial copolymers of alkylated 4-vinylpyridine. *Biomacromolecules* **2007**, *8*, 2995–2999. [CrossRef]
30. Halpenny, G.M.; Steinhardt, R.C.; Okialda, K.A.; Mascharak, P.K. Characterization of phema-based hydrogels that exhibit light-induced bactericidal effect via release of NO. *J. Mater. Sci. Mater. Med.* **2009**, *20*, 2353–2360. [CrossRef]
31. Ma, L.; Feng, S.; Fuente-Nunez, C.; Hancock, R.E.W.; Lu, X. Development of molecularly imprinted polymers to block quorum sensing and inhibit bacterial biofilm formation. *ACS Appl. Mater. Interfaces* **2018**, *10*, 18450–18457. [CrossRef]

32. Vieira, A.P.; Pimenta, A.F.R.; Silva, D.; Gil, M.H.; Alves, P.; Coimbra, P.; Mata, J.; Bozukova, D.; Correia, T.R.; Correia, I.J.; et al. Surface modification of an intraocular lens material by plasma-assisted grafting with 2-hydroxyethyl methacrylate (HEMA), for controlled release of moxifloxacin. *Eur. J. Pharm. Biopharm.* **2017**, *120*, 52–62. [CrossRef] [PubMed]
33. Katritzky, A.R.; Ramsden, C.A.; Joule, J.A.; Zhdankin, V.V. *Handbook of Heterocyclic Chemistry*; Elsevier Science: Amsterdam, The Netherlands, 2010.
34. Bovey, F.A.; Mirau, P.A. (Eds.) 3—The solution characterization of polymers. In *NMR of Polymers*; Academic Press: San Diego, CA, USA, 1996; pp. 155–241.
35. Kuroda, K.; Caputo, G.A.; DeGrado, W.F. The role of hydrophobicity in the antimicrobial and hemolytic activities of polymethacrylate derivatives. *Chem. Eur. J.* **2009**, *15*, 1123–1133. [CrossRef] [PubMed]
36. Muñoz-Bonilla, A.; Fernández-García, M. The roadmap of antimicrobial polymeric materials in macromolecular nanotechnology. *Eur. Polym. J.* **2015**, *65*, 46–62. [CrossRef]
37. Çaykara, T.; Özyürek, C.; Kantoğlu, Ö. Investigation of thermal behavior of poly(2-hydroxyethyl methacrylate-*co*-itaconic acid) networks. *J. Appl. Polym. Sci.* **2006**, *103*, 1602–1607. [CrossRef]
38. Demirelli, K.; Coşkun, M.; Kaya, E. A detailed study of thermal degradation of poly(2-hydroxyethyl methacrylate). *Polym. Degrad. Stab.* **2001**, *72*, 75–80. [CrossRef]
39. Vargün, E.; Usanmaz, A. Degradation of poly(2-hydroxyethyl methacrylate) obtained by radiation in aqueous solution. *J. Macromol. Sci. Part A* **2010**, *47*, 882–891. [CrossRef]
40. Fernandez-Garcia, M.; Torrado, M.F.; Martinez, G.; Sanchez-Chaves, M.; Madruga, E.L. Free radical copolymerization of 2-hydroxyethyl methacrylate with butyl methacrylate: Determination of monomer reactivity ratios and glass transition temperatures. *Polymer* **2000**, *41*, 8001–8008. [CrossRef]
41. CLSI. *Methods for Dilution Antimicrobial Susceptibility Tests for Bacteria That Grow Aerobically*; Approved Standard-Ninth Edition; CLSI Document M07-A9; Clinical and Laboratory Standards Institute: Wayne, PA, USA, 2012.
42. CLSI. *Performance Standards for Antimicrobial Susceptibility Testing*; Twenty-Second Informational Supplement; CLSI Document M100-S22; Clinical and Laboratory Standards Institute: Wayne, PA, USA, 2012.
43. Kong, H.; Jang, J. Synthesis and antimicrobial properties of novel silver/polyrhodanine nanofibers. *Biomacromolecules* **2008**, *9*, 2677–2681. [CrossRef]
44. Takahashi, H.; Palermo, E.F.; Yasuhara, K.; Caputo, G.A.; Kuroda, K. Molecular design, structures, and activity of antimicrobial peptide-mimetic polymers. *Macromol. Biosci.* **2013**, *13*, 1285–1299. [CrossRef]
45. Takahashi, H.; Caputo, G.A.; Vemparala, S.; Kuroda, K. Synthetic random copolymers as a molecular platform to mimic host-defense antimicrobial peptides. *Bioconjug. Chem.* **2017**, *28*, 1340–1350. [CrossRef] [PubMed]
46. CLSI. *Reference Method for Broth Dilution Antifungal Susceptibility Testing of Yeasts, Fourth Informational Supplement*; CLSI Document M27-S4; Clinical and Laboratory Standards Institute: Wayne, PA, USA, 2012.
47. Alvarez-Paino, M.; Munoz-Bonilla, A.; Lopez-Fabal, F.; Gomez-Garces, J.L.; Heuts, J.P.; Fernandez-Garcia, M. Effect of glycounits on the antimicrobial properties and toxicity behavior of polymers based on quaternized DMAEMA. *Biomacromolecules* **2015**, *16*, 295–303. [CrossRef] [PubMed]

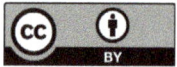

© 2018 by the authors. Licensee MDPI, Basel, Switzerland. This article is an open access article distributed under the terms and conditions of the Creative Commons Attribution (CC BY) license (http://creativecommons.org/licenses/by/4.0/).

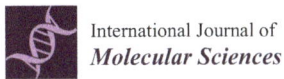

Article

New Polymeric Films with Antibacterial Activity Obtained by UV-induced Copolymerization of Acryloyloxyalkyltriethylammonium Salts with 2-Hydroxyethyl Methacrylate

Francesco Galiano [1], Raffaella Mancuso [2], Maria Grazia Guzzo [3], Fabrizio Lucente [3], Ephraim Gukelberger [2,4], Maria Adele Losso [3,*], Alberto Figoli [1,*], Jan Hoinkis [4] and Bartolo Gabriele [2,*]

[1] Institute on Membrane Technologies (ITM-CNR), Via Pietro Bucci 17/C, 87036 Arcavacata di Rende (CS), Italy; f.galiano@itm.cnr.it

[2] Laboratory of Industrial and Synthetic Organic Chemistry (LISOC), Department of Chemistry and Chemical Technologies, University of Calabria, 87036 Arcavacata di Rende (CS), Italy; raffaella.mancuso@unical.it (R.M.); ephraim.gukelberger@hs-karlsruhe.de (E.G.)

[3] Department of Biology, Ecology, and Earth Sciences (DiBEST), University of Calabria, 87036 Arcavacata di Rende (CS), Italy; mariagraziaguzzo22@gmail.com (M.G.G.); fabrizio.lucente93@gmail.com (F.L.)

[4] University of Applied Sciences Karlsruhe, Center of Applied Research (CAR), Moltkestraße 30, 76133 Karlsruhe, Germany; jan.hoinkis@hs-karlsruhe.de

* Correspondence: losso@unical.it (M.A.L.); a.figoli@itm.cnr.it (A.F.); bartolo.gabriele@unical.it (B.G.); Tel.: +39-0984-492-815 (B.G.)

Received: 7 May 2019; Accepted: 30 May 2019; Published: 31 May 2019

Abstract: New polymeric films with antibacterial activity have been prepared, by simple UV-induced copolymerization of readily available ω-(acryloyloxy)-*N*,*N*,*N*-triethylalcan-1-aminium bromides (or acryloyloxyalkyltriethylammonium bromides, AATEABs) with commercially available 2-hydroxyethyl methacrylate (HEMA), at different relative amounts. In particular, the antibacterial activity of polymeric films derived from 11-(acryloyloxy)-*N*,*N*,*N*-triethylundecan-1-aminium bromide (or acryloyloxyundecyltriethylammonium bromide, AUTEAB; bearing a C-11 alkyl chain linker between the acrylate polymerization function and the quaternary ammonium moiety) and 12-(acryloyloxy)-*N*,*N*,*N*-triethyldodecan-1-aminium bromide (or acryloyloxydodecyltriethylammonium bromide, ADTEB, bearing a C-12 alkyl chain linker) has been assessed against Gram-negative *Escherichia Coli* and Gram-positive *Staphylococcus aureus* cells. The results obtained have shown a clear concentration-dependent activity against both bacterial strains, the films obtained from homopolymerization of pure AUTEAB and ADTEAB being the most effective. Moreover, ADTEAB-based films showed a higher antibacterial activity with respect to the AUTEAB-based ones. Interestingly, however, both types of films presented a significant activity not only toward Gram-positive *S. aureus*, but also toward Gram-negative *E. Coli* cells.

Keywords: acrylates; antibacterial activity; copolymerization; polymeric films; polymerizable quaternary ammonium salts; quaternary ammonium salts; UV-induced polymerization

1. Introduction

The importance of developing new antimicrobial systems is becoming more and more important, owing to the well-known increasing phenomena of resistance to antibiotics associated with an augmented virulence of several pathogenic microbial species [1–5]. In particular, antimicrobial polymers have recently attracted high interest, in view of their significant, efficient, and broad-spectrum activity against resistant microorganisms [6–14]. Moreover, antimicrobial polymers can find extensive applications in several applicative fields [15], including health care and biomedical applications [16–20], food conservation and packaging [21–24], and industry (membrane [25–28] and textile industry [29–32], in particular).

It is well known that quaternary ammonium salts (QASs) present a strong antimicrobial activity (against fungi, bacteria, and viruses, in particular) [33–40], which is mainly related to their ability to promote an ionic exchange between the membrane cell and the positively charged group, thus leading to the loss of membrane integrity and cell death [41,42]. Polymerizable quaternary ammonium salts (PQASs) are a particularly interesting subclass of QASs, which is characterized by the presence, besides the quaternary group, of a suitable polymerizable function. This may allow their incorporation into a polymeric framework by means of copolymerization techniques, thus leading to polymeric materials with antimicrobial properties [43–45].

In this field, we recently reported a novel and practical synthetic approach to a particularly interesting class of polymerizable quaternary ammonium salts (PQASs), which are ω-(acryloyloxy)-N,N,N-triethylalcan-1-aminium bromides (or acryloyloxyalkyltriethylammonium bromides, AATEABs), as shown in Scheme 1 [46].

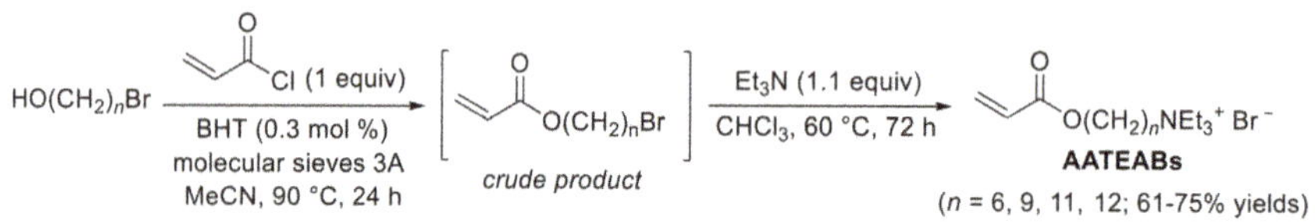

Scheme 1. Synthesis of acryloyloxyalkyltriethylammonium bromides (AATEABs) [46].

These compounds are characterized by the presence, on one hand, of a quaternary ammonium moiety, which confers them a significant antimicrobial activity, and, on the other hand, of an acryloyloxy function, which make these compounds easily polymerizable either by radical- [47,48] or UV-induced [49] polymerization. The two active terminal moieties are distanced through a suitable alkyl chain linker. We previously assessed the antimicrobial activity of the newly synthetized AATEABs against several Gram-positive and Gram-negative bacteria and yeast strains [46]. The results obtained showed that the AATEABs bearing a C-11 and a C-12 alkyl chain linker (11-(acryloyloxy)-N,N,N-triethylundecan-1-aminium bromide or acryloyloxyundecyltriethylammonium bromide, AUTEAB, and 12-(acryloyloxy)-N,N,N-triethyldodecan-1-aminium bromide (or acryloyloxydodecyltriethylammonium bromide, ADTEB, respectively) were the most active, in particular, against Gram-positive bacteria *Staphylococcus aureus* and *Streptococcus pyogenes* [46]. The higher bioactivity of AUTEAB and ADTEAB with respect to the other derivatives with shorter alkyl chain linkers was also recently theoretically interpreted by ab initio modeling calculations [50].

Considering the promising antibacterial activity of AUTEAB and ADTEAB [46,50], and the possibility to easily copolymerize them for obtaining new antibacterial materials [47–49], in this work we have studied the development of new polymeric films chemically incorporating these PQASs, for potential applications in biomedical, food packaging and textile field. In particular, we have prepared polymeric films based on the UV-induced copolymerization of AUTEAB as well as ADTEAB with commercially available 2-hydroxyethyl methacrylate (HEMA), at different relative amounts. The new films thus obtained were assessed for their antibacterial activity, at different concentrations, towards the two bacteria strains *E. coli* and *S. aureus*. The possibility to copolymerize antimicrobial AUTEAB and ADTEAB with HEMA is of particular interest, considering that the homopolymer obtained by polymerization of HEMA (pHEMA) is very well appreciated for its transparency and biocompatibility, properties that make pHEMA an ideal candidate for the production of contact lenses and other products in the biomedical field [51].

2. Results and Discussion

The new antimicrobial polymeric films developed in this work were obtained by UV-induced copolymerizazion of the PQASs AUTEAB or ADTEAB with commercially available HEMA, at different relative amounts. In particular, a proper amount of the PQAS (15.0, 35.0, 50.0 and 100 wt%) and HEMA (85, 65, 50, and 0 wt%, respectively) were mixed until a transparent solution was obtained. A small amount of the UV initiator 2,2-dimethoxy-2-phenylacetophenone (DMPA) was then added, and the mixture was poured in a glass petri dish and exposed to 500 W UV light irradiation (lamp emission from 180 nm to visible light). Polymerization was quite fast, and after 10 min transparent films were obtained (Figure 1a), which were detached form the petri dish in water and washed in water overnight, ready to be used for the subsequent antibacterial tests. As shown in scanning electron microscope (SEM) picture (Figure 1b), the film surface appeared characterized by a uniform, dense, and compact morphology. The morphology was practically the same for all the prepared films. The films presented an overall thickness of about 0.432 mm.

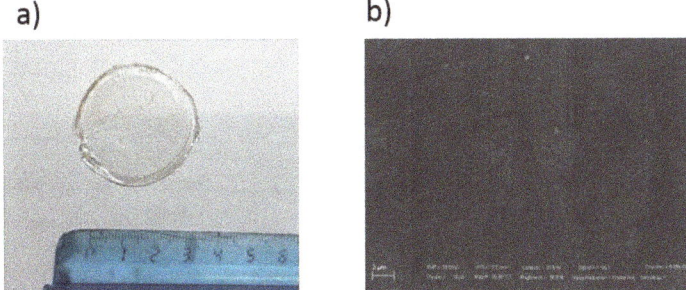

Figure 1. Image (a) and SEM picture (b) of a typical film obtained by copolymerization of acryloyloxyundecyltriethylammonium bromide (AUTEAB) with 2-hydroxyethyl methacrylate (HEMA).

An exemplificative Fourier transform infrared spectroscopy (FT-IR) spectrum of a film prepared with 15.0 wt% of ADTEAB and HEMA is reported in Figure 2. The wide and intense band at 3375 cm^{-1} can be assigned to the O-H stretching vibrations of pHEMA [52]. At 1718 cm^{-1}, it can be observed the stretching vibrations of the carbonyl C=O group (from both ADTEAB and pHEMA), which is generally found in the region of 1650–1800 cm^{-1} [53]. The region between 2900 and 3000 cm^{-1} is associated with the symmetric and anti-symmetric C-H vibrations of CH_2 and CH_3 groups of ADTEAB and pHEMA [52]. For comparison, the FT-IR spectra of AUEAB, ADTEAB, and HEMA are shown in Figure 3.

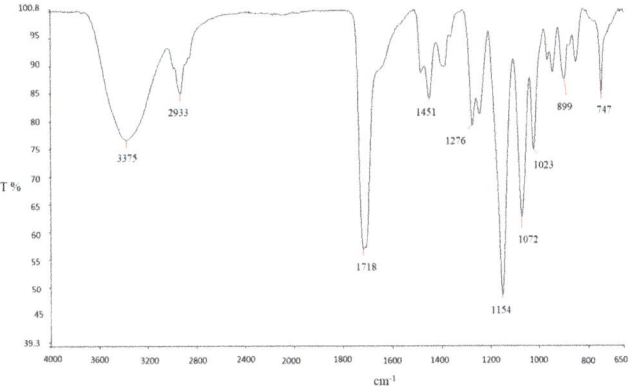

Figure 2. FT-IR spectrum of the polymeric film prepared with 15 wt% ADTEAB and 85 wt% HEMA.

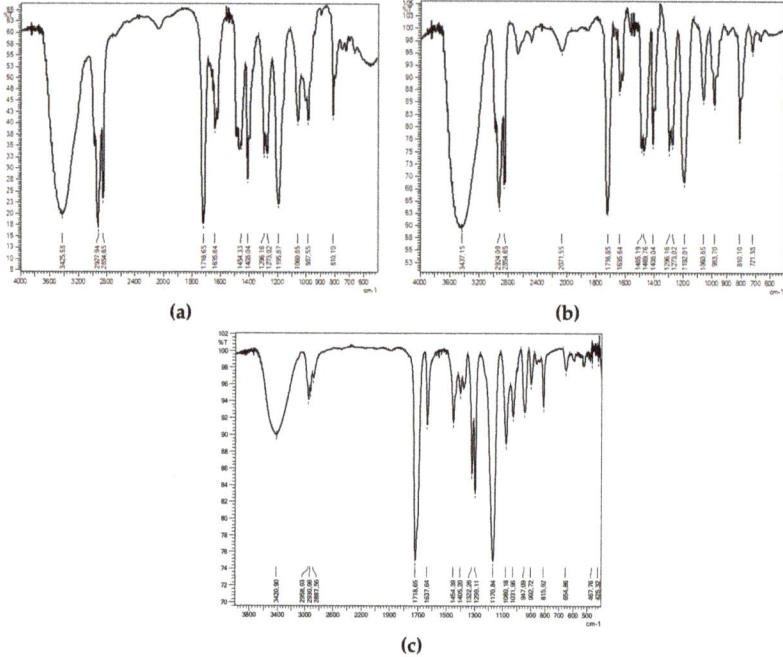

Figure 3. FT-IR spectra of AUTEAB (**a**), ADTEAB (**b**), and HEMA (**c**).

The antibacterial efficacy of the AUTEAB-HEMA and ADTEAB-HEMA polymeric films thus obtained, and of pHEMA as blank reference, was assessed on the basis of cell viability of *E. coli* TG1 (Gram-negative) and *Staphilococcus aureus* (Gram-positive) cultures, after being in contact with the films at different times (0, 1.5, 3, and 6 h). Figure 4a shows a comparison between the cell viability of *E. coli* TG1 in presence of AUTEAB-HEMA films at different incubation times. No loss of viable bacteria was detected in the cells control (no film exposure) and in the blank reference pHEMA (histograms in red and dark green, respectively). On the other hand, a clear concentration-dependent effect was observed with AUTEAB-HEMA polymeric films. While no antibacterial activity was obtained after 6 h with the 15% AUTEAB film (purple histogram, Figure 4a), a bacteriostatic effect was evident with the 35% AUTEAB film (light green histogram, Figure 4a), and a bactericidal activity with the 50% AUTEAB film (orange histogram, Figure 4a). As expected, the bactericidal effect was dramatic in the case of the homopolymeric film obtained from AUTEAB only (light blue histogram, Figure 4a). In fact, in this latter case, no viable cells could be detected after 1.5 h contact (light blue histogram, Figure 4a), while with the 50% AUTEAB film at the same incubation time, we observed a reduction of cell viability of about two orders of magnitude, and cell viability reached 0 only after 6 h of incubation (orange histogram, Figure 4a). The antimicrobial activity against the Gram-positive *S. aureus*, shown in Figure 4b, was more pronounced, as the bactericidal effect was reached either after only 1.5 h contact with the 50% AUTEAB film (orange histogram, Figure 4b) or after 3 h with the 15% AUTEAB film (purple histogram, Figure 4b).

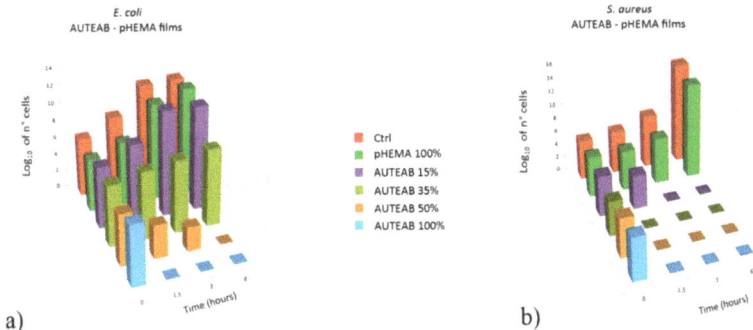

Figure 4. Comparison of viable cell number of *E. coli* TG1 (**a**) and *S. aureus* (**b**) as a function of time in the presence of control (no film, red histogram), blank reference (pHEMA, dark green histogram), 15% AUTEAB film (purple histogram), 35% AUTEAB film (light green histogram), 50% AUTEAB film (orange histogram) and 100% AUTEAB film (light blue histogram). Bacteria cells were grown in Luria-Bertani broth and the cell number was determined by surface spread plate technique, as described in the Materials and Methods Section.

Figure 5 shows the reduction of turbidity of the *E. coli* cultures in presence of AUTEAB-based films after 3 h contact with the film. It is evident that the degree of cell population in the medium (as evidenced by the culture turbidity) decreases by increasing the % of AUTAB in the AUTEAB-HEMA polymeric film. With the film obtained by homopolymerization of AUTEAB, the mixture is clear, confirming that no cell population is present.

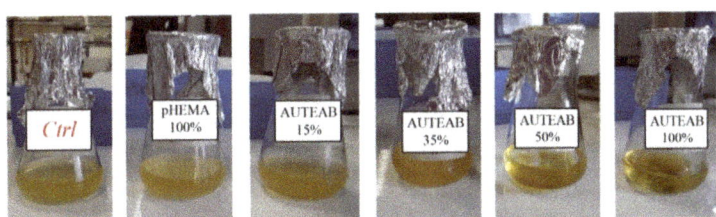

Figure 5. *E. coli* cultures maintained in contact with AUTEAB-HEMA polymeric films obtained with 15, 35, 50, and 100% AUTEAB. Control (no film exposure) and blank reference (pHEMA) are also shown for comparison.

It is known that the antibacterial mechanism of QASs is mainly related to their strong interaction with the cell membrane which causes its disorganization. This leads to the degradation of nucleic acids and proteins with consequent lysis of the bacterial cell wall by autolytic enzymes [41,42]. Usually, QASs present a significant different antibacterial efficiency toward Gram-positive and Gram-negative bacteria, due to the additional outer membrane in the Gram-negative bacteria, which is absent in the Gram-positive ones [52]. For this reason, the multilayer structure of the membrane makes the Gram-negative bacteria more resistant toward the access and the internalization in the cytoplasm of QASs. Our results, obtained with AUTEAB-HEMA polymeric films, while confirming a higher antimicrobial activity against the Gram-positive *S. aureus* with respect to the Gram-negative *E. coli* (compare Figure 4a with Figure 4b), also demonstrate that a significant concentration-dependent antimicrobial effect is exerted on the latter, with a bactericidal effect being observed after 6 h with the 50% AUTEAB film and after only 1.5 h with 100% AUTEAB film (Figure 4a).

We also prepared and tested polymeric films using acryloyloxydodecyltriethylammonium bromide (ADTEAB), bearing a C-12 rather than a C-11 alkyl linker. This derivative, in fact, presented a higher antimicrobial activity compared to the C-11 compound (AUTEAB) [46], which was also in agreement with ab initio modeling calculations [50]. In this latter theoretical work, it was demonstrated that the increase in the antimicrobial activity of QAS molecules could be mainly attributed to their "aspect ratio" [50]. QAS with a longer alkyl chain bonded to nitrogen, in fact, exhibited a lower aspect ratio resulting in a higher shielding effect on the quaternary ammonium group [50], which is known to cause a higher antimicrobial activity [53]. Interestingly, the "shielding" effect increases with the alkyl chain length but only up to a certain limit. For example, He et al. [54] found that the optimum alkyl chain length for the antimicrobial effect against *S. mutans* cells was between C-11 and C-16, while the effect tended to lower with longer alkyl chains.

The results obtained with ADTEAB-HEMA polymeric films are shown in Figure 6, together with the control (no film exposure) and the blank reference pHEMA. As expected (Figure 6a), no loss of viable *E. coli* cells was detected in the cells control and with pHEMA (histograms in red and dark green, respectively). Additionally, no activity was observed with the 15% ADTEAB film (purple histogram, Figure 6a). On the other hand, an evident bactericidal effect was obtained with 35 and 50% ADTEAB film after 3 and 1.5 h contact, respectively (light green and orange histograms, Figure 6a). As seen for AUTEAB-based films (Figure 4), the antimicrobial activity of ADTEAB-based films on the Gram-positive *S. aureus* was higher (Figure 6b). In fact, the bactericidal effect was reached after either 1.5 h with 35% and 50% ADTEAB film (Figure 6b, light green and orange histograms, respectively). Moreover, a viable cells decrease, of about 2 order of magnitude, was already seen with 15% ADTEAB after 1.5 h and no viable cells were detected at 3 h contact (Figure 6b, purple histogram), while no activity was observed with the same film against *E. coli* (purple histogram, Figure 6a). These results also confirmed a higher antimicrobial activity for ADTEAB-based films (Figure 6) in comparison to the ones prepared with AUTEAB (Figure 4). Rather interestingly, this was particularly evident in the Gram-negative *E. coli*.

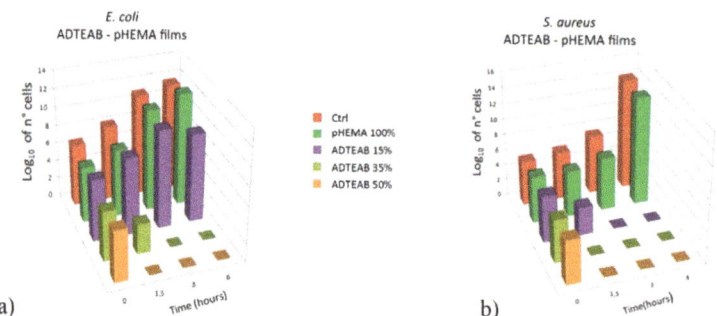

Figure 6. Comparison of viable cell number of *E. coli* TG1 (**a**) and *S. aureus* (**b**) as a function of time in the presence of control (no film, red histogram), blank reference (pHEMA, dark green histogram), 15% ADTEAB film (purple histogram), 35% ADTEAB film (light green histogram) and 50% ADTEAB film (orange histogram). Bacteria cells were grown in Luria-Bertani broth and the cell number was determined by surface spread plate technique, as described in the Materials and Methods Section.

3. Materials and Methods

3.1. Preparation of Polymeric Films

Antimicrobial films were prepared by mixing a proper amount of AUTEAB or ADTEAB (prepared as we already reported [46]) (15.0, 35.0, 50.0 and 100 wt%) with HEMA (purchased by Sigma-Aldrich Italia, Milan, Italy) (85, 65, 50, and 0 wt%, respectively). Films containing 100 wt% of antimicrobial agent were prepared by dissolving AUTEAB in water with a ratio of 75:25 AUTEAB/water. Solid films containing 100 wt% ADTEAB could not be prepared due to the high fragility of the polymerized material. The mixtures (1 g) were, then, stirred for 1 h until complete dissolution. The UV initiator 2,2-dimethoxy-2-phenylacetophenone DMPA (2,2-dimethoxy-1,2-diphenylethan-1-one; purchased by Sigma-Aldrich Italia, Milan, Italy) (0.6 wt% with respect to the total amount of the mixture) was then added. After 1 h stirring, the solutions were poured in a glass petri dish (3 cm in diameter) and exposed for polymerization to UV light irradiation (lamp emission from 180 nm to visible light, 500W; purchased from Helios Italquarz, Cambiago, Milan, Italy) for 10 min. The polymerized films were then detached form the petri dish in water and washed in water overnight. A blank film, not containing any antimicrobial agent, was also prepared through the polymerization of pure HEMA with 0.6 wt% of DMPA. Table 1 shows the composition of the prepared films.

Table 1. Relative amounts of the components used for preparing the polymeric films.

Film	AATEAB (wt%)	HEMA (wt%)	Water (wt%)
AUTEAB 15%	AUTEAB (15)	(85)	(0)
AUTEAB 35%	AUTEAB (35)	(65)	(0)
AUTEAB 50%	AUTEAB (50)	(50)	(0)
AUTEAB 100%	AUTEAB (75)	(0)	(25) [1]
ADTEAB 15%	ADTEAB (15)	(85)	(0)
ADTEAB 35%	ADTEAB (35)	(65)	(0)
ADTEAB 50%	ADTEAB (50)	(50)	(0)
pHEMA	(0)	(100)	(0)

[1] The final polymeric film contained only polymerized AUTEAB, since water evaporated completely during the polymerization process.

Fourier transform infrared spectroscopy (FT-IR) analysis was performed by using a Perkin Elmer Instrument (New York, NY, USA) in the range 4000–650 cm^{-1}; for the polymeric films, Attenuated Total Reflection (ATR) mode was used, while for HEMA, AUTEB and ADTEAB, KBr pellets were prepared. SEM image was acquired by means of Zeiss-EVO MA10 (thermal emission tungsten firing unit equipped with a secondary electron detector) instrument using an Electron High Tension (EHT) of 20 kV and with a probe current of 18 pA. Prior to analyses, the sample was coated with a thin layer of gold (sputter current of 20 mA and a sputter time of 240 s) using a sputter coater machine (Quorum Q150 RS) in order to make the sample conductive.

3.2. Microorganisms and General Growth Conditions

E. coli TG1 and *Staphilococcus aureus*, kindly provided by Prof. Michele Galluccio (Department of Ecology, Biology and Earth Sciences, University of Calabria, Rende, Italy), were selected as Gram-negative and Gram-positive bacteria, respectively. The two strains were grown aerobically, at 37 °C and 200 rpm in a thermostatic orbital shaking incubator (Sanyo Gallenkamp IOX400.XX1.C, Analitica De Mori, Milan, Italy), in sterile Luria Bertani (LB) broth, a rich growth medium (containing sodium chloride 5 g/L; yeast extract 5 g/L; trypton, 10 g/L at pH = 6.8). Oxoid Italia (Rodano, Milan, Italy) supplied the powders for medium preparation.

3.3. Antibacterial Assessment of Polymeric Films

An overnight culture of *E. coli* TG1 or *S. aureus* was diluted 1:100 (v/v) in 20 mL of fresh LB liquid medium to restart the cell cycle and incubated for circa 3 h at 37 °C until the exponential growth phase was reached. Then, the culture was diluted 1:10 (v/v) in 20 mL of LB liquid medium, in an Erlenmeyer flask, to reach a final density of circa 10^6 CFU/mL with an optical density, at 600 nm (OD$_{600}$), of about 0.06 [55]. This value was chosen on the basis of our preliminary data on growth curves of *E. coli* TG1 performed to correlate OD measurements and number of cells by plate counting. Finally, each different preparation of film was immersed in the bacterial suspension and shaken at 37 °C for 6 h. A same assay procedure was used for bacterial suspensions without films used as control.

The effect of antimicrobial films at different concentration on the bacterial growth has been assessed after 0, 1.5, 3, and 6 h, by OD_{600} and cell viability assays. To calculate the Colony Forming Unit (CFU) at the predetermined time, 100 µL of bacteria culture was taken from the flasks with and without film and decimal serial dilutions in LB were performed. 50 µL of the diluted sample were then spread onto sterile LB agar plates (LB broth with the addition of 16 g/L of agar). After incubation of the plates at 37 °C for 20–24 h, the number of viable cells (colonies) was counted manually to get the corresponding concentration of living bacteria. The log of N (cell number) was calculated using the formula: CFU/mL = n° of colonies × dilution factor/volume of culture spread. CFU for every time was calculated on the average of three different dilutions.

4. Conclusions

In conclusion, we have developed novel polymeric films based on UV-induced copolymerization of some readily available polymerizable quaternary ammonium salts (QASs), in particular, 11-(acryloyloxy)-N,N,N-triethylundecan-1-aminium bromide or acryloyloxyundecyltriethylammonium bromide, AUTEAB, and 12-(acryloyloxy)-N,N,N-triethyldodecan-1-aminium bromide or acryloyloxydodecyltriethylammonium bromide, ADTEB, with commercially available 2-hydroxyethyl methacrylate (HEMA). The antibacterial tests, conducted on typical Gram-negative (*E. Coli*) and Gram-positive (*S. aureus*) strains, have confirmed a significant antibacterial activity, not only against the Gram-positive cells, but also on the Gram-negative ones (which are known to be usually much more resistant toward QASs), although the activity was higher in the first case. Moreover, the results obtained have shown that the activity depended on the QAS concentration in the film and that is was higher for the films obtained from ADTEAB with respect to AUTEAB.

The possible application of the newly prepared films in various fields (biomedical, textile, and membrane technology, in particular) is underway in our laboratories and the results will be reported in due course.

Author Contributions: Conceptualization, F.G., M.A.L., A.F., and B.G.; Methodology, all authors; Validation, F.G., R.M., M.G.G., F.L., and J.H.; Investigation, F.G., R.M., M.G.G., F.L., and E.G.; resources, M.A.L., A.F., and B.G.; Writing—original draft preparation, F.G. and M.A.L.; Writing—review and editing, B.G.; Supervision, B.G.; Project administration, M.A.L., A.F., and B.G.; Funding acquisition, J.H.

Funding: This research has received funding from the European Union's Horizon 2020 research and innovation programme under grant agreement No. 689427 for the project VicInAqua.

Acknowledgments: We thank Michele Galluccio (Department of Ecology, Biology and Earth Sciences, University of Calabria, Rende, Italy) for providing microorganisms.

Conflicts of Interest: The authors declare no conflict of interest.

Abbreviations

AATEABs	acryloyloxydodecyltriethylammonium bromide (ω-(acryloyloxy)-N,N,N-triethylalcan-1-aminium bromides)
ADTEAB	acryloyloxydodecyltriethylammonium bromide (12-(acryloyloxy)-N,N,N-triethylundecan-1-aminium bromide)
AUTEAB	acryloyloxyundecyltriethylammonium bromide(11-(acryloyloxy)-N,N,N-triethyldodecan-1-aminium bromide)
CFU	colony-forming unit
DMPA	2,2-dimethoxy-2-phenylacetophenone (2,2-dimethoxy-1,2-diphenylethan-1-one)
HEMA	2-hydroxyethyl methacrylate
LB	Luria-Bertani
OD	optical density
pHEMA	poly-2-hydroxyethyl methacrylate
PQASs	polymerizable quaternary ammonium salts
QASs	quaternary ammonium salts

References

1. Almakki, A.; Jumas-Bilak, E.; Marchandin, H.; Licznar-Fajardo, P. Antibiotic resistance in urban runoff. *Sci. Total Environ.* **2019**, *667*, 64–76. [CrossRef] [PubMed]
2. Canica, M.; Manageiro, V.; Abriouel, H.; Moran-Gilad, J.; Franz, C.M.A.P. Antibiotic resistance in foodborne bacteria. *Trends Food Sci. Technol.* **2019**, *84*, 41–44. [CrossRef]
3. Li, R.; Jay, J.A.; Stenstrom, M.K. Fate of antibiotic resistance genes and antibiotic-resistant bacteria in water resource recovery facilities. *Water Environ. Res.* **2019**, *91*, 5–20. [CrossRef]
4. Peterson, E.; Kaur, P. Antibiotic resistance mechanisms in bacteria: Relationships between resistance determinants of antibiotic producers, environmental Bacteria, and clinical pathogens. *Front. Microbiol.* **2018**, *9*, 2928. [CrossRef] [PubMed]
5. Babakhani, S.; Oloomi, M. Transposons: The agents of antibiotic resistance in bacteria. *J. Basic Microbiol.* **2018**, *58*, 905–917. [CrossRef]
6. Xing, H.; Lu, M.; Yang, T.; Liu, H.; Sun, Y.; Zhao, X.; Xu, H.; Yang, L.; Ding, P. Structure-function relationships of nonviral gene vectors: Lessons from antimicrobial polymers. *Acta Biomater.* **2019**, *86*, 15–20. [CrossRef]
7. Munoz-Bonilla, A.; Echeverria, C.; Sonseca, A.; Arrieta, M.P.; Fernandez-Garcia, M. Bio-based polymers with antimicrobial properties towards sustainable development. *Materials* **2019**, *12*, 641. [CrossRef]
8. Konai, M.M.; Bhattacharjee, B.; Ghosh, S.; Haldar, J. Recent progress in polymer research to tackle infections and antimicrobial resistance. *Biomacromolecules* **2018**, *19*, 1888–1917. [CrossRef] [PubMed]
9. Ergene, C.; Yasuhara, K.; Palermo, E.F. Biomimetic antimicrobial polymers: Recent advances in molecular design. *Polym. Chem.* **2018**, *9*, 2407–2427. [CrossRef]
10. Al-Jumaili, A.; Kumar, A.; Bazaka, K.; Jacon, M.V. Plant secondary metabolite-derived polymers: A potential approach to develop antimicrobial films. *Polymers* **2018**, *10*, 515. [CrossRef] [PubMed]
11. Ergene, C.; Palermo, E.F. Antimicrobial synthetic polymers: An update on structure-activity relationships. *Curr. Pharm. Des.* **2018**, *24*, 855–865. [CrossRef]
12. Yang, Y.; Cai, Z.; Huang, Z.; Tang, X.; Zhang, X. Antimicrobial cationic polymers: From structural design to functional control. *Polym. J.* **2018**, *50*, 33–44. [CrossRef]
13. Lam, S.J.; Wong, E.H.H.; Boyer, C.; Qiao, G.G. Antimicrobial polymeric nanoparticles. *Progr. Polym. Sci.* **2018**, *76*, 40–64. [CrossRef]
14. Alvarez-Paino, M.; Munoz-Bonilla, A.; Fernandez-Garcia, M. Antimicrobial polymers in the nano-world. *Nanomaterials* **2017**, *7*, 48. [CrossRef]
15. Huang, K.-S.; Yang, C.-H.; Huang, S.-L.; Chan, C.-Y.; Lu, Y.-Y.; Lin, Y.-S. Recent advances in antimicrobial polymers: A mini-review. *Int. J. Mol. Sci.* **2016**, *17*, 1578. [CrossRef]
16. Gonzalez-Henriquez, C.M.; Sarabia-Vallejos, M.A.; Rodriguez Hernandez, J. Antimicrobial polymers for additive manufacturing. *Int. J. Mol. Sci.* **2019**, *20*, 1210. [CrossRef]
17. Feldman, D. Polymer nanocomposites for tissue engineering, antimicrobials and drug delivery. *Biointerface Res. Appl. Chem.* **2018**, *8*, 3153–3160.
18. Gahruie, H.H.; Niakousari, M. Antioxidant, antimicrobial, cell viability and enzymatic inhibitory of antioxidant polymers as biological macromolecules. *Int. J. Biol. Part A Macromol.* **2017**, *104*, 606–617.
19. Hartlieb, M.; Williams, E.G.L.; Kuroki, A.; Perrier, S.; Locock, K.E.S. Antimicrobial polymers: Mimicking amino acid functionality, sequence control and three-dimensional structure of host-defense peptides. *Curr. Med. Chem.* **2017**, *24*, 2115–2140. [CrossRef]
20. Wo, Y.; Brisbois, E.J.; Bartlett, R.H.; Meyerhoff, M.E. Recent advances in thromboresistant and antimicrobial polymers for biomedical applications: Just say yes to nitric oxide (NO). *Biomater. Sci.* **2016**, *4*, 1161–1183. [CrossRef]
21. Mujtaba, M.; Morsi, R.E.; Kerch, G.; Elsabee, M.Z.; Kaya, M.; Labidi, J.; Khawar, K.M. Current advancements in chitosan-based film production for food technology; A review. *Int. J. Biol. Macromol.* **2019**, *121*, 889–904. [CrossRef] [PubMed]
22. Vasile, C. Polymeric nanocomposites and nanocoatings for food packaging: A review. *Materials* **2018**, *11*, 1834. [CrossRef] [PubMed]

23. Santos, J.C.P.; Sousa, R.C.S.; Otoni, C.G.; Moraes, A.R.F.; Souza, V.G.L.; Medeiros, E.A.A.; Espita, P.J.P.; Pires, A.C.S.; Coimbra, J.S.R.; Soares, N.F.F. Nisin and other antimicrobial peptides: Production, mechanisms of action, and application in active food packaging. *Innov. Food Sci. Emerg. Technol.* **2018**, *48*, 179–194. [CrossRef]
24. Galie, S.; Garcia-Gutierrez, C.; Miguelez, E.M.; Villar, C.J.; Lombo, F. Biofilms in the food industry: Health aspects and control methods. *Front. Microbiol.* **2018**, *9*, 898. [CrossRef] [PubMed]
25. Gafri, H.F.S.; Zuki, F.M.; Aroua, M.K.; Hashim, N.A. Mechanism of bacterial adhesion on ultrafiltration membrane modified by natural antimicrobial polymers (Chitosan) and combination with activated carbon (PAC). *Rev. Chem. Eng.* **2019**, *35*, 421–443. [CrossRef]
26. Zhu, J.; Hou, J.; Zhang, Y.; Tian, M.; He, T.; Liu, J.; Chen, V. Polymeric antimicrobial membranes enabled by nanomaterials for water treatment. *J. Membr. Sci.* **2018**, *550*, 173–197. [CrossRef]
27. Mukherjee, M.; De, S. Antibacterial polymeric membranes: A short review. *Environm. Sci. Water Res. Technol.* **2018**, *4*, 1078–1104. [CrossRef]
28. Zhu, Y.; Wang, J.; Hou, J.; Zhang, Y.; Liu, J.; Ven der Bruggen, B. Graphene-based antimicrobial polymeric membranes: A review. *J. Mater. Sci. A* **2017**, *5*, 6776–6793. [CrossRef]
29. Akbari, S.; Kozlowski, R.M. A review of application of amine-terminated dendritic materials in textile engineering. *J. Text. Inst.* **2019**, *110*, 460–467. [CrossRef]
30. Emam, H.E. Antimicrobial cellulosic textiles based on organic compounds. *3 Biothech.* **2019**, *9*, 29. [CrossRef] [PubMed]
31. Ul-Islam, S.; Butola, B.S. Recent advances in chitosan polysaccharide and its derivatives in antimicrobial modification of textile materials. *Int. J. Biol. Macromol.* **2019**, *121*, 905–912. [CrossRef] [PubMed]
32. Morais, D.S.; Guedes, R.M.; Lopes, M.A. Antimicrobial approaches for textiles: From research to market. *Materials* **2016**, *9*, 498. [CrossRef]
33. Oblak, E.; Piecuch, A.; Rewak-Soroczynska, A.; Paluch, E. Activity of gemini quaternary ammonium aalts against microorganisms. *Appl. Microbiol. Biotechnol.* **2019**, *103*, 625–632. [CrossRef] [PubMed]
34. Fait, M.E.; Bakas, L.; Garrote, G.L.; Morcelle, S.R.; Saparrat, M.C.N. Cationic surfactants as antifungal agents. *Appl. Microbiol. Biothechnol.* **2019**, *103*, 97–112. [CrossRef]
35. Makvandi, P.; Jamaledin, R.; Jabbari, M.; Nikfarjam, N.; Borzacchiello, A. Antibacterial quaternary ammonium compounds in dental materials: A systematic review. *Dent. Mater.* **2018**, *34*, 851–867. [CrossRef] [PubMed]
36. Mulder, I.; Siemens, J.; Sentek, V.; Amelung, W.; Smalla, K.; Jachalke, S. Quaternary ammonium compounds in soil: Implications for antibiotic resistance development. *Rev. Environ. Sci. Bio-Technol.* **2018**, *17*, 159–185. [CrossRef]
37. Jiao, Y.; Niu, L.-n.; Ma, S.; Li, J.; Tay, F.R.; Chen, J.-h. Quaternary ammonium-based biomedical materials: State-of-the-art, toxicological aspects and antimicrobial resistance. *Progr. Polym. Sci.* **2017**, *71*, 53–90. [CrossRef]
38. Jennings, M.C.; Minbiole, K.P.C.; Wuest, W.M. Quaternary ammonium compounds: An antimicrobial mainstay and platform for innovation to address bacterial resistance. *Acs Infect. Dis.* **2015**, *1*, 288–303. [CrossRef]
39. Gerba, C.P. Quaternary ammonium biocides: Efficacy in application. *Appl. Environ. Microbiol.* **2015**, *81*, 464–469. [CrossRef] [PubMed]
40. Buffet-Bataillon, S.; Tattevin, P.; Bonnaure-Mallet, M.; Jolivet-Gougeon, A. Emergence of resistance to antibacterial agents: The role of quaternary ammonium compounds-a critical review. *Int. J. Antimicrob. Agents* **2012**, *39*, 381–389. [CrossRef]
41. Yoo, J.H. Review of disinfection and sterilization – Back to the basics. *Infect Chemother.* **2018**, *50*, 101–109. [CrossRef]
42. Inacio, A.S.; Domingues, N.S.; Nunes, A.; Martins, P.T.; Moreno, M.J.; Estronca, L.M.; Fernandes, R.; Moreno, A.J.M.; Borrego, M.J.; Gomes, J.P.; Vaz, W.L.C.; Vieira, O.V. Quaternary ammonium surfactant structure determines selective toxicity towards bacteria: Mechanisms of action and clinical implications in antibacterial prophylaxis. *J. Antimicrob. Chemother.* **2016**, *71*, 641–654. [CrossRef]
43. Zubris, D.L.; Minbiole, K.P.C.; Wuest, W.M. Polymeric quaternary ammonium compounds: Versatile antimicrobial materials. *Curr. Top. Med. Chem.* **2017**, *17*, 305–318. [CrossRef]
44. Zhang, W.; Zhou, J.J.; Dai, X.L. Preparation and characterization of reactive chitosan quaternary ammonium salt and its application in antibacterial finishing of cotton fabric. *Text. Res. J.* **2017**, *87*, 759–765. [CrossRef]

45. Xue, Y.; Xiao, H.N.; Zhang, Y. Antimicrobial polymeric materials with quaternary ammonium and phosphonium salts. *Int. J. Mol. Sci.* **2015**, *16*, 3626–3655. [CrossRef]
46. Mancuso, R.; Amuso, R.; Armentano, B.; Grasso, G.; Rago, V.; Cappello, A.R.; Galiano, F.; Figoli, A.; De Luca, G.; Hoinkis, J.; Gabriele, B. Synthesis and antibacterial activity of plymerizable acryloyloxytriethyl ammonium salts. *ChemPlusChem* **2017**, *82*, 1235–1244. [CrossRef]
47. Deowan, S.A.; Galiano, F.; Hoinkis, J.; Johnson, D.; Altinkaya, S.A.; Gabriele, B.; Hilal, N.; Drioli, E.; Figoli, A. Novel low-fouling membrane bioreactor (MBR) for industrial wastewater treatment. *J. Membr. Sci.* **2016**, *510*, 524–532. [CrossRef]
48. Galiano, F.; Figoli, A.; Deowan, S.A.; Johnson, D.; Altinkaya, S.A.; Veltri, L.; De Luca, G.; Mancuso, R.; Hilal, N.; Gabriele, B.; Hoinkis, J. A step forward to a more efficient wastewater treatment by membrane surface modification via polymerizable biocontinuous microemulsion. *J. Membr. Sci.* **2015**, *482*, 103–114. [CrossRef]
49. Galiano, F.; Schmidt, S.A.; Ye, X.; Kumar, R.; Mancuso, R.; Curcio, E.; Gabriele, B.; Hoinkis, J.; Figoli, A. UV-LED induced bicontinuous microemulsion polymerisation for surface modification of commercial membranes – Enhancing the antifouling properties. *Sep. Pur. Technol.* **2018**, *194*, 149–160. [CrossRef]
50. De Luca, G.; Amuso, R.; Figoli, A.; Mancuso, R.; Lucadamo, L.; Gabriele, B. Modeling of structure-property relashionships of polymerizable surfactants with antimicrobial activity. *Appl. Sci.* **2018**, *8*, 1972. [CrossRef]
51. Tomar, N.; Tomar, M.; Gulati, N.; Nagaich, U. pHEMA hydrogels: Devices for ocular drug delivery. *Int. J. Heal. Allied Sci.* **2012**, *1*, 224. [CrossRef]
52. Silhavy, T.J.; Kahne, D.; Walker, S. The bacterial cell envelope. *Cold Spring Harb. Perspect. Biol.* **2010**, *2*, a000414. [CrossRef] [PubMed]
53. Sundararaman, M.; Kumar, R.R.; Venkatesan, P.; Ilangovan, A. 1-Alkyl-(N,N-dimethylamino)pyridinium bromides: Inhibitory effect on virulence factors of Candida Albicans and on the growth of bacterial pathogens. *J. Med. Microbiol.* **2013**, *62*, 241–248. [CrossRef] [PubMed]
54. He, J.; Söderling, E.; Österblad, M.; Vallittu, P.K.; Lassila, L.V.J. Synthesis of methacrylate monomers with antibacterial effects against S. mutans. *Molecules* **2011**, *16*, 9755–9763. [CrossRef] [PubMed]
55. Sezonov, G.; Joseleau-Petit, D.; D'Ari, R. Escherichia Coli physiology in Luria-Bertani broth. *J. Bacteriol.* **2007**, *189*, 8746–8749. [CrossRef] [PubMed]

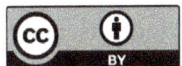

© 2019 by the authors. Licensee MDPI, Basel, Switzerland. This article is an open access article distributed under the terms and conditions of the Creative Commons Attribution (CC BY) license (http://creativecommons.org/licenses/by/4.0/).

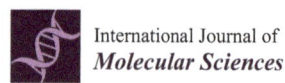

Article

Antimicrobial Coatings from Hybrid Nanoparticles of Biocompatible and Antimicrobial Polymers

Carolina Nascimento Galvão [1], Luccas Missfeldt Sanches [1], Beatriz Ideriha Mathiazzi [1], Rodrigo Tadeu Ribeiro [1], Denise Freitas Siqueira Petri [2] and Ana Maria Carmona-Ribeiro [1,*]

[1] Biocolloids Laboratory, Departamento de Bioquímica, Instituto de Química, Universidade de São Paulo, Av. Prof. Lineu Prestes 748, 05508-000 São Paulo, Brazil; carolinagalvao@usp.br (C.N.G.); luccas.sanches@hotmail.com (L.M.S.); bemathi@usp.br (B.I.M.); rodrigo@iq.usp.br (R.T.R.)
[2] Departamento de Química Fundamental, Instituto de Química, Universidade de São Paulo, Av. Prof. Lineu Prestes 748, 05508-000 São Paulo, Brazil; dfsp@usp.br
* Correspondence: amcr@usp.br; Tel.: +55-011-3091-1887

Received: 17 August 2018; Accepted: 26 September 2018; Published: 28 September 2018

Abstract: Hybrid nanoparticles of poly(methylmethacrylate) synthesized in the presence of poly (diallyldimethyl ammonium) chloride by emulsion polymerization exhibited good colloidal stability, physical properties, and antimicrobial activity but their synthesis yielded poor conversion. Here we create antimicrobial coatings from casting and drying of the nanoparticles dispersions onto model surfaces such as those of silicon wafers, glass coverslips, or polystyrene sheets and optimize conversion using additional stabilizers such as cetyltrimethyl ammonium bromide, dioctadecyldimethyl ammonium bromide, or soybean lecithin during nanoparticles synthesis. Methodology included dynamic light scattering, determination of wettability, ellipsometry of spin-coated films, scanning electron microscopy, and determination of colony forming unities (log CFU/mL) of bacteria after 1 h interaction with the coatings. The additional lipids and surfactants indeed improved nanoparticle synthesis, substantially increasing the conversion rates by stabilizing the monomer droplets in dispersion during the polymerization. The coatings obtained by spin-coating or casting of the nanoparticles dispersions onto silicon wafers were hydrophilic with contact angles increasing with the amount of the cationic polymer in the nanoparticles. Against *Escherichia coli* and *Staphylococcus aureus*, bacteria cell counts were reduced by approximately 7 logs upon interaction with the coatings, revealing their potential for several biotechnological and biomedical applications.

Keywords: coatings from nanoparticles; biocompatible polymer; antimicrobial polymer; dynamic light scattering; coatings wettability; microbicidal coatings; bacteria viability; bactericidal coatings; *Escherichia coli*; *Staphylococcus aureus*

1. Introduction

Biomimetic hybrid coatings have often been used as antibacterial materials [1–4]. For example, silver nanoparticles (NPs) embedded on dextran films or on a lysozyme/dextran network of natural polymers can be grafted onto a variety of surfaces with several biomedical applications possible from coating implants to catheters [5–7]. Biocompatible and antimicrobial polymers can be combined to yield a variety of nanostructures, among them, the popular and very useful NPs, which may further form coatings and films [8–10]. Antimicrobial polymeric NPs of poly(methylmethacrylate) (PMMA) synthesized in the presence of the cationic antimicrobial polymer poly(diallyldimethyl ammonium) chloride (PDDA) were first obtained in 2015 joining the biocompatible character of PMMA with the microbicide character of the cationic PDDA [11]. PMMA belongs to the Eudragit trademark that includes a diverse range of poly(methacrylate) and polyacrylate-based copolymers which are non-biodegradable, non-absorbable, and nontoxic with several applications in drug delivery [12]. The pharmaceutical applications of polyacrylates for coatings and films were recently and comprehensively reviewed [13].

On the other hand, PDDA was first described as a cationic antimicrobial polymer about 10 years ago, displaying outstanding activity as a microbicide and fungicide [7,14–16]. However, the synthesis of hybrid PMMA/PDDA NPs by emulsion polymerization in absence of surfactant yielded low conversion percentiles [11]. This was consistent with previously described and not very successful attempts to polymerize methyl acrylate (MA) or methyl methacrylate (MMA) using large amounts of monomer (>1.9 wt %) in oil-in-water microemulsions for which phase separation during polymerization took place [17–19]. The two major steps in emulsion polymerization are nucleation and particle growth. In the presence of surfactant, if the monomer has high affinity for the micelle core, nucleation occurs in the micelles where the monomers are. If the monomer is polar to a certain extent, there will be some affinity for the water phase so that polymerization also occurs in monomer droplets [20,21]. The initiator generates free radicals that react with MMA in the micelles and with MMA inside the droplets in the aqueous phase, yielding oligo radicals that colocalize with the monomers and proceeding with the polymerization. Apparently, the presence of PDDA during NPs synthesis in the absence of surfactant stabilized the smaller droplets of MMA yielding PMMA/PDDA hybrid and very small NPs [11]. Coatings prepared by spin-coating of PMMA and dioctadecyldimethyl ammonium bromide (DODAB) cationic lipid revealed a good compatibility between DODAB and PMMA leading to good antimicrobial activity against bacteria upon contact [22]. The dependence of the antimicrobial activity on the quaternary ammonium compound structure for combinations of PMMA and DODAB, cetyl trimethylammonium bromide (CTAB), or tetra propyl bromide (TPAB) for spin-coated films also yielded interesting results [23]. DODAB remained associated with PMMA films and killed bacteria upon contact, in contrast to CTAB that diffused out of the films killing bacteria in the outer medium [23]. In dispersion, PMMA/DODAB or PMMA/CTAB NPs prepared by emulsion polymerization over a range of high concentration of the quaternary ammonium amphiphiles showed remarkable antimicrobial activity over a range of micromolar concentrations [24].

Here we present some novel antimicrobial coatings based on hybrid NPs of PMMA and PDDA and solve the problem of low conversion during emulsion polymerization for PMMA/PDDA NPs synthesis by adding amphiphiles such as DODAB, CTAB, and lecithin in the reaction mixture. The results revealed remarkable microbicidal activity for the PMMA/PDDA coatings obtained from casting and drying PMMA/PDDA NPs and a substantial increase in conversion due to the presence of the amphiphiles during PMMA/PDDA NPs synthesis.

2. Results and Discussion

2.1. Physical Properties and Microbicidal Activity of Coatings from PMMA/PDDA Dispersions

The synthesis of PMMA/PDDA NPs, described previously by Sanches et al. [11], yielded monodisperse and cationic NPs in water dispersion named in accordance with MMA and PDDA concentrations used in the particles synthesis. For the dispersions A4, the concentrations used were 0.56 M MMA and 4 mg/mL PDDA; for A5, they were 0.56 M MMA and 5 mg/mL PDDA; and for B4, they were 1.32 M MMA and 4 mg/mL PDDA.

NPs in A4 have a mean diameter of 112 ± 17 nm as determined by Scanning Electron Microscopy (SEM) [11]. Casting and drying the original A4 dispersion on silicon wafers yielded the coating shown on the SEM micrograph (Figure 1), with the macroscopic features for the film seen on Figure 2. The coatings were homogeneous on the hydrophilic surfaces such as the silicon wafers and the glass coverslips. However, cracks and discontinuities were visible for those on the hydrophobic polystyrene substrates (Figure 2). The NPs structure was shown to involve a PMMA core surrounded by a PDDA shell [11] proving that the outer cationic and hydrophilic layer clearly interacted better with the hydrophilic surfaces such as those of the silicon wafer or the glass. The coating adhesion to the hydrophilic and anionic substrates was clearly better for A5 and A4-derived coatings than for those derived from B4 (Figure 2). The reason for this can be related to the higher relative ratio of PDDA to PMMA in A5 and A4-derived coatings than in the B4-derived ones. The interpretation for the ring appearing after casting B4 dispersion was related to the coffee-ring effect; such ring deposition occurs when liquid evaporation from the edge is replenished by liquid from the interior so that the resulting outward flow can carry most of the dispersed material to the edge [25]. This took place for the most hydrophobic NPs, namely, those with the lowest PDDA:PMMA molar ratios represented by the B4 dispersion. Similar ring deposition pattern was also observed for hydrophobic polystyrene particles deposited on glass from a water droplet and explained from the coffee ring effect [26]. The crack patterns visible for A4-derived coating on the polystyrene substrate were radial and similar to the ones previously described in the literature for similar systems [27]. The poor adhesion of the hydrophilic NPs of the A4 derived-coating to the hydrophobic polystyrene sheet might also have contributed to cracks in the coating (Figure 2).

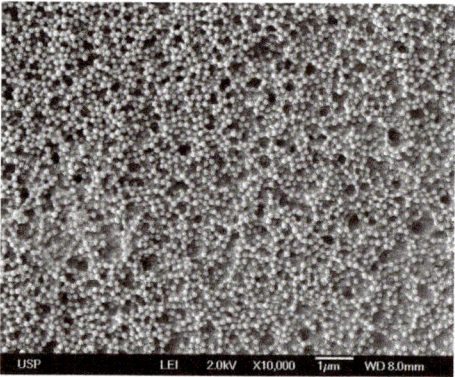

Figure 1. Scanning electron micrograph of the poly(methylmethacrylate) (PMMA)/poly(diallyldimethyl ammonium) chloride (PDDA) coating obtained by casting 0.050 mL of the original A4 nanoparticles dispersion (10 mg/mL) onto silicon wafers.

PMMA/PDDA coatings on silicon wafers are derived from two different procedures: (1) spin-coating of lyophilized A5 in 1:1 dichloromethane: ethanol; (2) casting of A5, A4, or B4 dispersions of NPs followed by drying under vacuum.

Spin-coating allows for the preparation of lipid [28–30] or polymer films [22] on very smooth surfaces such as those of the silicon wafers. In the present case, the composition of a hydrophobic polymer, such as PMMA, and a hydrophilic one, such as PDDA, required a special combination of solvents in order to obtain solubilization of both in the solvents mixture. Figure 3a–e shows the evaluation of solubilization of both polymers from the lyophilized A5 dispersion in ethanol (E):dichloromethane (D) over a range of E:D proportions. The complete solubilization only took place at 50:50% E:D. This allowed obtaining the coatings of PMMA: PDDA onto silicon wafers for evaluation of thickness, refractive index and contact angles (Table 1). These characteristics of the hybrid films compared to those of pure PMMA coatings revealed similar thicknesses and refractive indices but higher wettability for the hybrid coatings than those determined for the pure PMMA film (Table 1).

For coatings obtained by casting the PMMA/PDDA dispersions onto the silicon wafers, there was a consistent decrease of the contact angle upon increasing the PDDA relative amount in the dispersions from 35 ± 6 to 9 ± 2 degrees (Table 1). Coatings obtained by casting the dispersions yielded lower contact angles than those obtained by spin-coating, reconfirming that the hydrophilic PDDA immobilized as an outer layer of the PMMA/PDDA nanoparticle imparted a more hydrophilic character to the film surface than the one of the spin-coated PMMA/PDDA (Table 1).

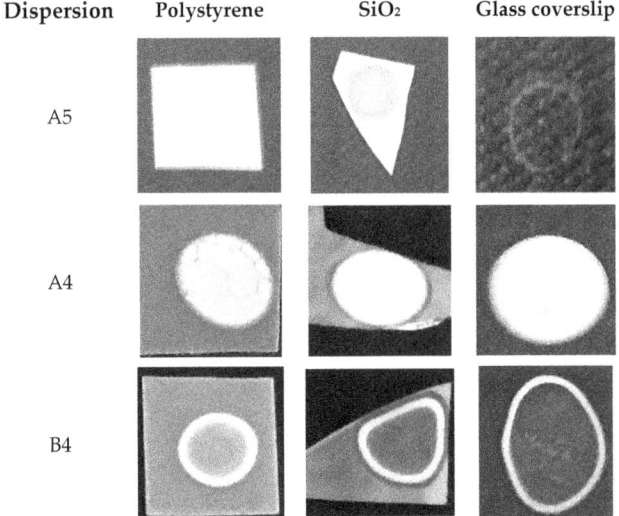

Figure 2. PMMA/PDDA films casted from 50 µL droplets of A5 (4.4 mg/mL), A4 (10 mg/mL), and B4 (5.8 mg/mL) dispersions on polystyrene sheets, silicon wafers, or glass coverslips.

The antimicrobial activity of the hybrid PMMA/PDDA coatings derived from A5, A4, and B4 casted onto glass coverslips revealed a remarkable microbicidal effect against *Escherichia coli* and *Staphylococcus aureus* (Table 2). In this case, the real potency of the coatings was established over orders of magnitude by determining bacteria viability from the log of CFU/mL. Bacteria viability decreased by 10^7–10^8 colony forming units (CFU) upon interaction with the coatings for 1 h (Table 2).

Table 1. Physical properties of PMMA/PDDA coatings on silicon wafers. The procedures for coating were: (1) spin-coating of lyophilized A5 in 1: 1 dichloromethane: ethanol; (2) casting of A5, A4, or B4 NPs dispersions followed by drying under vacuum.

Materials	Procedure	Composition	Thickness/nm	Refractive Index	Contact Angle θ_A/degrees
PMMA/PDDA	Spin-coating	Lyophilized A5	94 ± 3	1.495 ± 0.004	15 ± 1
PMMA/PDDA	Casting	A5	-	-	9 ± 2
PMMA/PDDA	Casting	A4	-	-	19 ± 2
PMMA/PDDA	Casting	B4	-	-	35 ± 6
PMMA [1]	Spin-coating	PMMA	91 ± 1	1.499 ± 0.004	76 ± 5

[1] Data from reference [22].

Table 2. Microbicidal activity of PMMA/PDDA coatings obtained from casting and drying under vacuum A5, A4, or B4 dispersions (0.2 mL) onto glass coverslips. Since 4 or 5 mg/mL of PDDA were the concentrations used for particle synthesis, in 0.2 mL of each dispersion used for the coatings there will be 0.8 to 1.0 mg of PDDA acting against the bacteria.

Dispersion Used for Coating	Microorganism	Initial Cell Viability/log (CFU/mL)	Final Cell Viability/log (CFU/mL)
A5	E. coli	7.2	0
A5	S. aureus	7.9	0
A4	E. coli	7.1	0
A4	S. aureus	8.2	0
B4	E. coli	7.1	0
B4	S. aureus	8.2	0

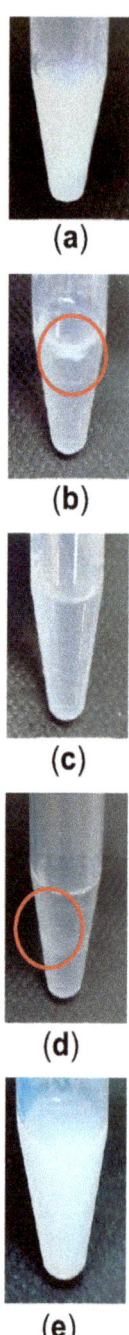

Figure 3. Checking solvent mixtures for the solubilization of lyophilized PMMA/PDDA A5 dispersion (1 mL) aiming at the preparation of coatings by spin-coating. Solvents were dichloromethane (**a**); 75% dichloromethane: 25% ethanol (**b**); 50% dichloromethane: 50% ethanol (**c**); 25% dichloromethane: 75% ethanol (**d**); and ethanol (**e**). The red circles emphasize the fact that some insoluble polymer still remained in the solvents mixture.

2.2. Optimization of Nanoparticles Synthesis and Conversion Percentiles

The synthesis of PMMA/PDDA NPs as dispersion A5 in absence of surfactants displayed low monomer-into-polymer conversion since only approximately 10% of the monomer mass added was converted into polymer [11]. In order to improve conversion percentiles, the effect of monomer concentration on conversion was determined (Figure 4; Table 3). At 5 mg/mL PDDA, decreasing the methylmethacrylate (MMA) concentration [MMA] improved conversion, and possible reasons for this would be the relative increase in PDDA capable of stabilizing the droplet/water interface and the increased average distance between MMA droplets reducing coalescence. One should note that NPs size could also be reduced by decreasing [MMA] meaning that polymerization from smaller droplets yielded smaller NPs. At this point, stabilizing the droplet/water interface seemed crucial for improving conversion. Therefore, CTAB, DODAB, and lecithin were introduced in the reaction mixture for further stabilization of the monomer droplets.

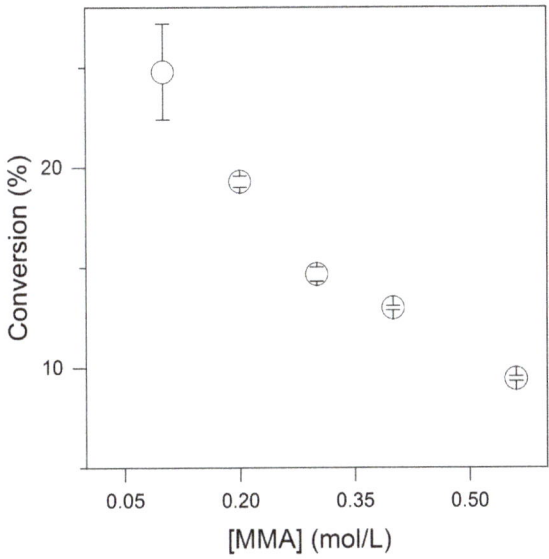

Figure 4. The effect of methyl methacrylate (MMA) concentration on conversion (%) of MMA into PMMA in the presence of PDDA (5 mg/mL) and AIBN (0.36 mg/mL) as initiator. The nanoparticles synthesis proceeded for 2 h at 70 to 80 °C and was followed by extensive dialysis before performing the dispersions characterization by dynamic light-scattering shown on Table 3.

Table 3. Effect of MMA concentration on physical properties of the PMMA/PDDA dispersions obtained by emulsion polymerization of MMA at 5 mg/mL PDDA in 1 mM NaCl using 0.36 mg/mL of AIBN.

[MMA] (M)	Dz (nm)	P	ζ (mV)	Solid Contents (mg/mL)
0.10	153 ± 1	0.04 ± 0.01	+46 ± 5	3.1 ± 0.3
0.20	188 ± 1	0.05 ± 0.01	+52 ± 3	3.4 ± 0.1
0.30	153 ± 1	0.04 ± 0.02	+47 ± 3	4.1 ± 0.1
0.40	244 ± 1	0.02 ± 0.00	+51 ± 2	5.8 ± 0.1
0.56	213 ± 3	0.03 ± 0.02	+54 ± 2	3.8 ± 0.1

In fact, all amphiphiles employed improved conversion (Table 4). The most efficacious amphiphile was CTAB, followed by DODAB and lecithin. Since lecithin corresponds to a mixture of lipids and fatty acids with a net negative charge [31,32], at 2 mM lecithin, the NPs became negatively charged;

all other NPs exhibited high and positive zeta-potentials (Table 4). In the presence of two stabilizers (amphiphile and PDDA), conversion was substantially increased in comparison to the one in the presence of a single stabilizer. Another interesting observation refers to the lower zeta-potential for PMMA/CTAB in comparison to the one for PMMA/DODAB; this is consistent with the reported immobilization of DODAB in the PMMA polymeric matrix which is absent for CTAB, since CTAB was reported to be more mobile than DODAB easily diffusing to the outer medium from PMMA films [22,23]. In summary, although amphiphiles indeed improved conversion, PDDA as a second stabilizer possibly provided an additional stabilizing factor, which was the electrosteric repulsion between the MMA droplets during NP synthesis. This also represented an important stabilizing factor for the final polymeric NPs.

Table 4. The effect of PDDA, surfactants, and lipids on NPs size (Dz), polydispersity (P), and zeta-potential (ζ) on the stabilization of MMA droplets in water and the improvement of solid contents and conversion percentiles for NPs synthesis.

Dispersion *	Dz (nm)	P	m(V)	Solids (mg/mL)	Conversion (%)
PMMA/PDDA	226 ± 3	0.01 ± 0.01	+51 ± 1	6 ± 1	11 ± 1
PMMA/CTAB	97 ± 0	0.05 ± 0.01	+25 ± 1	38 ± 1	66 ± 1
PMMA/CTAB/PDDA	91 ± 0	0.04 ± 0.01	+47 ± 3	26 ± 1	79 ± 1
PMMA/DODAB	177 ± 1	0.07 ± 0.01	+65 ± 1	16 ± 1	28 ± 1
PMMA/DODAB/PDDA	229 ± 2	0.03 ± 0.02	+45 ± 3	17 ± 1	47 ± 1
PMMA/Lecithin	178 ± 1	0.10 ± 0.01	-27 ± 2	13 ± 1	23 ± 1
PMMA/Lecithin/PDDA	233 ± 1	0.04 ± 0.02	+54 ± 1	8 ± 1	24 ± 1

* Concentrations used for NPs synthesis were: [MMA] = 0.56 M; [PDDA] = 5 mg/ mL; [CTAB] = [DODAB] = [Lecithin] = 2 mM.

Figure 5 and Table 5 show the remarkable colloidal stability of the NPs characterized by the physical properties on Table 4. The photos taken one day and 4 months after synthesis revealed very similar macroscopic features and absence of precipitates. The analysis of sizes, polydispersities, and zeta-potentials also revealed maintenance of these physical properties of the NPs over time (Table 5).

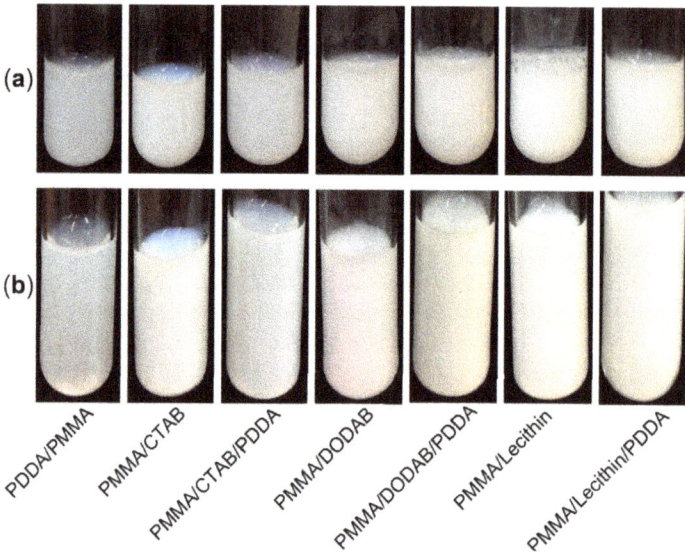

Figure 5. (a) Photos of dispersions just after synthesis and dialysis; (b) photos of the same dispersions approximately 4 months later. Details on composition and physical properties of the dispersions just after synthesis are on Table 5.

Table 5. The colloidal stability of NPs dispersions from sizing (Dz), polydispersity (P), and zeta-potential (ζ) for dispersions aged 1 and 120 days after synthesis.

Dispersion *	Dz/nm		P		ζ/mV	
	Day 1	Day 120	Day 1	Day 120	Day 1	Day 120
PMMA/PDDA	226 ± 3	211 ± 3	0.01 ± 0.01	0.05 ± 0.01	+51 ± 1	+55 ± 1
PMMA/CTAB	97 ± 0	95 ± 0	0.05 ± 0.01	0.08 ± 0.01	+25 ± 1	+26 ± 1
PMMA/CTAB/PDDA	91 ± 0	90 ± 1	0.04 ± 0.01	0.04 ± 0.01	+47 ± 3	+50 ± 2
PMMA/DODAB	177 ± 1	176 ± 1	0.07 ± 0.01	0.09 ± 0.02	+65 ± 1	+50 ± 1
PMMA/DODAB/PDDA	229 ± 2	226 ± 1	0.03 ± 0.02	0.04 ± 0.02	+45 ± 3	+54 ± 1
PMMA/Lecithin	178 ± 1	176 ± 1	0.10 ± 0.01	0.16 ± 0.02	−27 ± 2	−21 ± 1
PMMA/Lecithin/PDDA	233 ± 1	217 ± 2	0.04 ± 0.02	0.03 ± 0.02	+54 ± 1	+55 ± 1

* Concentrations used for NPs synthesis were: [MMA] = 0.56 M; [PDDA] = 5 mg/mL; [CTAB] = [DODAB] = [Lecithin] = 2 mM.

As compared to other similar systems in the literature, the present NPs use the self-assembly of biocompatible PMMA and the antimicrobial polymer PDDA instead of synthesizing block copolymers incorporating both functions. For example, glycosylated block copolymers were used as surfactants in butyl methacrylate emulsion polymerization [33]. However, the antimicrobial activity was not as high as the one obtained for the coatings described in this work (Table 2). The higher hydrophobicity inherent to the two methyl groups on the quaternary nitrogen of the PDDA molecule, as compared to the cationic glycosylated moieties, was an advantage for efficient microbicide activity. Indeed, several derivatives of PDDA evaluated for their antimicrobial activity revealed that these cationic polymers exhibit the highest activity when their chemical structure bears high frequency of hydrophobic methyl moieties [11,34]. The hydrophilic character of cationic antimicrobial polymers does not contribute to improvement of the antimicrobial action, although the NPs synthesis certainly benefits from their use as surfactants.

A major drawback of PMMA/PDDA NPs synthesis was the low conversion due to the relatively poor function of PDDA at the interface of MMA droplets and the surrounding water medium during NP synthesis (Figure 4). In this work, we solved this problem by adding amphiphiles such as CTAB, DODAB, and lecithin as surfactants active as stabilizers during the NPs synthesis. In addition, we must recognize the excellent perspective of these ternary systems as antimicrobials since PDDA, DODAB, and CTAB have already being described in separate as good antimicrobial agents [3,8,10,14,24,35–37]. The antimicrobial properties of these ternary systems both as latexes dispersions in water and as coatings still have to be determined.

3. Materials and Methods

3.1. Materials

MMA, PDDA, azobisisobutyronitrile (AIBN), NaCl, CTAB, DODAB, soybean lecithin, chloroform, ethanol, dichloromethane, and Mueller–Hinton agar (MHA) were purchased from Sigma-Aldrich (Darmstadt, Germany) and used without further purification. The composition of soybean lecithin includes several fatty acids and phospholipids [31,32]. Silicon (100) wafers were from Silicon Quest (Santa Clara, CA, USA) with a native oxide layer approximately 2 nm thick and used as substrates for casting the dispersions. These Si wafers with a native SiO_2 layer were cut into small pieces of ca 1 cm^2, cleaned with acetone, and dried under a N_2 stream; they are smooth substrates for the coatings. The syntheses in 1 mM NaCl solution prepared with Milli-Q water yielded NPs dispersions by emulsion polymerization that underwent dialysis for purification using a cellulose acetate dialysis bag with molecular weight cut-off around 12,400 g/mol. All other reagents were analytical grade and used without further purification.

3.2. Preparation of NPs by Emulsion Polymerization

A variety of hybrid and polymeric NPs were obtained by polymerization of MMA at 70 to 80 °C for 1 h using 10 mL of aqueous solutions of NaCl 1 mM and PDDA and/or CTAB, DODAB, or lecithin in accordance with compositions shown in Table 6 [11]. Briefly, a weak flux of nitrogen was applied to the solution during a few minutes before adding 3.6 mg of AIBN initiator and MMA. For dispersions containing surfactants or lipids, DODAB or lecithin were previously dissolved in chloroform in order to prepare lipid films under a nitrogen flux to evaporate the chloroform solvent [38,39]. Ten milliliters of the NaCl 1 mM solution was then added to the dried lipid films before proceeding with NP synthesis. In the case of CTAB, the required amount of CTAB in the NPs dispersion was directly added to the 1 mM NaCl solution before starting the NPs synthesis. The NP dispersions obtained were further purified by dialysis against Milli-Q water until water conductivity reached 5 µS/cm.

Table 6. Concentrations of MMA, PDDA, cetyl trimethylammonium bromide (CTAB), dioctadecyldimethyl ammonium bromide (DODAB), and/or lecithin used to synthesize hybrid NPs by emulsion polymerization.

Dispersion	[MMA] (M)	[PDDA] (mg/mL)	[CTAB] (mM)	[DODAB] (mM)	[Lecithin] (mM)
A5	0.56	5	-	-	-
A4	0.56	4	-	-	-
B4	1.32	4	-	-	-
PMMA/CTAB	0.56	-	2	-	-
PMMA/CTAB/PDDA	0.56	5	2	-	-
PMMA/DODAB	0.56	-	-	2	-
PMMA/DODAB/PDDA	0.56	5	-	2	-
PMMA/lecithin	0.56	-	-	-	2
PMMA/lecithin/PDDA	0.56	5	-	-	2

3.3. Determination of Zeta-Average Diameter (Dz), Polydispersity (P), Zeta-Potential (ζ), and Colloidal Stability of NPs Dispersions

Size distributions, Dz, ζ, and P were obtained by dynamic light-scattering (DLS) using a Zeta Plus Zeta Potential Analyzer (Brookhaven Instruments Corporation, Holtsville, NY, USA) equipped with a laser of 677 nm with measurements at 90°. P of the dispersions was determined by DLS following well defined mathematic equation [40]. Dz values were obtained from the log normal distribution of the light-scattered intensity curve against the diameter. ζ values were determined from the electrophoretic mobility (μ) and Smoluchowski equation $\zeta = \mu\eta/\varepsilon$, where η and ε are the viscosity and the dielectric constant of the medium, respectively. Samples were diluted 1:30 with a 1 mM NaCl water solution for performing the measurements at (25 ± 1) °C.

The colloidal stability of the dispersions was followed by two procedures: (1) from photographs of the dispersions; (2) from the physical properties (Dz, P, and ζ), both procedures performed at days one and 120.

3.4. Preparation of Coatings from the NPs Dispersions by Spin-coating or Casting

For preparing spin-coated films, 1 mL of the A5 dispersion was lyophilized and a 10 mg/mL solution in the solvents mixture (1:1 dichloromethane: ethanol) was prepared; 0.1 mL of this solution was then spin-coated onto silicon wafers using a Headway PWM32-PS-R790 spinner (Garland, TX, USA), operated at 3000 rpm during 40 s, at (24 ± 1) °C, and $(50 \pm 5)\%$ of relative humidity. Thereafter, the film was characterized by ellipsometry [41] which allowed us to obtain the thickness and refractive index of the film independently [22].

Films prepared by casting employed 0.05 mL of A5, A4, or B4 original dispersions casted onto three different surfaces: polystyrene, silicon wafers, or glass coverslips. After drying overnight under vacuum the films were photographed, observed by SEM, characterized regarding their wettability, and used for determining antimicrobial activity.

3.5. Physical Characterization of Coatings by SEM, Macroscopic Features from Photographs and Contact Angle Determinations

SEM for the coatings employed Jeol JSM-7401F equipment (JEOL Ltd., Akishima, Tokyo, Japan). In short, 2 µL of A5 dispersion on silicon wafers dried in a desiccator before coverage with a thin gold layer as required for contrast and visualization by SEM.

Coatings from A5, A4, or B4 onto different substrates (polystyrene sheet, silicon wafers, and glass coverslip) were obtained by casting 50 µL onto the substrates and allowing the material to dry overnight in a desiccator before taking pictures or determining wettability by using a home built apparatus, as previously described [29,30]. Photos of sessile water droplets of 10 µL allowed for the determining of the advancing contact angle (θ_A) over the first 5 min after depositing the droplet on the films. Each determination was taken as a mean ± the standard deviation of at least 4 measurements.

3.6. Microorganisms Growth and Determination of Cell Viability in the Presence of the Coatings

E. coli ATCC (American Type Culture Collection) 25322 and *S. aureus* ATCC 29213 growths were purchased from previously frozen stocks and kept at −20 °C in appropriate storage medium. The bacterial strains plated onto MHA were incubated at 37 °C/18–24 h before transferring some isolated colonies to an isotonic 0.264 M D-glucose solution and adjusting turbidity to 0.5 of the McFarland scale [42]. The 0.264 M D-glucose solution was used instead of any culture medium because cationic molecules are inactivated by the relatively high ionic strength or negatively charged molecules such as amino acids and polysaccharides. For determination of cell viability after interaction with the PMMA/PDDA NPs coatings, final bacteria cell concentrations in the suspensions were around 10^8 CFU/mL.

Sixty microliters of the bacterial suspensions were deposited on the coatings (obtained by casting of A5, A4, or B4 dispersions onto glass coverslips) and left in a water-vapor-saturated chamber for 1 h to prevent water evaporation from the droplet. Thereafter, the glass coverslips were transferred to 10 mL of 0.264 M D-glucose isotonic solution in Falcon tubes and vigorously stirred by vortexing before withdrawing 0.1 mL aliquots and preparing their 1:10 and 1:100 dilutions for plating on MHA plates, incubating the plates (37 °C/24 h), and reading the CFU. These readings were converted into CFU/mL and log (CFU/mL). When no counting was obtained, since the log function does not exist for zero, the CFU/mL counting was taken as 1 so that log CFU/mL could be taken as zero. Controls were bare glass coverslips.

4. Conclusions

PMMA/PDDA nanoparticles coated three different substrates by two different procedures: (1) spin-coating; (2) casting followed by drying of the casted dispersions. Macroscopically homogeneous films without cracks coated the hydrophilic substrates such as silicon wafers or glass coverslips. On hydrophobic substrates such as polystyrene surfaces, the coatings showed cracks after drying. The most homogeneous coatings occurred at the highest relative contents of PDDA:PMMA. Upon lowering PDDA contents in the NPs, the NPs accumulated at the periphery of the droplets casted on the substrates. This was due to the coffee ring effect, since the more hydrophobic NPs followed the capillary flow to the periphery of the droplet. The contact angles for the coatings showed a clear dependence of wettability on the PDDA content of the NPs. The higher the PDDA content, the lower the contact angle and the better the adhesion to oppositely charged hydrophilic substrates. Comparing films obtained by spin-coating with those obtained by casting of the NPs onto the substrates showed that spin-coated coatings had larger contact angles than coatings obtained by casting, suggesting that some PDDA molecules might have migrated to the silicon wafer–water interface hiding from the film surface and therefore becoming somewhat unavailable to kill bacteria at the film surface. There was a remarkable microbicide activity due to 0.8–1.0 mg of PDDA distributed in the coatings: after 1 h interaction with bacteria, their viability decreased by approximately 7 to 8 logs as tested against *E. coli* or *S. aureus* cells. This was possibly due to the more hydrophobic nature of PDDA in comparison with other hydrophilic cationic polymers.

CTAB, DODAB, or lecithin as additional stabilizers for the PMMA/PDDA NPs synthesis substantially improved conversion of MMA into PMMA. These ternary systems were stable and maintained their macroscopic and microscopic physical characteristics with time (checked for 4 months). The use of these ternary systems as microbicides still needs systematic evaluation.

Author Contributions: Conceptualization, A.M.C.-R.; Methodology, C.N.G., L.M.S., B.I.M., R.T.R., D.F.S.P., and A.M.C.-R.; Formal Analysis, C.N.G., L.M.S., D.F.S.P., and A.M.C.-R.; Investigation, C.N.G., L.M.S., B.I.M., R.T.R.; D.F.S.P. and A.M.C.-R.; Resources, A.M.C.-R.; Writing—Original Draft Preparation, A.M.C.-R.; Writing—Review & Editing, D.F.S.P. and A.M.C.-R.; Supervision, A.M.C.-R.; Project Administration, A.M.C.-R.; Funding Acquisition, A.M.C.-R.

Funding: Research support was from the Conselho Nacional de Desenvolvimento Científico e Tecnológico (CNPq) grant number 302352/2014-7 to the Project "Bioactive Supramolecular Assemblies" by A.M.C-R. CNPq also funded D.F.S.P. grant number 306848/2017. The APC was also from CNPq grant number 302352/2014-7. C.N.G. and B.I.M. were recipients of undergraduate fellowships of the Programa Unificado de Bolsas da Universidade de São Paulo granted to the Project "Cationic Supramolecular Assemblies and their Films" by A.M.C.-R., L.M.S. was recipient of several undergraduate fellowships from PIBIC–CNPq granted to the project "Antimicrobial Nanoparticles Synthesis from MMA in the Presence of PDDA" by A.M.C.-R.

Conflicts of Interest: The authors declare no conflict of interest. The funders had no role in the design of the study; in the collection, analyses, or interpretation of data; in the writing of the manuscript, and in the decision to publish the results.

Abbreviations

θ_A	Advancing Contact Angle
ATCC	American Type Culture Collection
AIBN	Azobisisobutyronitrile
CTAB	Cetyltrimethylammonium Bromide
CFU	Colony Forming Unities
D	Dichloromethane
ε	Dielectric Constant of the Medium
DODAB	Dioctadecyldimethylammonium Bromide
DLS	Dynamic Light Scattering
μ	Electrophoretic Mobility
E	Ethanol
MA	Methyl acrylate
MMA	Methyl methacrylate
MHA	Mueller-Hinton Agar
NPs	Nanoparticles
P	Polydispersity
PMMA	Poly(methyl methacrylate)
PDDA	Poly(diallyldimethylammonium) chloride
SEM	Scanning Electron Microscopy
η	Viscosity of the Medium
Dz	Zeta-average Diameter
ζ	Zeta-potential

References

1. Carmona-Ribeiro, A.M.; Barbassa, L.; Melo, L.D. Antimicrobial Biomimetics. In *Biomimetic Based Applications*; George, A., Ed.; InTechOpen: Rijeka, Croatia, 2011; Volume 1, pp. 227–284. ISBN 978-953-307-195-4.

2. Carmona-Ribeiro, A.M. The Versatile Dioctadecyldimethylammonium Bromide. In *Application and Characterization of Surfactants*; Najjar, R., Ed.; InTechOpen: Rijeka, Croatia, 2017; Volume 1, pp. 157–181. ISBN 978-953-51-3325-4.
3. Carmona-Ribeiro, A.M. Self-Assembled Antimicrobial Nanomaterials. *Int. J. Environ. Res. Public Health* **2018**, *15*, 1408. [CrossRef] [PubMed]
4. Vitiello, G.; Silvestri, B.; Luciani, G. Learning from Nature: Bioinspired Strategies towards Antimicrobial Nanostructured Systems. *Curr. Top. Med. Chem.* **2018**, *18*, 22–41. [CrossRef] [PubMed]
5. Coll Ferrer, M.C.; Hickok, N.J.; Eckmann, D.M.; Composto, R.J. Antibacterial Biomimetic Hybrid Films. *Soft Matter* **2013**, *8*, 2423–2431. [CrossRef] [PubMed]
6. Coll Ferrer, M.C.; Eckmann, U.N.; Composto, R.J.; Eckmann, D.M. Hemocompatibility and Biocompatibility of Antibacterial Biomimetic Hybrid Films. *Toxicol. Appl. Pharmacol.* **2013**, *272*, 703–712. [CrossRef] [PubMed]
7. Coll Ferrer, M.C.; Dastgheyb, S.; Hickok, N.J.; Eckmann, D.M.; Composto, R.J. Designing Nanogel Carriers for Antibacterial Applications. *Acta Biomater.* **2014**, *10*, 2105–2111. [CrossRef] [PubMed]
8. Melo, L.D.; Mamizuka, E.M.; Carmona-Ribeiro, A.M. Antimicrobial Particles from Cationic Lipid and Polyelectrolytes. *Langmuir* **2010**, *26*, 12300–12306. [CrossRef] [PubMed]
9. Xavier, G.R.S.; Carmona-Ribeiro, A.M. Cationic Biomimetic Particles of Polystyrene/Cationic Bilayer/Gramicidin for Optimal Bactericidal Activity. *Nanomaterials* **2017**, *7*, 422. [CrossRef] [PubMed]
10. Carrasco, L.D.M.; Sampaio, J.L.M.; Carmona-Ribeiro, A.M. Supramolecular Cationic Assemblies against Multidrug-Resistant Microorganisms: Activity and Mechanism of Action. *Int. J. Mol. Sci.* **2015**, *16*, 6337–6352. [CrossRef] [PubMed]
11. Sanches, L.M.; Petri, D.F.S.; Carrasco, L.D.M.; Carmona-Ribeiro, A.M. The Antimicrobial Activity of Free and Immobilized Poly (diallyldimethylammonium) Chloride in Nanoparticles of Poly (methylmethacrylate). *J. Nanobiotechnology* **2015**, *13*, 58. [CrossRef] [PubMed]
12. Thakral, S.; Thakral, N.K.; Majumdar, D.K. Eudragit®: A Technology Evaluation. *Expert Opin. Drug Deliv.* **2013**, *10*, 131–149. [CrossRef] [PubMed]
13. Patra, C.N.; Priya, R.; Swain, S.; Kumar Jena, G.; Panigrahi, K.C.; Ghose, D. Pharmaceutical Significance of Eudragit: A Review. *Future J. Pharm. Sci.* **2017**, *3*, 33–45. [CrossRef]
14. Carmona-Ribeiro, A.M.; Carrasco, L.D.M. Fungicidal Assemblies and Their Mode of Action. *OA Biotechnol.* **2013**, *2*, 25. [CrossRef]
15. Vieira, D.B.; Carmona-Ribeiro, A.M. Cationic Nanoparticles for Delivery of Amphotericin B: Preparation, Characterization and Activity in vitro. *J. Nanobiotechnol.* **2008**, *6*, 6. [CrossRef] [PubMed]
16. Carmona-Ribeiro, A.M.; Carrasco, L.D.M. Cationic Antimicrobial Polymers and Their Assemblies. *Int. J. Mol. Sci.* **2013**, *14*, 9906–9946. [CrossRef] [PubMed]
17. Atik, S.S.; Thomas, J.K. Polymerized Microemulsions. *J. Am. Chem. Soc.* **1981**, *103*, 4279–4280. [CrossRef]
18. Stoffer, J.O.; Bone, T. Polymerization in Water-in-Oil Microemulsion Systems II: SEM Investigation of Structure. *J. Disper. Sci. Technol.* **1980**, *1*, 393–412. [CrossRef]
19. Jayakrishnan, A.; Shah, D.O. Polymerization of Oil-in-water Microemulsions: Polymerization of Styrene and Methyl Methacrylate. *J. Polym. Sci. Pol. Lett.* **1984**, *22*, 31–38. [CrossRef]
20. Daniels, E.S.; Sudol, D.E.; El-Aasser, M.S. Overview of Polymer Colloids: Preparation, Characterization, and Applications. In *Polymer Colloids*; Daniels, E.S., Sudol, D.E., El-Aasser, M.S., Eds.; ACS Symposium Series; American Chemical Society: Washington, DC, USA, 2001; Volume 801, pp. 1–12. ISBN 13 9780841237599.
21. Lichti, G.; Gilbert, R.G.; Napper, D.H. The Mechanisms of Latex Particle Formation and Growth in the Emulsion Polymerization of Styrene Using the Surfactant Sodium Dodecyl sulfate. *J. Polym. Sci. Pol. Chem.* **1983**, *21*, 269–291. [CrossRef]
22. Pereira, E.M.A.; Kosaka, P.M.; Rosa, H.; Vieira, D.B.; Kawano, Y.; Petri, D.F.S.; Carmona-Ribeiro, A.M. Hybrid Materials from Intermolecular Associations between Cationic Lipid and Polymers. *J. Phys. Chem. B* **2008**, *112*, 9301–9310. [CrossRef] [PubMed]
23. Melo, L.D.; Palombo, R.R.; Petri, D.F.S.; Bruns, M.; Pereira, E.M.A.; Carmona-Ribeiro, A.M. Structure–Activity Relationship for Quaternary Ammonium Compounds Hybridized with Poly (methyl methacrylate). *ACS Appl. Mater. Interfaces* **2011**, *3*, 1933–1939. [CrossRef] [PubMed]
24. Naves, A.F.; Palombo, R.R.; Carrasco, L.D.M.; Carmona-Ribeiro, A.M. Antimicrobial Particles from Emulsion Polymerization of Methyl Methacrylate in the Presence of Quaternary Ammonium Surfactants. *Langmuir* **2013**, *29*, 9677–9684. [CrossRef] [PubMed]

25. Deegan, R.D.; Bakajin, O.; Dupont, T.F.; Huber, G.; Nagel, S.R.; Witten, T.A. Capillary Flow as the Cause of Ring Stains from Dried Liquid Drops. *Nature* **1997**, *389*, 827–829. [CrossRef]
26. Hu, H.; Larson, R.G. Marangoni Effect Reverses Coffee-Ring Depositions. *J. Phys. Chem. B* **2006**, *110*, 7090–7094. [CrossRef] [PubMed]
27. Pauchard, L.; Parisse, F.; Allain, C. Influence of Salt Contents on Crack Patterns Formed through Colloidal Suspension Desiccation. *Phys. Rev. E* **1999**, *59*, 3737–3740. [CrossRef]
28. Mennicke, U.; Salditt, T. Preparation of Solid-Supported Lipid Bilayers by Spin-Coating. *Langmuir* **2002**, *18*, 8172–8177. [CrossRef]
29. Pereira, E.M.A.; Petri, D.F.S.; Carmona-Ribeiro, A.M. Adsorption of Cationic Lipid Bilayer onto Flat Silicon Wafers: Effect of Ion Nature and Concentration. *J. Phys. Chem. B* **2006**, *110*, 10070–10074. [CrossRef] [PubMed]
30. Pereira, E.M.A.; Petri, D.F.S.; Carmona-Ribeiro, A.M. Synthetic Vesicles at Hydrophobic Surfaces. *J. Phys. Chem. B* **2002**, *106*, 8762–8767. [CrossRef]
31. Augusto, O.; Carmona-Ribeiro, A.M. Introducing Model Membranes and Lipoperoxidation. *Biochem. Educ.* **1989**, *17*, 209–210. [CrossRef]
32. Kagawa, Y.; Racker, E. Partial Resolution of the Enzymes Catalyzing Oxidative Phosphorylation VIII. Properties of a Factor Conferring Oligomycin Sensitivity on Mitochondrial Adenosine Trifosfatase. *J. Biol. Chem.* **1966**, *241*, 2461–2466. [PubMed]
33. Álvarez-Paino, M.; Muñoz-Bonilla, A.; López-Fabal, F.; Gómez-Garcés, J.L.; Heuts, J.P.A.; Fernández-García, M. Functional Surfaces Obtained from Emulsion Polymerization Using Antimicrobial Glycosylated Block Copolymers as Surfactants. *Polym. Chem.* **2015**, *6*, 6171–6181. [CrossRef]
34. Timofeeva, L.M.; Kleshcheva, N.A.; Moroz, A.F.; Didenko, L.V. Secondary and Tertiary Polydiallylammonium Salts: Novel Polymers with High Antimicrobial Activity. *Biomacromolecules* **2009**, *10*, 2976–2986. [CrossRef] [PubMed]
35. Campanhã, M.T.N.; Mamizuka, E.M.; Carmona-Ribeiro, A.M. Interactions between cationic liposomes and bacteria: the physical-chemistry of the bactericidal action. *J. Lipid Res.* **1999**, *40*, 1495–1500. [PubMed]
36. Martins, L.M.S.; Mamizuka, E.M.; Carmona-Ribeiro, A.M. Cationic Vesicles as Bactericides. *Langmuir* **1997**, *13*, 5583–5587. [CrossRef]
37. Vieira, D.B.; Carmona-Ribeiro, A.M. Cationic Lipids and Surfactants as Antifungal Agents: Mode of Action. *J. Antimicrob. Chemother.* **2006**, *58*, 760–767. [CrossRef] [PubMed]
38. Ribeiro, R.T.; Braga, V.H.A.; Carmona-Ribeiro, A.M. Biomimetic Cationic Nanoparticles Based on Silica: Optimizing Bilayer Deposition from Lipid Films. *Biomimetics* **2017**, *2*, 20. [CrossRef]
39. Sobral, C.N.C.; Soto, M.A.; Carmona-Ribeiro, A.M. Characterization of DODAB/DPPC Vesicles. *Chem. Phys. Lipids* **2008**, *152*, 38–45. [CrossRef] [PubMed]
40. Grabowski, E.; Morrison, I. Particle Size Distribution from Analysis of Quasi-elastic Light Scattering Data. In *Measurement of Suspended Particles by Quasi-elastic Light Scattering*, 1st ed.; Dahneke, B.E., Ed.; John Wiley & Sons: New York, NY, USA, 1983; Volume 21, pp. 199–236. ISBN 0-471-87289-X.
41. Azzam, R.M.A.; Bashara, N.M. *Ellipsometry and Polarized Light*; North Holland Amsterdam: Amsterdam, The Netherlands, 1987; ISBN 0-444-87016-4.
42. Chapin, K.; Lauderdale, T.L. Comparison of Bactec 9240 and Difco ESP Blood Culture Systems for Detection of Organisms from Vials whose Entry Was Delayed. *J. Clin. Microbiol.* **1996**, *34*, 543–549. [PubMed]

© 2018 by the authors. Licensee MDPI, Basel, Switzerland. This article is an open access article distributed under the terms and conditions of the Creative Commons Attribution (CC BY) license (http://creativecommons.org/licenses/by/4.0/).

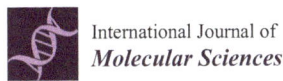

Article
Antibacterial Composites of Cuprous Oxide Nanoparticles and Polyethylene

Yanna Gurianov, Faina Nakonechny, Yael Albo and Marina Nisnevitch *

Department of Chemical Engineering, Biotechnology and Materials, Ariel University, Kyriat-ha-Mada, Ariel 4070000, Israel; yannag@ariel.ac.il (Y.G.); fainan@ariel.ac.il (F.N.); yaelyt@ariel.ac.il (Y.A.)
* Correspondence: marinan@ariel.ac.il; Tel.: +972-391-430-42

Received: 28 December 2018; Accepted: 18 January 2019; Published: 21 January 2019

Abstract: Cuprous oxide nanoparticles (Cu_2ONPs) were used for preparing composites with linear low-density polyethylene (LLDPE) by co-extrusion, thermal adhesion, and attachment using ethyl cyanoacrylate, trimethoxyvinylsilane, and epoxy resin. The composites were examined by Scanning electron microscope and tested for their antibacterial activity against Gram-positive *Staphylococcus aureus* and Gram-negative *Escherichia coli*. All of these composites—except for the one obtained by extrusion—eradicated cells of both bacteria within half an hour. The composite prepared by thermal adhesion of Cu_2ONPs on LLDPE had the highest external exposure of nanoparticles and exhibited the highest activity against the bacteria. This composite and the one obtained using ethyl cyanoacrylate showed no leaching of copper ions into the aqueous phase. Copper ion leaching from composites prepared with trimethoxyvinylsilane and epoxy resin was very low. The antibacterial activity of the composites can be rated as follows: obtained by thermal adhesion > obtained using ethyl cyanoacrylate > obtained using trimethoxyvinylsilane > obtained using epoxy resin > obtained by extrusion. The composites with the highest activity are potential materials for tap water and wastewater disinfection.

Keywords: cuprous oxide nanoparticles; linear low-density polyethylene; composites; adhesives; antibacterial activity; water disinfection

---

1. Introduction

Polymeric materials have long become an integral part of our lives. They are used in most industrial fields, including the textile industry, food packaging, medical device production, and water supply and purification systems [1]. In the latter, piping for water transportation is made from polyolefins, such as polyvinylchloride [2], different kinds of polyethylene [3], polypropylene, and polybutylene [4,5]. Polyolefins do not possess antibacterial properties, and this is the cause for various problems that accompany water transportation, such as contamination by microorganisms, biofilm formation [6], and adherence of fungi and viruses to pipe walls. These problems may lead to the propagation of serious infections among humans. According to the World Health Organization (WHO), waterborne diseases lead to the deaths of 3.4 million people annually, most of whom are children, as a result of inaccessibility to clean water [7]. It is thus necessary to carry out effective water disinfection in order to combat and prevent water contamination.

The most common treatment for water purification from harmful microorganisms is chlorination. This treatment has been demonstrated to be efficacious for destroying microorganisms. However, it has several disadvantages, including the production of toxic, mutagenic, and carcinogenic disinfection byproducts [8,9].

It is possible to replace conventional water treatment methods by methods that are as effective but less toxic in order to improve the drinking water quality. One alternative method is to treat water in plumbing systems by antibacterial materials such as embedding heavy metals into the pipelines, thus eradicating pathogens before they reach the tap faucet. The most widely used heavy metals with proven efficacy against various microorganisms are silver, copper, and zinc [10]. These metals have been applied for years as antibacterial agents in industries, healthcare institutions, and agriculture [11]. Moreover, copper also possesses antiviral [12] and antifungal [13,14] properties. The exact mechanism of the antimicrobial action of these metals is still not totally clear due to many factors. The main suggested mechanism of copper activity against pathogens relates to the ability of copper ions to penetrate through the bacterial cell wall or outer membrane and bind to DNA, thus blocking the cell replication process [15]. In addition, high concentrations of copper ions stimulate oxidative stress, such as the generation of reactive oxygen species (ROS) [16–18], lipid peroxidation, [19,20] and protein oxidation [21].

Several studies show that copper nanoparticles (CuNPs) are more effective antibacterial agents than the same quantity of copper microparticles [22]. Copper oxide nanoparticles (NPs) also exhibit strong antibacterial activity by suppressing bacterial cell growth [23], and this activity even exceeds that of the metal copper NPs [24]. Both copper oxides (CuO and Cu_2O) embedded into polyvinyl chloride (PVC) demonstrated high ability to inhibit bacterial adhesion to PVC when tested against *Escherichia coli* (*E. coli*) cells. It should be mentioned that Cu_2O-PVC composites were more effective than CuO-PVC in preventing *E. coli* biofilm formation [25].

There are two approaches for the production of metal/polymer composites using NPs—in situ, where polymer matrices serve as reaction media for NP synthesis, and ex situ, where NPs are obtained beforehand and are later incorporated into a polymer [11]. The latter approach enables more precise dosing and distribution of NPs in polymers.

The aim of the present study is to propose simple approaches for immobilization of cuprous oxide nanoparticles (Cu_2ONPs) for preparing composites with polyethylene that exhibit antibacterial properties for water disinfection.

2. Results and Discussion

2.1. Immobilization of Cu_2ONPs onto A Solid Phase

Domestic water piping is made of polymers. Linear low density polyethylene (LLDPE) was therefore chosen as a support for immobilization of Cu_2ONPs. The use of LLDPE enabled application of various approaches for immobilization of Cu_2ONPs and easy handling of the prepared composites. Several methods were used for NP immobilization.

The first method was based on extrusion of a mixture of LLDPE beads with Cu_2ONPs. As a result, polymeric strips with Cu_2O impregnated into the entire volume of polyethylene (PE) were obtained. The strips were evenly colored in brown-red, which is characteristic for Cu_2ONPs, and seemed to have a homogeneous distribution of NPs. However, Scanning electron microscope (SEM) examination of the strips showed that their surface was composed mostly of PE (Figure 1a), while inside the strips, rare clusters of Cu_2ONPs were surrounded by massive polymeric parts, as can be seen in the cross-section of the strip (Figure 1b and the inset in Figure 1b). It can be assumed that practically no NPs were exposed on the surface of the strips and that the Cu_2ONPs were distributed very unevenly inside the polymer.

The second method of immobilization was thermal adhesion of Cu_2ONPs distributed onto a surface of the heated, melting LLDPE and pressed into the melted polymer under slight pressure. This approach led to results that were different from those obtained by the extrusion method. Figure 1c shows that after this treatment, the polymeric surface was covered with clearly distinguishable Cu_2ONPs (Figure 1c), and imaging of the polymer cross-section indicated a distinct two-layer structure of the obtained composite where the external layer composed of Cu_2ONPs had a thickness of 72.7 ± 0.3 μm (Figure 1d).

Other immobilization methods were based on attaching Cu_2ONPs onto the LLDPE surface using three types of adhesives: ethyl cyanoacrylate, epoxy resin, and trimethoxyvinylsilane. In the case of the ethyl cyanoacrylate, the attached NPs were distributed over the entire polymeric surface and were partially exposed on the external side (Figure 1e). The layer of the attached NPs was quite even and had a thickness of 97.2 ± 2.2 μm (Figure 1f). Epoxy resin yielded a rather even distribution of Cu_2ONPs on the polymer surface, but the NPs were mostly covered by a film of the adhesive (Figure 1g). The layer thickness in this case was 89.7 ± 0.2 μm (Figure 1h). Cu_2ONPs attachment using trimethoxyvinylsilane yielded an uneven surface distribution of the NPs, which were mostly covered by an adhesive film. However, in some areas, good exposure of NPs was clearly evident (Figure 1i). The adhesive layer containing NPs had a thickness of 152.1 ± 1.5 μm (Figure 1j).

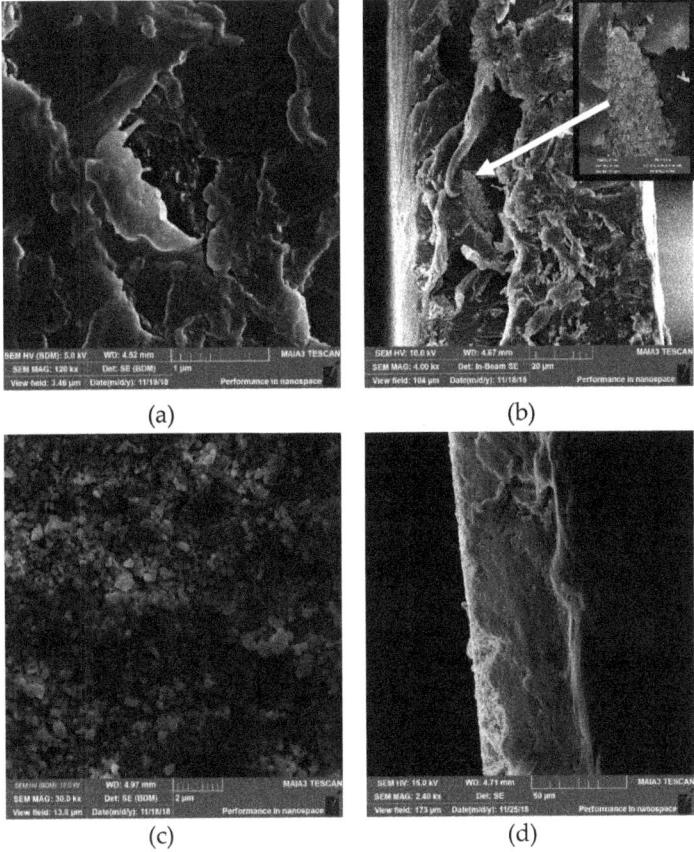

Figure 1. *Cont.*

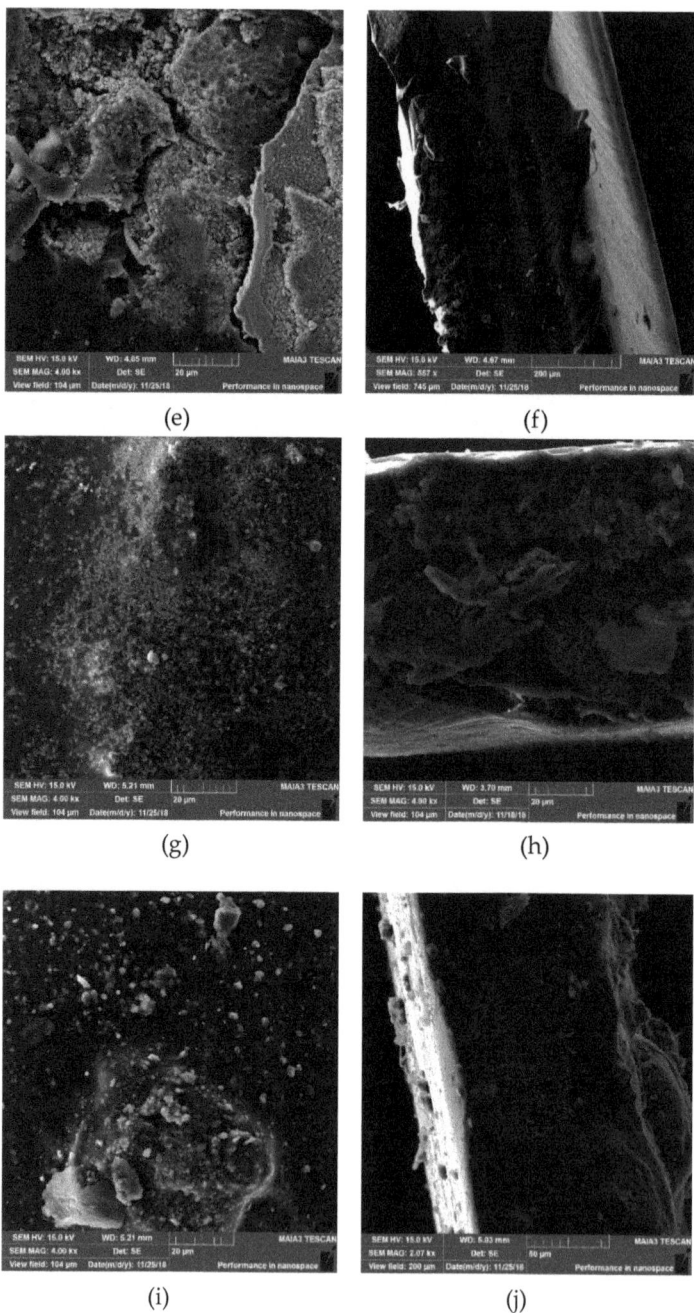

Figure 1. Scanning electron microscope (SEM) micrographs of Cu_2ONPs immobilized onto linear low-density polyethylene (LLDPE) by extrusion: (**a**) surface and (**b**) cross-section images; by thermal adhesion: (**c**) surface and (**d**) cross-section images; using ethyl cyanoacrylate: (**e**) surface and (**f**) cross-section images; using epoxy resin: (**g**) surface and (**h**) cross-section images; using trimethoxyvinylsilane: (**i**) surface and (**j**) cross-section images.

The surfaces of all the composites were characterized by elemental mapping. Figure 2 shows that unbound Cu$_2$ONPs exposed only copper and oxygen atoms (Figure 2a), whereas all composites showed the presence of carbon, copper, and oxygen, as expected (Figure 2b–e). In the composite prepared by extrusion (Figure 2b), practically no copper and oxygen atoms were found on the surface. This supports our previous observation that Cu$_2$ONPs are located inside the polymer and are not exhibited on the surface of the composite (Figure 1a). For the rest of the composites, the molar fraction of oxygen was higher than expected for Cu$_2$O, which can be explained by the presence of oxygen atoms in the adhesives, and probably also by partial oxidation of Cu^{+1} to Cu^{+2} in the external layer of the NPs, which was exposed to air. X-ray diffraction (XRD) analysis of the composite obtained using trimethoxyvinylsilane showed the presence of three copper species—Cu^0, Cu^{+1}, and Cu^{+2} (Figure 3)—where Cu^{+1} was the prevalent form for both powder Cu$_2$ONPs (Figure 3a) and immobilized Cu$_2$ONPs (Figure 3b). We therefore concluded that the bulk of Cu$_2$ONPs retain their chemical structure.

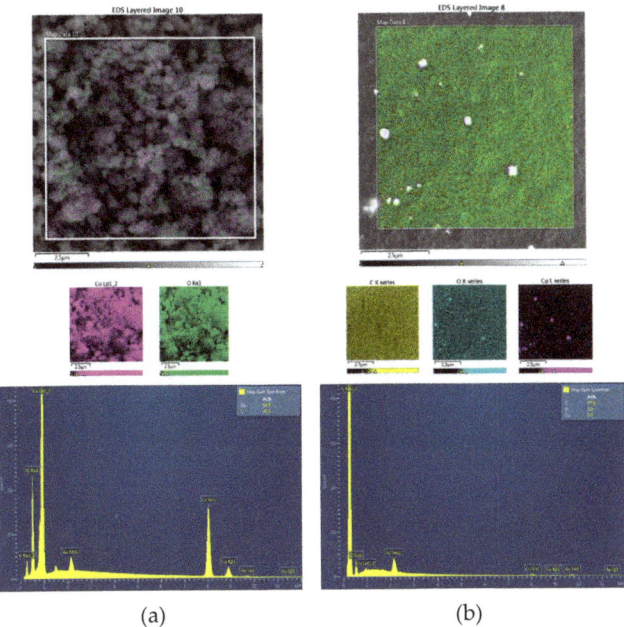

(a)   (b)

Figure 2. *Cont.*

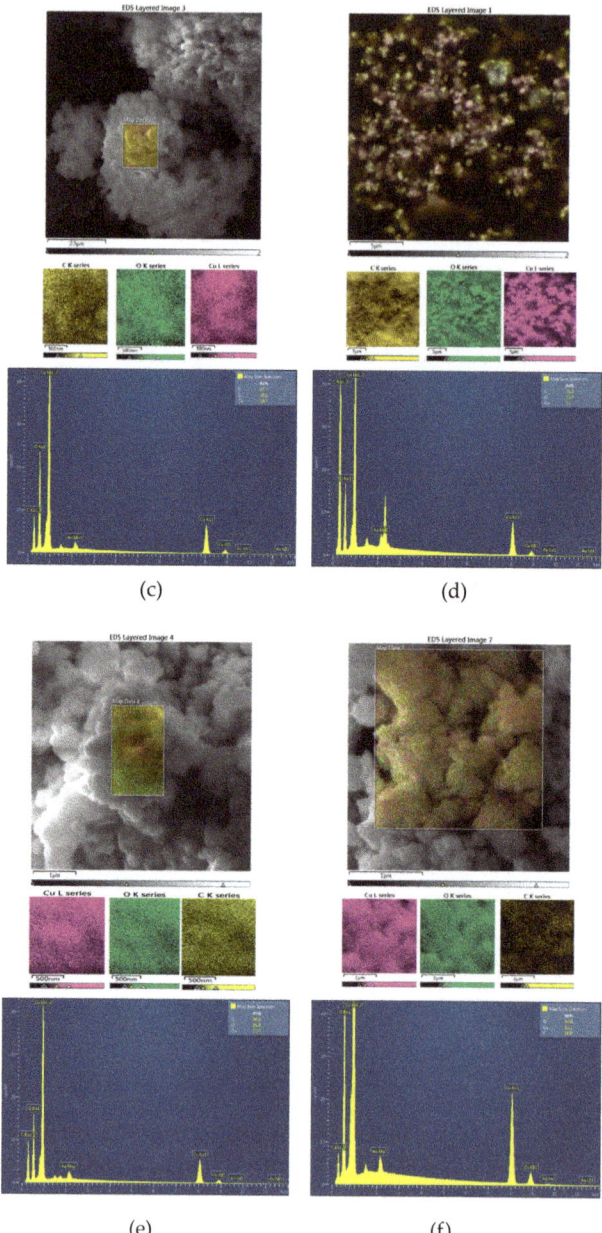

Figure 2. Surface elemental mapping of gold-coated (**a**) powder Cu_2ONPs; (**b**) Cu_2ONPs immobilized onto LLDPE by extrusion; (**c**) Cu_2ONPs immobilized onto LLDPE using ethyl cyanoacrylate; (**d**) Cu_2ONPs immobilized onto LLDPE using epoxy resin; (**e**) Cu_2ONPs immobilized onto LLDPE using trimethoxyvinylsilane; (**f**) Cu_2ONPs immobilized onto LLDPE by thermal adhesion. Each sample is characterized by an energy dispersive X-ray spectroscopy (EDS) layered image (upper panel) with individual elemental mapping showing oxygen as green, copper as purple, and carbon as yellow (middle panel), and EDS spectrum (bottom panel).

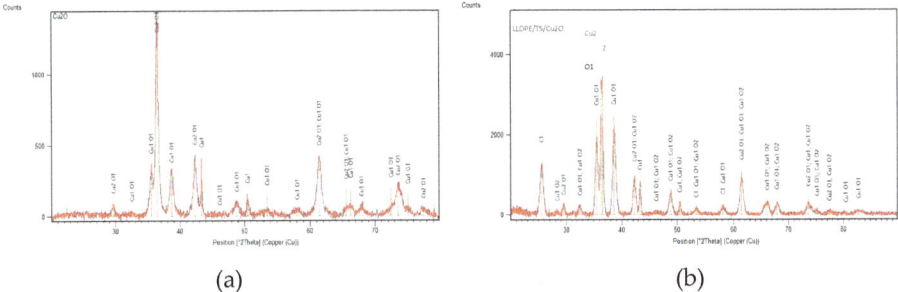

Figure 3. X-ray diffraction (XRD) analysis of (**a**) powder Cu_2ONPs and (**b**) immobilized using trimethoxyvinylsilane Cu_2ONPs (LLDPE/TS/Cu_2O).

2.2. Leaching of Copper from Immobilized Cu_2ONPs

Copper ions are well known for their antibacterial activity. However, they are toxic to humans (even at low concentrations), causing gastrointestinal distress and liver or kidney damage [26,27]. Standards for copper ions in tap water are therefore very strict, and the maximum permitted copper concentration in drinking water is 1.4–2 ppm [28,29]. The copper ion concentration cannot exceed 2–15 ppm in sanitary and combined waste discharges [30,31].

Since the probability of copper leaching into water from the Cu_2ONPs-polymer composites in the case of immobilization by surface attachment seemed to be high, we tested the copper ion concentration of the composite samples after immersing them in tap water for one month under the following conditions: temperature 20.1 ± 1.0 °C, pH 8.2 ± 0.1, dissolved oxygen concentration 5.4 ± 0.3 mg/L, and salinity 0.301 ± 0.034 mS.

The results of this test are presented in Figure 4. The copper concentration in the control tap water was 0.24 ± 0.02 ppm. Thus, it did not exceed the maximum permitted concentration. No leaching of copper ions into the aqueous phase was detected when Cu_2ONPs were immobilized with ethyl cyanoacrylate and thermal adhesion, and the average copper concentration was 0.35 ± 0.06 ppm and 0.25 ± 0.05 ppm, respectively. These results were similar to the tap water control series, with a P-value of 0.15 for ethyl cyanoacrylate and 0.48 for thermal adhesion. The picture was quite different for the two other adhesives where the copper concentration in water increased with time (Figure 4).

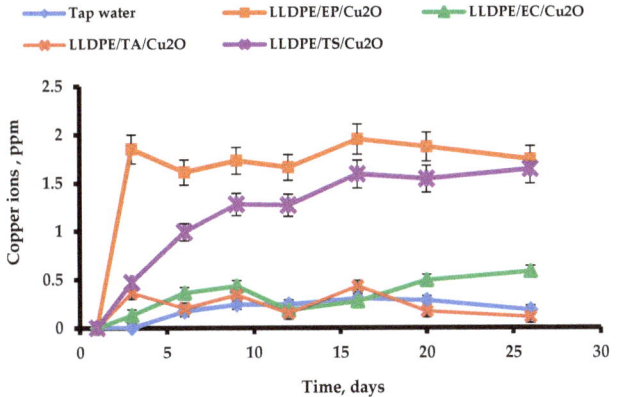

Figure 4. Testing the leaching of copper ions into tap water from LLDPE with Cu_2ONPs attached to the surface using ethyl cyanoacrylate (EC), trimethoxyvinylsilane (TS), epoxy resin (EP), and thermal adhesion (TA). Control—tap water.

In both cases, the copper leaching curve could be described as a saturation curve; for the composite produced with epoxy resin, saturation at ca. 1.9 ppm was already reached after three days, and for the trimethoxyvinylsilane-based composite, saturation at ca. 1.6 ppm was reached after 16 days. These values were significantly different from the tap water. For the former composite, the P-value was 0.0032, and for the latter, it was 0.010. Small amounts of Cu_2ONPs were probably not attached well enough to the polymer support and leached upon contact with water. It should be emphasized that the experiment was performed in a batch mode, i.e., the leached copper ions accumulated in the aqueous phase during the experiment. In a continuous regime, the concentration of the leached copper is considered to be lower, since the leached ions will be removed by the water flow.

Average rates of copper leaching from the composites prepared by various methods and total amount of leached copper are presented in Table 1. It can be seen that the rate of leaching and the percent of leached copper were very low in the case of the composites prepared by thermal attachment and using ethyl cyanoacrylate. In the case of the two other methods, these parameters were higher but leached copper still comprised only ca. 1% from the applied amount. These findings indicate that copper leaching can be regarded as being either negligible or very low in all cases.

Table 1. Rate and amount of copper leaching from composites of Cu_2ONPs and LLDPE.

Composite	Rate of Copper Leaching, $\mu g\ cm^{-2}\ day^{-1}$	Percent of Leached Copper
Obtained by thermal adhesion	0.019	0.15
Obtained using ethyl cyanoacrylate	0.025	0.17
Obtained using epoxy resin	1.32	1.11
Obtained using trimethoxyvinylsilane	0.166	1.06

2.3. Antibacterial Activity of Immobilized Cu_2ONPs

Firstly, antibacterial activity of free suspended Cu_2ONPs was tested against Gram-positive *Staphylococcus aureus* (*S. aureus*) and Gram-negative *E. coli*. Figure 5 shows that the NPs were very active and eradicated the cells of both bacteria after 15 min.

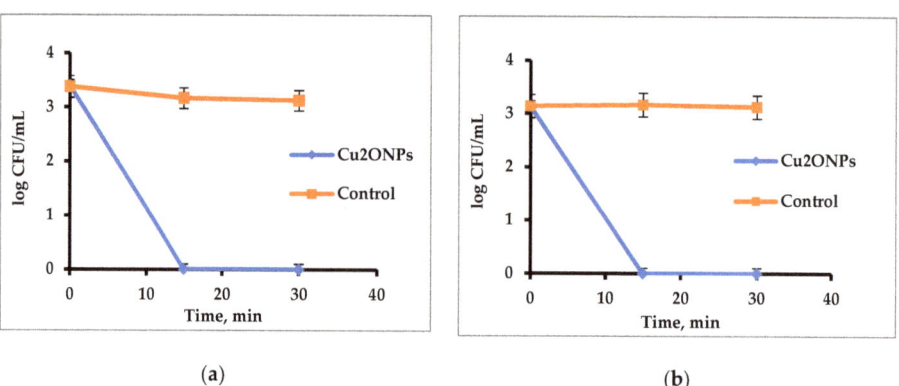

Figure 5. Activity of free Cu_2ONPs against (**a**) *Staphylococcus aureus* and (**b**) *Escherichia coli* cells. Control—untreated bacterial cells.

After that, we studied the ability of immobilized Cu_2ONPs to eradicate the same bacteria. For this purpose, the samples of LLDPE bearing Cu_2ONPs were placed into bacterial suspensions with known concentrations and incubated for half an hour. After short washing, the polymeric samples were then transferred into a dish with a new portion of fresh suspension with the same initial concentration. This procedure was repeated several times. Each time, the bacterial concentration was analyzed before and after the incubation. In the control series, bacteria were incubated in the absence of any polymer and in the presence of samples of LLDPE and LLDPE coated with adhesives without the addition of Cu_2ONPs.

The results of testing the activity of immobilized Cu_2ONPs against *S. aureus* are presented in Figure 6. It can be seen that Cu_2ONPs immobilized by extrusion did not exhibit any toxicity against the cells (Figure 6a), whereas all other LLDPE samples bearing Cu_2ONPs on the surface were active against *S. aureus* and totally eradicated the cells within half an hour (Figure 6b–e).

The highest activity was demonstrated by the sample obtained by thermal adhesion of Cu_2ONPs onto the LLDPE surface. This sample demonstrated an ability to kill the cells over the course of 10 cycles of re-use (Figure 6b). Other composites were less active against *S. aureus*; Cu_2ONPs attached to the LLDPE surface by ethyl cyanoacrylate totally destroyed the cells over the course of five cycles of re-use and decreased the cell concentration by 1.5–2 log_{10} during cycles six through 10 (Figure 6c). The Cu_2ONPs-LLDPE composites obtained with epoxy resin and trimethoxyvinylsilane were active only for a single use, caused only a 2 log_{10} decrease in the *S. aureus* concentration during the second re-use, and were inactive during the third re-use (Figure 6d,e, respectively).

No decrease in the *S. aureus* concentration was observed in the control experiments in the absence of the composites and in the presence of uncoated LLDPE or LLDPE coated with each of the adhesives (Figure 6) except the LLDPE coated with epoxy resin, which was toxic for bacteria in the first cycle (Figure 6d).

The results of the experiments of testing the antibacterial activity of the composites against Gram-negative *E. coli* were very similar to those found for *S. aureus*. The Cu_2ONPs-LLDPE composite obtained by extrusion was also inactive against *E. coli* (Figure 7a). The composite obtained by thermal adhesion exhibited the highest activity, which was retained for ten cycles of re-use (Figure 7b). The composite obtained using ethyl cyanoacrylate was active for seven re-use cycles, and in the eighth cycle, the concentration of *E. coli* decreased by 2.5 log_{10} (Figure 7c). Contrary to *S. aureus*, the composite produced with epoxy resin was inactive—even in the first use (Figure 7d). The composite obtained using trimethoxyvinylsilane was active against *E. coli* during two cycles of use, but in the third re-use, the cell concentration dropped by 2 log_{10} only (Figure 7e). No decrease in *E. coli* cell concentration was registered in the control experiments (Figure 7).

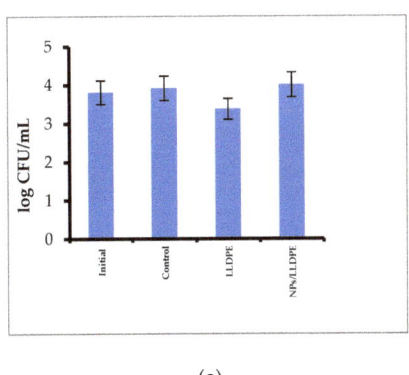

(a)

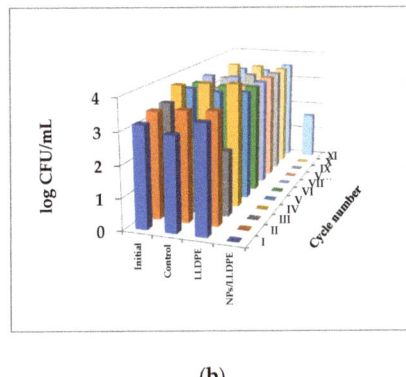

(b)

Figure 6. *Cont.*

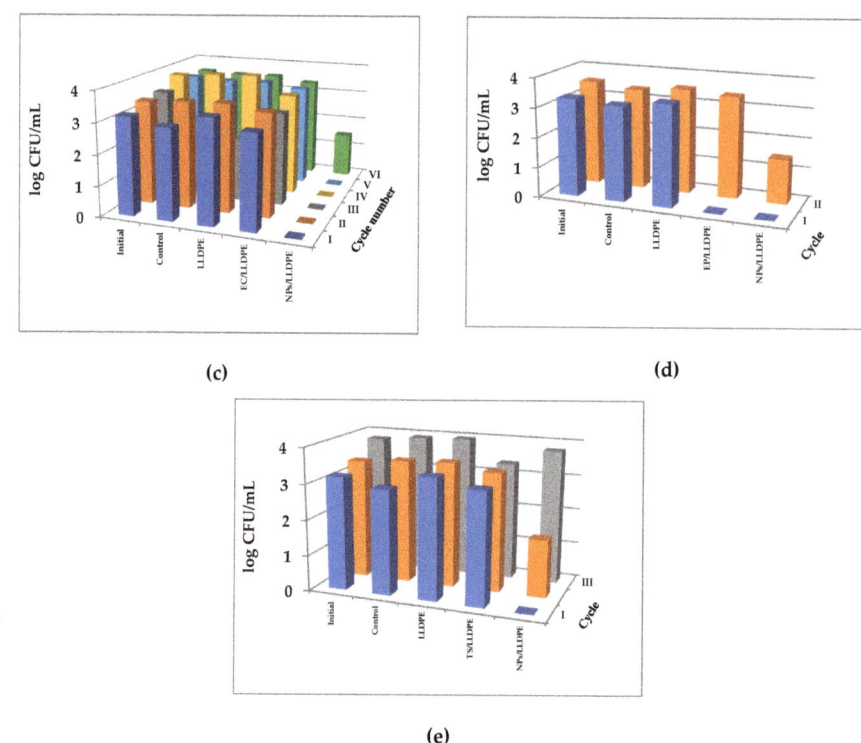

(c)   (d)

(e)

Figure 6. Activity of the Cu$_2$ONPs-LLDPE composites against *S. aureus* cells of composites obtained by: (**a**) extrusion; (**b**) thermal adhesion; (**c**) using ethyl cyanoacrylate; (**d**) using epoxy resin; (**e**) using trimethoxyvinylsilane. Roman figures show the number of re-use cycles. Initial—*S. aureus* cells before the incubation, control—*S. aureus* cells after 30 min incubation, LLDPE—*S. aureus* cells after 30 min incubation with LLDPE, EC/LLDPE—*S. aureus* cells after 30 min incubation with LLDPE coated with an ethyl cyanoacrylate layer, TS/LLDPE—*S. aureus* cells after 30 min incubation with LLDPE coated with a trimethoxyvinylsilane layer, EP/LLDPE—*S. aureus* cells after 30 min incubation with LLDPE coated with an epoxy resin layer, NPs/LLDPE—*S. aureus* cells after 30 min incubation with the Cu$_2$ONPs-LLDPE composite. In all cases, relative standard errors did not exceed 10%.

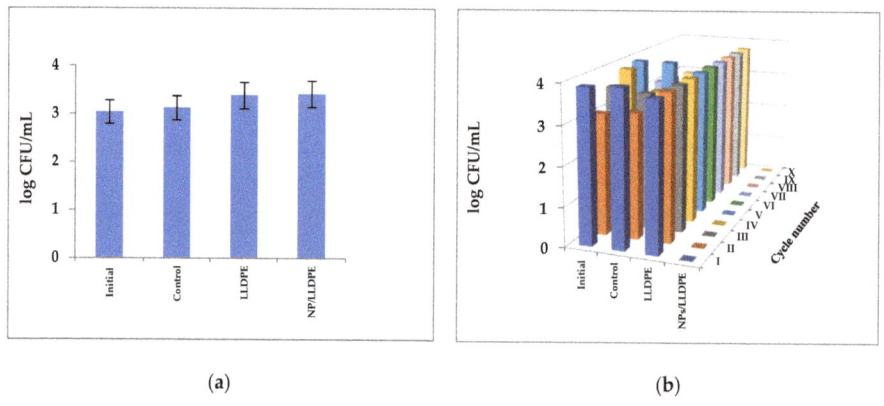

(a)   (b)

Figure 7. *Cont.*

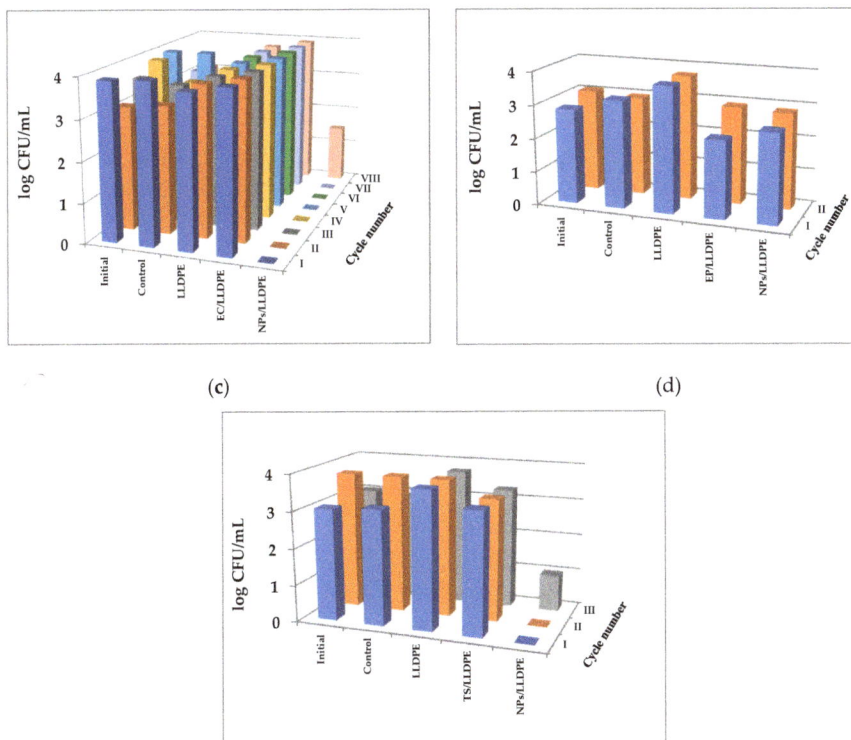

Figure 7. Activity of the Cu$_2$ONPs-LLDPE composites against *E. coli* cells of composites obtained by: (**a**) extrusion; (**b**) thermal adhesion; (**c**) using ethyl cyanoacrylate; (**d**) using epoxy resin (**e**) using trimethoxyvinylsilane. Roman figures show the number of re-use cycles. Initial—*E. coli* cells before the incubation, control—*E. coli* cells after 30 min incubation, LLDPE—*E. coli* cells after 30 min incubation with LLDPE, EC/LLDPE—*E. coli* cells after 30 min incubation with LLDPE coated with an ethyl cyanoacrylate layer, TS/LLDPE—*E. coli* cells after 30 min incubation with LLDPE coated with a trimethoxyvinylsilane layer, EP/LLDPE—*E. coli* cells after 30 min incubation with LLDPE coated with an epoxy resin layer, NPs/LLDPE—*E. coli* cells after 30 min incubation with the Cu$_2$ONPs-LLDPE composite. In all cases, relative standard errors did not exceed 10%.

Taking the results of Gram-positive and Gram-negative bacteria eradication into account, the overall antibacterial activity of the obtained composites can be rated as follows: obtained by thermal adhesion > attached using ethyl cyanoacrylate > attached using trimethoxyvinylsilane > attached using epoxy resin > obtained by extrusion. The different antimicrobial activities of the obtained composites can be explained by different exposure rates of Cu$_2$ONPs to the aqueous phase, as demonstrated in Figure 1, and by different degrees of leaching of copper ions from the polymer surface. The Cu$_2$ONPs were highly exposed in the case of thermal adhesion to the polymer, and in this case, copper leaching was zero. This composite also demonstrated the highest activity against the bacterial cells. In the case of ethyl cyanoacrylate, the rate of Cu$_2$ONPs exposure was less than in the former case but still high enough, and no leaching of copper ions was observed. These features explain the second position of this composite in the antibacterial rating. The composites produced using trimethoxyvinylsilane and epoxy resin had a very low rate of Cu$_2$ONPs exposure and showed leaching of copper ions into the water. Thus, contact between bacterial cells and immobilized Cu$_2$ONPs was very poor and probably even decreased with time since copper leached into the aqueous phase.

The high antibacterial activity of the composites obtained by thermal adhesion and using the ethyl cyanoacrylate makes them potential materials for application in tap or waste water disinfection in batch or continuous regimes. Since these composites showed no leaching of copper ions into the aqueous phase (Figure 4), it can be concluded that cell killing occurs upon direct contact between the cells and the Cu$_2$ONPs found on the surface. The absence of copper ions in the aqueous environment supports this conclusion.

3. Materials and Methods

3.1. Materials

The LLDPE was purchased from Sigma-Aldrich, Israel Ltd. Cu$_2$ONPs of 18 nm size were purchased from US Research Materials (Houston, TX, USA). Ethyl cyanoacrylate ("super glue") was purchased from Loctite® (Westlake, OH, USA), trimethoxyvinylsilane (Hybrifix Super 7) was purchased from Den Braven Sealants B.V (Oosterhout, Netherlands), and epoxy resin and polyamine hardener were purchased from Evobond® (Kaohsiung City, Taiwan).

3.2. Immobilization of Cu$_2$ONPs onto LLDPE Polymer by Thermal Adhesion

Three grams of LLDPE pellets were melted at 130 °C on a Kapton polyimide film (Shagal Marketing Solutions Ltd., Modiin, Israel). The melted polymer was coated with another polyimide film and a thick stainless steel plate and pressed under moderate pressure to obtain a 1 mm thick layer. After removal of the plate and the upper polyimide film, 0.15 g of Cu$_2$ONPs were dispersed on the molten polymer using a sieve, covered with another polyimide film and the plate and slightly pressed in. The samples were cooled to room temperature.

3.3. Attachment of Cu$_2$ONPs to the LLDPE Polymer

The LLDPE sample was prepared as described in Section 3.2. After cooling the sample to room temperature, a layer of one of the adhesives (ethyl cyanoacrylate, trimethoxyvinylsilane, or epoxy resin) was applied to the polymer by a draw down technique, and 0.15 g of cuprous oxide NPs were dispersed on the adhesives immediately using a sieve. The samples were air-dried for 24 h under sterile conditions.

3.4. Immobilization of Cu$_2$ONPs into A LLDPE Matrix by Extrusion

Immobilization of the Cu$_2$ONPs into LLDPE was performed by a co-extrusion technique using an extruder (Allspeeds Ltd., Accrington, England) under an inlet temperature of 170 °C and an outlet temperature of 210 °C. For this purpose, a mixture of 50 g of polymer beads and 2.5 g of Cu$_2$ONPs was placed in a feed, and the extruder was activated to melt the mixture at 30 rpm. The resulting fluid composition was pushed through a die with a flat 1 × 19.6 mm section. This procedure yielded polymeric rods with the incorporated Cu$_2$ONPs. The rods were chopped into 5 cm-long pieces.

3.5. Bacterial Growth

Inoculums of Gram-positive S. aureus (ATCC 25923) and Gram-negative E. coli (ATCC 10798) were grown in brain heart infusion broth (BH; Acumedia, Lansing, MI, USA) and Luria Bertani broth (LB; Acumedia, Lansing, MI, USA), respectively, at 37 ± 1°C under shaking at 150 rpm for 24 h, diluted 1:100 with the corresponding medium, and incubated again for ca. 2 h at 37 ± 1°C until reaching OD$_{660nm}$ = 0.1. The bacterial suspensions were diluted with sterile saline to a final concentration of 10^3 or 10^4 CFU/mL.

3.6. Testing of Antibacterial Activity

The antibacterial activity of free and immobilized Cu_2ONPs samples was tested against *S. aureus* and *E. coli*; 0.15 g of Cu_2ONPs (powder) or 3 g of Cu_2ONPs-LLDPE composites were added to 20 mL of bacterial culture and incubated at $37 \pm 1\,^\circ C$ by shaking at 120 rpm for 30 min. The samples were then diluted by one and two decimal dilutions and 100 µL of these samples were distributed onto BH or LB agar plates in the cases of *S. aureus* and *E. coli*, respectively. The plates were incubated overnight at $37 \pm 1\,^\circ C$, and the bacterial colony forming units (CFU) were counted using a colony counter Scan 500 (Interscience, Saint Nom la Bretèche, France). The bacterial concentration was determined while taking the appropriate dilutions into account.

3.7. Leaching of Copper Ions from Samples of Immobilized Cu_2ONPs into Tap Water

Six grams of LLDPE with 0.3 g of immobilized Cu_2ONPs were added to 100 mL of tap water and stirred at 120 rpm with a magnetic stirrer for one month under sampling twice a week. One mL samples were diluted by 9 mL of distilled water and filtered through Polyvinylidene fluoride (PVDF) filters with 0.45 µm pore size (Membrane Solutions, Kent, WA, USA). The copper ion concentration in the samples was measured using an ICP-AES (Spectro Arcos, Ametek®, Berwyn, PA, USA) instrument. The pH and temperature were tested with a HI 2211 pH/OPR meter (HANNA Instruments, Woonsocket, RI, USA). Dissolved oxygen concentration was measured by a DO-5510 oxygen meter (Lutron, Taiwan). Salinity was measured with a CD-4303HA conductivity meter (Lutron, Taiwan).

3.8. SEM Imaging and EDS Analysis of Immobilized Cu_2ONPs

Imaging of surfaces and cross-sections of immobilized Cu_2ONPs was performed with an SEM microscope (Tescan MAIA3, Triglav™, Brno, Czech Republic). The samples were placed onto a carbon tape and covered with a 10 nm gold layer using a Q150T ES Quorum coater (Quorum Technologies Ltd., Lewes, UK) under a sputter current of 12 mA for 30 s. SEM measurements were performed at operating voltages of 5, 10, and 15 kV and at magnifications of ×557, ×2.07 k, ×2.40 k, ×4.00 k, ×30.0 k, and ×120 k. The samples were detected with In-beam SE (secondary electrons) and SE-BDM (beam deceleration mode) detectors. Elemental analysis of the samples was performed by energy dispersive X-ray analysis in SEM mode under the resolution of 127 eV using a X-Max^N SDD detector 51-xmx1010 (Oxford Instruments NanoAnalysis, High Wycombe, UK).

3.9. XRD Analysis of Powder and Immobilized Cu_2ONPs

Phase analysis of the samples was carried out using a Panalytical X'Pert Pro X-ray powder diffractometer (Malvern Panalytical Ltd., Malvern, UK) with Cu Kα radiation ($\lambda = 0.154$ nm) for phase identification. Full pattern identification was performed by the X'Pert HighScore Plus software package, version 2.2e (2.2.5) (Malvern Panalytical Ltd., Malvern, UK). XRD patterns were obtained at 40 kV and 40 mA. For immobilized Cu_2ONPs, the grazing incidence geometry with an incident angle of -5° was applied. The XRD patterns were recorded in the 2θ range of $20-80^\circ$ with a step size of 0.02° and time per step of 1 s. For powder Cu_2ONPs, Bragg-Brentano geometry was applied. The XRD patterns were recorded in the 2θ range of $20-80^\circ$ with a step size of 0.03° and time per step of 2 s.

3.10. Statistical Analysis

The results obtained from at least three independent experiments carried out in duplicates were analyzed by single-factor Analysis of Variance (ANOVA). The difference between the results was considered significant when the *P*-value was less than 0.05. Quantitative results are presented as the mean $\pm$ standard error.

4. Conclusions

Composites of cuprous oxide nanoparticles with linear low-density polyethylene showed no or very low leaching of copper ions into the aqueous phase and exhibited good antibacterial activity against *S. aureus* and *E. coli*.

Author Contributions: Conceptualization: M.N.; methodology: F.N. and Y.A.; investigation: Y.G.; resources: M.N. and Y.A.; data curation: F.N. and Y.A.; writing—original draft preparation: Y.G. and M.N.; writing—review and editing: M.N.; supervision: M.N.; project administration: M.N.

Funding: This research was supported by the Research Authority of the Ariel University, Israel and by the Cherna Moskowitz Foundation, California, USA.

Acknowledgments: We acknowledge Natalya Litvak and Olga Krichevski (Ariel University, Israel) for their assistance in SEM imaging and EDS analysis, Alexey Kossenko for his help in XRD analysis, Rami Kriger (Ariel University, Israel) for technical assistance in ICP measurements and for Efrat Emanuel for her help in interpretation of some results.

Conflicts of Interest: The authors declare no conflict of interest.

Abbreviations

NPs	Nanoparticles
Cu_2ONPs	Cuprous oxide nanoparticles
PE	Polyethylene
LLDPE	Linear low-density polyethylene
EDS	Energy-dispersive X-ray spectroscopy
SEM	Scanning electron microscope
XRD	X-ray diffraction

References

1. National Research Council. *Polymer Science and Engineering: The Shifting Research Frontiers*; National Academy Press: Washington, DC, USA, 1994; pp. 114–115.
2. Prest, E.I.; Hammes, F.; van Loosdrecht, M.C.M.; Vrouwenvelder, J.S. Biological stability of drinking water: Controlling factors, methods, and challenges. *Front. Microbiol.* **2016**, *7*, 1–24. [CrossRef] [PubMed]
3. Brocca, D.; Arvin, E.; Mosbaek, H. Identification of organic compounds migrating from polyethylene pipelines into drinking water. *Water Res.* **2002**, *36*, 3675–3680. [CrossRef]
4. Lee, Y. An evaluation of microbial and chemical contamination sources related to the deterioration of tap water quality in the household water supply system. *Int. J. Environ. Res. Public Health* **2013**, *10*, 4143–4160. [CrossRef] [PubMed]
5. *Health Aspects of Plumbing*; World Health Organization (WHO): Geneva, Switzerland, 2006; pp. 50–51. Available online: http://www.who.int/water_sanitation_health/publications/plumbinghealthasp.pdf (accessed on 24 December 2018).
6. Mahapatra, A.; Padhi, N.; Mahapatra, D.; Bhatt, M.; Sahoo, D.; Jena, S.; Dash, D.; Chayani, N. Study of Biofilm in bacteria from water pipelines. *J. Clin. Diagn. Res.* **2015**, *9*, 9–11. [CrossRef] [PubMed]
7. WHO World Water Day Report. 2014. Available online: https://www.who.int/water_sanitation_health/takingcharge.html (accessed on 24 December 2018).
8. Yan, M.; Han, M.L. Behavior of I/Br/Cl-THMs and their projected toxicities under simulated cooking conditions: Effects of heating, table salts and residual chlorine. *J. Hazard. Mater.* **2016**, *314*, 105–112. [CrossRef] [PubMed]
9. Adhikary, J.; Meistelman, M.; Burg, A.; Shamir, D.; Meyerstein, D.; Albo, Y. Reactive dehalogenation of monobromo- and tribromoacetic acid by sodium borohydride catalyzed by gold nanoparticles entrapped in sol-gel matrices follows different pathways. *Eur. J. Inorg. Chem.* **2017**, 1510–1515. [CrossRef]
10. Borkow, G.; Gabbay, J. Copper as a biocidal tool. *Curr. Med. Chem.* **2005**, *12*, 2163–2175. [CrossRef]

11. Palza, H. Antimicrobial polymers with metal nanoparticles. *Int. J. Mol. Sci.* **2015**, *16*, 2099–2116. [CrossRef]
12. Jordan, F.T.W.; Nassar, T.J. The survival of infections bronchitis (IB) virus in water. *Avian Pathol.* **1973**, *2*, 91–101. [CrossRef]
13. Kalatehjari, P.; Yousefian, M.; Khalilzadeh, M.A. Assessment of antifungal effects of copper nanoparticles on the growth of the fungus *Saprolegnia* sp. on white fish (*Rutilus frisii kutum*) eggs. *Egypt J. Aquat. Res.* **2015**, *41*, 303–306. [CrossRef]
14. Zatcoff, R.C.; Smith, M.S.; Borkow, G. Treatment of tinea pedis with socks containing copper-oxide impregnated fibers. *Foot* **2008**, *18*, 136–141. [CrossRef] [PubMed]
15. Mallick, S.; Sharma, S.; Banerjee, M.; Ghosh, S.S.; Chatopadhyay, A.; Paul, A. Iodine-stabilized Cu nanoparticle chitosan composite for antibacterial applications. *Appl. Mater. Interfaces* **2012**, *4*, 1313–1323. [CrossRef] [PubMed]
16. Warnes, S.L.; Keevil, C.V. Mechanism of copper surface toxicity in vancomycin-resistant enterococci following wet or dry surface contact. *Appl. Environ. Microb.* **2011**, *77*, 6049–6059. [CrossRef]
17. Warnes, S.L.; Caves, V.; Keevil, C.V. Mechanism of copper surface toxicity in *Escherichia coli* O157:H7 and *Salmonella* involves immediate membrane depolarization followed by slower rate of DNA destruction which differs from that observed for Gram-positive bacteria. *Environ. Microbiol.* **2012**, *14*, 1730–1743. [CrossRef] [PubMed]
18. Macomber, L.; Rensing, C.; Imlay, J.A. Intracellular copper does not catalyze the formation of oxidative DNA damage in *Escherichia coli*. *J. Bacteriol.* **2007**, *189*, 1616–1626. [CrossRef] [PubMed]
19. Hong, R.; Kang, T.Y.; Michels, C.A.; Gadura, N. Membrane lipid peroxidation in copper alloy-mediated contact killing of *Escherichia coli*. *Appl. Environ. Microb.* **2012**, *78*, 1776–1784. [CrossRef]
20. Howlett, N.G.; Avery, S.V. Induction of lipid peroxidation during heavy metal stress in *Saccharomyces cerevisiae* and influence of plasma membrane fatty acid unsaturation. *Appl. Environ. Microb.* **1997**, *63*, 2971–2976.
21. Stadtman, E.R.; Levine, R.L. Free radical-mediated oxidation of free amino acids and amino acid residues in proteins. *Amino Acids* **2003**, *25*, 207–218. [CrossRef]
22. Karllson, H.L.; Cronholm, P.; Hedberg, Y.; Tornberg, M.; Battice, L.D.; Svedhen, S.; Wallinder, I.O. Cell membrane damage and protein interaction induced by copper containing nanoparticles—Importance of the metal release process. *Toxicology* **2013**, *313*, 59–69. [CrossRef]
23. Gunawan, C.; Teoh, W.Y.; Marquis, C.P.; Amal, R. Cytotoxic origin of copper(II) oxide nanoparticles: Comparative studies with micron-sized particles, leachate, and metal salts. *ACS Nano* **2011**, *5*, 7214–7225. [CrossRef]
24. Delgado, K.; Quijada, R.; Palma, R.; Palza, H. Polypropylene with embedded copper metal or copper oxide nanoparticles as a novel plastic antimicrobial agent. *Lett. Appl. Microbiol.* **2011**, *53*, 50–54. [CrossRef] [PubMed]
25. Rodriguez-Llamazares, S.; Mondaca, M.; Badilla, C.; Maldonado, A. PVC/copper oxide composites and their effect on bacterial adherence. *J. Child. Chem. Soc.* **2012**, *57*, 1163–1165. [CrossRef]
26. Araújo, C.S.T.; Carvalho, D.C.; Rezende, H.C.; Almeida, I.L.S.; Coelho, L.M.; Coelho, N.M.M.; Marques, T.L.; Alves, V.N. Bioremediation of waters contaminated with heavy metals using *Moringa oleifera* seeds as biosorbent. In *Applied bioremediation—Active and Passive Approaches*; Patil, Y.B., Rao, P., Eds.; InTech Open Access Publisher: Rijeka, Croatia, 2013; pp. 227–255.
27. US EPA. Water Regulations. Basic Information about Regulated Drinking Water Contaminants. Basic Information about Copper in Drinking Water. 2013. Available online: http://water.epa.gov/drink/contaminants/basicinformation/copper.cfm (accessed on 24 December 2018).
28. *Guidelines for Drinking-Water Quality*, 4th ed.; WHO Press: Geneva, Switzerland, 2011; pp. 340–341, ISBN 978 92 4 154815 1. Available online: http://apps.who.int/iris/bitstream/handle/10665/44584/9789241548151_eng.pdf;jsessionid=B1CEC2F9092D877380BECBFE2B075603?sequence=1 (accessed on 24 December 2018).
29. Public Health Regulations. The sanitary quality of drinking water and drinking water facilities. *Collect. Regul.* **2013**, *7262*, 24. Available online: https://www.health.gov.il/Subjects/Environmental_Health/drinking_water/Documents/Briut47-Eng.pdf (accessed on 24 December 2018).

30. Sewerage and Drainage Act. 1999. Available online: https://sso.agc.gov.sg/SL/SDA1999-RG5?DocDate=20161003 (accessed on 24 December 2018).
31. Sewer Use Program of Utilities Board. *Regulations for Wastewater Discharge Limits for Sewer Wastewater*; The City of Sylacauga: Sylacauga, AL, USA, 2011. Available online: http://www.sylacauga.net/utilities/wastewater/Sewer_Use_Regulations%20August%202011.pdf (accessed on 24 December 2018).

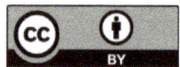

© 2019 by the authors. Licensee MDPI, Basel, Switzerland. This article is an open access article distributed under the terms and conditions of the Creative Commons Attribution (CC BY) license (http://creativecommons.org/licenses/by/4.0/).

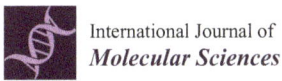

International Journal of
Molecular Sciences

Article

Use of Materials Based on Polymeric Silica as Bone-Targeted Drug Delivery Systems for Metronidazole

Katarzyna Czarnobaj, Magdalena Prokopowicz and Katarzyna Greber *

Department of Physical Chemistry, Medical University of Gdańsk, al. gen. J. Hallera 107, 80-416 Gdańsk, Poland; kczar@gumed.edu.pl (K.C.); mprokop@gumed.edu.pl (M.P.)
* Correspondence: greber@gumed.edu.pl; Tel.: +48-58-349-14-59

Received: 26 February 2019; Accepted: 11 March 2019; Published: 15 March 2019

Abstract: Mesostructured ordered silica-based materials are the promising candidates for local drug delivery systems in bone disease due to their uniform pore size and distribution, and high surface area which affect their excellent adsorption properties, good biocompatibility and bioactivity, and versatile functionalization so that their properties can be controlled. Ordered mesoporous silica (MCM-41 type) was synthesized by a surfactant-assisted sol-gel process using tetraethoxysilane as a silica precursor and hexadecyltrimethylammonium bromide as the structure-directing agent. Functionalized silica materials containing various types of organic groups (3-aminopropyl, 3-mercaptopropyl, or 3-glycidyloxypropyl groups) were synthesized by the post-grafting method onto pre-made mesoporous silica. Comparative studies of their structural characteristics, the surface mineralization activity and release properties for the model drug Metronidazole (MT) were then conducted. It has been found that porosity parameters, mineralization activity and adsorption/release of metronidazole from mesoporous channels of silica can be regulated using functional groups which are chemically bounded with an outer silica surface. The preferential mineral nucleation was found on negatively charged surfaces—MCM-41, and mercaptopropyl and glycidyloxypropyl functionalized silica (MCM-SH and MCM-epoxy, respectively) in simulated body fluid (SBF solution), as well as a sustained release of MT. In contrast to them, aminopropyl-functionalized samples (MCM-NH$_2$) achieved a high MT release rate. These results confirm the potential of silica-based materials for local therapeutic applications (as drug carriers and bone substitutes) in bone disease.

Keywords: amorphous materials; ordered mesoporous silica; sol-gel preparation; drug carrier

---

1. Introduction

Currently, the most common ways of delivering drugs to the body are oral and parenteral administration. However, these manners have lower efficiency for some therapies, e.g., treatment of bone diseases/infections.

Therefore, local delivery systems are more effective for such types of disease. The desired carrier in the local treatment of bones diseases should demonstrate the possibility to simultaneously introduce in situ drug release in combination with the filling and regeneration of the tissue defect, for example to stimulate the growth of the natural tissue helping in its replacement or complementation [1–3].

The ordered mesoporous silica-based materials are the leading candidates in tissue reconstruction technology. Their characteristic features include a low susceptibility to bacterial colonization, and absolute resistance to corrosion, unlike metallic implants. Upon implantation, silica materials exhibit bioactive properties—by hydroxyapatite formation on a surface they are able to bond with the living bone, which makes them biocompatible. In addition, because of their high surface area, controllable pore size, narrow pore size distribution, thermal and mechanical stability and easy surface functionalization, they may be used as carrier designated for the controlled release of therapeutic drugs [4–10].

MCM-41 silica (Mobil Composition of Matter No. 41) is a mesoporous material with a hierarchical structure that was first developed by researchers at Mobil Oil Corporation and that was initially introduced as adsorbent and catalyst [11]. After the first utilization of mesoporous silica in delivering drugs by Vallet-Regı' and co-workers [12], this material has also acquired a lot of interest in pharmaceutical applications. Therapeutic formulations of various compounds like anti-inflammatory agents (i.e., ibuprofen, metronidazole), antibiotics (i.e., vancomycin, amoxicillin, gentamicin) and anticancer agents (i.e., doxorubicin, carboplatin) have been developed using MCM-41 formulations [13–20].

Generally, mesoporous silica-based materials are synthesized via a template-directed method in the presence of a surfactant, which is either neutral or charged, and that serves as a structure-directing agent for the in situ polymerization of orthosilicic acid [11].

In the case of MCM-41, silica has a hexagonal arrangement with a pore diameter of 2.5 nm to 6 nm wherein cationic surfactants, in particular hexadecyltrimethylammonium bromide—CTAB, are used as templates. The most common silica source for the synthesis of MCM-41 is tetraethyl orthosilicate (TEOS) using the sol-gel process (called inorganic polymerization). It involves the hydrolysis and condensation of the TEOS monomers into a colloidal solution (sol), which acts as a precursor to the formation of the ordered polysilicate ($\equiv$Si$-$O$-$Si$\equiv$) network around the surfactant micelles [12].

In recent years some researchers have demonstrated the usefulness of functionalized ordered mesoporous silica materials for the adsorption release of drugs such as famotidine, amoxicillin, itraconazole, methotrexate, and so on [21].

The many, possible surface modifications of silica materials allow the precise control of surface chemistry to modify drug loading and release characteristics.

Surface modification of silica is achieved by reaction with organoalkoxysilanes. Organoalkoxysilanes form Si–O–Si bonds to the surface in a condensation reaction with the residual silanol groups on the silica surface. Usually, silica is functionalized with alkyl-/aryl, 3-aminopropyl-, 3-mercaptopropyl-, and glycidyloxypropyl-silanes.

Usually, functionalization of mesoporous silica can be accomplished by co-condensation, and by post-synthetic grafting. Since the organosilanes are introduced during the one-step synthesis procedure (co-condensation), the organic groups are generally more homogeneously distributed in the framework compared to material external surface-functionalized by a grafting method. However, in the co-condensation synthesis, the structurally different precursors having different hydrolysis and condensation rates lead to a decreased degree of ordered mesoporous structures, and a reduction in the pore diameter, pore volume, and specific surface areas compared to that synthesized via the grafting approach [22,23].

Thus, the objective of this paper is to study the physicochemical properties and mineralization potential of ordered silica-based materials to assess the usefulness of these types of material in the construction of bioactive implants to reconstruct the bone structure. Next, the loading and release of Metronidazole (MT)—a nonsteroidal anti-inflammatory drug acting in the diseased bone area—from obtained carrier matrices based on functionalized mesoporous silica were compared.

Therefore, a cetyltrimethylammoniumbromide (CTAB)-templated, mesoporous silica MCM-41 synthesized under basic conditions was chosen as support. Functional groups including 3-aminopropyl, 3-mercaptopropyl, and glycidyloxypropyl groups were used to functionalize the mesoporous MCM-41 via grafting approach to maintain a mesoscopic order while metronidazole was used as model molecule to investigate the surface-drug interactions, and to explain an effect of the structural differences between the carriers on in vitro drug release.

The obtained carriers were subjected to pre-formulation studies necessary for a thorough investigation of silica materials structure (e.g., porosity and surface area measurements through the Brunauer, Elmer and Teller method (BET) using spectroscopic tools such as Fourier transform infrared (FTIR), powder X-ray diffraction (XRPD) and electron microscopy (TEM and SEM) analyzes). Drug release studies were performed using a USP Type IV, comprising a UV-VIS spectroscopy for monitoring drug concentrations in the acceptor fluid.

2. Results and Discussion

2.1. Characterization of Functionalized Mesoporous Materials

Figure 1a shows the small-angle XRD pattern of MCM-41. The measurements of the silica sample revealed three diffraction peaks, which were indexed to the (100), (110) and (200) diffraction peaks confirming a highly ordered 2D-hexagonal mesoporous structure. Figure 1b shows the TEM image of the hexagonal arrangements of the porous system and the uniformity of the pores of silica. TEM measurement of the silica structure shows silica wall thickness ~5 nm, pore size ~3.3 nm (Figure 1c). The functionalized mesoporous materials also characterized by ordered mesostructures (not shown), they differ only slightly in pore size, which has been confirmed by BET studies (Table 1).

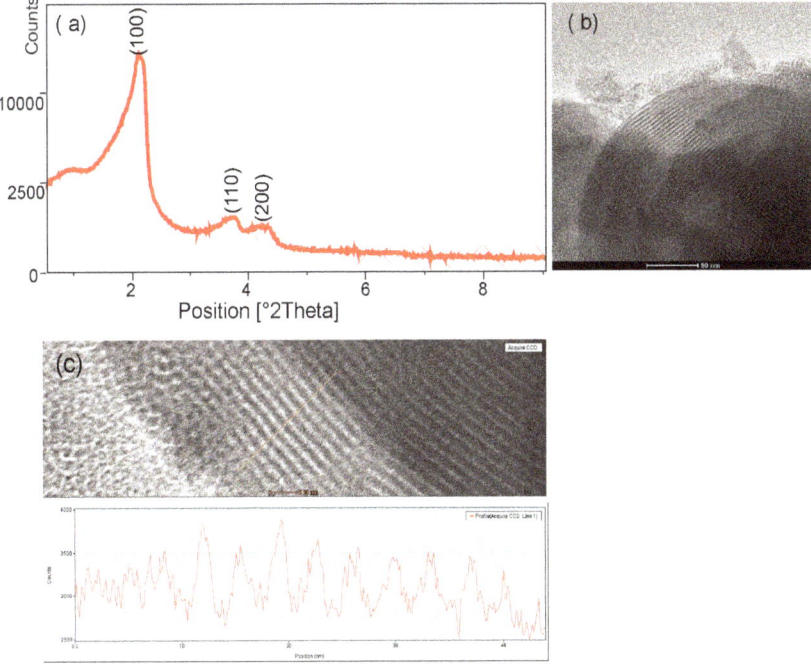

Figure 1. (a) X-ray diffraction pattern of MCM-41, (b) Transmission electron micrographs of MCM-41 in the (100) direction, (c) TEM measurement of the silica wall thickness and pore size.

Table 1. Physical data of the silica-based materials.

Sample	Pore Diameter (nm)	BET Surface Area ($m^2\ g^{-1}$)	Total Pore Volume ($cm^3\ g^{-1}$)	MT Loading (mg MT g^{-1} Sample)
MCM-41	3.51	743	0.72	18
MCM-epoxy	3.44	659	0.57	17
MCM-SH	3.42	662	0.54	20
MCM-NH$_2$	2.93	553	0.38	12

The mesoporous structures of MCM-41 and functionalized MCMs were investigated by N_2 adsorption-desorption analyses. The specific surface area and pore sizes of the materials are reported in Table 1. All the samples showed high surface areas between 743–553 m2 g^{-1}. The results reveal that these materials have average mesopore diameters between 2.93–3.51 nm and the pore volumes between 0.72–0.38 cm3 g^{-1}. Among the samples tested, MCM-NH$_2$ was characterized by smallest the specific surface areas, pore volumes and pore sizes.

FTIR spectroscopy provided qualitative information about the chemical structure of the synthesized drug carriers. As shown in Figure 2 (spectrum a), no characteristic peaks of CTAB were detected, indicating the complete removal of surfactant from the pores of the synthesized MCM-41 material during the high-temperature calcination process. The resulting FTIR spectrum for the MCM-41 material showed bands derived only from bonds present in the silica. The strong bands were caused by the vibrations of Si–O–Si groups at 1076 and 800 cm^{-1}, which is indicative of a high degree of polymerization. Two broad bands, one at 3450 cm^{-1} and the other at 1631 cm^{-1}, were caused by O–H vibrations of Si–OH groups and the water molecule retained in the pores of the oxide network [24]. Figure 2 (spectra b, c, d) illustrate the FTIR spectra for functionalized MCM samples: MCM-NH2, MCM-SH and MCM-epoxy. Compared to the MCM-41, the all functionalized MCM samples exhibited additional absorption peaks of C–H bonds at 2900–2800 cm^{-1} region derived from alkyl chains of used organosiloxanes. For the MCM-NH2, additional absorption bands were observed at 1563 cm^{-1} and 689 cm^{-1}, which were attributed to the vibration of N–H bonds. The MCM-SH exhibited characteristic absorption peaks of thiol group: S–H band at 2567 cm^{-1} and C-S band at 688 cm^{-1}. For the MCM-epoxy, the peak at around 908 cm^{-1} was assigned to the vibration of C–O–C bonds. These observations demonstrated that organic groups were successfully grafted onto the MCM material [25,26].

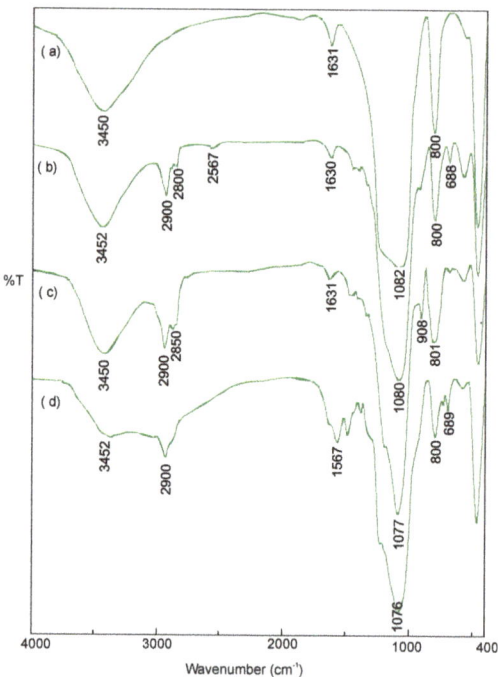

Figure 2. FTIR spectra of (**a**) MCM-41, (**b**) MCM-NH$_2$, (**c**) MCM-SH, and (**d**) MCM-epoxy.

2.2. Adsorption and Release of Metronidazole

The differences in surface area and pore size (Table 1) between the MCM-41 and three functionalized MCM samples cause the pure silica, and samples functionalized with mercaptopropyl and glycidyloxypropyl groups, to adsorb significantly more metronidazole than the samples functionalized with aminopropyl groups. This indicates that the porosity parameters (surface area, volume and pore size) are mainly responsible for differences in the adsorption capacity of materials.

The differences in adsorption properties of the samples to metronidazole could be partially attributed to the differences in the type of the functional groups and possible degree of interaction between the surface groups and MT molecules.

In the case of MCM-41, the surface of silica is negatively charged by the ionization of silanol groups in aqueous solution. The surface has an acidic character due to the possibility of proton displacement (-Si-O- + H+). Since metronidazole is a weak base that appears to have an affinity to the acidic surface of silica [27].

The silica surface modifications cause its hydrophobization but at the same time functionalization: -SH groups have the acidic character (stronger than -OH groups); -NH2 groups—basic character, the -epoxide groups easily open to the reactive diols, that are capable of complexing various compounds. The adsorption of MT appears to be more favorable on MCM-SH and MCM-epoxy carriers. The reduced adsorption of MT on MCM-NH$_2$ carrier reflects the increase of repulsive forces between basic groups of surface and drug.

All obtained silica carriers with metronidazole have two-stage release profiles characterized by a faster initial release (0–10 min) followed by a constant slow-release. As shown in Figure 3, MT release from MCM-NH$_2$ and MCM-41 was clearly higher compared to that from MCM-epoxy and MCM-SH. This study showed that 50% of the drug was released within the first 5 min from MCM-NH$_2$, 15, 50 and 60 min from MCM-41, MCM-epoxy and MCM-SH, respectively. A complete release of the drug (95%) occurred within 2.5 hr from MCM-NH$_2$, and 3.25 hr from MCM-41. In contrast, in the same time period only about 70% of MT from MCM-epoxy and MCM-SH was found to be released. A further release of MT from these carriers proceeded in a linear and slow manner. Complete amount of MT was released after 7 h and 7.2 h from MCM-SH and MCM-epoxy, respectively.

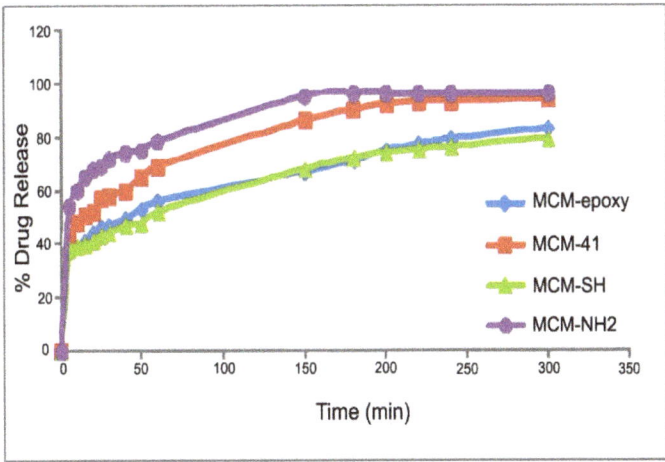

Figure 3. Mean cumulative release of MT (wt.%) from silica carriers during the 5 h of the experiment.

Based on the Korsmeyer-Peppas model [28], the release exponent, n, for the all drug-loaded carriers was between 0.40 and 0.53. These values are close to 0.5 and indicate a diffusion-controlled release.

This study shows that the type of organic modification of SiO_2 determines the release rate of the drug. A much more rapid release was demonstrated in MT-MCM-NH_2 system. The rapid release of the drug may be related to the smallest pore size and surface area of this material, therefore the lowest drug loading. MCM-NH_2 samples holding low amounts of MT keep it on the outer surface of the matrix or close to the surface of the matrix and release it easily; however, release of the higher amount of MT from pure MCM-41 and MCM-SH and MCM-epoxy (having higher porosity parameters compared to MCM-NH_2) takes longer and release does not occur easily. Another reason that may cause this phenomenon is the interactions between the drug substance and the matrix. The most important role in MT release is the hydrogen bonding between MT and the silica matrices. The MCM-41 has hydroxyl groups on the surface of the pores through which they can interact (through hydrogen bonds) with the drug and thus slow down its release. The addition of organic groups to the silica surface can cause changes in these interactions by: (i) increasing the hydrophobicity of the surface by the presence of alkyl groups; (ii) reducing the amount of surface hydroxyl groups as a result of the grafting reaction, and (iii) the surface functionalization through the presence of -NH2, -SH and epoxy-groups.

The addition of organosiloxanes hydrophobizes of surface and at the same time replaces the part of -OH groups with the alkyl groups which do not interact electrostatically with the drug; therefore, these matrices may have facilitated the release of the drug through its weaker interactions with drug. However, the hydrophobic carrier can hinder the penetration of the dissolution medium into the pores, which may slow drug release. Nevertheless, because this hydrophobization affects all carriers, it has no effect on the differences in drug release.

The functional groups, the most distant from the silica surface, most easily can interact with the drug molecule, causing its stronger binding in the pores (-SH and epoxy groups) or its repulsion (amine groups). The mentioned first can affect the slowdown of the release of the drug, in contrast to the amine groups, which may cause its easier release.

2.3. Evaluation of In Vitro Mineralization

The ceramic and glass oxide materials are considered bioactive if form a bone-like apatite layer on their surfaces after being implanted in bone. The ability of biomaterials to integrate with bone tissue can be evaluated using the simulated body fluid (SBF) test to study the in vitro formation of bone-like apatite at the surface of such materials when immersed in SBF [29]. SBF has almost equal compositions of inorganic ions to human blood plasma and does not contain any cells or proteins. In such an environment, bone-like apatite is created by the chemical reactions of the biomaterial components with the SBF ions. The mineralization activity of oxide materials decides both the chemical composition and the surface properties, especially the porosity (the presence of pores larger than 2 nm) and hydrophilicity of the surface [30]. These aspects suggest that ordered mesoporous silica materials, such as MCM-41 or functionalized MCM-41, thanks to high surface area, appropriate size of pores and the occurrence of reactive groups (-OH, -NH2, -SH, -epoxy), are the promising candidates as bioactive bone tissue substitutes.

To confirm the mineralization activity of the MCM-based materials, the samples of silica were soaked in SBF and then the formation of apatite phase was detected by FTIR, XRD, and SEM techniques.

The changes of FTIR spectra along with soaking time in SBF solution are illustrated in Figure 4B(a) taking MCM-41 as an example. After one week of experiment, the new absorption peaks appeared, and became stronger and stronger with longer soaking time. The existence of PO_4^{3-} group was shown by the sharp doublet at about 564 cm^{-1} and 602 cm^{-1} wavenumbers (the major absorption mode of the phosphate groups—the O–P–O bending mode), and also 885 cm^{-1} (the P–OH stretching mode). In addition, carbonate groups CO_3^{2-} can be detected in samples by the appearance of bands at 1400–1460 cm^{-1}. Clearly, these peaks appearing in arrange of 500–1600 cm^{-1} indicates the formation of crystalline apatite with doping of some carbonate [31].

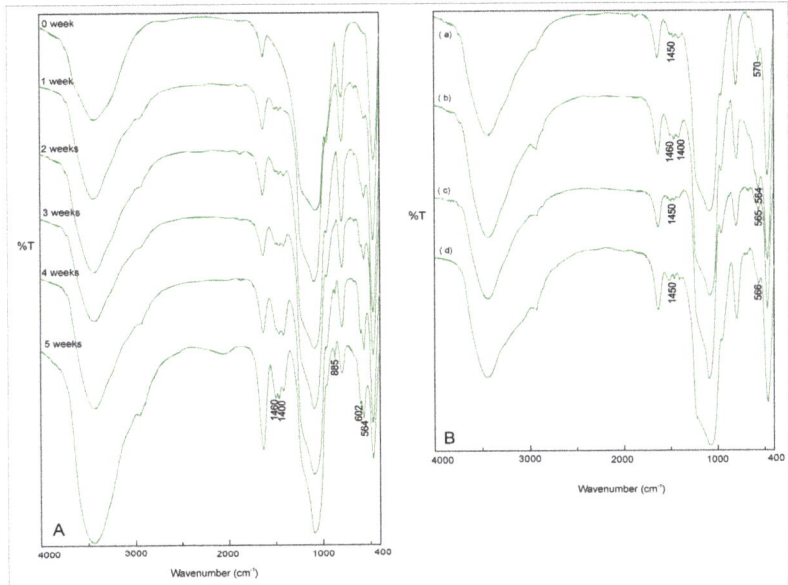

Figure 4. FTIR spectra of (**A**) MCM-41 during the 5 weeks of mineralization studies in simulated body fluid and (**B**) (a) MCM-41, (b) MCM-epoxy, (c) MCM-SH, and (d) MCM-NH$_2$ after 2 weeks of mineralization studies in simulated body fluid.

The induction period for the crystallinity of HA is different for various types of silicas. It was observed that the incubation of pure MCM-41 in SBF solution results in the fast growth of hydroxyapatite on its surface (1 week). In case of MCM-SH and MCM-epoxy, the appearance of HA on their surface was also after 1 week of the experiment, but the FTIR peaks were less intense. In case of MCM-NH2, the formation of HA on their surface was observed after two weeks of the experiment. In Figure 4B(b), the FT-IR spectra of all the four samples were put together and compared for apatite depositions after two weeks. The differences in the HA growth on the samples surface are related to its formation mechanism. Kokubo formulated a theory of the mechanism of in vitro apatite formation in bioactive materials (by immersion experiments in a simulated physiological solution—SBF) [32]. According to this, when silica-based material is soaked in SBF, a hydrated silica gel layer is formed. This layer, which is abundant in silanol (Si–OH) groups, provides favourable sites for the apatite nucleation, thanks to silanols complexation with Ca2+ ions. The absorbed Ca2+ ions may subsequently attract PO43- ions and form apatite layers on the surface of the material. This demonstrates that the surface functional groups, which are capable of binding Ca ions, may become sites for the surface nucleation. This applies especially to negatively charged groups (strong ion-ion interactions), followed by nonionic-polar (ion-polar interactions) and positively charged groups (repulsion of ions). The effective apatite formation ability observed for negatively charged group-bearing surfaces (with -OH, -SH and -epoxy groups) apparently proceeds by its strong ion-ion interactions with calcium ions and its subsequent phosphate ion adsorption.

Evaluation of the characteristic peaks of HA crystals by X-ray diffraction and the observation of surface morphology by SEM further confirmed the existence of HA.

After in vitro mineralization experiment, the XRD analysis showed that all samples produced new peaks demonstrating the surface crystallization. The most intense peaks occur at 2θ 32°, 26° that are 2 1 1 and 0 0 2 diffractions respectively of the apatite (according to the standard JCPDS cards (09-0432)). As apparent from the diffraction pattern, the content of crystalline phase decreases for NH$_2$-modified silica sample as shown by previous studies FTIR (Figure 5).

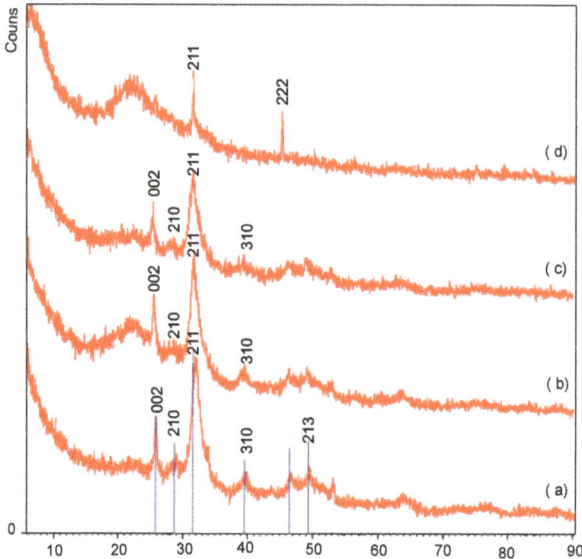

Figure 5. X-ray diffraction (XRD) patterns of (**a**) MCM-41 (**b**) MCM-epoxy, (**c**) MCM-SH, and (**d**) MCM-NH$_2$ after 2 weeks of mineralization studies in simulated body fluid.

The formation of HA deposition was further proved by SEM analysis. Because of the similarity in SEM images, only images for MCM-41 sample was presented in Figure 6 to show silica surface before the experiment and then the deposited apatite on silica soaked in SBF for one month. Before the silica-based samples were soaked in SBF, all materials show smooth surfaces (Figure 6a for silica). After soaking for one month, the HA precipitates can be induced on the surfaces of all obtained types of silica. SEM images reveal that a large number of tiny plate-like crystals—characteristic for apatite—was deposited on the surface of these materials after mineralization experiment (Figure 6b,c).

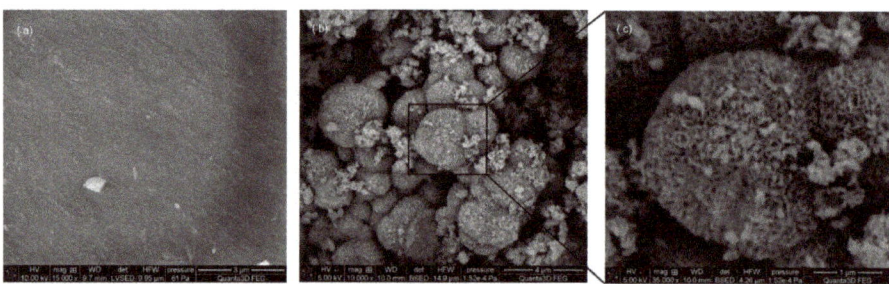

Figure 6. Scanning electron microscope (SEM) of (**a**) MCM-41 before mineralization studies, and (**b**,**c**) MCM-41 after 1 month of mineralization studies in simulated body fluid.

3. Materials and Methods

3.1. Materials and Reagents

Tetraethoxysilane (TEOS), 3-aminopropyltriethoxysilane (APTS), 3-mercaptopropyltrimethoxysilane (MPTS), 3-glycidyloxypropyltrimethoxysilane (GPTMS), cetyltrimethyammoniumbromide (CTAB), tris(hydroxymethyl)aminomethane) (TRIZMA) were obtained from Sigma-Aldrich, Poznań, Poland.

NaCl, NaHCO3, KCl, K2HPO4 3H2O, MgCl2 6H2O, CaCl2 2H2O, Na2SO4 hydrochloric acid (36.5%), ethanol (analytical grade purity), 25% aqueous ammonia and anhydrous toluene were purchased from POCh Co., Gliwice, Poland.

3.2. Synthesis of Functionalized Mesoporous Materials via Post-Grafting Method

First, MCM-41 silica was prepared and then functionalized with different organic groups.

MCM-41 was prepared according to the procedure reported by Grün et al. [33]. Typically, CTAB (2.39 g) was first dissolved in a polypropylene beaker containing a mixture of de-ionized water (125 g), 25% aqueous ammonia (9.18 g), and ethanol (12.5 g) for 1 h under stirring (200 rpm). Then, TEOS (10.03 g) was added dropwise with continuous stirring. After 2 h of stirring, the white precipitate was allowed to heat in an oven at 100 °C for 5 days. The obtained solid product was separated via filtration, washed with ethanol and water, and dried at 50 °C for 24 h. Synthesized material was calcined at 550 °C for 5 h (Muffle Furnace, M-525, USA, heating rate 1 K min^{-1}) to remove the CTAB surfactant. Finally, silica polymer was obtained as a white powder.

The dry MCM-41 was grafted with 3-aminopropyl, 3-mercaptopropyl, and 3-glycidyloxypropyl groups by stirring 1.2 g MCM-41 with 4.4 mmol of APTS, MPTS, or GPTMS, respectively, in 200 mL toluene for 24 h. The selected MCM-41 to organosilane ratio is optimum for obtaining the maximum possible grafted groups in the materials, as reported by the scientific research [34]. The samples were then washed with a substantial amount of ethanol and dried at 100 °C.

3.3. Drug-Loading Efficiency

Metronidazole was loaded into MCM-41 by immersion with water solution of MT (the incipient wetness method) [35]. The drug loading experiment was performed by adding 50 mL of water solution of MT (1 mg mL^{-1}) to a flask containing 1 g of MCM-41.

This mixture was shaken for 24 h at room temperature (25 ± 0.5 °C) under light-sealed conditions. Next, the supernatant was separated from the silica by centrifugation, and the residual MT content was determined using a UV–VIS spectrophotometer (Shimadzu UV-1800 spectrometer, Kyoto, Japan) by reading the absorbance at 320 nm. The percentage of drug adsorption versus initial concentration was plotted, allowing determination of the loading efficiency of the silica samples. The amount of absorbed MT in the sample was 18 mg MT g^{-1} MCM-41.

The loading of MT into organically modified silica samples was in a similar way as in the case of MCM-41. The loading efficiency obtained was 17, 20 and 11 mg MT g^{-1} sample, for MCM-epoxy, MCM-SH and MCM-NH$_2$, respectively.

3.4. Metronidazole Release Experiments

Drug release studies were performed using the Flow-Through-Cell USP Apparatus 4 (closed loop) (Erweka, DZT-770, Heusenstamm, Germany). Typically, 100 mg of the carrier samples with drugs were placed on glass beads in a 22.6 mm flow-through cell. The SBF solution was used as an acceptor fluid. The experiment was carried out for 5 h in 100 mL of acceptor fluid with a flow rate of fluid of 4 mL min^{-1} at 37 °C.

At predetermined time intervals, 3 mL of release fluid was taken out for analysis of the release drug concentration with UV–VIS spectrophotometer, at λmax of 320 nm. Taken aliquot was replenished with fresh SBF (3 mL). All experiments were repeated in triplicate. Drug-elution data were plotted as the cumulative mass amount of drug released as a function of time.

The Korsmeyer-Peppas power law model was used as a mathematical description of drug release, expressed by the following Equation [28]

$$M_t/M_\infty = kt^n \qquad (1)$$

where M_t/M_∞ is a fraction of drug released at time t, k is the release rate constant, and n is the release exponent. The value of n characterizes the mechanism of drug release. The exponent n value close to 1 corresponds to zero-order release kinetics (the drug release rate is time-independent), $n \leq 0.5$ to a Fickian diffusion mechanism, and $0.5 < n < 1$ to non-Fickian transport (the drug release is considered as anomalous). Generally, an early portion of a release profile (to 60%) is used in the Korsmeyer-Peppas model.

3.5. Characterization

The molecular structure of samples was determined using a Fourier transform infrared (FT/IR) spectrometer (410 Spectrometer, Jasco), using the potassium bromide (KBr) disk technique. The spectra were collected over a range of 4000–400 cm^{-1} (64 scans, resolution 4 cm^{-1}).

The specific surface area and pore size distribution were determined by N2 adsorption using a Micromeritics ASAP 2405N instrument (Micromeritics, Norcross, GA, USA) and the Barret–Joyner–Halenda (BJH) methods, respectively.

The X-ray diffraction (XRD) spectra of samples were taken with an Empyrean/PANalytical XRPD diffractometer using CuKα1 radiation, operating at 20 kV and 40 mA.

The morphology of the silica was characterized using transmission electron microscope (TEM) (Tecnai G2 20X-TWIN, FEI Company, Hillsboro, OR, USA) and scanning electron microscope (SEM) (Quanta 3D FEG, FEI Company, Hillsboro, OR, USA).

3.6. Evaluation of In Vitro Mineralization

In vitro mineralization (ability to apatite formation on the silica surface) was performed as follows: 0.5 g of sample was incubated in 50 mL of SBF solution in the thermostated shaking water bath (Julabo, Seelbach, Germany, 50 rpm) at 37 °C ($\pm$ 0.5 °C) for five weeks. The samples were tested daily using FTIR, XRD, and SEM techniques to detect apatite.

4. Conclusions

We studied the three important aspects of mesoporous silica implantable drug delivery systems: porosity, surface chemistry and ability for mineralization.

The results indicated that the functionalization of the silica surface significantly affects adsorption/release behaviour and mineralization activity, and also modifies the porosity parameters.

Among the tested carriers, pure silica and silica modified with MPTS and GPTMS have similar porosity parameters and the ability to mineralize the surface, in contrast to APTS modified silica, which exhibits smaller pores and a weaker ability for apatite nucleation. The modification of silica surface with SH and epoxy groups also influenced the slowdown of metronidazole release (compared to pure silica and especially silica modified with amine groups) due to the ability to create strong electrostatic interactions with the drug.

These results confirm the potential of silica-based materials for local therapeutic applications, as drug carriers and bone substitutes in bone disease.

Author Contributions: K.C. designed the study, performed the experiments, analysed the data and wrote the paper, M.P. helped with data analysis and preparation of the manuscript for publication, K.G. helped with preparation of the manuscript for publication.

Funding: This work was partly financed by the Ministry of Science and Higher Education to maintain the research potential from funds for statutory activity ST3 02-0003/07/518.

Conflicts of Interest: The authors declare that they have no conflict of interest.

References

1. Goodman, S.B.; Gómez Barrena, E.; Takagi, M.; Konttinen, Y.T. Biocompatibility of total joint replacements: A review. *J. Biomed. Mater. Res. Part A* **2009**, *90A*, 603–618. [CrossRef] [PubMed]
2. Pan, H.; Zhao, X.; Darvell, B.W.; Lu, W.W. Apatite-formation ability—Predictor of "bioactivity"? *Acta Biomater.* **2010**, *6*, 4181–4188. [CrossRef] [PubMed]
3. Ragelle, H.; Danhier, F.; Préat, V.; Langer, R.; Anderson, D.G. Nanoparticle-based drug delivery systems: A commercial and regulatory outlook as the field matures. *Expert Opin. Drug Deliv.* **2017**, *4*, 851–864. [CrossRef]
4. Vallet-Regí, M.; Ragel, C.V.; Salinas, A.J. Glasses with Medical Applications. *Eur. J. Inorg. Chem.* **2003**, *2003*, 1029–1042. [CrossRef]
5. Yan, X.; Yu, C.; Zhou, X.; Tang, J.; Zhao, D. Highly Ordered Mesoporous Bioactive Glasses with Superior In Vitro Bone-Forming Bioactivities. *Angew. Chem. Int. Ed.* **2004**, *43*, 5980–5984. [CrossRef] [PubMed]
6. Vallet-Regí, M.; Balas, F.; Arcos, D. Mesoporous Materials for Drug Delivery. *Angew. Chem. Int. Ed.* **2007**, *46*, 7548–7558. [CrossRef]
7. Vallet-Regí, M.; Colilla, M.; Izquierdo-Barba, I.; Manzano, M. Mesoporous Silica Nanoparticles for Drug Delivery: Current Insights. *Molecules* **2018**, *23*, 47. [CrossRef]
8. Castillo, R.R.; Colilla, M.; Vallet-Regí, M. Advances in mesoporous silica-based nanocarriers for co-delivery and combination therapy against cancer. *Expert Opin. Drug Deliv.* **2017**, *14*, 229–243. [CrossRef]
9. Martínez-Carmona, M.; Lozano, D.; Colilla, M.; Vallet-Regí, M. Lectin-conjugated pH-responsive mesoporous silica nanoparticles for targeted bone cancer treatment. *Acta Biomater.* **2017**, *65*, 393–404. [CrossRef]
10. Manzano, M.; Vallet-Regí, M. Mesoporous silica nanoparticles in nanomedicine applications. *J. Mater. Sci. Mater. Med.* **2018**, *29*, 65–79. [CrossRef] [PubMed]
11. Kresge, C.T.; Leonowicz, M.E.; Roth, W.J.; Vartuli, J.C.; Beck, J.S. Ordered mesoporous molecular sieves synthesized by a liquid-crystal template mechanism. *Nature* **1992**, *359*, 710–712. [CrossRef]
12. Vallet-Regi, M.; Rámila, A.; del Real, R.P.; Pérez-Pariente, J. A New Property of MCM-41. *Drug Deliv. Syst.* **2000**. [CrossRef]
13. Di Pasqua, A.J.; Wallner, S.; Kerwood, D.J.; Dabrowiak, J.C. Adsorption of the Pt^{II} Anticancer Drug Carboplatin by Mesoporous Silica. *Chem. Biodivers.* **2009**, *6*, 1343–1349. [CrossRef] [PubMed]
14. Lai, C.-Y.; Trewyn, B.G.; Jeftinija, D.M.; Jeftinija, K.; Xu, S.; Jeftinija, S.; Lin, V.S.-Y. A Mesoporous Silica Nanosphere-Based Carrier System with Chemically Removable CdS Nanoparticle Caps for Stimuli-Responsive Controlled Release of Neurotransmitters and Drug. *Molecules* **2003**. [CrossRef] [PubMed]
15. Halamová, D.; Zeleňák, V. NSAID naproxen in mesoporous matrix MCM-41: Drug uptake and release properties. *J. Incl. Phenom. Macrocycl. Chem.* **2012**, *72*, 15–23. [CrossRef]
16. Koneru, B.; Shi, Y.; Wang, Y.-C.; Chavala, S.H.; Miller, M.L.; Holbert, B.; Conson, M.; Ni, A.; Di Pasqua, A.J. Tetracycline-Containing MCM-41 Mesoporous Silica Nanoparticles for the Treatment of *Escherichia coli*. *Molecules* **2015**, *20*, 19690–19698. [CrossRef] [PubMed]
17. Czarnobaj, K.; Prokopowicz, M.; Sawicki, W. Formulation and In Vitro Characterization of Bioactive Mesoporous Silica with Doxorubicin and Metronidazole Intended for Bone Treatment and Regeneration. *AAPS PharmSciTech* **2017**, *18*, 3163–3171. [CrossRef] [PubMed]
18. Prokopowicz, M. Characterization of low-dose doxorubicin-loaded silica-based nanocomposites. *Appl. Surf. Sci.* **2018**, *427 Pt A*, 55–63. [CrossRef]
19. Choi, E.; Kim, S. How Can Doxorubicin Loading Orchestrate in Vitro Degradation Behaviors of Mesoporous Silica Nanoparticles under a Physiological Condition? *Langmuir* **2017**, *33*, 4974–4980. [CrossRef]
20. Anirudhan, T.S.; Nair, A.S. Temperature and ultrasound sensitive gatekeepers for the controlled release of chemotherapeutic drugs from mesoporous silica nanoparticles. *J. Mater. Chem. B* **2018**, *6*, 428–439. [CrossRef]
21. Sun, R.; Wang, W.; Wen, Y.; Zhang, X. Recent Advance on Mesoporous Silica Nanoparticles-Based Controlled Release System: Intelligent Switches Open up New Horizon. *Nanomaterials* **2015**, *5*, 2019–2053. [CrossRef]
22. Wang, G.; Otuonye, A.N.; Blair, E.A.; Denton, K.; Tao, Z.; Asefa, T. Functionalized mesoporous materials for adsorption and release of different drug molecules: A comparative study. *J. Solid State Chem.* **2009**, *182*, 1649–1660. [CrossRef]
23. Croissant, J.C.; Fatieiev, Y.; Almalik, A.; Khashab, N.M. Mesoporous silica and organosilica nanoparticles: Physical chemistry, biosafety, delivery strategies, and biomedical applications. *Adv. Healthc. Mater.* **2017**, *7*, 1700831. [CrossRef]

24. Aguiar, H.; Serra, J.; González, P.; León, B. Structural study of sol–gel silicate glasses by IR and Raman spectroscopies. *J. Non-Cryst. Solids* **2009**, *355*, 475–480. [CrossRef]
25. Capeletti, L.B.; Baibich, I.M.; Butler, I.S.; dos Santos, J.H.Z. Infrared and Raman spectroscopic characterization of some organic substituted hybrid silicas. *Spectrochim. Acta Part A Mol. Biomol. Spectrosc.* **2014**, *133*, 619–625. [CrossRef]
26. Zhang, X.; Zhao, Y.; Xie, S.; Sun, L. Fabrication of functionalized porous silica nanoparticles and their controlled release behavior. *J. Drug Deliv. Sci. Technol.* **2017**, *37*, 38–45. [CrossRef]
27. Wu, Y.; Fassihi, R. Stability of metronidazole, tetracycline HCl and famotidine alone and in combination. *Int. J. Pharm.* **2005**, *290*, 1–13. [CrossRef]
28. Peppas, N.A. Analysis of Fickian and non-Fickian drug release from polymers. *Pharm. Acta Helv.* **1985**, *60*, 110–118.
29. Kokubo, T.; Takadama, H. How useful is SBF in predicting in vivo bone bioactivity? *Biomaterials* **2006**, *27*, 2907–2915. [CrossRef]
30. Gaharwar, A.K.; Detamore, M.S.; Khademhosseini, A. Emerging Trends in Biomaterials Research. *Ann. Biomed. Eng.* **2016**, *44*, 1861–1862. [CrossRef]
31. Byrappa, K.; Ohachi, T. *Crystal Growth Technology*; William Andrew co-published with Springer: Norwich, NY, USA, 2003; ISBN 9780815516804.
32. Kokubo, T. Design of bioactive bone substitutes based on biomineralization process. *Mater. Sci. Eng. C* **2005**, *25*, 97–104. [CrossRef]
33. Grün, M.; Lauer, I.; Unger, K.K. The synthesis of micrometer- and submicrometer-size spheres of ordered mesoporous oxide MCM-41. *Adv. Mater.* **1997**, *9*, 254–257. [CrossRef]
34. Horcajada, P.; Rámila, A.; Férey, G.; Vallet-Regí, M. Influence of superficial organic modification of MCM-41 matrices on drug delivery rate. *Solid State Sci.* **2006**, *8*, 1243–1249. [CrossRef]
35. Prokopowicz, M.; Czarnobaj, K.; Szewczyk, A.; Sawicki, W. Preparation and in vitro characterisation of bioactive mesoporous silica microparticles for drug delivery applications. *Mater. Sci. Eng. C* **2016**, *60*, 7–18. [CrossRef]

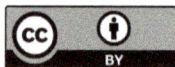

© 2019 by the authors. Licensee MDPI, Basel, Switzerland. This article is an open access article distributed under the terms and conditions of the Creative Commons Attribution (CC BY) license (http://creativecommons.org/licenses/by/4.0/).

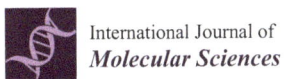

Article

Olive Mill Wastewater Valorization in Multifunctional Biopolymer Composites for Antibacterial Packaging Application

Laura Sisti [1], Grazia Totaro [1,*], Nicole Bozzi Cionci [2], Diana Di Gioia [2], Annamaria Celli [1], Vincent Verney [3] and Fabrice Leroux [3]

1. Dipartimento di Ingegneria Civile, Chimica, Ambientale e dei Materiali, Università di Bologna, Via Terracini 28, 40131 Bologna, Italy; laura.sisti@unibo.it (L.S.); annamaria.celli@unibo.it (A.C.)
2. Department of Agricultural and Food Sciences, Università di Bologna, viale Fanin 42, 40127 Bologna, Italy; nicole.bozzicionci@unibo.it (N.B.C.); diana.digioia@unibo.it (D.D.G.)
3. Institut de Chimie de Clermont Ferrand (ICCF)—UMR 6296 Clermont-Auvergne Université, CNRS, 24 Avenue Blaise Pascal, 63177 Aubiere (CEDEX), France; vincent.verney@uca.fr (V.V.); fabrice.leroux@uca.fr (F.L.)
* Correspondence: grazia.totaro@unibo.it; Tel.: +39-(0)51-2090425

Received: 4 April 2019; Accepted: 11 May 2019; Published: 14 May 2019

Abstract: Olive mill wastewater (OMW) is the aqueous waste derived from the production of virgin olive oil. OMW typically contains a wide range of phenol-type molecules, which are natural antioxidants and/or antibacterials. In order to exploit the bioactive molecules and simultaneously decrease the environmental impact of such a food waste stream, OMW has been intercalated into the host structure of ZnAl layered double hydroxide (LDH) and employed as an integrative filler for the preparation of poly(butylene succinate) (PBS) composites by in situ polymerization. From the view point of the polymer continuous phase as well as from the side of the hybrid filler, an investigation was performed in terms of molecular and morphological characteristics by gel permeation chromatography (GPC) and X-ray diffraction (XRD); also, the thermal and mechanical properties were evaluated by thermogravimetric analysis (TGA), differential scanning calorimetry (DSC), and dynamic thermomechanical analysis (DMTA). Antibacterial properties have been assessed against a Gram-positive and a Gram-negative bacterium, *Staphylococcus aureus* and *Escherichia coli*, respectively, as representatives of potential agents of foodborne illnesses.

Keywords: multifunctional hybrid systems; olive mill wastewater; antibacterial properties; layered double hydroxides; bionanocomposites

1. Introduction

High-added-value compounds, such as pectin and polyphenols, can be recovered from agro-wastes and reused as food ingredients, cosmetics, or even in pharmaceutical preparation [1,2]. Many recent studies have been devoted to the valorization of agro-food by-products in order to address sustainable and environmental requirements [3–5]. However, the recovery of target components from waste implies the use of downstream and purification processes which are time consuming and costly as well as not environmentally friendly due to the use of huge amounts of water. An alternative approach consists of exploiting agro-wastes without any pretreatment, with the aim of preparing multifunctional materials, the development of which is indeed of great interest now for the industry, which is always looking for high-performance products obtainable through simple and low-cost processes. In the field of packaging, for example, where preserving the quality and increasing the safety of the products is of crucial importance, antibacterial, antioxidant, and/or anti-UV properties are greatly required.

At the same time, in the packaging sector, biopolymers (from natural sources and/or biodegradable) are emerging on the market because of growing global pressure deriving from the extensively publicized effects of climate change, price increases of fossil materials, as well as depletion of global fossil resources [6]. However, bio-based materials do not achieve technical performance comparable to their fossil counterparts.

A straightforward strategy that allows for obtaining high-performance and multifunctional materials involves the use of organo-modified layered double hydroxides (LDHs) dispersed in polymeric matrices. LDHs are a class of anionic clays consisting of stacked brucite-type [$Mg(OH)_2$] octahedral layers with water molecules and exchangeable anions in the interlayer region, offering a large variety of heterostructured materials [7]. Thanks to their great versatility as well as simple preparation, LDH host structures are often considered as a toolbox and their applications are strongly diversified, ranging from catalysis to biomedicine, cosmetics, functional additives, and/or stabilizers in polymer formulations, sorbents, and scavengers for pollutants [8,9].

Our research group is profoundly concerned with targeting green fillers in association with bio-based and biodegradable polymer. Our previous studies have demonstrated that the use of organo-modified LDHs may provoke a significant chain extension effect on polymer matrices with consequent improvement of their processability [10–14]. Moreover, suitable properties, such as antioxidant/antibacterial/anti-UV, due to the tethered/intercalated anions into the LDH, can be exploited, leading to multifunctional fillers. LDH acts as inorganic cargo hosting bioactive molecules and it protects them from thermal degradation, thus enhancing their thermal stability as well as allowing the preservation of their bioactivity, which is well-maintained under such a protective layer against injection/extrusion during polymer composite processing [15,16]. Therefore, multifunctional composite materials with antioxidant/antibacterial/anti-UV properties can be achieved.

In a previous work [17], olive mill wastewater (OMW), without any pretreatment, was successfully intercalated into a Zn_2Al-LDH with the aim of enhancing the durability of polypropylene (PP) and poly(butylene succinate) (PBS) melt-blended composites. In the current study, the antibacterial and thermomechanical properties of similar systems have been further investigated. Therefore, the materials prepared can be suitable for antibacterial/antioxidant coating and packaging, as well as medical devices and household products.

OMW is a high-organic-load and recalcitrant waste stream of great environmental concern and its management is a very important issue in Mediterranean countries because of the huge amount of olives: more than 2.4 million tons/year, 90% of which is meant for olive oil production, thus generating up to 30 million m^3 per year of OMW [17,18]. The composition of OMW consists of 80–90% water, 4–16% organic compounds (such as tyrosol, hydroxytyrosol, p-coumaric acid, ferulic acid, syringic acid, protocatechuic acid, vanillic acid tannins, anthocyanins, etc.), and 0.4–2.5% mineral salts (K, Ca, and Na). Due to their low partition coefficients, olive phenols are more soluble in water than in the oil phase. Thus, polyphenols are found in OMW at concentrations ranging from 0.03–11.5 g/L according to the processing system used for olive oil production [1].

Among bio-based polyesters, PBS is of particular interest. It is a biodegradable semicrystalline polymer, the pristine monomers of which (1,4-butanediol and succinic acid) can both be obtained from sugar fermentation. PBS is emerging in agriculture, consumer goods, and especially in the flexible packaging market [6]. Due to its thermal and mechanical characteristics, PBS ranks similar to PP for its strength (tensile strength of 34 MPa for PBS and 33 MPa for PP) and between low-density (LDPE) and high-density polyethylene (HDPE) for its stiffness (flexural modulus of 656 MPa for PBS, 176 MPa for LDPE, and 1070 MPa for HDPE) [19,20].

In detail, OMW was here used as an intercalating agent in layered Zn_2Al-LDH (i.e., between its organo-modified platelets). Some phenol model molecules, as typical chemical structures of the main components present in OMW (namely, vanillic acid (VA), ferulic acid (FA), and protocatechuic acid (PA)), were also employed for comparison. Mixed systems were also prepared by simultaneous coprecipitation of two or three biomolecules to simulate a medium containing more than one bioactive compound, as in OMW. The organo-modified LDHs (5 wt%) were employed for the preparation of PBS composites through in situ polymerization. Both the organo-modified LDHs and the obtained composite samples were tested for their antimicrobial action against *Escherichia coli* and *Staphylococcus aureus*. Thermal and thermomechanical properties were investigated by thermogravimetric analysis (TGA), differential scanning calorimetry (DSC), and dynamic thermomechanical analysis (DMTA).

2. Results and Discussion

A full characterization of the prepared LDH samples, as well as the total organic compound (TOC) of the biowaste (4.51 ± 0.65 g GA eq/L, GA = gallic acid) were reported elsewhere [17]. Briefly, HPLC analysis revealed the presence of protocatechuic acid, vanillic acid, trans-cinnamic acid, gallic acid, and chlorogenic acid in OMW. FT-IR and X-ray analyses of the LDHs containing vanillic acid (Zn_2Al/VA), ferulic acid (Zn_2Al/FA), and protocatechuic acid (Zn_2Al/PA) demonstrated the intercalation of the anions between the lamellae. Mixed systems were also prepared by simultaneous coprecipitation of FA and PA (Zn_2Al/FA-PA) or VA, FA, and PA (Zn_2Al/VA-FA-PA) to simulate a medium containing more than one bioactive molecule, as in OMW. Concerning such systems and the sample intercalated with OMW (Zn_2Al/OMW), a selective interaction with some molecules was evident from FT-IR, but from X-ray diffraction analysis, it was concluded that the coprecipitation of LDH in the presence of OMW was not 100% efficient in yielding the LDH structure, giving rise to another inorganic material (γ-AlOOH) unable to trap organic guests. This was confirmed by a lower organic weight loss percentage from TGA in Zn_2Al/OMW. Therefore, in such a sample (Zn_2Al/OMW), the two structures (LDH and γ-AlOOH) were concomitantly present. The thermal protecting role of the LDH towards the anions was clear from TGA analysis because the thermal stability was enhanced after intercalation. This is a key point in this strategy because it allows the preservation of the bioactivity, which is well-maintained under such a protective layer during polymer composite processing.

In the current study, 5 wt% of the organic/inorganic (O/I) hybrid fillers was employed to prepare PBS bionanocomposites by in situ polymerization, which is an effective method to reach a good state of dispersion for the LDH filler. Such loading was reported to be appropriate, in similar systems, to assure the persistence of bioactivity [16,17,21]. Scheme 1 shows the monomers employed and the conditions of the in situ polymerization process. The bionanocomposites have been labeled PBS:Zn_2Al/X, according to the LDH employed.

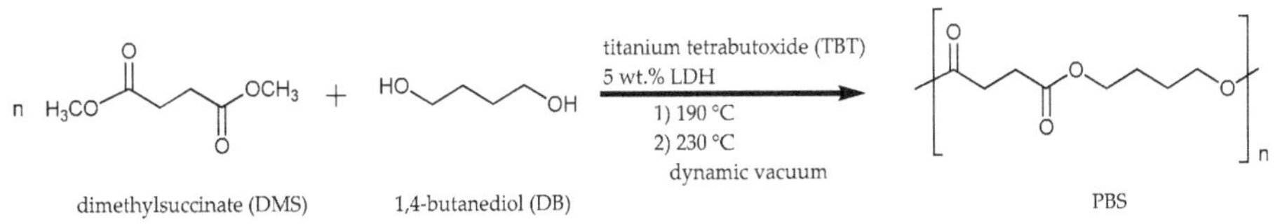

Scheme 1. In situ polymerization of poly(butylene succinate) (PBS) bionanocomposites.

The molecular weights of all composites, obtained by gel permeation chromatography (GPC) analysis, were high, into the range of $50 \times 10^3 < M_w < 90 \times 10^3$ g/mol with polydispersity values coherent to common polyesters ($M_w/M_n \approx 2$) (Table 1).

Table 1. Gel permeation chromatography (GPC) and thermogravimetric analysis (TGA) results of PBS, PBS:ferulic acid (FA)/protocatechuic acid (PA) and PBS:Zn$_2$Al/X composites.

Sample	M$_w$ (× 10^{-3} g mol^{-1}) [a]	M$_w$/M$_n$ [a]	T$_{onset}$ (°C) [b]	T^{10}$_D$ (°C) [b]	T$_{max}$ (°C) [b]
PBS	69	2.4	380	363	406
PBS:Zn$_2$Al/VA	91	2.4	353	344	393
PBS:Zn$_2$Al/FA	47	2.2	357	340	393
PBS:Zn$_2$Al/PA	49	2.3	355	347	389
PBS:Zn$_2$Al/FA-PA	61	2.3	355	338	395
PBS:Zn$_2$Al/VA-FA-PA	68	2.5	345	341	387
PBS:Zn$_2$Al/OMW	61	2.4	355	347	387
PBS:FA/PA	8	2.7	376	360	403

[a] Determined by GPC in CHCl$_3$; [b] Determined by TGA under air flow.

PBS:FA/PA, without LDH, with 1 wt% of FA and 1 wt% of PA with respect to the polymer theoretical yield, was also prepared in order to better understand the beneficial role of LDH. Of course, during the polymerization, FA and PA competed with dimethyl succinate (DMS) in the condensation reaction with 1,4-butanediol (BD); therefore, a copolymer was formed. ^{1}H NMR showed that only 0.32 mol% of both FA and PA had copolymerized. The results of GPC analysis indicated that oligomers were formed (M$_w$ = 8 × 10^3 g/mol) because FA and PA possess only one reactive functional group; therefore, they act as a chain stopper during macromolecular growth.

The degree of dispersion of the organo-modified LDHs in the PBS matrix was evaluated by XRD analysis. In Figure 1, since the same results were obtained for all the samples, only some representative composite XRD patterns are reported, showing the diffraction lines characteristic of PBS and the absence of the diffraction peaks of the associated filler. This can be explained by a low crystallinity of the filler or a potential exfoliation occurring during thermal processing. All the characteristic peaks ascribable to the crystalline structure of PBS (020) (021) (110) (111) can be found in the 2θ range of 18°–30°, and no significant difference can be depicted with PBS free of filler. The copolymer presented narrow diffraction lines due to PBS crystallinity.

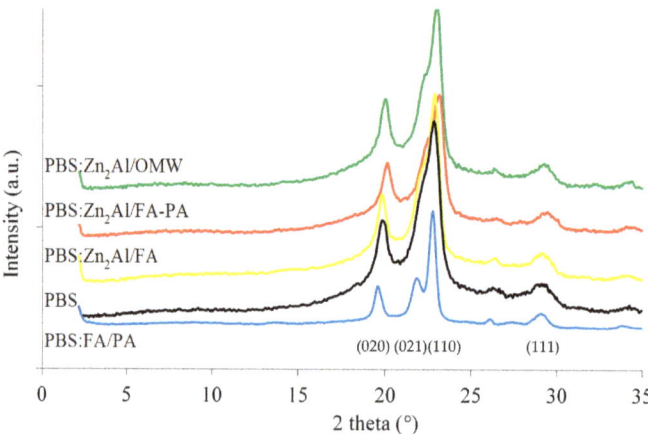

Figure 1. XRD profiles of PBS and some PBS:Zn$_2$Al/X composites with indexing of the main reflections due to the crystalline structure of PBS.

Tables 1 and 2 list all the results from TGA and DSC analyses of the nanocomposites. From Figure 2, reporting the TGA thermograms of all the samples, a main decomposition process is depicted in the temperature range of 360–375 °C. Concerning the nanocomposites, the filler did not exert thermal stabilization upon the matrix because of the catalyzing effect of metals, as well as the polyester hydrolysis promoted by the water released during its thermal degradation. In any case, the thermal data reported (onset degradation (T_{onset}), 10% mass loss ($T^{10}{}_D$), and maximum degradation temperatures (T_{max})) were consistently higher than the melting temperature of PBS (116 °C); therefore, such expected thermal degradation was overcome during processing. This is consistent with the literature [12,13]. As expected, the copolymer showed initial and maximum degradation temperatures close to PBS.

Table 2. Thermomechanical results of PBS, PBS:FA/PA, and PBS:Zn$_2$Al/X.

Sample	T_g (°C) [a]	T_g (°C) [b]	T_c (°C) [c]	ΔH_c (J·g^{-1}) [c]	T_m (°C) [b]	ΔH_m (J·g^{-1}) [b]
PBS	−16.3	−33	70	72	116	77
PBS:Zn$_2$Al/VA	−14.4	−35	73	64	113	64
PBS:Zn$_2$Al/FA	−8.9	−36	73	52	113	47
PBS:Zn$_2$Al/PA	−8.9	−34	76	53	115	48
PBS:Zn$_2$Al/FA-PA	−8.9	−36	77	55	114	51
PBS:Zn$_2$Al/VA-FA-PA	−13.4	−36	77	61	114	58
PBS:Zn$_2$Al/OMW	−13.4	−36	66	51	114	57
PBS:FA/PA	/	−30	66	62	110	67

[a] Determined by dynamic thermomechanical analysis (DMTA); [b] Determined by differential scanning calorimetry (DSC) during the second heating scan; [c] Determined by DSC during the cooling scan from the melt at 10 °C min^{-1}.

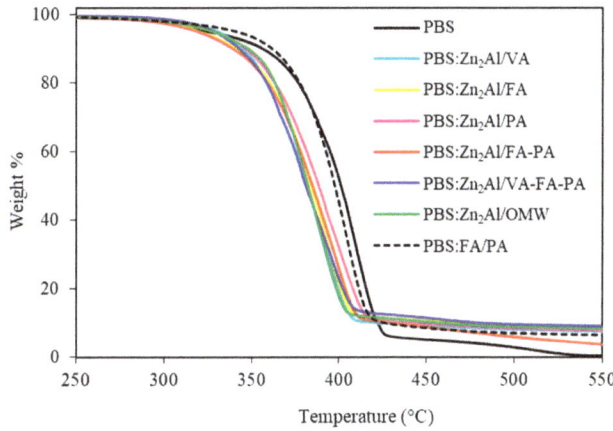

Figure 2. TGA profiles of PBS, PBS:FA/PA, and PBS:Zn$_2$Al/X composites.

From the DSC analysis reported in Table 2, it can be noted that melting temperature (T_m) values of the nanocomposites slightly decreased with respect to 116 °C (the melting temperature of PBS). Moreover, the peak shapes were complex and multiple endothermic peaks were present due to the melting–recrystallization process that generally occurs in polyesters (Figure 3) [22]. Concerning the cooling scan, most of the composites crystallized at higher temperatures with respect to PBS, while PBS:Zn$_2$Al/OMW had a lower crystallization temperature (T_c). However, all the composites presented lower enthalpy of crystallization (ΔH_c) with respect to PBS; therefore, the motion of the polymer chains in the melt were restricted by the platelets and the crystallization process was somehow hindered. Indirectly, this behavior confirmed a good degree of dispersion of the LDHs in the PBS matrix.

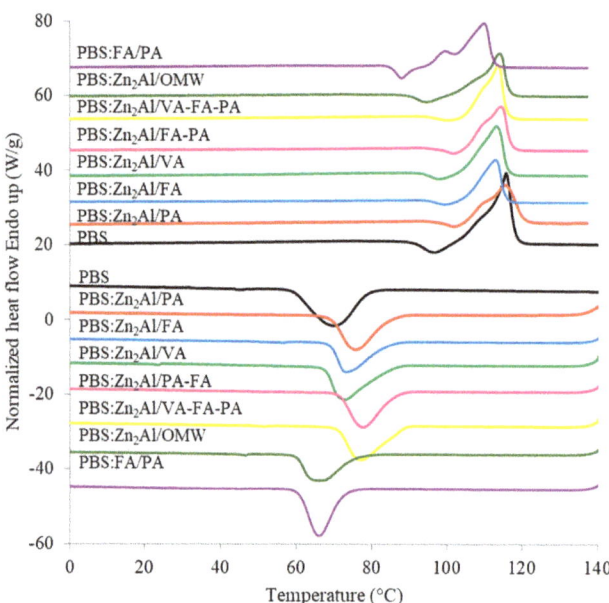

Figure 3. DSC profiles of PBS, PBS:FA/PA, and PBS:Zn$_2$Al/X composites.

In order to evaluate the mechanical properties of the samples prepared, DMTA, which measures the response of a material to a cyclic deformation as a function of the temperature, was performed. Figure 4 shows the storage modulus E' and tan δ, which is the ratio of the loss modulus to storage modulus, as a function of temperature. The nanocomposites, with respect to the homopolymer, presented superimposable curves, with E' values slightly higher than PBS within the entire temperature range, which revealed the reinforcing role of the O/I hybrid filler upon PBS. Additionally, it highlighted an efficient interface interaction between the filler and the polymer, as well as a good state of dispersion of LDH platelets. The reinforcement effect of the fillers became more important above the glass transition temperature, when materials become soft, due to the restricted movement of the polymer chains [23]. At 20 °C, the fillers showed a medium E' enhancement of 40%, and the maximum value was related to PBS:Zn$_2$Al/PA (51%). With respect to DSC analysis, DMTA is a more sensitive technique to evaluate the glass transition temperature (T_g) (Table 2). The bionanocomposites showed higher T_g values with respect to PBS (−16.3 °C), which was due to the restriction of the movements of the macromolecular chains because of their interaction with the nanosheets of organo-modified LDH fillers.

The antibacterial properties of both O/I hybrid fillers and nanocomposites were checked against a Gram-positive bacterium, *S. aureus*, and a Gram-negative one, *E. coli*, which are potential agents of foodborne illnesses causing serious infections [15] and ubiquitous widespread bacteria [24,25] (Figure 5). The activity was calculated using Equation (1), expressed as a percentage of the reduction of viable cells in the assayed sample compared with a negative control consisting of a bacterial culture grown in the absence of any material. As a prerequisite for the whole set of experiments, reference materials (PuralMg61 and PBS) were assayed for the antimicrobial evaluation tests, showing no antibacterial effectiveness for PuralMg61 and an antimicrobial activity of 10% and 18% for PBS in the presence of *E. coli* and *S. aureus*, respectively. Hybrid LDH powders were characterized by a strong antibacterial activity (cell mortality rate = 100%) against *S. aureus* and *E. coli*. Slightly lower values were recorded for Zn$_2$Al/VA versus *S. aureus* (87%) and Zn$_2$Al/OMW (94% and 91% versus *E. coli* and *S. aureus*, respectively). In the latter case, the presence in the waste of different phenolic compounds, as well as of other substances, might have somehow interfered with the antibacterial activity, causing a slightly lower mortality with respect to the use of the pure compounds. However, the percentage of mortality was also high (>90%) with the OMW-containing samples. These results are in agreement with literature data [26–28] and confirm the strong antimicrobial activity associated with OMW phenolic compounds.

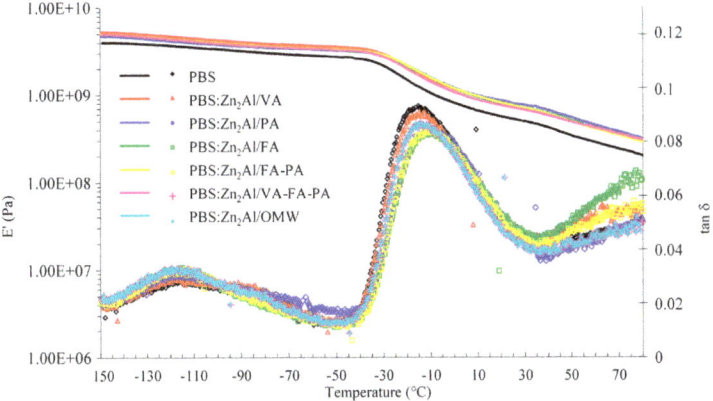

Figure 4. DMTA profiles of PBS and PBS:Zn$_2$Al/X composites.

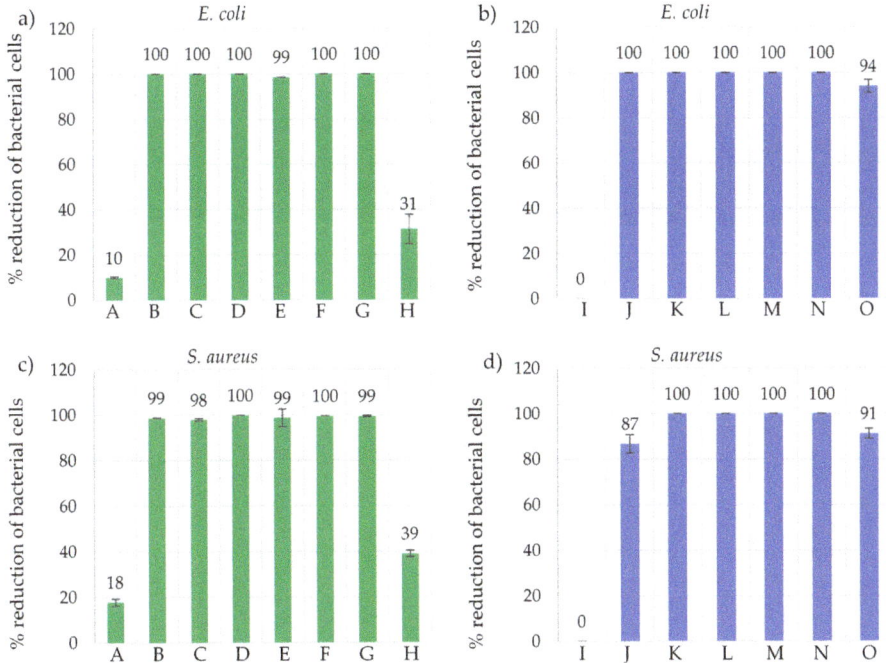

Figure 5. Antibacterial properties of PBS, PBS:FA/PA, bionanocomposites (left side), and layered double hydroxides (LDHs) (right side) against *Escherichia coli* (a,b) and *Staphylococcus aureus* (c,d). A = PBS, B = PBS:Zn$_2$Al/VA, C = PBS:Zn$_2$Al/FA, D = PBS:Zn$_2$Al/PA, E = PBS:Zn$_2$Al/FA-PA, F = PBS:Zn$_2$Al/VA-FA-PA, G = PBS:Zn$_2$Al/OMW, H = PBS:FA/PA, I = PuralMg61, J = Zn$_2$Al/VA, K = Zn$_2$Al/FA, L = Zn$_2$Al/PA, M = Zn$_2$Al/FA-PA, N = Zn$_2$Al/VA-FA-PA, and O = Zn$_2$Al/OMW.

Considering the PBS nanocomposites, the results obtained using 50 mg of each sample on 500 µL of bacterial cells (10^5 colony forming units (CFU)/mL) (Figure 5a,c) highlight that the antimicrobial activity was maintained in the final products, reaching values of 100% of mortality against *E. coli* and close to 100% against *S. aureus*. In addition, two amounts of PBS:Zn$_2$Al/OMW (50 and 10 mg) were tested using the same suspension of *E. coli* cells (500 µL), reaching in both cases a cell mortality rate of 100%. The slight differences in the antibacterial properties could be due to the different architectures of the outer layers of Gram-positive and -negative bacteria that may favor the antibacterial action of lipophilic molecules in Gram-negative cells. Indeed, *E. coli* has an extra lipopolysaccharide membrane outside a thin cell wall layer, while a thick peptidoglycan wall represents the external envelope in Gram-positive bacteria [15]. Phenols are reported both to destroy the external Gram-negative layers and to pass through this layer, thus exerting their biocidal activity in the cytoplasm [29]. Indeed, they act specifically on the cell membrane and inactivate intracytoplasm enzymes by forming unstable complexes.

On the other hand, as expected, the copolymer PBS:FA/PA did not present any significant antibacterial activity, thus highlighting the role of LDH in protecting the bioactivity of the organic modifiers during the polymerization process. Indeed, the inorganic host thermally protected the intercalated molecules, thus preserving their bioactivity.

To evaluate if such high activity in the case of the hybrid LDH materials could have been due to phenolic acids potentially released from the LDH surface into the test medium, release studies of VA (as a target bioactive molecule) from Zn$_2$Al/VA and PBS:Zn$_2$Al/VA were carried out (Figure 6). The results show a maximum release of 300 mg/L from Zn$_2$Al/VA in saline but, most importantly, a negligible release was obtained for the corresponding nanocomposite (maximum 9 mg/L). The released VA could not be responsible for the inhibitory activity against the target microorganisms, considering that the minimal inhibitory concentration (MIC) of VA is 500 mg/L versus *E. coli* (although a partial inhibition can also be seen at 300 mg/L) and higher than 500 mg/L versus *S. aureus* (i.e., higher amounts with respect to those released from the specimens (Table 3)).

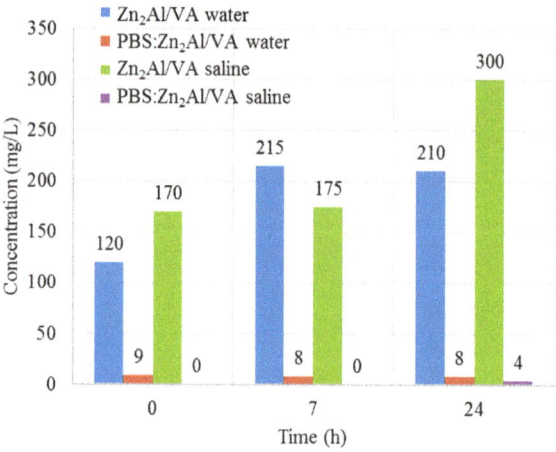

Figure 6. Concentration of vanillic acid evaluated by HPLC analyses in water or saline in which samples have been immersed.

Table 3. Minimal inhibitory concentration (MIC) of vanillic acid (taken as a target bioactive molecule) vs. *E. coli* and *S. aureus*. Strain growth is reported as turbidity in the McFarland scale. Values represent the difference between the turbidity measured after 24 h of incubation at 37 °C and that detected at the beginning of the incubation.

Vanillic Acid (mg/L)	Growth after 24 h of Incubation	
	E. coli	*S. aureus*
500	0.175 ± 0.025	1.385 ± 0.016
300	0.495 ± 0.015	3.235 ± 0.031
150	1.240 ± 0.023	3.585 ± 0.021
75	2.800 ± 0.018	4.24 ± 0.017
0	3.250 ± 0.026	4.935 ± 0.024

The potential of using OMW as an antimicrobial agent was confirmed by the data obtained with LDH and PBS nanocomposites containing the waste as it is. These results demonstrated that it is possible to obtain optimal antimicrobial performances also by using OMW without any pretreatment, potentially leading to a true recycling and valorization of this biowaste in the development of multifunctional materials.

3. Materials and Methods

3.1. Materials

BD, DMS, sodium hydroxide, aluminum nitrate $Al(NO_3)_3 \cdot 9H_2O$, zinc nitrate $Zn(NO_3)_2 \cdot 6H_2O$, VA, FA, PA, ethanol, and titanium tetrabutoxide (TBT) were purchased from Aldrich Chemical (Darmstadt, Germany). All the materials were used as received. Nutrient broth and plate count agar were from Oxoid, Basingstoke, UK. McFarland turbidity standards were from Biolife, Milano, Italy. The OMW was furnished by Sant'Agata d'Oneglia (Imperia, Italia) and concentrated prior to use: from 10 L, 1 L was obtained. Its main chemical features were: chemical oxygen demand (COD) of 43.5 ± 1.6 g/L; TOC of 4.51 ± 0.65 g GA eq/L; and total suspended solids (TSS) of 39,200 ± 4,808 mg/L.

3.2. LDH Synthesis

The LDHs were prepared by coprecipitation following a procedure described elsewhere [17] with OMW, VA, FA, and PA. Two co-intercalated LDHs with mixtures of FA + PA and VA + FA + PA were also prepared. Briefly, 50 mL of deionized water solution containing 31.2 mmol of $Zn(NO_3)_2 \cdot 6H_2O$ and 15.6 mmol of $Al(NO_3)_3 \cdot 9H_2O$ was added dropwise for 3 h in a reactor containing 62.4 mmol of the anion in 100 mL of ethanol/deionized water (60/40) under vigorous stirring. In the case of OMW, 60 mL was used. The pH was maintained at 9.5 (±0.1) through the addition of NaOH solution. The reaction was carried out under nitrogen atmosphere and stirred for 3 h at room temperature. The solid material was separated and submitted to three cycles of deionized washing/ethanol centrifugation. The samples were labeled as Zn_2Al/X, where X is the anion. A full characterization of the LDHs (X-ray diffraction, FT-IR, and TGA analysis) is reported elsewhere [17].

3.3. Bionanocomposite Preparation

Bionanocomposites with 5 wt% loading of the organo-modified LDHs were prepared by in situ polymerization following a common procedure already reported [30]. As an example, the procedure for preparing $PBS:Zn_2Al/VA$ was as follows: a round-bottomed, wide-neck glass reactor (250-mL capacity) was loaded with BD (29.6 g, 328 mmol), TBT (0.0585 g, 0.172 mmol), and 2.35 g of Zn_2Al/VA (previously dried overnight at 105 °C), corresponding to 5 wt% with respect to the polymer theoretical yield. The reactor was closed with a three-necked flat flange lid equipped with a mechanical stirrer and a torque meter which gave an indication of the viscosity of the reaction melt. The system was then connected to a water-cooled condenser and immersed in a thermostatic salt-bath at 190 °C under vigorous stirring. After 1 h, DMS (40.0 g, 274 mmol) was added and the mixture was kept at 190 °C until all the methanol distilled off. Then, the reactor was connected to a liquid-nitrogen-cooled condenser and a dynamic vacuum was applied down to 0.5 mbar while the temperature was increased up to 230 °C. When the torque of the melt was around 7–8 mN, a highly viscous, light-brown, and transparent melt was discharged from the reactor. For comparison, a PBS homopolymer was also synthesized, as well as PBS:FA/PA, without LDH with 1 wt% of FA + 1 wt% of PA. The molecular structure of PBS was confirmed by ^{1}H NMR. ^{1}H NMR on PBS:FA/PA was conducted on a purified sample.

3.4. Antibacterial Properties

The antimicrobial properties were assessed by evaluating the survival of bacterial cells exposed to the prepared samples: LDHs intercalated with phenolic acids or OMW, in order to check the antibacterial activity of the active principles, and PBS with 5 wt% LDHs, to test the efficacy of the final bionanocomposites. The two microorganisms used were E. coli ATCC 8739 and S. aureus ATCC 6538. Bacteria were grown aerobically in nutrient broth for 16 h at 37 °C. The bacterial culture obtained was centrifuged at 7000 rpm for 10 min, washed in sterile saline (0.9% w/v NaCl), and resuspended in the same solution in order to obtain ≈10^5 CFU/mL.

The experiments on both LDHs and composites were performed using 50 mg of powder of each sample, which were put in contact with 500 µL of cells (≈10^5 CFU/mL in saline) at room temperature (about 23 ± 1 °C) for 24 h. The same experiment was preliminarily done with a commercial LDH sample (PuralMg61) and a commercial PBS (i.e., with no added compounds). The composites were sieved in order to achieve a homogeneous, fine particle size. After the incubation, each sample was serially diluted (1:10) and the dilutions were plated on plate count agar. After incubation of the plates at 37 °C for 24 h, the number of colonies corresponding to the number of viable cells was determined, after averaging using triplicates, through a modification of the equation reported by Lala et al. [31]:

$$R \% = [(B-A)/B] \times 100 \qquad (1)$$

where R % is the percentage of reduction of viable cells, A is the average number of viable cells obtained after 24 h of contact with sample powders, and B is the average number of viable cells after 24 h of incubation of a bacterial cell suspension in the absence of any material. As already mentioned, the commercial powders with no added compounds were also tested for their antimicrobial activity against the same strains.

An additional experiment was carried out only on the bionanocomposite intercalated with OMW (PBS:Zn_2Al/OMW) in order to evaluate the antimicrobial activity with a less concentrated amount of sample: 10 mg of powder was put in contact with 500 µL of E. coli cells (≈10^5 CFU/mL in saline) and incubated like the previous experiment.

3.4.1. MIC of Vanillic Acid as a Target Compound

Different concentrations of vanillic acid were tested in order to evaluate the minimal concentration that inhibits the growth of E. coli and S. aureus. A stock solution of the assayed compound was prepared at a concentration of 10,000 mg/L in ethanol 70% (v/v of water). The concentrations tested were: 500, 300, 150, and 0 mg/L. Bacterial growth in the presence of vanillic acid at different concentrations was monitored by evaluating the turbidity of the culture after 24 h of incubation at 37 °C using a densitometer (DEN1-Biosan, Riga, Latvia), which evaluated turbidity using the MacFarland scale. Commercial McFarland standards (0.0–0.6 McFarland units) were used for calibrating the densitometer. The sample for MIC testing consists of 3 mL of nutrient broth, to which 100 µL of a culture grown overnight (10^8 CFU/mL) and the appropriate volume of vanillic acid from the stock solution were added. The assay was performed in duplicate.

3.4.2. Release Study

Release studies of vanillic acid from LDH and nanocomposite to the surrounding environment were conducted in water and saline on samples containing Zn_2Al/VA and the corresponding composite (50 mg/500 µL) under stirring for 24 h at room temperature. Small aliquots of the supernatants were analyzed by HPLC at 0, 8, and 24 h of incubation.

3.5. Measurements

^1H NMR spectra were recorded on a Varian Mercury 400 spectrometer (chemical shifts are in part per million downfield from tetramethylsilane; the solvent used was $CDCl_3$.

GPC measurements were performed on a HP 1100 Series using a PL gel 5-µm Minimixed-C column with chloroform as the eluent and solvent for polymer samples. A refractive index detector was used and a calibration plot was constructed with polystyrene standards.

TGA was performed in air atmosphere using a TGA7 apparatus (gas flow of 30 mL/min, Perkin Elmer, Waltham, Massachusetts, USA) at a 10 °C min^{-1} heating rate from 50 to 900 °C for all the samples. The T_{onset}, $T^{10}{}_D$, and T_{max} were measured.

DSC was carried out, under nitrogen flow, using a DSC6 (Perkin Elmer, Waltham, Massachusetts, MA, USA). To erase any previous thermal history, the samples (ca. 10 mg) were first heated at 20 °C min^{-1} to 140 °C, kept at a high temperature for 2 min, cooled down to −60 °C at 10 °C min^{-1}, and heated from −60 to 150 °C at 10 °C min^{-1} (second scan). During the cooling scan, the T_c and ΔH_c were measured. During the second heating scan, the T_g, T_m, and corresponding enthalpy (ΔH_m) were measured.

Nanocomposite powder samples were analyzed by XRD in steps of 0.07° over a 2θ range of 2.1°–35° at room temperature with a Bragg/Brentano diffractometer (XPERT-PRO, PANalytical, Royston, United Kingdom) with Cu Kα radiation (λ = 0.154 nm, monochromatization by primary graphite crystal) generated at 40 mA and 40 kV.

Physical and mechanical properties were determined using a DMTA IV Dynamic Mechanic Thermo analysis instrument (Rheometric Scientific, Reichelsheim Germany) with a dual cantilever testing geometry. Typical test samples were bars (33 mm × 8 mm × 2 mm) obtained by injection molding at 140 °C using a Minimix Molder. The analysis was carried out from −150 to 80 °C (heating rate of 3 °C min^{-1}, frequency of 3 Hz, and strain of 0.01%).

4. Conclusions

Layered double hydroxides intercalated by vanillic acid, ferulic acid, protocatechuic acid, and olive mill wastewater were dispersed in PBS through in situ polymerization. The thermal protecting role of the inorganic host towards the bioactive molecules was here confirmed. DMTA demonstrated that all the fillers endowed PBS with a pronounced reinforcing effect. In particular, the nanocomposite with Zn_2Al/PA at 20 °C displayed an elastic modulus E′ enhanced by more than 50% compared with PBS free of filler.

All the nanocomposites presented impressive antibacterial activity as well as negligible release of the active agent under the tested conditions. Therefore, these preliminary results highlight the possibility of using OMW as a potential agent to confer antimicrobial activity to nanocomposites, with an important additional value of decreasing the environmental impact of an offensive food stream. In addition, besides the pronounced antimicrobial properties, the phenolic compounds in OMW have proved to exert beneficial effects on human health: PA is reported to be an anticancer agent [32] as well as FA, which has anti-inflammatory, antiviral, and immunoprotective properties. Both molecules can inhibit cancer by scavenging reactive oxygen species or being involved in the cell cycle upon cellular uptake [33]. These points further support the use of OMW phenolic compounds for applications addressed to human health and care, taking also into account their previously demonstrated antioxidant properties [17].

Reminiscent of the use of other biowastes, such as lignosulfonated LDH blends with plasticized starch and thermoplastics [34], this could represent a general strategy that is potentially employable with other biowastes.

Author Contributions: Conceptualization, L.S. and A.C.; methodology, L.S., A.C., D.D.G., V.V., and F.L.; investigation, G.T. and N.B.C.; writing—original draft preparation, G.T.; writing—review and editing, all authors.

Funding: This research received no external funding.

Acknowledgments: The authors wish to thank Lorenzo Bertin for providing OMW and Andrea Negroni for HPLC analysis.

Conflicts of Interest: The authors declare no conflicts of interests.

References

1. El-Abbassi, A.; Saadaoui, N.; Kiai, H.; Raiti, J.; Hafidi, A. Potential applications of olive mill wastewater as biopesticide for crops protection. *Sci. Total Environ.* **2017**, *576*, 10–21. [CrossRef] [PubMed]
2. Fritsch, C.; Staebler, A.; Happel, A.; Cubero Márquez, M.A.; Aguiló-Aguayo, I.; Abadias, M.; Gallur, M.; Cigognini, I.M.; Montanari, A.; Jose López, M.; et al. Processing, Valorization and Application of Bio-Waste Derived Compounds from Potato, Tomato, Olive and Cereals: A Review. *Sustainability* **2017**, *9*, 1492. [CrossRef]
3. Scoma, A.; Pintucci, C.; Bertin, L.; Carlozzi, P.; Fava, F. Increasing the large scale feasibility of a solid phase extraction procedure for the recovery of natural antioxidants from olive mill wastewaters. *Chem. Eng. J.* **2012**, *198*, 103–109. [CrossRef]
4. Zhu, W.F.; Wang, C.L.; Ye, F.; Sun, H.P.; Ma, C.Y.; Liu, W.Y.; Feng, F.; Abe, M.; Akihisa, T.; Zhang, J. Chemical Constituents of the Seed Cake of *Camellia oleifera* and Their Antioxidant and Antimelanogenic Activities. *Chem. Biodivers.* **2018**, *15*, e1800137. [CrossRef] [PubMed]
5. Waldron, K. *Handbook of Waste Management and Co-Product Recovery in Food Processing*, 1st ed.; Woodhead Publishing Limited: Cambridge, UK, 2007; pp. 1–662.
6. Market Drivers and Development. Available online: https://www.european-bioplastics.org/market/market-drivers/ (accessed on 13 November 2018).
7. Park, D.H.; Hwang, S.J.; Oh, J.M.; Yang, J.H.; Choy, J.H. Polymer–inorganic supramolecular nanohybrids for red, white, green, and blue applications. *Prog. Polymer. Sci.* **2013**, *38*, 1442–1486. [CrossRef]
8. Rossi, C.; Schoubben, A.; Ricci, M.; Perioli, L.; Ambrogi, V.; Latterini, L.; Aloisi, G.G.; Rossi, A. Intercalation of the radical scavenger ferulic acid in hydrotalcite-like anionic clays. *Int. J. Pharm.* **2005**, *295*, 47–55. [CrossRef] [PubMed]
9. Yamada, H.; Tamura, K.; Watanabe, Y.; Iyi, N.; Morimoto, K. Geomaterials: their application to environmental remediation. *Sci. Technol. Adv. Mater.* **2011**, *12*, 064705. [CrossRef]
10. Sisti, L.; Totaro, G.; Fiorini, M.; Celli, A.; Coelho, C.; Hennous, M.; Verney, V.; Leroux, F. Poly(butylene succinate)/layered double hydroxide bionanocomposites: Relationships between chemical structure of LDH anion, delamination strategy, and final properties. *J. Appl. Polym. Sci.* **2013**, *130*, 1931–1940. [CrossRef]
11. Leroux, F.; Dalod, A.; Hennous, M.; Sisti, L.; Totaro, G.; Celli, A.; Coelho, C.; Verney, V. X-ray diffraction and rheology cross-study of polymer chain penetrating surfactant tethered layered double hydroxide resulting into intermixed structure with polypropylene, poly(butylene)succinate and poly(dimethyl)siloxane. *Appl. Clay Sci.* **2014**, *100*, 102–111. [CrossRef]
12. Totaro, G.; Sisti, L.; Celli, A.; Askanian, H.; Verney, V.; Leroux, F. Poly(butylene succinate) bionanocomposites: a novel bio-organo-modified layered double hydroxide for superior mechanical properties. *RSC Adv.* **2016**, *6*, 4780–4791. [CrossRef]
13. Totaro, G.; Sisti, L.; Celli, A.; Hennous, M.; Askanian, H.; Verney, V.; Leroux, F. Chain extender effect of 3-(4-hydroxyphenyl)propionic acid/layered double hydroxide in PBS bionanocomposites. *Europ. Polym. J.* **2017**, *94*, 20–32. [CrossRef]
14. Leroux, F.; Verney, V.; Sisti, L.; Celli, A.; Totaro, G. Organo-modified layered double hydroxides and composite polymer materials comprising same. U.S. Patent US 20180208739 A1, 26 July 2018.

15. Totaro, G.; Sisti, L.; Celli, A.; Aloisio, I.; Di Gioia, D.; Marek, A.; Verney, V.; Leroux, F. Dual chain extension effect and antibacterial properties of biomolecules interleaved within LDH dispersed into PBS by in situ polymerization. *Dalton Trans.* **2018**, *47*, 3155–3165. [CrossRef] [PubMed]
16. Marek, A.A.; Verney, V.; Totaro, G.; Sisti, L.; Celli, A.; Leroux, F. Composites for « white and green » solutions: Coupling UV resistance and chain extension effect from poly(butylene succinate) and layered double hydroxides composites. *J. Solid State Chem.* **2018**, *268*, 9–15. [CrossRef]
17. Sisti, L.; Totaro, G.; Celli, A.; Diouf-Lewis, A.; Verney, V.; Leroux, F. A new valorization route for Olive Mill wastewater: Improvement of durability of PP and PBS composites through multifunctional hybrid systems. *J. Environ. Chem. Eng.* **2019**, *7*, 103026. [CrossRef]
18. Goula, A.M.; Lazarides, H.N. Integrated processes can turn industrial food waste into valuable food by-products and/or ingredients: The cases of olive mill and pomegranate wastes. *J. Food Eng.* **2015**, *167*, 45–50. [CrossRef]
19. Totaro, G.; Sisti, L.; Vannini, M.; Marchese, P.; Tassoni, A.; Lenucci, M.S.; Lamborghini, M.; Kalia, S.; Celli, A. A new route of valorization of rice endosperm by-product: production of polymeric biocomposites. *Composites B* **2018**, *139*, 195–202. [CrossRef]
20. Jiang, L.; Zhang, J. *Biodegradable and Biobased Polymers in Applied Plastics Engineering Handbook: Processing and Materials*; Kutz, M., Andrew, W., Eds.; Elsevier: Oxford, UK, 2011.
21. Coelho, C.; Hennous, M.; Verney, V.; Leroux, F. Functionalisation of polybutylene succinate nanocomposites: From structure to reinforcement of UV-absorbing and mechanical properties. *RSC Adv.* **2012**, *2*, 5430–5438. [CrossRef]
22. Yoo, E.S.; Im, S.S. Melting Behavior of Poly(butylene succinate) during Heating Scan by DSC. *J. Polym. Sci. B Polym. Phys.* **1999**, *37*, 1357–1366. [CrossRef]
23. Pavlidou, S.; Papaspyrides, C.D. A review on polymer–layered silicate nanocomposites. *Prog. Polym. Sci.* **2008**, *33*, 1119–1198. [CrossRef]
24. Sisti, L.; Cruciani, L.; Totaro, G.; Vannini, M.; Berti, C.; Tobaldi, D.M.; Tucci, A.; Di Gioia, D.; Aloisio, I.; Commereuc, S. TiO_2 deposition on the surface of activated fluoropolymer substrate. *Thin Solid Films* **2012**, *520*, 2824–2828. [CrossRef]
25. Sisti, L.; Cruciani, L.; Totaro, G.; Vannini, M.; Berti, C.; Aloisio, I.; Di Gioia, D. Antibacterial coatings on poly(fluoroethylenepropylene) films via grafting of 3-hexadecyl-1-vinyl imidazolium bromide. *Prog. Org. Coat.* **2012**, *73*, 257–263. [CrossRef]
26. Carraro, L.; Fasolato, L.; Montemurro, F.; Martino, M.E.; Balzan, S.; Servili, M.; Novelli, E.; Cardazzo, B. Polyphenols from olive mill waste affect biofilm formation and motility in *Escherichia coli* K-12. *Microb. Biotechnol.* **2014**, *7*, 265–275. [CrossRef]
27. Yakhlef, W.; Arhab, R.; Romero, C.; Brenes, M.; de Castro, A.; Medina, E. Phenolic composition and antimicrobial activity of Algerian olive products and by-products. *LWT* **2018**, *93*, 323–328. [CrossRef]
28. Leouifoudi, I.; Harnafi, H.; Zyad, A. Olive mill waste extracts: polyphenols content, antioxidant, and antimicrobial activities. *Adv. Pharmacol. Sci.* **2015**, *2015*, 714138. [CrossRef]
29. Maris, P. Modes of action of disinfectants. *Rev. Sci. Tech. Off. Int. Epiz.* **1995**, *14*, 47–55. [CrossRef]
30. Totaro, G.; Marchese, P.; Sisti, L.; Celli, A. Use of ionic liquids based on phosphonium salts for preparing biocomposites by in situ polymerization. *J. Appl. Polym. Sci.* **2015**, *132*, 42467–42475. [CrossRef]
31. Lala, N.L.; Ramaseshan, R.; Bojun, L.; Sundarrajan, S.; Barhate, R.S.; Ying-jun, L.; Ramakrishna, S. Fabrication of nanofibers with antimicrobial functionality used as filters: protection against bacterial contaminants. *Biotechnol. Bioeng.* **2007**, *97*, 1357–1365. [CrossRef]
32. Barahuie, F.; Hussein, M.Z.; Gani, S.A.; Fakurazi, S.; Zaina, Z. Synthesis of protocatechuic acid–zinc/aluminium–layered double hydroxide nanocomposite as an anticancer nanodelivery system. *J. Solid State Chem.* **2015**, *221*, 21–31. [CrossRef]

33. Kim, H.J.; Ryu, K.; Kang, J.H.; Choi, A.J.; Kim, T.I.; Oh, J.M. Anticancer Activity of Ferulic Acid-Inorganic Nanohybrids Synthesized via Two Different Hybridization Routes, Reconstruction and Exfoliation-Reassembly. *Sci. World J.* **2013**, *2013*, 421967. [CrossRef]
34. Privas, E.; Leroux, F.; Navard, P. Preparation and properties of blends composed of lignosulfonated layered double hydroxide/plasticized starch and thermoplastics. *Carbohydr. Polym.* **2013**, *96*, 91–100. [CrossRef] [PubMed]

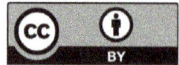

© 2019 by the authors. Licensee MDPI, Basel, Switzerland. This article is an open access article distributed under the terms and conditions of the Creative Commons Attribution (CC BY) license (http://creativecommons.org/licenses/by/4.0/).

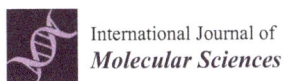

Article

Synthesis, Characterization, and Bacterial Fouling-Resistance Properties of Polyethylene Glycol-Grafted Polyurethane Elastomers

Iolanda Francolini *, Ilaria Silvestro, Valerio Di Lisio, Andrea Martinelli and Antonella Piozzi *

Department of Chemistry, Sapienza University of Rome, 00185 Rome, Italy; ilaria.silvestro@uniroma1.it (I.S.); valerio.dilisio@uniroma1.it (V.D.L.); andrea.martinelli@uniroma1.it (A.M.)
* Correspondence: iolanda.francolini@uniroma1.it (I.F.); antonella.piozzi@uniroma.it (A.P.)

Received: 25 January 2019; Accepted: 20 February 2019; Published: 25 February 2019

Abstract: Despite advances in material sciences and clinical procedures for surgical hygiene, medical device implantation still exposes patients to the risk of developing local or systemic infections. The development of efficacious antimicrobial/antifouling materials may help with addressing such an issue. In this framework, polyethylene glycol (PEG)-grafted segmented polyurethanes were synthesized, physico-chemically characterized, and evaluated with respect to their bacterial fouling-resistance properties. PEG grafting significantly altered the polymer bulk and surface properties. Specifically, the PEG-grafted polyurethanes possessed a more pronounced *hard/soft* phase segregated microstructure, which contributed to improving the mechanical resistance of the polymers. The better flexibility of the *soft* phase in the PEG-functionalized polyurethanes compared to the pristine polyurethane (PU) was presumably also responsible for the higher ability of the polymer to uptake water. Additionally, dynamic contact angle measurements evidenced phenomena of surface reorganization of the PEG-functionalized polyurethanes, presumably involving the exposition of the polar PEG chains towards water. As a consequence, *Staphylococcus epidermidis* initial adhesion onto the surface of the PEG-functionalized PU was essentially inhibited. That was not true for the pristine PU. Biofilm formation was also strongly reduced.

Keywords: segmented polyurethanes; polyethylene glycol; microbial biofilm; antifouling materials; medical device-related infections; wound dressings

1. Introduction

Polymeric materials have a prominent place in biomedical applications, due to their broad range of physico-chemical properties that can be tailored to fit a wide plethora of applications [1–3]. Segmented polyurethanes (PUs) are among the most important classes of biomedical polymers, mainly due to their excellent hemocompatibility and unique mechanical properties deriving from the presence of *hard* segment-rich and *soft* segment-rich domains in a phase-separated microstructure. Such *hard/soft*-phase segregation in the polymer permits the combination of elastomeric properties that are typical of rubbers, with high mechanical resistance properties typical of thermoplastic materials [4]. A large variety of biomedical-grade PUs with different compositions, such as Biomer®, Pellethane®, and Cardiothane, are on the market, and their applications cover mainly cardiovascular devices, including central venous catheters and heart valves, but also artificial organs, scaffolds for tissue engineering, and wound dressings [5].

Despite the benefits of using PUs for intravascular devices manufacturing, complications are still associated with their use. Especially, these materials do not protect patients from the risk of developing localized or systemic bloodstream infections [6,7]. For this reason, considerable efforts have been made over the years to improve the bacterial fouling resistance of polyurethanes, in order to reduce the incidence of bloodstream infections [8]. Traditionally, antimicrobial or antifouling polyurethanes were obtained by the adsorption/conjugation of drugs or antiseptics [9–13]. More recently, research efforts have been focused on either the use of natural compounds with anti-biofilm properties [14–17], or on the development of intrinsically antimicrobial and antifouling materials, by either physical or chemical technological approaches [17–20]. Physical approaches mainly consist of developing micro- or nano-scale surface texturing in order to affect bacterial adhesiveness, growth, and more in general, biofilm formation [21–24]. Chemical approaches, instead, mainly involve the functionalization of material surfaces, to meet some criteria that are well-recognized to confer repelling activities, which include strong hydrophilicity, neutral charge, and the presence of groups that are able to establish hydrogen bonds [25].

Polyethylene glycol (PEG) is undoubtedly, the most closely investigated antifouling polymer, as it meets all of the criteria listed above [26]. The ability of such a polymer to resist the adsorption of proteins and bacteria has been related to both hydration and steric hindrance effects [27]. Specifically, in aqueous environment, the hydration of PEG chains occurs resulting in the formation of a layer consisting of tightly bound water molecules, which acts as a physical barrier (steric repulsion) against the approach of proteins and bacteria to the polymer itself [28]. Measurements of forces of interaction between bacteria and PEG chains anchored onto glass surfaces showed that PEG brushes not only blocked the long-range attractive forces, but also introduced repulsive steric effects between the bacteria and the substrate. Presumably, the repulsive forces resulted from the compression of the highly flexible PEG chains, which would involve the removal of water molecules from the hydrated polymer, and is not a thermodynamically favorable process [29].

As for polyurethanes, PEG was either introduced in the backbone as a *soft* segment [30–32], or grafted in the polymer side chain [33,34]. Most of such PEG-containing PUs were studied in terms of bio- and hemo-compatibility properties, through the study of polymer affinity towards biomolecules such as albumin, fibrinogen, or heparin [35–39]. Only recently, a series of studies has been carried out to investigate the influence of PEG-containing PUs on microbial adhesiveness [22,40,41]. The few positive datasets available so far encourage further experimentations in order to uniquely confirm PEG as a potent antibacterial fouling agent for polyurethane surfaces.

In this study, a segmented carboxylated polyurethane, obtained by the polymerization of an aromatic di-isocianate, an ether macrodiol, and a low molecular weight diol displaying a carboxylic group, was functionalized with PEG by a Steglich esterification reaction, in order to improve polymer-antifouling abilities. Specifically, PEG was grafted onto the polymer aromatic *hard* segments, which, being hydrophobic, were supposed to be the domains that were more susceptible to bacterial colonization. We hypothesized that the reduction in the *hard* domains' hydrophobicity by PEG grafting could be a potential strategy to confer antifouling features to the polymer without changing the polymer backbone composition, neither in terms of monomer type (aliphatic vs. aromatic) nor in *hard/soft* segment ratio, which could have had a negative effect on the polymer physico-mechanical properties, as previously reported [42]. The obtained PEG-grafted PUs were fully characterized, to assess the effect of PEG-grafting on the thermal and mechanical properties of the polymer itself. Additionally, contact angle measurements and experiments with water uptake were carried out to verify the influence of the polymer bulk and surface hydrophilicity on the adhesiveness and biofilm formation of *Staphylococcus epidermidis*, a bacterial strain chosen because of its implication in the pathogenesis of intravascular device-related infections.

2. Results and Discussion

In this study, a segmented polyurethane (PEUA, Figure 1)-containing polypropylene oxide (PPO) as a *soft* phase, and the aromatic methylene bis-phenyl-diisocyanate (MDI), plus di-hydroxymethyl propionic acid (DHMPA) as a *hard* phase, were synthesized and functionalized with poly(ethylene glycol), with the aim of obtaining polymers (PEUA-PEG, Figure 1) that were resistant to bacterial adhesion. PEUA is a hemo-compatible polymer, which was synthesized for the first time by our group [43], and it contains interesting elastomeric properties and biocompatibilities. This polymer was also shown to be able to bind antibiotics [44] and complex antiseptic metal ions [45], thanks to the presence of a reactive carboxylic group per repeat unit. Such a group was now exploited for the grafting of PEG by a Steglich reaction mediated by di-cyclohexylcarbodiimide and 4-dimethylaminopyridine (DMAP) activation.

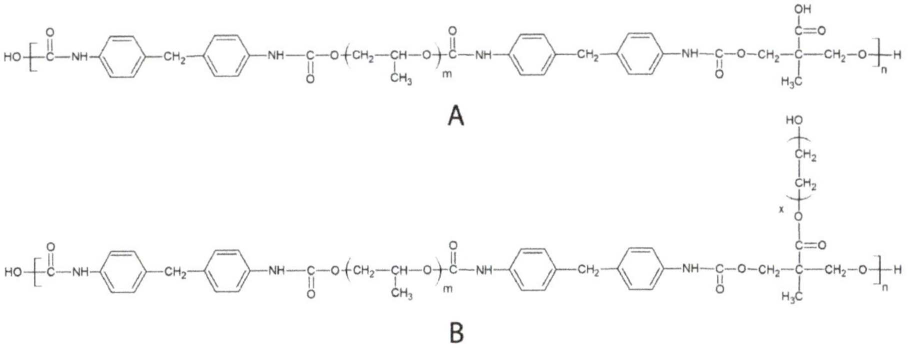

Figure 1. Chemical structure of the repeat unit of PEUA (A) and PEUA-PEG (B).

Specifically, three PEG:PEUA molar ratios (2:1, 3:1, and 5:1) were employed during synthesis, and an excess of PEG was chosen to reduce the probability of PEUA cross-linking by the bi-functional PEG. Among the three obtained PEG-functionalized polymers, the one resulting from a 2:1 PEG:PEUA molar ratio was found to be insoluble in organic solvents, and it also precipitated during functionalization, suggesting a high degree of polymer cross-linking. In contrast, a good degree of solubility in all common organic solvents (tetrahydrofurane, dimethyl formamide, and dimethyl sulfoxide) was shown by the polymer obtained from a 5:1 molar ratio while the polymer obtained with a 3:1 molar ratio showed intermediate behavior, resulting in only partial solubility in some solvents, specifically in di-methylformamide.

Nuclear magnetic resonance spectroscopy was used to evaluate the success of polymer synthesis and functionalization with PEG. In Figure 2, the ^{13}C-NMR spectra of pure PEUA and PEUA-PEG obtained with a 5:1 molar ratio are reported.

As far as the ^{13}C-NMR spectrum of PEUA is concerned, the signal at 153 ppm was attributed to the urethanic C=O, the signal at 136 ppm to MDI-C_1 and MDI-C_4, the signals at 120 ppm and 130 ppm to MDI-C_2 and MDI-C_3, respectively, and the signal at 41 ppm to the CH_2 between the phenyl groups. The signals of the PPO *soft* phase were found at 18 ppm (methyl), 77 ppm (methine) and 73–75 ppm (methylene). The signals of DHMPA were at 46 ppm (quaternary carbon), 72 ppm (–CH_2–), and ca. 20 ppm (–CH_3). Finally, at 175 ppm, the signal of the carboxylic group was observed. As far as the ^{13}C-NMR spectrum of PEUA-PEG is concerned, even if it was not possible to observe the peak related to the ester C=O, a new signal at 62 ppm was present, specifically the ester CH_2 of the linked PEG. Additionally, the peak of the DHMPA quaternary carbon shifted from 46 ppm to 50 ppm, presumably due to the different chemical environments.

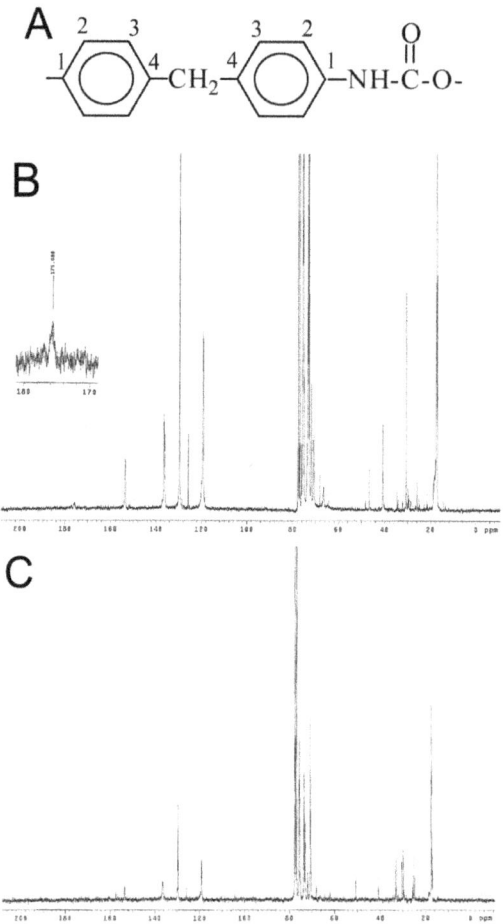

Figure 2. Numeration of methylene bis-phenyl-diisocyanate (MDI) carbons in PEUA (**A**); ^{13}C-NMR spectrum of PEUA (**B**) and PEUA-PEG obtained with a 5:1 PEG:PEUA molar ratio (**C**). In the inset of B, the magnification of the signal at 175 ppm, attributed to the PEUA carboxylic group, is reported.

In Figure 3A, the ^{1}H-NMR spectrum of PEUA is reported. The peaks at 9.6 and 10 ppm were attributed to urethane (NH), and the signal splitting was presumably due to the different linkers (PPO or DHMPA). The signals in the range of 7–8.0 ppm were attributed to the MDI aromatic ring, and the signal at 3.8 ppm was related to –CH$_2$– between the two phenyls. The PPO methine and methylene groups showed a wide peak at 3.4 ppm when linked to the ether oxygen, and at 4.9 ppm when linked to the urethane NH. The signal at 3.5 ppm was attributed to the DHMPA methylene groups while the signal at 1.1 ppm was related to the methyl groups of DHMPA and PPO.

The signals of the PEG –CH$_2$– groups in PEUA-PEG are in the same spectral range (ca. 3.6 ppm) as the protons of PPO (Figure 3B). The yield of functionalization was calculated by the ratio of the intensity of the peak at 7 ppm (aromatic ring), and that of the peak at 3.6 ppm (methylene groups), from which the contribution of PPO was subtracted. The resulting yield of esterification was ca. 30% in the case of the polymer obtained with a 5:1 PEG:PEUA molar ratio, and 20% for the soluble portion of the polymer obtained with a 3:1 molar ratio.

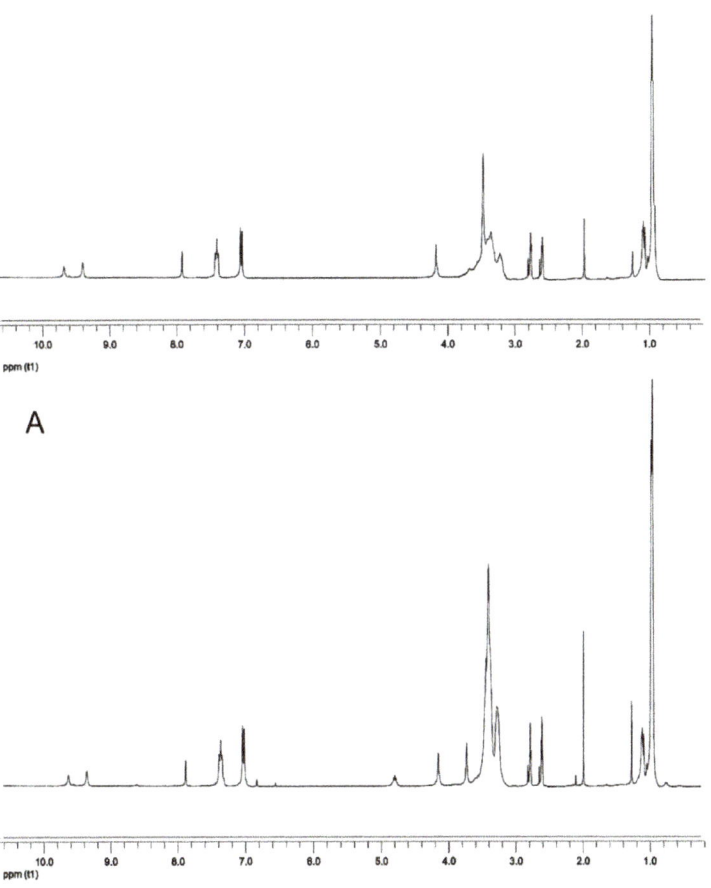

Figure 3. ^{1}H-NMR spectrum of PEUA (**A**) and PEUA-PEG obtained with a 5:1 PEG:PEUA molar ratio (**B**).

In segmented polyurethanes, differential scanning calorimetry can allow for not only the determination of the polymer transition temperatures, but also the estimation of polymer *hard/soft* phase segregation. Specifically, information on polymer phase segregation can be extrapolated by the glass transition temperature (T_g), which, being characteristic of the *soft* phase of the polymer, depends on the *soft* phase mobility, and is affected by the interaction of the *soft* phase with the *hard* phase. An increase in the T_g value usually suggests low mobility of the *soft* phase, as a consequence of an increase in *hard/soft* phase mixing [46]. In Figure 4, as an example, the thermograms of PEUA and PEUA-PEG$_{30}$ in cycles I and II of heating are reported, while in Table 1, the values of the glass transition temperature, and the variation of the specific heat (ΔC_p) at T_g for all of the polymers are reported. The T_g value of free PPO, found in the literature [47], is also reported in Table 1 for comparison.

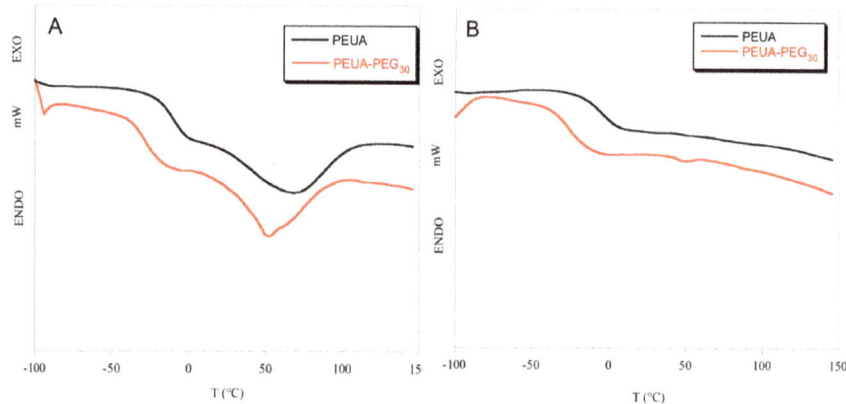

Figure 4. Thermograms of PEUA and PEUA-PEG$_{30}$ in the I cycle (**A**) and the II cycle (**B**) of heating.

In the first cycle of heating, a flex, corresponding to the glass transition of the *soft* phase, and a broad endothermic band, corresponding to the melting of *hard* microdomains, can be observed in the thermograms of all polymers. Such an endothermic transition was no longer observable in the II cycle of heating. The T$_g$ values of the PEG-functionalized polyurethanes were similar and lower than that of PEUA (Table 1). That suggests a greater phase segregation in the PEG-functionalized polyurethanes, compared to pristine PEUA. Presumably, PEG chains introduced in the *hard* phase of PEUA favored the cohesion of the *hard* domains by hindering the establishment of H-bonds among the urethane –NH groups of the *hard* phase and the ether oxygens of the *soft* phase. Additionally, some cross-linking between the polymer *hard* segments could occur, and further contribute to the segregation of the PEG-functionalized polymers. The variation in specific heat in correspondence with glass transition is also lower in the PEG-functionalized polymers compared to PEUA (Table 1), suggesting that a lower amount of the *soft* phase is involved in the glass transition. Presumably, a higher cohesion of the *hard* micro-domains, or the partial cross-linking of *hard* segments in the PEG-functionalized polymers can reduce the amount of the mobile portion of the *soft* phase. Such a phenomenon has already been described in the literature for segmented polyurethanes functionalized with carboxylate or sulfonate ions [48].

Table 1. Glass transition temperature (T$_g$) and variation of specific heat (ΔC_p) at the glass transition temperature for PEUA and PEG-functionalized polyurethanes. The glass transition temperature of the free *soft* phase (PPO) is also reported, for comparison. $^{(*)}$ The subscript indicates that the PEUA:PEG molar ratio employed during functionalization. Indeed, it was not possible to determine the functionalization degree for this polymer, as it is insoluble in common solvents.

Polymer	T$_g$ (°C)	ΔC_p (J/g*K)
PEUA	−11 ± 2	0.50 ± 0.02
PEUA-PEG$_{1:2}$ $^{(*)}$	−33 ± 2	0.39 ± 0.02
PEUA-PEG$_{20}$	−29 ± 2	0.40 ± 0.03
PEUA-PEG$_{30}$	−27 ± 2	0.43 ± 0.03
Soft phase (PPO)	−67	-

In Figure 5, the thermogravimetric curves of the pristine and functionalized polymers are reported. The first derivative of the weight vs. temperature is also reported. As it can be observed, PEUA-PEG$_{1:2}$ (obtained with a PEG:PEUA molar ratio 2:1) was the most thermally stable polymer, presumably because of the higher crosslinking content. Pristine PEUA degraded mainly in one step from 250 to 400 °C, while the PEG-functionalized polymers showed two steps of degradation. The first one was attributed to PEG weight loss, and the second one to the degradation of the polyurethane backbone. By taking into consideration the weight of the PEUA repeat unit, a good agreement between the PEG weight loss and the 30% esterification yield determined by ^{1}H-NMR was found for PEUA-PEG$_{30}$. That was not true for PEUA-PEG$_{20}$, presumably because of the chemical heterogeneity between the polymer soluble portion submitted to ^{1}H-NMR, and the whole-polymer sample (soluble portion + insoluble portion) submitted to thermogravimetric analysis.

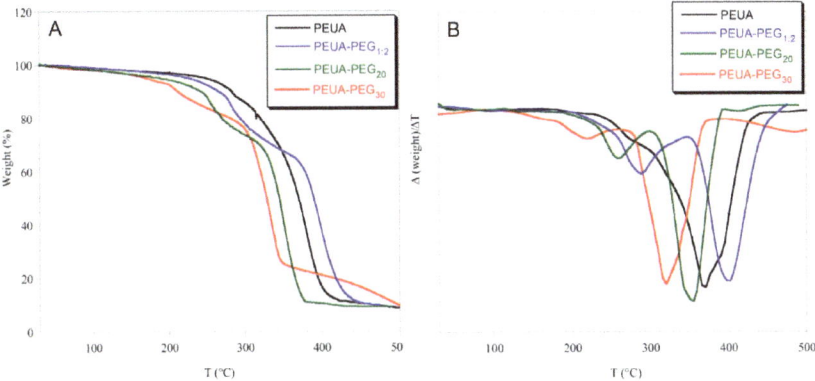

Figure 5. Thermogravimetric curves of PEUA, PEUA-PEG$_{1:2}$, PEUA-PEG$_{20}$, and PEUA-PEG$_{30}$ (**A**); first derivative (Δ(weight)/ΔT) of the thermogravimetric curves (**B**). The subscript 1:2 on PEUA:PEG$_{1:2}$ indicates the molar ratio employed during functionalization.

Material surface hydrophilicity/hydrophobicity is a very important feature that affects bacterial adhesion to the material itself. In general, it has been recently shown that superhydrophobic and superhydrophilic surfaces can both prevent microbial adhesion [49]. Superhydrophobic surfaces are those resembling the lotus leaf, which has been shown to have a water contact angle that is higher than 150°, and self-cleaning properties, thanks to its hierarchical micro/nanostructured surface covered with a low surface energy waxy hydrophobic film [50]. On the other side, very hydrophilic surfaces have intrinsic antifouling properties, due to the formation of a dense layer of water molecules, which weakens the interaction between the bacterial cell surface and the material surface [29,51].

To evaluate the effect of PEG-grafting on polymer hydrophilicity, polymer swelling in water and the dynamic contact angle were evaluated. Since these analyses, as well as the subsequent mechanical and biological tests, were performed on polymer films obtained by solvent casting (see Experimental Section), only the soluble polymers PEUA and PEUA-PEG$_{30}$ will be subsequently characterized.

In Figure 6A, the swelling curves for the two polymers are reported.

As it can be observed, PEUA-PEG$_{30}$ was more strongly hydrophilic than PEUA, reaching a swelling degree at an equilibrium of ca. 150%, compared to ca. 25% of PEUA. Such a big increase in polymer hydrophilicity after PEUA functionalization with PEG is surely due to the PEG intrinsic hydrophilic properties, but presumably also to the good *hard/soft* phase segregation of PEUA-PEG$_{30}$, which makes the polymer *soft* phase free to move and interact with water molecules. This hypothesis was confirmed by the calculation of the Diffusion Coefficient (D) of water in each of the two polymeric matrices. Specifically, in a diffusional regime in which the Fick's first law is valid, D can be calculated by the following equation [52]: $\frac{W_t}{W_{tot}^{\infty}} = \frac{4t^{1/2}D^{1/2}}{L\pi^{1/2}}$ where W_{eq} is the amount of water adsorbed at the equilibrium, W_t is the amount of water that is adsorbed at the specific time t, and L is the polymer film thickness (which was assumed to be constant during swelling). This expression describing the transport behavior of the penetrant into the polymer can be applied only to the initial stages of swelling, i.e., up to a 60 % increase in the mass of the polymer ($W_t/W_{eq.} \leq 0.6$) [53]. The values of D were obtained from the plot of the ratio of the swollen polymer mass at time t, and t = eq. (W_t/W_{eq}), as a function of the ratio of the square root of time ($t^{1/2}$), by following the initial slope method (Figure 6B). The following D values were extrapolated: $D_{PEUA} = (1.7 \pm 0.1) \times 10^{-9}$ cm$^2 \cdot$s^{-1}, and $D_{PEUA-PEG30} = (5.0 \pm 0.2) \times 10^{-9}$ cm$^2 \cdot$s^{-1}. The higher D value of water in PEUA-PEG$_{30}$ compared to PEUA suggests a higher ability of water molecules to diffuse into the polymer matrix, presumably due to a higher mobility of the hydrophilic *soft* phase achieved by the higher polymer *hard/soft* phase segregation.

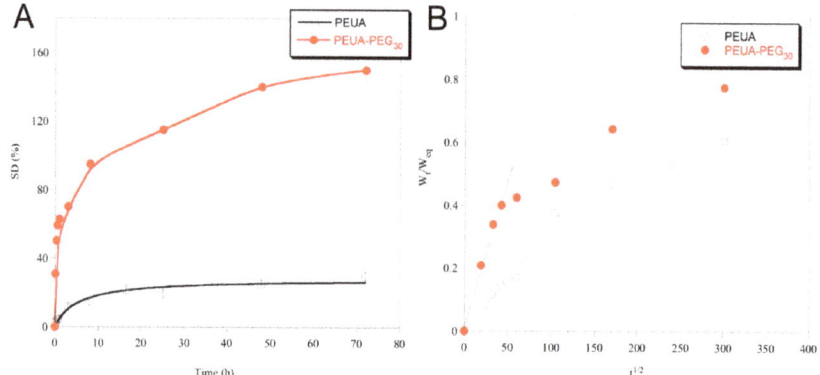

Figure 6. Swelling curves of PEUA and PEUA-PEG$_{30}$ (**A**); Ratio between the swollen polymer mass at time t, and at the equilibrium (W_t/W_{eq}), as a function of the ratio of the square root of time (**B**). The diffusion coefficient was extrapolated by the slope of the linear fitting of the initial points.

Measurements of dynamic contact angle confirmed the higher hydrophilicity of PEUA-PEG$_{30}$, compared to PEUA. In such an analysis, the surface hydrophilicity (or wettability) can be evaluated [54]. In Figure 7, as an example, the profile of the two immersion cycles for PEUA-PEG$_{30}$ is shown, and in Table 2, the values of the contact angles, in advancing and in receding, and the contact angle hysteresis, are reported. As observed in Table 2, in the first cycle of immersion, the two polymers showed similar θ_{av}, suggesting a similar wettability. However, PEUA-PEG$_{30}$ showed a significantly lower θ_{rec} than PEUA (35 ° vs. 47 °) and, as a consequence, a higher hysteresis.

Such a finding is presumably related to the surface chemical heterogeneity of PEUA-PEG$_{30}$ (greater than PEUA). Additionally, in the second immersion cycle, PEUA-PEG$_{30}$ showed a kinetic contact angle hysteresis, evidenced by the decrease of θ_{adv} from 94 ° to 83 °, suggesting a molecular rearrangement of the polymer surface on wetting, which presumably involved the exposition of the polar PEG chains towards water.

Langmuir firstly observed the flipping of the surfactant molecules, as polar head groups migrated towards hydrophilic environments [55]. It was, later demonstrated that such re-organization was driven by the minimization of the surface free energy at the interface [56].

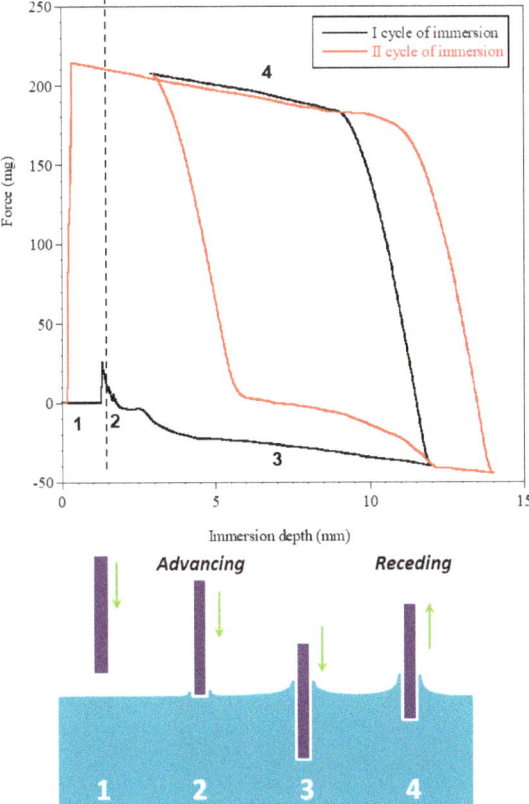

Figure 7. DCA cycles of immersion for PEUA-PEG$_{30}$ by using the Wilhelmy plate method. In the figure, numbers 1 to 4 indicate the position of the plate with respect to the liquid, as shown in the image below the figure. 1—Out of the liquid; 2—point of touch of the sample with the liquid; 3—Immersion into the liquid (θ_{adv}); 4—Emersion from the liquid (θ_{rec}).

Table 2. Contact angle values (θ_{adv} and θ_{rec}) and hysteresis (H) for PEUA and PEUA-PEG$_{30}$ in the first and second cycles of immersion.

Polymer	I cycle		II cycle		H (I cycle)	H (II cycle)
	Θ_{adv}	Θ_{rec}	Θ_{adv}	Θ_{rec}		
PEUA	93 ± 3	47 ± 3	92 ± 1	50 ± 3	46	42
PEUA-PEG$_{30}$	94 ± 2	35 ± 3	83 ± 2	37 ± 1	59	46

The two polymers also showed significantly different mechanical properties, as shown by INSTRON analysis. In Figure 8, the stress–strain curves of PEUA and PEUA-PEG$_{30}$ are reported.

As it can be observed, both polymers showed an elongation at a break of ca. 10. The Young Modulus, determined from the slope of the initial linear trend, was also similar for the two polymers (E_{PEUA} = 0.9 MPa e $E_{PEUA-PEG30}$ = 0.7 MPa). However, the trend of the two stress–strain curves was very different. Indeed, PEUA showed a Yield Point at an elongation of ca. 0.7, in correspondence with which a collapse of the material resistance was observed. In contrast, PEUA-PEG$_{30}$ showed a typical trend of elastomeric materials, in which the Yield Point was not really clear, and the stress increased with the elongation up to material break. The stress at break of PEUA-PEG$_{30}$ (0.5 MPa) is also ca. one order of magnitude higher than that of PEUA (0.06 MPa). Overall, the mechanical properties of PEUA-PEG$_{30}$ are coherent, with a marked *hard/soft* phase segregation in this polymer as evidenced by DSC analysis. Presumably, the presence of strong chain–chain interactions hinders chain slippage, and make the material resistant to big deformations. In addition, the occurrence of chemical cross-linkages between the *hard* segments cannot be excluded, even if the solubility of the sample suggests a case of low cross-linking. Of course, if present, *hard–hard* segment cross-linkages can further justify the elastomeric properties of the polymer.

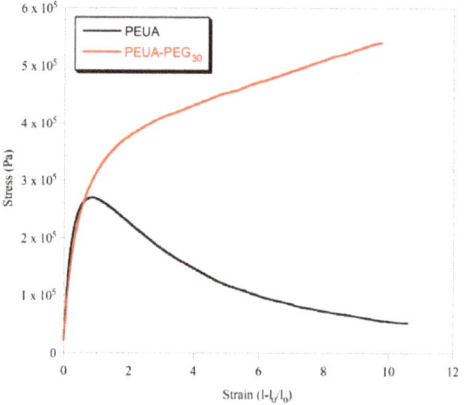

Figure 8. Stress-strain curves of PEUA and PEUA-PEG$_{30}$.

Finally, the abilities of PEUA and PEUA-PEG$_{30}$ to prevent microbial adhesion and biofilm formation was evaluated. In Figure 9, SEM micrographs showing the surface of PEUA and PEUA-PEG$_{30}$ after 30 min (Figure 9A,B) or 24 hr (Figure 9C,D) incubation with *S. epidermidis* suspensions are reported.

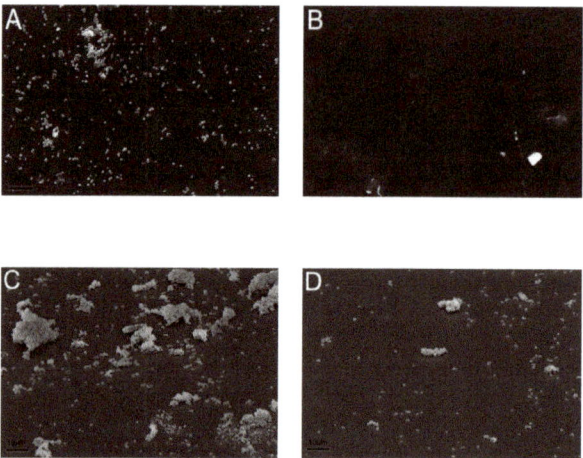

Figure 9. Initial bacterial adhesion after 30 min incubation on PEUA (**A**) and PEUA-PEG$_{30}$ (**B**). Biofilm formation after 24 h incubation on PEUA (**C**) and PEUA-PEG$_{30}$ (**D**). Scale bar = 10 µm.

As it can be noted, *S. epidermidis* can easily adhere to PEUA. Indeed, the presence of *S. epidermidis* colonies in the first stages of adhesion could be observed on the PEUA surface (Figure 9A). In contrast, PEUA-PEG$_{30}$ was essentially free from colonization (Figure 9B). Such different initial bacterial adhesion rates were reflected in the biofilm formations on the two polymer surfaces.

Indeed, heavy colonization of the PEUA surface was observed with the presence of large biofilm structures (Figure 9C) after 24 h incubation, while just a few sporadic adhering cells and small bacterial aggregates were present on PEUA-PEG$_{30}$ (Figure 9D). Such difference in biofilm formation was confirmed by the cell count, the number of CFU per surface unit (CFU/cm^2) being 4×10^8 and 7×10^5 for PEUA and PEUA-PEG$_{30}$, respectively.

The excellent ability of PEUA-PEG$_{30}$ to reduce bacterial adhesion and biofilm formation is definitely related to its higher bulk and surface hydrophilicity which also presumably involve the exposition of PEG chains at the material/water interface, as shown by dynamic contact angle analysis. However, since the polymer does not completely inhibit bacterial adhesion, such a system should be used in combination with other anti-biofilm molecules, to maximize its performance [15,57,58]. Unexpectedly, the mechanical resistance of the PEG-functionalized polymer also improved because the presence of PEG, with benefits for the application.

3. Materials and Methods

3.1. Materials

Polyethylene glycol (PEG, M$_n$ = 1000 g/mol) (Sigma Aldrich s.r.l., Milan, Italy) was used as received. Methylene bis-phenyl-diisocyanate (MDI) (Sigma Aldrich s.r.l.) was distilled before use. Polypropylene oxide (PPO) (1200 g·mol^{-1}, Sigma Aldrich s.r.l.) was degassed under vacuum at 60 °C for 12 h. Di-hydroxymethyl propionic acid (DHMPA) (Sigma Aldrich s.r.l.), dicyclohexylcarbodiimide (DCC) (Sigma Aldrich s.r.l.) and 4-dimethylaminopyridine (DMAP) (Sigma Aldrich s.r.l.) were used as received.

3.2. Polymer Synthesis and Functionalization

A carboxylated segmented polyurethane, PEUA (one carboxyl group per repetitive unit, Mw = 40,000 g·mol^{-1}, M$_w$/M$_n$ = 1.6, Figure 1) was synthesized by a two-step condensation of MDI, PPO, and DHMPA in a 2:1:1 stoichiometric ratio, as previously described [43].

Functionalization of PEUA with PEG was achieved by a DCC-activated esterification of polymer carboxylic acids, by using DMAP as an accelerator [59]. Specifically, DMAP and DCC, in equimolecular amounts with respect to the polymer carboxyl groups, were added to a 5% (w/v) solution of PEUA in dichloromethane at 0 °C. After 20 min, PEG was added in molar excess (2:1, 3:1 and 5:1) with respect to PEUA to avoid polymer crosslinking. Temperature was then raised to 25 °C and the solution was left under stirring for 24 h. After the reaction, dicyclohexylurea precipitate during polymer functionalization was filtered. Then, the polymer was recovered by precipitation in hexane, and washed in water to eliminate the unreacted PEG. The polymer, whose repetitive unit is reported in Figure 1, was named PEUA-PEG$_X$, where x is the functionalization degree.

3.3. Polymer Characterization

^{1}H-NMR and ^{13}C-NMR spectra were performed, employing a Varian XL 300 instrument (Varian Inc., Palo Alto, CA, USA) and deuterated di-methylformamide (DMF-d7) as the solvent.

Differential scanning calorimetry (DSC) was performed from −100 to +150 °C under N$_2$ flux by using a Mettler TA-3000 DSC apparatus (Mettler Toledo, Columbus, Ohio, US). The scan rate used for the experiments was 10 °C·min^{-1} and the sample weight was 6–7 mg. Thermo-gravimetric analysis (TGA) was carried out employing a Mettler TG 50 thermobalance at a heating rate of 10 °C·min^{-1} under N$_2$ flow in the temperature range 25–600 °C.

Swelling measurements of both the pristine and functionalized polyurethanes were performed at room temperature in water. For such experiments, circular test samples (1 cm in diameter and 100 µm in thickness) were obtained by cutting cast films of the polymers. Polymer films were obtained by dissolving the polymer in tetrahydrofuran (5% w/v) and layering such a solution on circular Teflon plates, 5 cm in diameter. After solvent evaporation at room temperature, polymer films were detached from the Teflon plates with the aid of tweezers. The polyurethane samples were then immersed in water. At the determined times, specimens were removed from the water and weighed, after removal of the excess of the solvent using filter paper. The analysis was repeated until a constant weight (equilibrium swelling) was reached. The swelling degree, SD, was calculated by applying the following equation:

$$SD\ (\%) = \frac{W_t - W_0}{W_0}$$

where W_t is the weight of the sample after swelling at time t, and W_0 was the initial weight of the film. Five parallel swelling experiments were performed for each sample, and data were reported as the average value ± standard deviation.

The dynamic contact angle was performed by using a Dynamic Contact Angle Analyzer Cahn DCA 312 (CAHN Instruments, Inc., South Carmenita Road, Cerritos, CA, USA), on the basis of the Wilhelmy balance method. Such a method consists of detecting by a balance the change in the weight of a thin vertical plate when it is brought in contact with a liquid. The detected weight change is a combination of the buoyancy and the wetting force, while the gravity force remains the same. Since the wetting force (F_w) is defined as:

$$F_w = \gamma_{lv}\ p\ \cos\theta$$

where γ_{lv} is the liquid surface tension, p is the perimeter of the sample, and θ is the contact angle, the force change (F) detected by the balance is:

$$F = \gamma_{lv}\ p\ \cos\theta - V\Delta\rho\ g$$

where V is the volume of the displaced liquid, $\Delta\rho$ is the difference in density between the liquid and air, and g is the acceleration of gravity. Thus, as long as γ_{lv} and the solid perimeter (p) are known, the contact angle value can be determined.

Contact angle measurements were performed with an immersion rate of 20 μm/s, carrying out two consecutive immersion cycles. In the second immersion cycle, the immerged area of the sample was greater than that of the first cycle, in order to verify the absence of the release of substances from the sample into water. The analyses were performed on samples obtained by layering the polymer on rectangular glass coverslide (1 cm × 2 cm) by solvent casting. When the sample was immersed into the liquid, the advancing contact angle (θ_{adv}) was recorded, while when the sample was emerging, the receding contact angle (θ_{rec}) was measured (Figure 8). The difference between the advancing and the receding angles is called the contact angle hysteresis (H = $\theta_{adv} - \theta_{rec}$), which mainly arises from surface roughness and/or chemical heterogeneity [60]. However, other factors, including liquid adsorption and retention, or molecular rearrangement on wetting, can contribute to hysteresis [61].

The mechanical properties of the pristine and functionalized polyurethanes were studied by tensile tests, which were carried out with an ISTRON 4502 instrument (Instorn Inc., Norwood, MA, USA). Measurements were performed on rectangular polymer films (50 mm long × 6 wide × 0.2 thick), by employing a 10 N load cell and a deformation rate of 50 mm·min^{-1}.

3.4. Bacterial Strains and Culture Medium

For an evaluation of the antifouling features of polymers, the oxacillin-resistant *Staphylococcus epidermidis* ATCC 35984, a strong exopolysaccharide producer [62], was routinely grown in tryptic soy agar (TSA) and tryptic soy broth (TSB). Biofilm production was assessed according to the protocol described by Francolini et al. [63].

3.5. Assessment of the Polymer Ability to Prevent Bacterial Adhesion and Biofilm Formation

To evaluate the effect of polyurethanes on bacterial adhesion and biofilm formation, test tubes were filled with 2.5 mL of a bacterial suspension (0.5 McFarland) and grown at 37 °C in TSB supplemented with 1% glucose, to promote massive exopolysaccharide production. One tube was used as a reference (control), while polymer discs (1 cm in diameter, 100 µm in thickness) were introduced into the other tubes. Tubes were incubated at 37 °C for 30 min to assess early bacterial adhesion, or for 24 h to assess late bacterial adhesion [64,65].

After incubation, bacterial adhesion and biofilm formation were assessed by scanning electron microscopy (SEM, Assing, Rome, Italy). Specifically, polymer discs were collected, washed twice with PBS (pH 7.4) to remove loosely adherent cells, fixed with 2.5% glutaraldehyde in 0.1 M cacodylate buffer (pH 7.4) at room temperature for 30 min, dehydrated through graded ethanol, treated with hexamethyldisilazane for 20 min, and gold-sputtered for SEM observation.

Polymer discs incubated with bacterial suspension for 24 h (biofilm formation) were also submitted to colony forming unit (CFU) counts. Specifically, disks were put into test tubes with 10 mL of phosphate buffer, and sonicated for 5 min to remove the adherent cells. Six 10-fold dilutions were prepared, and three 10 µL aliquots of each dilution were plated onto TSA plates. Plates were then incubated at 37 °C for 18 h, and CFUs were counted and referred to the polymer surface unit (CFUs/cm^2).

3.6. Statistics

Analysis of variance comparisons were performed using Mini-Tab. Differences were considered significant for $p < 0.05$. Data are reported as means $\pm$ SD.

4. Conclusions

This study confirms the strong antifouling ability of polyethylene glycol materials, and shows the great potential for PEG-grafting to confer bacterial resistance properties to segmented polyurethanes. Indeed, the functionalization of a thermoplastic polyurethane with PEG resulted in a material with superior elastomeric properties, and the ability to prevent the adhesion of the Gram-positive *S. epidermidis*, a microbial pathogen that is commonly isolated in medical device-related infections. Additionally, since the developed antifouling material is intrinsically active, it does not exhaust its activity over time, and it could provide long-term protection, at least in principle. Under an applicative point of view, the PEG-functionalized polyurethane obtained in this study could find a role in several biomedical applications, spanning from intravascular medical device manufacturing to wound dressings, where it could be applied as an antifouling coating, or incorporated within the bulk structure.

Author Contributions: Conceptualization, I.F. and A.P.; Methodology I.F., A.M. and A.P.; Formal Analysis, I.S. and V.D.L., Investigation, I.S. and V.D.L.; Data Curation, A.M. and V.D.L.; Writing—Original Draft Preparation, I.F.; Writing—Review & Editing, A.P.; Funding Acquisition, I.F. and A.P.

Funding: This research was funded by Sapienza University of Rome, through a grant to I.F.

Acknowledgments: The authors would like to thank Sapienza University for funding the research.

Conflicts of Interest: The authors declare no conflict of interest.

References

1. Shin, E.J.; Choi, S.M. Advances in Waterborne Polyurethane-Based Biomaterials for Biomedical Applications. *Adv. Exp. Med. Biol.* **2018**, *1077*, 251–283. [PubMed]
2. Guelcher, S.A. Biodegradable polyurethanes: Synthesis and applications in regenerative medicine. *Tissue Eng. Part B Rev.* **2008**, *14*, 3–17. [CrossRef] [PubMed]
3. Burke, A.; Hasirci, N. Polyurethanes in biomedical applications. *Adv. Exp. Med. Biol.* **2004**, *553*, 83–101. [PubMed]
4. Piozzi, A.; Francolini, I. Biomimetic polyurethanes. In *Polymeric Materials with Antimicrobial Activity from Synthesis to Applications*, 1st ed.; Muñoz-Bonilla, A., Cerrada, M., Fernández-García, M., Eds.; RSC Publishing: Cambridge, UK, 2014; pp. 224–264.

5. Zdrahala, R.J.; Zdrahala, I.J. Biomedical applications of polyurethanes: A review of past promises, present realities, and a vibrant future. *J. Biomater. Appl.* **1999**, *14*, 67–90. [CrossRef]
6. Bell, T.; O'Grady, N.P. Prevention of Central Line-Associated Bloodstream Infections. *Infect. Dis. Clin. N. Am.* **2017**, *31*, 551–559. [CrossRef] [PubMed]
7. Seckold, T.; Walker, S.; Dwyer, T. A comparison of silicone and polyurethane PICC lines and post-insertion complication rates: A systematic review. *J. Vasc. Access* **2015**, *16*, 167–177. [CrossRef] [PubMed]
8. Francolini, I.; Piozzi, A. Antimicrobial polyurethanes for intravascular medical devices. In *Advances in Polyurethane Biomaterials*; Cooper, S.L., Guan, J., Eds.; Woodhead Publishing (Elsevier Ltd.): Sawston, UK, 2016; Chapter 12; pp. 349–385.
9. Sheng, W.H.; Ko, W.J.; Wang, J.T.; Chang, S.C.; Hsueh, P.R.; Luh, K.T. Evaluation of antiseptic-impregnated central venous catheters for prevention of catheter-related infection in intensive care unit patients. *Diagn. Microbiol. Infect. Dis.* **2000**, *38*, 1–5. [CrossRef]
10. Yorganci, K.; Krepel, C.; Weigelt, J.A.; Edmiston, C.E. In vitro evaluation of the antibacterial activity of three different central venous catheters against gram-positive bacteria. *Eur. J. Clin. Microbiol. Infect. Dis.* **2002**, *21*, 379–384. [PubMed]
11. Donelli, G.; Francolini, I.; Ruggeri, V.; Guaglianone, E.; D'Ilario, L.; Piozzi, A. Pore formers promoted release of an antifungal drug from functionalized polyurethanes to inhibit Candida colonization. *J. Appl. Microbiol.* **2006**, *100*, 615–622. [CrossRef] [PubMed]
12. Nowatzki, P.J.; Koepsel, R.R.; Stoodley, P.; Min, K.; Harper, A.; Murata, H.; Donfack, J.; Hortelano, E.R.; Ehrlich, G.D.; Russell, A.J. Salicylic acid-releasing polyurethane acrylate polymers as anti-biofilm urological catheter coatings. *Acta Biomater.* **2012**, *8*, 1869–1880. [CrossRef] [PubMed]
13. Francolini, I.; Donelli, G.; Crisante, F.; Taresco, V.; Piozzi, A. Antimicrobial polymers for anti-biofilm medical devices: State-of-art and perspectives. *Adv. Exp. Med. Biol.* **2015**, *831*, 93–117. [PubMed]
14. Huang, K.S.; Yang, C.H.; Huang, S.L.; Chen, C.Y.; Lu, Y.Y.; Lin, Y.S. Recent Advances in Antimicrobial Polymers: A Mini-Review. *Int. J. Mol. Sci.* **2016**, *17*, 1578. [CrossRef] [PubMed]
15. Cattò, C.; Villa, F.; Cappitelli, F. Recent progress in bio-inspired biofilm-resistant polymeric surfaces. *Crit. Rev. Microbiol.* **2018**, *44*, 633–652. [CrossRef] [PubMed]
16. Adlhart, C.; Verran, J.; Azevedo, N.F.; Olmez, H.; Keinänen-Toivola, M.M.; Gouveia, I.; Melo, L.F.; Crijns, F. Surface modifications for antimicrobial effects in the healthcare setting: A critical overview. *J. Hosp. Infect.* **2018**, *99*, 239–249. [CrossRef] [PubMed]
17. Muñoz-Bonilla, A.; Fernández-García, M. Polymeric materials with antimicrobial activity. *Prog. Polym. Sci.* **2012**, *37*, 281–339. [CrossRef]
18. Campoccia, D.; Montanaro, L.; Arciola, C.R. A review of the biomaterials technologies for infection-resistant surfaces. *Biomaterials* **2013**, *34*, 8533–8554. [CrossRef] [PubMed]
19. Francolini, I.; Vuotto, C.; Piozzi, A.; Donelli, G. Antifouling and antimicrobial biomaterials: An overview. *APMIS* **2017**, *125*, 392–417. [CrossRef] [PubMed]
20. Carmona-Ribeiro, A.M.; de Melo Carrasco, L.D. Cationic antimicrobial polymers and their assemblies. *Int. J. Mol. Sci.* **2013**, *14*, 9906–9946. [CrossRef] [PubMed]
21. Vargas-Alfredo, N.; Rodríguez Hernández, J. Microstructured polymer blend surfaces produced by spraying functional copolymers and their blends. *Materials* **2016**, *9*, 431. [CrossRef] [PubMed]
22. Xu, L.C.; Siedlecki, C.A. Protein adsorption, platelet adhesion, and bacterial adhesion to polyethylene-glycol-textured polyurethane biomaterial surfaces. *J. Biomed. Mater. Res. B Appl. Biomater.* **2017**, *105*, 668–678. [CrossRef] [PubMed]
23. Mendez, A.R.; Tan, T.Y.; Low, H.Y.; Otto, K.H.; Tan, H.; Khoo, X. Micro-textured films for reducing microbial colonization in a clinical setting. *J. Hosp. Infect.* **2018**, *98*, 83–89. [CrossRef] [PubMed]
24. Vargas-Alfredo, N.; Martínez-Campos, E.; Santos-Coquillat, A.; Dorronsoro, A.; Cortajarena, A.L.; Del Campo, A.; Rodríguez-Hernández, J. Fabrication of biocompatible and efficient antimicrobial porous polymer surfaces by the Breath Figures approach. *J. Colloid Interface Sci.* **2018**, *513*, 820–830. [CrossRef] [PubMed]
25. Ostuni, E.; Chapman, R.G.; Holmlin, E.; Takayama, S.; Whitesides, G.M. A survey of structure-property relationships of surfaces that resist the adsorption of protein. *Langmuir* **2001**, *17*, 5605–5620. [CrossRef]
26. Desai, N.P.; Hossainya, S.F.A.; Hubbell, J.A. Surface-immobilized polyethylene oxide for bacterial repellence. *Biomaterials* **1992**, *13*, 417–420. [CrossRef]

27. Chen, S.F.; Li, L.Y.; Zhao, C.; Zheng, J. Surface hydration: Principles and applications toward low-fouling/nonfouling biomaterials. *Polymer* **2010**, *51*, 5283–5293. [CrossRef]
28. Jeon, S.I.; Lee, J.H.; Andrade, J.D.; De Gennes, P.G. Protein-surface interactions in the presence of polyethylene oxide ii. Effect of protein size. *J. Colloid Interface Sci.* **1991**, *142*, 159–166. [CrossRef]
29. Razatos, A.; Ong, Y.; Boulay, F.; Elbert, D.L.; Hubbell, J.A.; Sharma, M.M.; Georgiou, G. Force measurements between bacteria and poly(ethylene glycol)-coated surfaces. *Langmuir* **2000**, *16*, 9155–9158. [CrossRef]
30. Corneillie, S.; Lan, P.N.; Schacht, E.; Davies, M.; Shard, A.; Green, R.; Denyer, S.; Wassall, M.; Whitfield, H.; Choong, S. Polyethylene glycol-containing polyurethanes for biomedical applications. *Polym. Int.* **1998**, *46*, 251–259. [CrossRef]
31. Chen, X.; Liu, W.; Zhao, Y.; Jiang, L.; Xu, H.; Yang, X. Preparation and characterization of PEG-modified polyurethane pressure-sensitive adhesives for transdermal drug delivery. *Drug Dev. Ind. Pharm.* **2009**, *35*, 704–711. [CrossRef] [PubMed]
32. Rana, S.; Lee, S.Y.; Cho, J.W. Synthesis and characterization of biocompatible poly(ethylene glycol)-functionalized polyurethane using click chemistry. *Polym. Bull.* **2010**, *64*, 401–411. [CrossRef]
33. Orban, J.M.; Chapman, T.M.; Wagner, W.R.; Jankowski, R. Easily grafted polyurethanes with reactive main chain functional groups. Synthesis, characterization, and antithrombogenicity of poly(ethylene glycol)-grafted poly(urethanes). *J. Polym. Sci. A Polym. Chem.* **1999**, *37*, 3441–3448. [CrossRef]
34. Park, K.D.; Suzuki, K.; Lee, W.K.; Lee, J.E.; Kim, Y.H.; Sakurai, Y.; Okano, T. Platelet adhesion and activation on polyethylene glycol modified polyurethane surfaces. Measurement of cytoplasmic calcium. *ASAIO J.* **1996**, *42*, M876–M880. [CrossRef] [PubMed]
35. Han, D.K.; Park, K.; Park, K.D.; Ahn, K.D.; Kim, Y.H. In vivo biocompatibility of sulfonated PEO-grafted polyurethanes for polymer heart valve and vascular graft. *Artif. Organs* **2006**, *30*, 955–959. [CrossRef] [PubMed]
36. Chen, H.; Hu, X.; Zhang, Y.; Li, D.; Wu, Z.; Zhang, T. Effect of chain density and conformation on protein adsorption at PEG-grafted polyurethane surfaces. *Colloids Surf. B Biointerfaces* **2008**, *61*, 237–243. [CrossRef] [PubMed]
37. Choi, H.S.; Suh, H.; Lee, J.H.; Park, S.N.; Shin, S.H.; Kim, Y.H.; Chung, S.M.; Kim, H.K.; Lim, J.Y.; Kim, H.S. A polyethylene glycol grafted bi-layered polyurethane scaffold: Preliminary study of a new candidate prosthesis for repair of a partial tracheal defect. *Eur. Arch. Oto-Rhino-Laryngol.* **2008**, *265*, 809–816. [CrossRef] [PubMed]
38. Rao, L.; Zhou, H.; Li, T.; Li, C.; Duan, Y.Y. Polyethylene glycol-containing polyurethane hydrogel coatings for improving the biocompatibility of neural electrodes. *Acta Biomater.* **2012**, *8*, 2233–2242. [CrossRef] [PubMed]
39. Mei, T.; Zhu, Y.; Ma, T.; He, T.; Li, L.; Wei, C.; Xu, K. Synthesis, characterization, and biocompatibility of alternating block polyurethanes based on PLA and PEG. *J. Biomed. Mater. Res. A* **2014**, *102*, 3243–3254. [CrossRef] [PubMed]
40. Park, J.H.; Cho, Y.W.; Kwon, I.C.; Jeong, S.Y.; Bae, Y.H. Assessment of PEO/PTMO multiblock copolymer/segmented polyurethane blends as coating materials for urinary catheters: In vitro bacterial adhesion and encrustation behavior. *Biomaterials* **2002**, *23*, 3991–4000. [CrossRef]
41. Patel, J.D.; Ebert, M.; Ward, R.; Anderson, J.M. S. epidermidis biofilm formation: Effects of biomaterial surface chemistry and serum proteins. *J. Biomed. Mater. Res. A* **2007**, *80*, 742–751. [CrossRef] [PubMed]
42. Francolini, I.; Donelli, G.; Vuotto, C.; Baroncini, F.A.; Stoodley, P.; Taresco, V.; Martinelli, A.; D'Ilario, L.; Piozzi, A. Antifouling polyurethanes to fight device-related staphylococcal infections: Synthesis, characterization, and antibiofilm efficacy. *Pathog. Dis.* **2014**, *70*, 401–407. [CrossRef] [PubMed]
43. Marconi, W.; Martinelli, A.; Piozzi, A.; Zane, D. Direct synthesis of carboxylated polyurethanes. *Europ. Polymer. J.* **1991**, *27*, 135–139. [CrossRef]
44. Piozzi, A.; Francolini, I.; Occhiaperti, L.; Di Rosa, R.; Ruggeri, V.; Donelli, G. Polyurethanes loaded with antibiotics: Influence of polymer-antibiotic interactions on in vitro activity against *Staphylococcus epidermidis*. *J. Chemother.* **2004**, *16*, 446–452. [CrossRef] [PubMed]
45. Francolini, I.; Ruggeri, V.; Martinelli, A.; D'Ilario, L.; Piozzi, A. Novel metal-polyurethane complexes with enhanced antimicrobial activity. *Macromol. Rapid. Commun.* **2006**, *27*, 233–237. [CrossRef]
46. Schneider, N.S.; Sung, C.S.P. Transition behavior and phase segregation in TDI polyurethanes. *Polym. Eng. Sci.* **1977**, *17*, 73–80. [CrossRef]

47. Faucheris, J.A. The dependence of glass transition temperature on molecular weight for poly(propylene oxide) and poly(butylene oxide). *Polym. Lett.* **1965**, *3*, 143–145. [CrossRef]
48. Okkema, A.Z.; Cooper, S.L. The effect of carboxylate and/or sulfonate ions on phase segregation in polyurethanes. *Biomaterials* **1991**, *12*, 668. [CrossRef]
49. Song, F.; Koo, H.; Ren, D. Effects of material properties on bacterial adhesion and biofilm formation. *J. Dent. Res.* **2015**, *94*, 1027–1034. [CrossRef] [PubMed]
50. Zhang, X.; Wang, L.; Levanen, E. Superhydrophobic surfaces for the reduction of bacterial adhesion. *RSC Adv.* **2013**, *3*, 12003–12020. [CrossRef]
51. Ko, J.; Cho, K.; Han, S.W.; Sung, H.K.; Baek, S.W.; Koh, W.G.; Yoon, J.S. Hydrophilic surface modification of poly(methyl methacrylate)-based ocular prostheses using poly(ethylene glycol) grafting. *Colloids Surf. B Biointerfaces* **2017**, *158*, 287–294. [CrossRef] [PubMed]
52. Pissis, P.; Apekis, L.; Christodoulides, C.; Niaounakis, M.; Kyritsis, A.; Nebdal, J. Water effects in polyurethane block copolymers. *J. Polym. Sci. Part B Polym. Phys.* **1996**, *34*, 1529–1539. [CrossRef]
53. Ritger, P.L.; Peppas, N.A. A simple equation for description of solute release. II Fickian and anomalous release from swellable devices. *J. Control. Release* **1987**, *5*, 37–42. [CrossRef]
54. Wang, C.; Nair, S.; Wynne, K.J. Wilhelmy balance characterization beyond contact angles: Differentiating leaching from nanosurface reorganization and optimizing surface modification. *Polymer* **2017**, *116*, 565–571. [CrossRef]
55. Blodgett, K.B.; Langmuir, I. Built-up films of barium stearate and their optical properties. *Phys. Rev.* **1937**, *51*, 964–982. [CrossRef]
56. Kaganer, V.M.; Mohwald, H.; Dutta, P. Structure and phase transitions in Langmuir monolayers. *Rev. Mod. Phys.* **1999**, *71*, 779–819.
57. Grassi, L.; Maisetta, G.; Esin, S.; Batoni, G. Combination strategies to enhance the efficacy antimicrobial peptides against bacterial biofilms. *Front. Microbiol.* **2017**, *8*, 2409. [CrossRef] [PubMed]
58. Blanchette, K.A.; Wenke, J.C. Current therapies in treatment and prevention of fracture wound biofilms: Why a multifaceted approach is essential for resolving persistent infections. *J. Bone Jt. Infect.* **2018**, *3*, 50–67. [CrossRef] [PubMed]
59. Neises, B.; Steglich, W. Simple method for the esterification of carboxylic acids. *Angew. Chem.* **1978**, *7*, 522–524. [CrossRef]
60. Long, J.; Hyder, M.N.; Huang, R.Y.M.; Chen, P. Thermodynamic modeling of contact angles on rough, heterogeneous surfaces. *Adv. Colloid Interface Sci.* **2005**, *118*, 173–190. [CrossRef] [PubMed]
61. De Gennes, P.G. Wetting: Statics and dynamics. *Rev. Mod. Phys.* **1985**, *57*, 827–863. [CrossRef]
62. Donelli, G.; Francolini, I.; Romoli, D.; Guaglianone, E.; Piozzi, A.; Ragunath, C.; Kaplan, J.B. Synergistic activity of dispersin B and cefamandole nafate in inhibition of staphylococcal biofilm growth on polyurethanes. *Antimicrob. Agents Chemother.* **2007**, *51*, 2733–2740. [CrossRef] [PubMed]
63. Francolini, I.; Piozzi, A.; Donelli, G. Efficacy evaluation of antimicrobial drug-releasing polymer matrices. In *Microbial Biofilms*; Humana Press: New York, NY, USA, 2014; Volume 1147, pp. 215–225.
64. Merritt, J.H.; Kadouri, D.E.; O'Toole, G.A. Growing and analyzing static biofilms. *Curr. Protoc. Microbiol.* **2005**, *22*. [CrossRef]
65. Azeredo, J.; Azevedo, N.F.; Briandet, R.; Cerca, N.; Coenye, T.; Costa, A.R.; Desvaux, M.; Di Bonaventura, G.; Hébraud, M.; Jaglic, Z.; et al. Critical review on biofilm methods. *Crit. Rev. Microbiol.* **2017**, *43*, 313–351. [CrossRef] [PubMed]

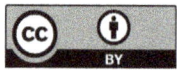

© 2019 by the authors. Licensee MDPI, Basel, Switzerland. This article is an open access article distributed under the terms and conditions of the Creative Commons Attribution (CC BY) license (http://creativecommons.org/licenses/by/4.0/).

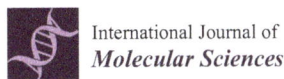

Article

α-Chymotrypsin Immobilized on a Low-Density Polyethylene Surface Successfully Weakens *Escherichia coli* Biofilm Formation

Cristina Cattò [1], Francesco Secundo [2], Garth James [3], Federica Villa [1] and Francesca Cappitelli [1,*]

[1] Department of Food, Environmental and Nutritional Sciences, Università degli Studi di Milano, Milano 20133, Italy; cristina.catto@unimi.it (C.C.); federica.villa@unimi.it (F.V.)
[2] Institute of Chemistry of Molecular Recognition, National Research Council, Milano 20131, Italy; francesco.secundo@icrm.cnr.it
[3] Center for Biofilm Engineering, Montana State University, Bozeman, MT 59717, USA; gjames@montana.edu
* Correspondence: francesca.cappitelli@unimi.it; Tel.: +39-02-5031-9121

Received: 5 November 2018; Accepted: 10 December 2018; Published: 12 December 2018

Abstract: The protease α-chymotrypsin (α-CT) was covalently immobilized on a low-density polyethylene (LDPE) surface, providing a new non-leaching material (LDPE-α-CT) able to preserve surfaces from biofilm growth over a long working timescale. The immobilized enzyme showed a transesterification activity of 1.24 nmol/h, confirming that the immobilization protocol did not negatively affect α-CT activity. Plate count viability assays, as well as confocal laser scanner microscopy (CLSM) analysis, showed that LDPE-α-CT significantly impacts *Escherichia coli* biofilm formation by (i) reducing the number of adhered cells ($-70.7 \pm 5.0\%$); (ii) significantly affecting biofilm thickness ($-81.8 \pm 16.7\%$), roughness ($-13.8 \pm 2.8\%$), substratum coverage ($-63.1 \pm 1.8\%$), and surface to bio-volume ratio ($+7.1 \pm 0.2$-fold); and (iii) decreasing the matrix polysaccharide bio-volume ($80.2 \pm 23.2\%$). Additionally, CLSM images showed a destabilized biofilm with many cells dispersing from it. Notably, biofilm stained for live and dead cells confirmed that the reduction in the biomass was achieved by a mechanism that did not affect bacterial viability, reducing the chances for the evolution of resistant strains.

Keywords: biofilm; anti-biofilm surface; surface functionalization; α-chymotrypsin; proteinase

1. Introduction

The main strategy for limiting bacterial loading in medical and industrial settings relies on regular cleaning and disinfection treatments aimed at killing the microbial cells on solid surfaces [1]. The incorporation of disinfectants, antiseptics, antibiotics, and metallic nanoparticles into several materials has also been proposed as a strategy to minimize pathogen growth on surfaces [2–5]. However, these strategies have shown limited efficacy and recurrent drawbacks, making their use questionable [2,6].

The major concern lies in the property of bacteria to coexist in a protective self-produced extracellular matrix within an extremely coordinated and structured surface-adhered community, known as biofilm [7]. It has been established that antibiotic overuse also triggers increased multidrug resistance in many microbial taxa [8,9]. Biofilms display high tolerance to antimicrobial agents as a result of the matrix itself, which acts as a protective barrier, and because of the reduced metabolic rate of bacteria and the presence of some dormant cells highly tolerant to a variety of drugs [10]. Additionally, most antimicrobial-releasing materials have shown a discontinuous release rate and short-term efficiency, typically no longer than 24 h, which make them less suitable for long-term applications [11,12].

In the last decade, researchers have concentrated their attention on approaches involving mechanisms of action that do not affect microbial life, including those that sabotage the biofilm lifestyle in a non-toxic way, and with modalities that decrease the selection pressure for drug-resistant mutations [13]. A straightforward approach is to target the biofilm matrix. Indeed, the deployment of enzymes that degrade the polymers that make up the biofilm matrix have been proposed as an effective approach to impact biofilm architecture while still preserving cell integrity [14]. Since a biofilm matrix encases bacterial cells within the biofilm colony, matrix degradation results in the destabilization of the biofilm organization and its physical integrity [15]. Therefore, the biofilm multicellular structure is compromised with a modality that does not affect cellular functions crucial for microbial survival [14]. For example, glycosidases as well as proteases or deoxyribonuclease have been reported to degrade bacterial matrix [16–19].

Despite these promising results, the real application of these molecules has been less feasible due to the lack of a suitable technology for efficiently retaining the anti-biofilm enzyme over a working timescale. Indeed, until now, attention has been mainly focused on the activity of enzymes in solution or as coatings. In addition, most of the effects studied occur during the initial surface attachment phase, which only partially involves matrix production by cells [13].

In the present work, the protease α-chymotrypsin (α-CT) was covalently immobilized on a low-density polyethylene (LDPE) surface to provide a new non-leaching material able to preserve surfaces from biofilm growth over a long working timescale. Immobilization makes enzymes more robust and more resistant to environmental changes in comparison to the counterpart free in solution [20]. More importantly, the heterogeneity of the immobilized enzyme systems allows continuous operation of enzymatic processes and rapid reactions [20]. As this strategy does not act by killing cells, it does not impose a selective pressure that would cause the onset of resistance [21]. Additionally, as the multicellularity of the biofilm is compromised, the planktonic state might be forced, restoring the efficacy of antimicrobial agents [22]. Notably, in this paper the anti-biofilm activity of immobilized enzymes was tested using a high-level and realistic approach by setting up an *Escherichia coli* laboratory-scale model system able to simulate the real conditions encountered in vivo, and provides information about the new material effect on the structure of a well-established mature biofilm [23].

2. Results

2.1. Immobilized α-CT Retains Its Activity

The possibility to link enzymes to plastics (e.g., polypropylene and polyethylene) was previously shown by our team [24]. The procedure indicates that the preventive plasma treatment of the surface is crucial for providing the plastic surface with functional groups exploitable for the covalent binding of the enzyme to the surface by glutaraldehyde (GA). Herein, on the basis of these previously reported results obtained with different proteases, α-CT immobilization was carried out by submitting LDPE coupons to a plasma treatment for 30 min and using GA as a linker. After washing (no leaching was observed on placing the coupons in water before their use) and drying, LDPE-α-CT showed transesterification activity in toluene of 1.24 nmol/h. Enzyme activity was measured in organic solvent as, in the immobilized form, the enzyme catalyzes the reaction in an insoluble form (heterogeneous solid/liquid catalysis), i.e., in the presence of mass transfer limitation conditions [25]. In this physical condition, the enzyme activity tested in organic solvent gave more reproducible results with respect to the methods carried out in aqueous media.

2.2. LDPE-α-CT Reduces Biofilm Biomass

Experiments showed that LDPE-α-CT had an optimal anti-biofilm performance, reducing viable adhered cells by 70.7 ± 5.0% in comparison to the LDPE control surface (Figure 1). Significant differences were also detected among the negative control samples, namely LDPE and

LDPE-GA (Figure 1). Indeed, the number of adhered cells on LDPE-GA was 31.0 ± 5.8% lower than those attached on LDPE.

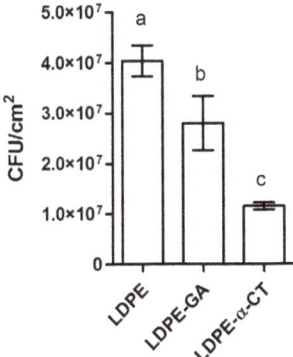

Figure 1. Biomass within the biofilm grown on non-functionalized (low-density polyethylene (LDPE) and LDPE-glutaraldehyde (GA)) and functionalized polyethylene surfaces (LDPE-α-chymotrypsin (α-CT)) by plate count viability assay. Data represent the mean ± standard deviation of four independent measurements. Letters a, b and c indicate significant differences (Tukey's honest significant different (HSD) test, $p \leq 0.05$) between the means of different surfaces.

2.3. LDPE-α-CT Reduces Biofilm Biomass without Affecting Cell Viability

Epifluorescence microscopic techniques were additionally used to provide image analysis and in situ quantification of bacterial cells. Figure 2 shows direct microscope visualizations of the total biofilm biomass on functionalized and non-functionalized coupons, stained for live and dead cells.

Microscope assay revealed that the biofilm displayed a number of dead cells lower than 1.9 ± 1.1%, with no significant differences in the percentage of stained area between the LDPE and LDPE-GA surfaces, whereas a lower number of dead cells were found on LDPE-α-CT (Figure 2) (dead cells: LDPE: 1.9 ± 1.1%; LDPE-GA: 1.3 ± 1.1%; LDPE-α-CT: 0.7 ± 0.5%).

Biofilm on LDPE-α-CT showed a decreased number of live cells compared to the LDPE control surface, by up to 66.4 ± 11.0%, confirming results obtained in the plate count viability assay (Figure 2) (live cells: LDPE: 73.0 ± 14.1%; LDPE-α-CT: 24.5 ± 6.6%). A reduction of 23.9 ± 2.9% in the percentage of live cells on LDPE-GA compared to LDPE cells was also detected (live cells: LDPE-GA: 56.2 ± 7.0%) (Figure 2).

Statistical analysis of relative viability revealed no significant difference between LDPE, LDPE-GA, and LDPE-α-CT materials (relative viability: LDPE: 39.3 ± 15.5; LDPE-GA: 42.6 ± 7.5; LDPE-α-CT: 36.3 ± 4.8).

Coupons without biofilm and stained with the same dye did not produce detectable fluorescence, therefore no false positive signals were produced (Figure 2E).

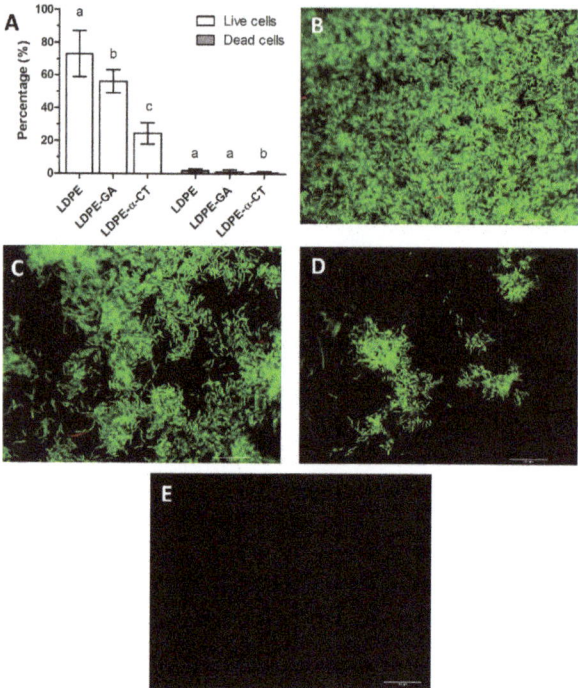

Figure 2. Epifluorescence microscope analysis. (**A**) Percentage of live and dead cells within the biofilm grown on non-functionalized (LDPE and LDPE-GA) and functionalized polyethylene surfaces (LDPE-α-CT). Data represent the mean ± standard deviation of four independent measurements. Letters a, b and c indicate significant differences (Tukey's HSD, $p \leq 0.05$) between the means of different surfaces. (**B–D**) Representative epifluorescence microscope images of *E. coli* biofilm stained with a Live/Dead BacLight viability kit and grown on LDPE (**B**), LDPE-GA (**C**), and LDPE-α-CT (**D**) surfaces (60×, 1.0 NA water immersion objective). Green fluorescence corresponds to *E. coli* live cells (λ_{ex}: 480 nm and λ_{em}: 516 nm) and red fluorescence corresponds to *E. coli* dead cells (λ_{ex}: 581 nm and λ_{em}: 644 nm). (**E**) Representative epifluorescence microscope image of LDPE, LDPE-GA, and LDPE-α-CT without biofilm and stained with a Live/Dead BacLight viability kit showing no detectable fluorescence. Scale bar = 20 µm.

2.4. LDPE-α-CT Affect Biofilm Morphology

Biofilm morphology was assessed by confocal laser scanner microscopy (CSLM) after staining with SYBR Green I and Texas Red-labeled concanavalin A. Projection analysis as well as three-dimensionally (3D) reconstructed CLSM images showed a complex biofilm on the LDPE biofilm with an intense red and green signal corresponding to multi-layers of cells (green signal) organized in macro-colonies inside a well-structured polysaccharide matrix (red signal) (Figure 3A–C). Interestingly, cells were mostly located at the bottom of the biofilm, in contact with the surface, whereas the matrix was generally found over the cellular component. On the contrary, biofilm growth on LDPE-α-CT resulted in a significant decrease of thickness with a mono-layer of dispersed cells and very low presence of polysaccharide matrix (Figure 2B–D). In addition, there were many cells dispersing from the biofilm.

No detectable fluorescence was observed when coupons without biofilm were stained with the same dyes, indicating that false positive signals were not produced (Figure 3E).

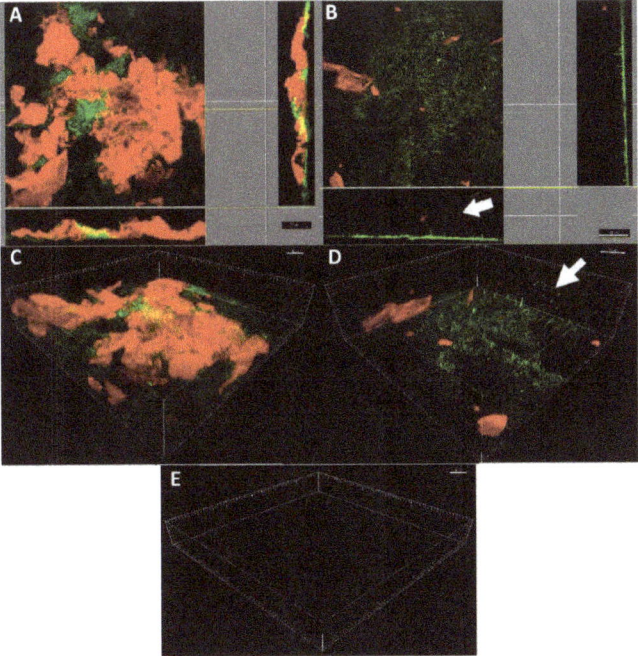

Figure 3. Confocal laser scanning microscopy analysis. Representative projection analysis (**A**,**B**) and three-dimensionally (3D) reconstructed CLSM images (**C**,**D**) of *E. coli* biofilm grown on non-functionalized LDPE surface (**A**,**C**) and LDPE-α-CT (**B**,**D**) functionalized surface (63×, 0.9 NA water immersion objective). The arrows indicate cells detaching from the biofilm. Live cells were stained green with SYBR Green I (λ_{ex} at 488 nm, λ_{em} at 520 nm), whereas the polysaccharide matrix was stained red with Texas Red-labeled concanavalin A (ConA) (λ_{ex} at 543 nm, λ_{em} at 615 nm). (**E**) Representative 3D reconstructed CLSM images of LDPE and LDPE-α-CT without biofilm and stained with SYBR Green I or Texas Red-labeled ConA showing no detectable fluorescence. Scale bar = 20, 30, or 40 µm.

Table 1 provides the morphological parameters of biofilm grown on LDPE, LDPE-GA, and LDPE-α-CT. CLSM image analysis showed that the biofilm grown on LDPE and LDPE-GA control surfaces reached about 20 µm in thickness. On the contrary, the biofilm on LDPE-α-CT displayed a thickness below 4 µm, with a decrease of up to 81.8 ± 16.7% with respect to the biofilm grown on LDPE. Additionally, biofilm roughness was slightly decreased in both LDPE-GA (−13.8 ± 1.7%) and LDPE-α-CT (−13.8 ± 2.8%), indicating a more uniform biofilm layer in comparison to the control LDPE biofilm. On LDPE-α-CT, the substratum covered by biofilm was significantly lower (−63.1 ± 1.8%) than that in the corresponding non-functionalized LDPE. Interestingly, a small reduction in the substratum coverage was also recorded for the biofilm grown on LDPE-GA (−13.8 ± 1.7%). Total bio-volume of the biofilm grown on LDPE-α-CT was found to be significantly decreased compared to both LDPE and LDPE-GA biofilms, with a reduction of up to the 78.0 ± 16.1% in comparison to the LDPE control surface. Indeed, LDPE-α-CT exhibited a reduced cellular bio-volume by 71.7 ± 3.4% and a reduced polysaccharide matrix bio-volume by 80.2 ± 23.2% compared to the LDPE surface. Additionally, a statistically significant reduction in the cellular bio-volume was found in the biofilm grown on LDPE-GA compared to that grown on LDPE (−21.8 ± 1.0%). The matrix/cell bio-volume ratio always displayed a value over 1.9 with no statistically significant differences among surfaces, which indicates a predominance of matrix with respect to the cellular component. The biofilm exposed surface/bio-volume ratio significantly increased when biofilm was grown on LDPE-α-CT

(7.1 ± 0.2-fold) whereas no significant differences were detected between biofilms grown on LDPE and LDPE-GA.

Table 1. Biofilm morphological parameters of biofilm grown on non-functionalized (LDPE, LDPE-GA) and functionalized polyethylene surfaces (LDPE-α-CT). In the brackets, percentage reduction/increase in comparison to the LDPE control sample is reported when significant. Data represent the mean ± standard deviation of four independent measurements.

Parameter	LDPE	LDPE-GA	LDPE-α-CT
Thickness (μm)	20.5 ± 5.0 [a]	19.1 ± 4.9 [a]	3.7 ± 1.1 [b] (−81.8 ± 16.7)
Roughness	0.25 ± 0.03 [a]	0.22 ± 0.02 [b] (−11.1 ± 1.0)	0.21 ± 0.04 [b] (−13.8 ± 2.8)
Substratum coverage (%)	72.3 ± 3.8 [a]	62.3 ± 1.2 [b] (−13.8 ± 1.7)	26.7 ± 1.3 [c] (−63.1 ± 1.8)
Total bio-volume ($\mu m^3\, \mu m^{-2}$)	89.4 ± 20.1 [a]	76.3 ± 21.2 [a]	19.7 ± 4.1 [b] (−78.0 ± 16.1)
Cells bio-volume ($\mu m^3\, \mu m^{-2}$)	23.7 ± 4.0 [a]	18.5 ± 0.9 [b] (−21.8 ± 1.0)	6.7 ± 0.3 [c] (−71.7 ± 3.4)
Polysaccharide matrix bio-volume ($\mu m^3\, \mu m^{-2}$)	65.8 ± 7.8 [a]	57.8 ± 14.9 [a]	13.0 ± 3.8 [b] (−80.2 ± 23.2)
Matrix/cells bio-volume ratio	2.8 ± 0.6 [a]	3.1 ± 0.8 [a]	1.9 ± 0.5 [a]
Surface/bio-volume ($\mu m^2\, \mu m^{-3}$) × 10^{-2}	1.1 ± 0.3 [a]	1.3 ± 0.4 [a]	8.7 ± 1.7 [b] (+7.8 ± 1.6-fold)

Superscript letters a, b and c indicate significant differences (Tukey's HSD, $p \leq 0.05$) between the means of different surfaces.

3. Discussion

In this study, the protease α-CT was covalently and irreversibly immobilized on an LDPE surface to provide a new material with anti-biofilm properties. LDPE was chosen as it is a polymer with excellent chemical resistance, low wetting properties in aqueous media, high impact strength, light weight, and high flexibility [26,27] and is currently used for many applications, e.g., biomedical devices [28] and food packaging [29].

Among others (e.g., subtilisin Carlsberg from *Bacillus licheniformis*, lipase from *Burkholderia cepacia* or pectinase from *Aspergillus niger*), α-CT was preferred as, in a previous work by these authors, this enzyme showed the highest transesterification activity once immobilized with GA [24,30]. Notably, the same authors observed an increase in the catalytic activity of α-CT after treatment with GA [31]. In addition, several studies confirmed the ability of α-CT to limit biofilm formation on solid surfaces, both free-in-solution treatment as well as in coatings [32–37].

Beside the previously promising results, the use of the free enzyme has drawbacks resulting from sensitivity to process conditions, low stability, or propensity to be inhibited by other molecules. Indeed, applications are limited by the lack of long-term operational stability and the technical challenge of enzyme recovery and reuse [38]. Additionally, enzyme coatings suffer decreased activity as degradation of the coating quickly occurs [39].

Compared to the enzyme used free in solution as well as in coatings, chemical immobilization ensures the retention of the catalytic activity, which allows the enzyme to be used repeatedly and continuously, as well as confining the protease activity where biofilm formation occurs [30,38]. Indeed, the nature of the covalent binding guarantees the long life of the material since molecules are permanently attached and integrated into the polymer scaffold structure [40], preserving the surrounding environment from enzyme contamination. This is especially useful in those fields where chemical contamination in the final product must be avoided for safety reasons, e.g., in food contact processing surfaces [41]. In addition, immobilization enhances the enzyme stability under both storage and operational conditions, e.g., by increasing its thermal stability, and therefore making it more attractive for diverse applications, especially when surfaces are subjected to harsh reaction conditions [24,31,42]. Recently, Spadoni-Andreani et al. [37] covalently linked α-CT on polypropylene, thus providing a new material able to preserve the surface from *Candida albicans* colonization. The authors carried out covalent enzyme immobilization by activating the surface with a plasma treatment and linking the enzyme with GA. Herein, a similar protocol was applied, and α-CT was immobilized on LDPE coupons after a plasma treatment of 30 min and using GA as a linker.

Plasma technology was previously employed to improve LDPE surface properties, leading to the generation of activated species including hydrophilic functional groups on the first molecular layers of the material [40]. Functional groups allowed the initiation of the surface enzyme immobilization using GA as a linker. Among various cross-linking agents, GA has been long used for protein immobilization, including a number of enzymes [43–45]. Indeed, GA has been successfully used to covalently immobilize α-CT onto modified polyvinyl chloride microspheres [46] as well as on silica beads [47]. Here, for the first time, the peculiar properties of plasma technology and GA were combined, giving the right condition for α-CT immobilization on the LDPE surface. Indeed, the plasma treatment was crucial for providing the plastic surface with functional groups exploitable for the covalent binding of the enzyme to the surface, whereas the inclusion of the spacer GA was essential to improve conformational flexibility, to restrict interaction among immobilized enzyme molecules, and to enhance enzymatic activity [37]. Previous literature also highlighted the role of GA in retaining much of the original activity of enzyme when used as linker in the immobilization process, allowing the new material to be reused more than six times without loss of efficacy [46]. The combination of plasma treatment with a linker seems also to be instrumental to retain the anti-biofilm activity over a long timescale. Indeed, in the past, the coupling of plasma treatment with the linker 2-hydroxyethyl methacrylate was used to functionalize LDPE surfaces with small molecules, providing new materials able to maintain their anti-biofilm performance after having been used for more than 10 times [40].

In a previous work by these authors, it was shown that α-CT activity was negligibly affected by the immobilization reaction with GA. Furthermore, it was shown that GA has an activating effect on α-CT [31]. In line with the previous work, α-CT immobilized on LDPE showed protease activity, confirming that immobilization did not affect the enzyme activity. This promising result opens up the possibility to extend the adopted immobilization protocol to other polymeric materials. Notably, the use of plasma technology coupled with GA makes all surfaces, including those that do not possess the required chemical features, suitable for covalent binding [45,48]. Plasma sources can be also used to modify three-dimensional structures and is therefore not limited to thin, flat samples [49]. Moreover, GA is not corrosive to various substrata, including stainless steel, soft metals, rubber, and glass [50]. In this paper, the ability of the new material to affect cell adhesion and biofilm structure was evaluated against *E. coli*, using a Center for Disease Control (CDC) biofilm reactor able to simulate the conditions to which surfaces of a wide range of applications are subjected during their use, according to previous literature [51,52]. Moreover, with the aim of transferring the technology to consumer products suitable for widespread application, standard procedures were used to evaluate the efficacy of the anti-biofilm material.

Experiments showed that the biofilm was significantly affected when grown on LDPE-α-CT. Plate count viability assays as well as CLSM analysis displayed a significant reduction in both the amount of adhered cells (over 70%) and matrix production (up to 80.2%). Biofilm stained for live and dead cells confirmed that the reduction in biomass was achieved by a mechanism that did not affect bacterial viability, reducing the chances for the evolution of resistant strains [22]. Morphology analysis displayed a statistically significant decrease of biofilm thickness on LDPE-α-CT (up to 81.8%), whereas the biofilm exposed surface/bio-volume ratio was found to be significantly increased (up to 7.1-fold). A high surface to bio-volume ratio usually corresponds to the presence of single cells and small cell clusters attached to the substratum [53]. Moreover, it is an indicative parameter of biofilm adaptation to the environment and it has been shown to increase in stress conditions [54]. Indeed, an increase in the specific surface area of the biofilm could optimize nutrient capture from the environment, especially when the role of the matrix to retain nutrient particles fails [55].

E. coli autotransporter adhesins, e.g., the outer membrane protein Antigen 43, were found to be instrumental in promoting cell-to-cell adhesion and aggregation at the initial stages of biofilm formation [56–58]. Moreover, E. coli proteinaceous amyloid curli fibers play important roles in the irreversible adhesion, enhance initial cell-cell interactions, and ensure the integrity of the three-dimensional biofilm architecture [59–65]. Notably, the inhibition of curli assembly has been found to result in a decrease of E. coli biofilm formation, with no apparent bactericidal or bacteriostatic effects [66]. Extracellular proteins also regulate biofilm detachment and dispersal through the enzymatic degradation of polysaccharides, proteins, and nucleic acids [67,68]. Serine proteases, including α-CT, have been reported to be effective in biofilm eradication via hydrolysis of both the proteinaceous component of the matrix and the proteins (e.g., adhesins) involved in cell adhesion to the surface [14,69,70]. Therefore, as proteins are essential for biofilm formation, their inactivation through the cleavage of their peptide bonds inevitably results in a weakened biofilm.

According to previous literature, in this study, 3D reconstructed CLSM images showed a seriously destabilized biofilm with many cells being dispersed from the substrate. Since the extracellular matrix holds the individual cells together, the enzymatic degradation of the matrix proteins inevitably causes a massive cellular dispersal event [14,22]. Once cells have returned to the planktonic lifestyle, they are more susceptible to both immune systems and the conventional antimicrobials as compared to those in intact biofilm [71]. Additionally, the increased values of the surface to bio-volume ratio leave more biofilm surface available for antibiotic action [72]. Therefore, the combination of a LDPE-α-CT surface with conventional antimicrobial treatments might be a step toward maximizing the anti-biofilm performance of this new material, making cleaning treatments and disinfection procedures effective at low doses. This allows a more potent control against the development of drug-resistant strains [73].

The effect of the introduction of a GA linker into the LDPE polymer backbone on biofilm formation was also evaluated. Indeed, the experiments showed that the linked GA alone contributed, though slightly, to decrease the biofilm formation on the surface (up to 31.0%) (Figure 2A,C), with a mechanism that did not affect cell viability. A weak GA effect on *Bacillus cereus*, *Pseudomonas fluorescens*, *Staphylococcus aureus*, and E. coli biofilm formation was previously reported in the literature [74–77]. However, these studies highlighted that GA had a significant effect on biofilm removal, inducing sloughing events, only under long-term exposure [75]. The anti-biofilm effect of GA could be attributed to its two aldehyde groups which can interact with microbial cell constituents, among these the amino groups of the proteins within the biofilm. Indeed, GA forms methylene bridges, which may play a part in subsequent reactions including cross-linking with another protein chain in the cells. This leads to the removal of water from the biofilm followed by a dehydration effect [77,78]. In addition, it is reported that GA causes the deformation of alpha-helix structures in proteins on the outer cellular layers [79], which may include some proteins important for bacterial adhesion and biofilm formation. Indeed, studies have shown the strong binding of GA to the outer membrane proteins of E. coli [80], and its role in E. coli biofilm formation is well known [81]. Other researchers have suggested that GA also reacts with proteins of the polymeric matrix, leading to the disruption of the matrix structure [74]. Notably, GA is reported to enhance enzyme activity in the immobilization process as it introduces intermolecular cross-linking in proteins or it improves the attachment of enzyme molecules to the support [31,82].

4. Materials and Methods

4.1. Polymeric Surface Preparation

LDPE coupons (Ø 1.3 cm) were functionalized with α-CT according to Spadoni-Andreani et al. [31]. Briefly, LDPE coupons were preventively washed with bi-deionized water and acetone and then dried. Next, they were activated by exposure to O_2 plasma for 30 min using a Harrick Plasma PDC-002 plasma cleaner (740 V, 40 mA, 29.6 W, Ithaca, NY, USA). This step is crucial for the chemical functionalization of the coupon surface (e.g., the formation of carboxyl and hydroxyl groups) [24]. Just after the plasma treatment, enzyme immobilization was carried out, loading onto the coupon 80 μL of α-CT solution (5 mg/mL) in buffer A (0.02 M potassium phosphate, pH 7.2), containing 0.005% (v/v) glutaraldehyde (GA). Then the solution was left to evaporate overnight at 25 °C and under vacuum. Control coupons were analogously prepared without α-CT.

4.2. Evaluation of Immobilized α-CT Activity

Activity of the immobilized α-CT was tested in toluene (0.5 mL) measuring the alcoholysis rate of N-acetyl phenylalanine ethyl ester (1 mg/mL) in the presence of 1-propanol (5%). Tests were carried out using 3-mL vials shaken at 150 rpm at 25 °C. At a scheduled time, product formation was analyzed by a GC-FID Agilent 6850 (Santa Clara, CA, USA) networked GC system and with a polydimethylsiloxane column (30 m, 0.32 mm, film thickness 0.25 μm) (Agilent Technologies 19091Z-413E) with H_2 as carrier gas and N_2 and air as support gases, split 80, constant flow 2.7 mL/min, injector and FID heated at 250 °C, with a temperature ramp of 10 °C/min from 160 °C, held for 0.5 min, further heated to 240 °C, and held for 1 min.

4.3. E. coli Strain and Growth Condition

E. coli strain MG1655 was used as a model system for bacterial biofilms, being a cosmopolitan bacterium that shares a core set of genes with clinically relevant serotypes and foodborne pathogen strains, including genes involved in biofilm formation [83]. The strain was stored at −80 °C in suspensions containing 20% glycerol and 2% peptone, and was routinely grown in Luria–Bertani broth (LB, Sigma-Aldrich, St. Louis, MO, USA) at 37 °C.

4.4. Biofilm Growth in the CDC Reactor

E. coli biofilm was grown on non-functionalized (LDPE and LDPE-GA) and functionalized (LDPE-α-CT) coupons in the CDC biofilm reactor (Biosurface Technologies, Bozeman, MT, USA) according to Cattò et al. [84]. Briefly, the bioreactor was inoculated with 400 mL of sterile LB medium with the addition of 1 mL of diluted pre-washed overnight culture containing 10^7 cells of *E. coli*. The culture was grown at 37 °C with continuous stirring for 24 h. When the 24-h adhesion phase was over, the peristaltic pump was started and sterile 10% LB medium was continuously pumped into the reactor at a rate of 8.3 mL/min. After 48 h of dynamic phase, functionalized and non-functionalized coupons were removed, gently washed with phosphate-buffered saline (PBS, 0.01 M phosphate buffer, 0.0027 M potassium chloride, pH 7.4) and processed for analysis.

4.5. Plate Count Viability Assay

Collected coupons were transferred to 5 mL of PBS, and sessile cells were removed from the coupon surface by 30 s vortex mixing and 2 min sonication (Branson 3510, Branson Ultrasonic Corporation, Dunburry, CT, USA) followed by another 30 s vortex mixing. Serial dilutions of the resulting cell suspensions were plated on Tryptic Soy Agar (TSA, Fisher Scientific, Pittsburgh, PA, USA) and incubated overnight at 37 °C. Colony forming units (CFUs) were determined by the standard colony counting method. Obtained data were reported as the number of viable bacterial cells normalized to the area and means were calculated. The efficacy of the anti-biofilm material was calculated as the percentage reduction of the CFUs with respect to the LDPE control. Four coupons for each surface were analyzed. The experiment was repeated four times for a total of 16 coupons analyzed.

4.6. Epifluorescence Microscopy Analysis

The percentage of live and dead cells in the biofilm biomass grown on both non-functionalized and functionalized coupons was determined using a Live/Dead BacLight viability kit (L7012, Molecular Probes-Life Technologies, Thermo Fisher Scientific, Waltham, MA, USA). Biofilm was incubated with 2 µL of each fluorescent probe per ml of sterile filtered PBS at room temperature in the dark for 25 min and then rinsed with sterile PBS, according to the manufacturer's instruction. Coupons without biofilm were also stained with the dyes in order to exclude any false positive signals. Biofilm samples were visualized using a Nikon Eclipse E800 epifluorescent microscope with excitation at 480 nm and emission at 516 nm for the green channel and excitation at 581 nm and emission at 644 nm for the red channel (Tokyo, Japan). Images were captured with a 60×, 1.0 NA water immersion objective and analyzed via MetaMorph 7.5 software (Molecular Devices, Sunnyvale, CA, USA). The percent area of stained cells was obtained by calculating at least 10 random images for each sample. The efficacy of the anti-biofilm material was calculated as the percentage reduction in the stained cell area with respect to the LDPE control images. Relative viability within the biofilm was determined by dividing the percent area of the live cells by the percent area of the dead cells in each sample. Four coupons of each surface were analyzed. The experiment was repeated four times for a total of 16 coupons analyzed.

4.7. Confocal Laser Scanning Microscopy (CLSM) Analysis

Three-dimensional morphology of biofilm growth on non-functionalized and functionalized surfaces was analyzed by CLSM according to Cattò et al. [85]. Biofilm was stained with 200 µg/mL lectin concanavalin A-Texas Red conjugate dye (C825, Molecular Probes-Life Technologies, Thermo Fisher Scientific) to visualize the polysaccharide component of the extracellular polymeric substances (EPS) and 1:1000 SYBR Green I fluorescent nucleic acid dye (S7563, Molecular Probes-Life Technologies, Thermo Fisher Scientific) to display biofilm cells, in the dark for 30 min. Coupons without biofilm were also stained in order to exclude any false positive signals. Biofilm samples were visualized using a Leica SP5 CLSM with excitation at 488 nm and emission at 520 nm for the green channel and excitation at 543 nm and emission at 615 nm for the red channel. Images were captured with a 63×, 0.9 NA water immersion objective and projections and 3D reconstructed images of biofilm were generated using the Imaris software package (Bitplane Scientific Software, Zurich, Switzerland).

Quantitative biofilm structural parameters were calculated, including (i) mean thickness, which identifies the mean distance from the substratum in the direction normal to the substrate where there is biofilm; (ii) roughness, a quantity calculated from the thickness distribution and that describes the heterogeneity of the biofilm; (iii) substratum coverage, the percentage of substrate area occupied by the biofilm; (iv) surface-to-volume ratio, which reflects the fraction of biofilm area that is exposed to nutrients; and (v) bio-volume, of both cells and the polysaccharide matrix, which provides an estimation of the biomass in the biofilm [86]. Biofilm morphological parameters were obtained via MetaMorph 7.5 (Molecular Devices, Sunnyvale, CA, USA) and COMSTAT software from at least five random images for each sample according to Heydorn et al. [53]. Four coupons of each surface were analyzed. The experiment was repeated four times for a total of 16 coupons analyzed.

4.8. Statistical Analysis

Two-tailed ANOVA analysis, via software run in a MATLAB environment (Version 7.0, The MathWorks Inc., Natick, MA, USA), was applied to statistically evaluate any significant differences among the samples and concentrations. The ANOVA analysis was carried out after verifying data independence (Pearson's Chi-square test), normal distribution (D'Agostino-Pearson normality test), and homogeneity of variance (Bartlett's test). Tukey's honest significant different test (HSD) was used

5. Conclusions

In this work, α-CT was successfully immobilized on an LDPE surface to provide a new material able to inhibit biofilm colonization. The multiple-target nature of the protease activity allows the new material to be used with a broad-spectrum activity against polymicrobial infections, including drug-resistant strains. Indeed, the use of drugs that impact multiple targets simultaneously is better at controlling complex disease systems, e.g., biofilms, and makes resistance development rather unlikely [87–89].

LDPE-α-CT may provide a solution to potentiate the anti-biofilm activity of conventional antimicrobials that are otherwise largely effective only against planktonic bacteria. Indeed, in many industrial and clinical sector surface treatments that retard biofilm formation could represent a great step forward against the challenge of biofilm formation [90]. Nowadays, the combination of antibiotics with anti-biofilm mechanisms leading to synergism is considered the best solution for the treatment of biofilm [91,92].

Both LDPE and α-CT are currently available at affordable prices, providing a positive foundation for the production of LDPE-α-CT at the industrial level at affordable cost. Additionally, the simple protocol for enzyme immobilization makes it suitable for application to other surfaces and complementary enzymes, e.g., those attacking other components of the biofilm matrix.

Author Contributions: All authors conceived and designed experiments; C.C. and F.V. performed microbiological experiments and collected data; F.S. performed biochemical experiments and collected data; C.C. and F.S. analyzed data; C.C. wrote the paper; all authors checked the content of the paper and revised the manuscript; F.C. was responsible for funding acquisition.

Funding: This research was funded by Fondazione Cariplo, grant number 2011-0277.

Acknowledgments: The Department of Food, Environmental and Nutritional Sciences, Università degli Studi di Milano, partially covered the open access APC.

Conflicts of Interest: The authors declare no conflict of interest. The funders had no role in the design of the study; in the collection, analyses, or interpretation of data; in the writing of the manuscript, or in the decision to publish the results.

References

1. Swan, J.S.; Deasy, E.C.; Boyle, M.A.; Russell, R.J.; O'Donnell, M.J.; Coleman, D.C. Elimination of biofilm and microbial contamination reservoirs in hospital washbasin U-bends by automated cleaning and disinfection with electrochemically activated solutions. *J. Hosp. Infect.* **2016**, *94*, 169–174. [CrossRef]
2. Chen, M.; Yu, Q.; Sun, H. Novel strategies for the prevention and treatment of biofilm related infections. *Int. J. Mol. Sci.* **2013**, *14*, 18488–18501. [CrossRef] [PubMed]
3. Lo, J.; Lange, D.; Chew, B.H. Ureteral stents and foley catheters-associated urinary tract infections: The role of coatings and materials in infection prevention. *Antibiotics* **2014**, *3*, 87–97. [CrossRef] [PubMed]
4. Ahire, J.J.; Hattingh, M.; Neveling, D.P.; Dicks, L.M.T. Copper-containing anti-biofilm nanofiber scaffolds as a wound dressing material. *PLoS ONE* **2016**, *11*, e0152755. [CrossRef] [PubMed]
5. Garuglieri, E.; Catto, C.; Villa, F.; Zanchi, R.; Cappitelli, F. Effects of sublethal concentrations of silver nanoparticles on *Escherichia coli* and *Bacillus subtilis* under aerobic and anaerobic conditions. *Biointerphases* **2016**, *11*, 04B308. [CrossRef] [PubMed]
6. Pechook, S.; Sudakov, K.; Polishchuk, I.; Ostrov, I.; Zakin, V.; Pokroy, B.; Shemesh, M. Bioinspired passive anti-biofouling surfaces preventing biofilm formation. *J. Mater. Chem. B* **2015**, *3*, 1371–1378. [CrossRef]
7. Costerton, J.W. Introduction to biofilm. *Int. J. Antimicrob. Agents* **1999**, *11*, 217–221; discussion 237–219. [CrossRef]
8. Ventola, C.L. The antibiotic resistance crisis: Part 1: Causes and threats. *Pharm. Ther.* **2015**, *40*, 277–283.
9. Frieri, M.; Kumar, K.; Boutin, A. Antibiotic resistance. *J. Infect. Public Health* **2017**, *10*, 369–378. [CrossRef]

10. Batoni, G.; Maisetta, G.; Esin, S. Antimicrobial peptides and their interaction with biofilms of medically relevant bacteria. *Biochim. Biophys. Acta* **2016**, *1858*, 1044–1060. [CrossRef]
11. Von Eiff, C.; Jansen, B.; Kohnen, W.; Becker, K. Infections associated with medical devices: Pathogenesis, management and prophylaxis. *Drugs* **2005**, *65*, 179–214. [CrossRef] [PubMed]
12. Gharbi, A.; Humblot, V.; Turpin, F.; Pradier, C.M.; Imbert, C.; Berjeaud, J.M. Elaboration of antibiofilm surfaces functionalized with antifungal-cyclodextrin inclusion complexes. *FEMS Immunol. Med. Microbiol.* **2012**, *65*, 257–269. [CrossRef] [PubMed]
13. Roy, R.; Tiwari, M.; Donelli, G.; Tiwari, V. Strategies for combating bacterial biofilms: A focus on anti-biofilm agents and their mechanisms of action. *Virulence* **2018**, *9*, 522–554. [CrossRef] [PubMed]
14. Fleming, D.; Rumbaugh, K.P. Approaches to dispersing medical biofilms. *Microorganisms* **2017**, *5*, 15. [CrossRef] [PubMed]
15. Kaplan, J.B. Biofilm matrix-degrading enzymes. *Methods Mol. Biol.* **2014**, *1147*, 203–213. [CrossRef] [PubMed]
16. Elchinger, P.H.; Delattre, C.; Faure, S.; Roy, O.; Badel, S.; Bernardi, T.; Taillefumier, C.; Michaud, P. Immobilization of proteases on chitosan for the development of films with anti-biofilm properties. *Int. J. Biol. Macromol.* **2015**, *72*, 1063–1068. [CrossRef]
17. Stiefel, P.; Mauerhofer, S.; Schneider, J.; Maniura-Weber, K.; Rosenberg, U.; Ren, Q. Enzymes enhance biofilm removal efficiency of cleaners. *Antimicrob. Agents Chemother.* **2016**, *60*, 3647–3652. [CrossRef]
18. Mitrofanova, O.; Mardanova, A.; Evtugyn, V.; Bogomolnaya, L.; Sharipova, M. Effects of Bacillus Serine Proteases on the Bacterial Biofilms. *BioMed Res. Int.* **2017**, *2017*, 8525912. [CrossRef]
19. Sharma, K.; Singh, A.P. Antibiofilm effect of dnase against single and mixed species biofilm. *Foods* **2018**, *7*, 42. [CrossRef]
20. Homaei, A.A.; Sariri, R.; Vianello, F.; Stevanato, R. Enzyme immobilization: An update. *J. Chem. Biol.* **2013**, *6*, 185–205. [CrossRef]
21. Villa, F.; Cappitelli, F. Plant-derived bioactive compounds at sub-lethal concentrations: Towards smart biocide-free antibiofilm strategies. *Phytochem. Rev.* **2013**, *12*, 245–254. [CrossRef]
22. Kaplan, J.B. Biofilm dispersal: Mechanisms, clinical implications, and potential therapeutic uses. *J. Dent. Res.* **2010**, *89*, 205–218. [CrossRef] [PubMed]
23. Azeredo, J.; Azevedo, N.F.; Briandet, R.; Cerca, N.; Coenye, T.; Costa, A.R.; Desvaux, M.; Di Bonaventura, G.; Hebraud, M.; Jaglic, Z.; et al. Critical review on biofilm methods. *Crit. Rev. Microbiol.* **2017**, *43*, 313–351. [CrossRef] [PubMed]
24. Spadoni-Andreani, E.S.; Magagnin, L.; Secundo, F. Preparation and comparison of hydrolase-coated plastics. *Chemistryselect* **2016**, *1*, 1490–1495. [CrossRef]
25. Stepankova, V.; Bidmanova, S.; Koudelakova, T.; Prokop, Z.; Chaloupkova, R.; Damborsky, J. Strategies for stabilization of enzymes in organic solvents. *ACS Catal.* **2013**, *3*, 2823–2836. [CrossRef]
26. Sastri, V.R. Commodity thermoplastics: Polyvinyl chloride, polyolefin, and polystyrene. In *Plastics in Medical Devices: Properties, Requirements, and Applications*, 2nd ed.; Sastri, V.R., Ed.; Elsevier Inc.: Amsterdam, The Netherlands, 2010; pp. 73–119, ISBN 9780323265638.
27. Jordan, J.L.; Casem, D.T.; Bradley, J.M.; Dwivedi, A.K.; Brown, E.N.; Jordan, C.W. Mechanical properties of low density polyethylene. *J. Dyn. Behav. Mater.* **2016**, *2*, 411–420. [CrossRef]
28. Unger, S.; Landis, A. Assessing the environmental, human health, and economic impacts of reprocessed medical devices in a Phoenix hospital's supply chain. *J. Clean. Prod.* **2016**, *112*, 1995–2003. [CrossRef]
29. Raj, B.; Sankar, U.K.; Siddaramaiah. Low density polyethylene/starch blend films for food packaging applications. *Adv. Polym. Technol.* **2004**, *23*, 32–45. [CrossRef]
30. Villa, F.; Secundo, F.; Polo, A.; Cappitelli, F. Immobilized hydrolytic enzymes exhibit antibiofilm activity against *Escherichia coli* at sub-lethal concentrations. *Curr. Microbiol.* **2015**, *71*, 106–114. [CrossRef]
31. Secundo, F.; Barletta, G.L.; Parini, G.; Roda, G. Effects of stabilizing additives on the activity of alpha-chymotrypsin in organic solvent. *J. Mol. Catal. B Enzym.* **2012**, *84*, 128–131. [CrossRef]
32. Novick, S.J.; Dordick, J.S. Protein-containing hydrophobic coatings and films. *Biomaterials* **2002**, *23*, 441–448. [CrossRef]
33. Zanaroli, G.; Negroni, A.; Calisti, C.; Ruzzi, M.; Fava, F. Selection of commercial hydrolytic enzymes with potential antifouling activity in marine environments. *Enzyme Microb. Technol.* **2011**, *49*, 574–579. [CrossRef] [PubMed]

34. Artini, M.; Papa, R.; Scoarughi, G.L.; Galano, E.; Barbato, G.; Pucci, P.; Selan, L. Comparison of the action of different proteases on virulence properties related to the staphylococcal surface. *J. Appl. Microbiol.* **2013**, *114*, 266–277. [CrossRef] [PubMed]
35. Harris, L.G.; Nigam, Y.; Sawyer, J.; Mack, D.; Pritchard, D.I. *Lucilia sericata* chymotrypsin disrupts protein adhesin-mediated staphylococcal biofilm formation. *Appl. Environ. Microbiol.* **2013**, *79*, 1393–1395. [CrossRef] [PubMed]
36. Leccese Terraf, M.C.; Tomas, M.S.J.; Rault, L.; Le Loir, Y.; Even, S.; Nader-Macias, M.E.F. Biofilms of vaginal *Lactobacillus reuteri* CRL 1324 and *Lactobacillus rhamnosus* CRL 1332: Kinetics of formation and matrix characterization. *Arch. Microbiol.* **2016**, *198*, 689–700. [CrossRef] [PubMed]
37. Spadoni-Andreani, E.S.; Villa, F.; Cappitelli, F.; Krasowska, A.; Biniarz, P.; Lukaszewicz, M.; Secundo, F. Coating polypropylene surfaces with protease weakens the adhesion and increases the dispersion of *Candida albicans* cells. *Biotechnol. Lett.* **2017**, *39*, 423–428. [CrossRef] [PubMed]
38. Mohamad, N.R.; Marzuki, N.H.; Buang, N.A.; Huyop, F.; Wahab, R.A. An overview of technologies for immobilization of enzymes and surface analysis techniques for immobilized enzymes. *Biotechnol. Equip.* **2015**, *29*, 205–220. [CrossRef]
39. Saldarriaga Fernández, I.C.S.; van der Mei, H.C.; Lochhead, M.J.; Grainger, D.W.; Busscher, H.J. The inhibition of the adhesion of clinically isolated bacterial strains on multi-component cross-linked poly(ethylene glycol)-based polymer coatings. *Biomaterials* **2007**, *28*, 4105–4112. [CrossRef]
40. Dell'orto, S.; Cattò, C.; Villa, F.; Forlani, F.; Vassallo, E.; Morra, M.; Cappitelli, F.; Villa, S.; Gelain, A. Low density polyethylene functionalized with antibiofilm compounds inhibits *Escherichia coli* cell adhesion. *J. Biomed. Mater. Res. A* **2017**, *105*, 3251–3261. [CrossRef]
41. Rather, I.A.; Koh, W.Y.; Paek, W.K.; Lim, J. The sources of chemical contaminants in food and their health implications. *Front. Pharmacol.* **2017**, *8*, 830. [CrossRef]
42. Garcia-Galan, C.; Berenguer-Murcia, A.; Fernandez-Lafuente, R.; Rodrigues, R.C. Potential of different enzyme immobilization strategies to improve enzyme performance. *Adv. Synth. Catal.* **2011**, *353*, 2885–2904. [CrossRef]
43. Chae, H.J.; In, M.J.; Kim, E.Y. Optimization of protease immobilization by covalent binding using glutaraldehyde. *Appl. Biochem. Biotechnol.* **1998**, *73*, 195–204. [CrossRef] [PubMed]
44. Lopez-Gallego, F.; Guisan, J.M.; Betancor, L. Glutaraldehyde-mediated protein immobilization. *Methods Mol. Biol.* **2013**, *1051*, 33–41. [CrossRef] [PubMed]
45. Barbosa, O.; Ortiz, C.; Berenguer-Murcia, A.; Torres, R.; Rodrigues, R.C.; Fernandez-Lafuente, R. Glutaraldehyde in bio-catalysts design: A useful crosslinker and a versatile tool in enzyme immobilization. *RSC Adv.* **2014**, *4*, 1583–1600. [CrossRef]
46. Li, D.F.; Ding, H.C.; Zhou, T. Covalent immobilization of mixed proteases, trypsin and chymotrypsin, onto modified polyvinyl chloride microspheres. *J. Agric. Food Chem.* **2013**, *61*, 10447–10453. [CrossRef] [PubMed]
47. Xiao, P.; Lv, X.F.; Deng, Y.L. Immobilization of chymotrypsin on silica beads based on high affinity and specificity aptamer and its applications. *Anal. Lett.* **2012**, *45*, 1264–1273. [CrossRef]
48. Onyshchenko, I.; De Geyter, N.; Nikiforov, A.Y.; Morent, R. Atmospheric pressure plasma penetration inside flexible polymeric tubes. *Plasma Process. Polym.* **2015**, *12*, 271–284. [CrossRef]
49. Pedroni, M.; Morandi, S.; Silvetti, T.; Cremona, A.; Gittini, G.; Nardone, A.; Pallotta, F.; Brasca, M.; Vassallo, E. Bacteria inactivation by atmospheric pressure plasma jet treatment. *J. Vac. Sci. Technol. B* **2018**, *36*, 01A107. [CrossRef]
50. Lin, W.S.; Niu, B.; Yi, J.L.; Deng, Z.R.; Song, J.; Chen, Q. Toxicity and metal corrosion of glutaraldehyde-didecyldimethylammonium bromide as a disinfectant agent. *Biomed Res. Int.* **2018**, *2018*, 9814209. [CrossRef]
51. Gilmore, B.F.; Hamill, T.M.; Jones, D.S.; Gorman, S.P. Validation of the CDC Biofilm reactor as a dynamic model for assessment of encrustation formation on urological device materials. *J. Biomed. Mater. Res. B* **2010**, *93B*, 128–140. [CrossRef]
52. Williams, D.L.; Woodbury, K.L.; Haymond, B.S.; Parker, A.E.; Bloebaum, R.D. A Modified CDC biofilm reactor to produce mature biofilms on the surface of peek membranes for an in vivo animal model application. *Curr. Microbiol.* **2011**, *62*, 1657–1663. [CrossRef] [PubMed]

53. Heydorn, A.; Nielsen, A.T.; Hentzer, M.; Sternberg, C.; Givskov, M.; Ersbøll, B.K.; Molin, S. Quantification of biofilm structures by the novel computer program COMSTAT. *Microbiology* **2000**, *146*, 2395–2407. [CrossRef] [PubMed]
54. Mangwani, N.; Shukla, S.K.; Kumari, S.; Das, S.; Rao, T.S. Effect of biofilm parameters and extracellular polymeric substance composition on polycyclic aromatic hydrocarbon degradation. *RSC Adv.* **2016**, *6*, S7540–S7551. [CrossRef]
55. Bester, E.; Kroukamp, O.; Hausner, M.; Edwards, E.A.; Wolfaardt, G.M. Biofilm form and function: Carbon availability affects biofilm architecture, metabolic activity and planktonic cell yield. *J. Appl. Microbiol.* **2011**, *110*, 387–398. [CrossRef] [PubMed]
56. Danese, P.N.; Pratt, L.A.; Dove, S.L.; Kolter, R. The outer membrane protein, antigen 43, mediates cell-to-cell interactions within Escherichia coli biofilms. *Mol. Microbiol.* **2000**, *37*, 424–432. [CrossRef] [PubMed]
57. Ulett, G.C.; Valle, J.; Beloin, C.; Sherlock, O.; Ghigo, J.M.; Schembri, M.A. Functional analysis of antigen 43 in uropathogenic *Escherichia coli* reveals a role in long-term persistence in the urinary tract. *Infect. Immun.* **2007**, *75*, 3233–3244. [CrossRef]
58. Vo, J.L.; Ortiz, G.C.M.; Subedi, P.; Keerthikumar, S.; Mathivanan, S.; Paxman, J.J.; Heras, B. Autotransporter Adhesins in *Escherichia coli* Pathogenesis. *Proteomics* **2017**, *17*, 1600431. [CrossRef]
59. Hobley, L.; Harkins, C.; MacPhee, C.E.; Stanley-Wall, N.R. Giving structure to the biofilm matrix: An overview of individual strategies and emerging common themes. *FEMS Microbiol. Rev.* **2015**, *39*, 649–669. [CrossRef]
60. Kikuchi, T.; Mizunoe, Y.; Takade, A.; Naito, S.; Yoshida, S. Curli fibers are required for development of biofilm architecture in *Escherichia coli* K-12 and enhance bacterial adherence to human uroepithelial cells. *Microbiol. Immunol.* **2005**, *49*, 875–884. [CrossRef]
61. Evans, M.L.; Chapman, M.R. Curli biogenesis: Order out of disorder. *Biochim. Biophys. Acta* **2014**, *1843*, 1551–1558. [CrossRef]
62. Hufnagel, D.A.; Depas, W.H.; Chapman, M.R. The biology of the *Escherichia coli* extracellular matrix. *Microbiol. Spectr.* **2015**, *3*. [CrossRef] [PubMed]
63. Taglialegna, A.; Lasa, I.; Valle, J. Amyloid structures as biofilm matrix scaffolds. *J. Bacteriol.* **2016**, *198*, 2579–2588. [CrossRef] [PubMed]
64. Reichhardt, C.; Cegelski, L. The Congo red derivative FSB binds to curli amyloid fibers and specifically stains curliated *E. coli*. *PLoS ONE* **2018**, *13*, e0203226. [CrossRef] [PubMed]
65. Li, B.Y.; Huang, Q.; Cui, A.L.; Liu, X.L.; Hou, B.; Zhang, L.Y.; Liu, M.; Meng, X.R.; Li, S.W. Overexpression of outer membrane protein X (OmpX) compensates for the effect of TolC inactivation on biofilm formation and curli production in extraintestinal pathogenic *Escherichia coli* (ExPEC). *Front. Cell. Infect. Microbiol.* **2018**, *8*, 208. [CrossRef] [PubMed]
66. Jain, N.; Aden, J.; Nagamatsu, K.; Evans, M.L.; Li, X.Y.; McMichael, B.; Ivanova, M.I.; Almqvist, F.; Buxbaum, J.N.; Chapman, M.R. Inhibition of curli assembly and *Escherichia coli* biofilm formation by the human systemic amyloid precursor transthyretin. *Proc. Natl. Acad. Sci. USA* **2017**, *114*, 12184–12189. [CrossRef] [PubMed]
67. Fong, J.N.C.; Yildiz, F.H. Biofilm matrix proteins. *Microbiol. Spectr.* **2015**, *3*, 2. [CrossRef] [PubMed]
68. Flemming, H.C.; Wingender, J. The biofilm matrix. *Nat. Rev. Microbiol.* **2010**, *8*, 623–633. [CrossRef]
69. Leroy, C.; Delbarre-Ladrat, C.; Ghillebaert, F.; Compere, C.; Combes, D. Effects of commercial enzymes on the adhesion of a marine biofilm-forming bacterium. *Biofouling* **2008**, *24*, 11–22. [CrossRef]
70. Lister, J.L.; Horswill, A.R. *Staphylococcus aureus* biofilms: Recent developments in biofilm dispersal. *Front. Cell. Infect. Microbiol.* **2014**, *4*, 178. [CrossRef]
71. Davey, M.E.; O'Toole, G.A. Microbial biofilms: From ecology to molecular genetics. *Microbiol. Mol. Biol. Rev.* **2000**, *64*, 847–867. [CrossRef]
72. Shukla, S.K.; Rao, T.S. *Staphylococcus aureus* biofilm removal by targeting biofilm-associated extracellular proteins. *Indian J. Med. Res.* **2017**, *146*, 1–8. [CrossRef]
73. Estrela, A.B.; Abraham, W.R. Combining biofilm-controlling compounds and antibiotics as a promising new way to control biofilm infections. *Pharmaceuticals* **2010**, *3*, 1374–1393. [CrossRef] [PubMed]
74. Pereira, M.O.; Vieira, M.J. Effects of the interactions between glutaraldehyde and the polymeric matrix on the efficacy of the biocide against Pseudomonas fluorescens biofilms. *Biofouling* **2001**, *17*, 93–101. [CrossRef]

75. Simoes, L.C.; Lemos, M.; Araujo, P.; Pereira, A.M.; Simoes, M. The effects of glutaraldehyde on the control of single and dual biofilms of *Bacillus cereus* and *Pseudomonas fluorescens*. *Biofouling* **2011**, *27*, 337–346. [CrossRef] [PubMed]
76. Sehmi, S.K.; Allan, E.; MacRobert, A.J.; Parkin, I. The bactericidal activity of glutaraldehyde-impregnated polyurethane. *Microbiologyopen* **2016**, *5*, 891–897. [CrossRef]
77. Tran, V.N.; Dasagrandhi, C.; Truong, V.G.; Kim, Y.M.; Kang, H.W. Antibacterial activity of *Staphylococcus aureus* biofilm under combined exposure of glutaraldehyde, near-infrared light, and 405-nm laser. *PLoS ONE* **2018**, *13*, e0202821. [CrossRef]
78. Migneault, I.; Dartiguenave, C.; Bertrand, M.J.; Waldron, K.C. Glutaraldehyde: Behavior in aqueous solution, reaction with proteins, and application to enzyme crosslinking. *Biotechniques* **2004**, *37*, 790–796. [CrossRef]
79. Silva, C.; Sousa, F.; Bitz, G.G.; Cavaco-Paulo, A. Chemical modifications on proteins using glutaraldehyde. *Food Technol. Biotechnol.* **2004**, *42*, 51–56.
80. Maillard, J.Y. Bacterial target sites for biocide action. *J. Appl. Microbiol.* **2002**, *92*, S16–S27. [CrossRef]
81. Van Houdt, R.; Michiels, C.W. Role of bacterial cell surface structures in *Escherichia coli* biofilm formation. *Res. Microbiol.* **2005**, *156*, 626–633. [CrossRef]
82. Bhushan, B.; Pal, A.; Jain, V. Improved enzyme catalytic characteristics upon glutaraldehyde cross-linking of alginate entrapped xylanase isolated from *Aspergillus flavus* MTCC 9390. *Enzyme Res.* **2015**, *2015*, 210784. [CrossRef] [PubMed]
83. Faucher, S.P.; Charette, S.J. Editorial on: Bacterial pathogens in the non-clinical environment. *Front. Microbiol.* **2015**, *6*, 331. [CrossRef] [PubMed]
84. Cattò, C.; Grazioso, G.; Dell'Orto, S.; Gelain, A.; Villa, S.; Marzano, V.; Vitali, A.; Villa, F.; Cappitelli, F.; Forlani, F. The response of *Escherichia coli* biofilm to salicylic acid. *Biofouling* **2017**, *33*, 235–251. [CrossRef] [PubMed]
85. Cattò, C.; James, G.; Villa, F.; Villa, S.; Cappitelli, F. Zosteric acid and salicylic acid bound to a low density polyethylene surface successfully control bacterial biofilm formation. *Biofouling* **2018**, *34*, 440–452. [CrossRef] [PubMed]
86. Chang, Y.W.; Fragkopoulos, A.A.; Marquez, S.M.; Kim, H.D.; Angelini, T.E.; Fernandez-Nieves, A. Biofilm formation in geometries with different surface curvature and oxygen availability. *New J. Phys.* **2015**, *17*, 033017. [CrossRef]
87. Talevi, A. Multi-target pharmacology: Possibilities and limitations of the "skeleton key approach" from a medicinal chemist perspective. *Front. Pharmacol.* **2015**, *6*, 205. [CrossRef]
88. Pfalzgraff, A.; Brandenburg, K.; Weindl, G. Antimicrobial peptides and their therapeutic potential for bacterial skin infections and wounds. *Front. Pharmacol.* **2018**, *9*, 281. [CrossRef]
89. Ramsay, R.R.; Popovic-Nikolic, M.R.; Nikolic, K.; Uliassi, E.; Bolognesi, M.L. A perspective on multi-target drug discovery and design for complex diseases. *Clin. Transl. Med.* **2018**, *7*. [CrossRef]
90. Cappitelli, F.; Polo, A.; Villa, F. Biofilm formation in food processing environments is still poorly understood and controlled. *Food Eng. Rev.* **2014**, *6*, 29–42. [CrossRef]
91. Cui, J.H.; Ren, B.; Tong, Y.J.; Dai, H.Q.; Zhang, L.X. Synergistic combinations of antifungals and anti-virulence agents to fight against *Candida albicans*. *Virulence* **2015**, *6*, 362–371. [CrossRef]
92. Miquel, S.; Lagrafeuille, R.; Souweine, B.; Forestier, C. Anti-biofilm Activity as a Health Issue. *Front. Microbiol.* **2016**, *7*, 592. [CrossRef] [PubMed]

© 2018 by the authors. Licensee MDPI, Basel, Switzerland. This article is an open access article distributed under the terms and conditions of the Creative Commons Attribution (CC BY) license (http://creativecommons.org/licenses/by/4.0/).

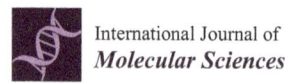

Communication

Additives for Efficient Biodegradable Antifouling Paints

Fabienne Faÿ *, Maëlle Gouessan, Isabelle Linossier and Karine Réhel

Université Bretagne Sud, EA 3884, LBCM, IUEM, F-56100 Lorient, France; maelle.gouessan@univ-ubs.fr (M.G.); isabelle.linossier@univ-ubs.fr (I.L.); karine.rehel@univ-ubs.fr (K.R.)
* Correspondence: fabienne.fay@univ-ubs.fr; Tel.: +33-029-787-4626

Received: 20 December 2018; Accepted: 13 January 2019; Published: 16 January 2019

Abstract: The evolution of regulations concerning biocidal products aims to increase protection of the environment (e.g., EU Regulation No 528/2012) and requires the development of new non-toxic anti-fouling (AF) systems. The development of these formulations implies the use of ingredients (polymers, active substances, additives) that are devoid of toxicity towards marine environments. In this context, the use of erodable antifouling paints based on biodegradable polymer and authorized biocides responds to this problem. However, the efficiency of paints could be improved by the use of specific additives. For this purpose, three additives acting as surface modifiers were studied (Tween 80, Span 85 and PEG-silane). Their effects on parameters involved in antifouling efficiency as hydrophobicity, hydration and copper release were studied. Results showed that the addition of 3% of additives modulated hydrophobicity and hydration without an increase of copper release and significantly reduced microfouling development. Efficient paints based on biodegradable polymer and with no organic biocide could be obtained by mixing copper thiocyanate and additives.

Keywords: antifouling; copper paint; additives; biofilm

1. Introduction

Biofouling can be defined as the accumulation of micro- and macro-organisms on artificial surfaces immersed in seawater. To control biofouling, antifouling (AF) paints have been developed and commonly used for several decades. They contain polymers as binders, toxic compounds, called biocides, which are leached from the paint matrix, and additives (thixotropic agents, pigments, viscosity modifiers). Biocides are based on copper compounds (copper oxide or copper thiocyanate) associated with booster biocides. These organic biocides are intended to be environmentally less harmful than the organotin biocides used in the 1970s. However, alternative strategies are researched because problems of toxicity for marine species and an accumulation of substances in seawater persist [1,2]. Among them, the use of natural antifouling compounds has received a lot of attention. For example, papain, butenolide or cardenolides recently showed an interesting efficiency against biofouling [3–5]. However, several restrictions limit the use of these products: large scale production, degradation, compatibility with paint matrix, release characteristics and costs are the main difficulties impeding their development [6]. Moreover, recent regulation concerning the use of biocides (EU Regulation No 528/2012) known as Biocide Product Regulation (BPR) also restricts their industrial development for reasons concerning costs. Actually, only a few biocides are authorized by European Union and commercialized: 3 copper derivatives (copper, copper thiocyanate and dicopper oxide), 5 booster biocides (DCOIT, Zineb, copper pyrithione, zinc pyrithione and a substituent of copper called Tralopyril). Currently, antifouling paint researchers have to look for a compromise between efficiency of coatings and their impact on the environment.

The aim of this work is to study paints based on a copper derivative such as copper thiocyanate, but devoid of booster biocides. Copper is an effective biocide against algae and mollusks. Moreover, a lower amount of copper thiocyanate is needed than copper oxide for the same level of efficiency [7]. However, to improve its efficiency and to enlarge the activity spectrum of paints, an additive acting as surface modifier could be added. Its role is not to produce a biocidal effect but instead the promotion of an anti-adhesive effect by modifying wettability of surface and paint surface/organisms interactions. Fouling release (FR) coatings based on poly(dimethylsiloxane) (PDMS) rely on this principle by decreasing surface energy [8]. However, several publications have mentioned the combination of antifouling and fouling release concepts to develop new hybrid materials effective in marine antifouling protection. Azemar and al. have proposed a hybrid system based on triblock copolymer poly(ε-caprolactone)-block-poly(dimethylsiloxane)-block-poly(ε-caprolactone) to mix the properties of erosion/biocide release used in antifouling systems and hydrophobicity properties through the use of PDMS [9]. Afterwards, Yang et al. have confirmed the need to combine the concepts of "antifouling" and "fouling release" [10].

The surface wettability plays a major role in antifouling performance [10]. It can be modulated by the use of surfactants. For example, Tween 20 has improved the antifouling characteristics of membranes by adsorption at interfaces [11,12]. In antifouling applications, we have previously shown that Tween 85 disturbed interactions between colonizing organisms and surfaces by decreasing their hydrophobicity and thus a physical repelling of Tween 85 has been hypothesized [13]. Another strategy concerns the use of grafted surfaces. Surface-grafted poly(ethylene glycol) (PEG) molecules are known to prevent protein adsorption and coatings based on PDMS-g-PEG have been studied in seawater [8,14,15]. In this study, bacteria and diatoms adhesion were inhibited. Recently, Jimenez-Pardo et al. have proposed hydrophilic self-replenishing coatings based on polycarbonate-poly(ethylene glycol) methyl ether polyurethane exhibiting low proteins adhesion values [16].

Hence, this work has studied the effect of three additives incorporated in a copper paint: Tween 80 and Span 85, two no ionic, hydrophilic and hydrophobic surfactant respectively and a PEG-silane. The last one is considered as a surface modifier because of its properties such as hydrophilicity, flexibility, high exclusion volume in water and non toxicity [17]. The paint had an additive free formulation. Parameters as surface hydrophobicity, paint hydration and copper release were evaluated. The anti-microfouling and anti-macrofouling efficiencies of paints were studied as well as their toxicity.

2. Results and Discussion

2.1. Effect of Additifs on Paints Characteristics

To study the effects of additives on hydrophobicity, hydration, and copper release, four paints were studied: three paints containing a surface modifier at 3% (w/w) (Figure 1) and one paint without additives. The same formulation was used for all the paints. Only the additive nature changed. Tween 80 is a hydrophilic surfactant (hydrophilic lipophilic balance (HLB 16.7), whereas Span 85 is a hydrophobic one (HLB 1.8). PEG-silane is a biocompatible polymer. Immobilized onto surfaces, it confers protein and cell resistance [18]. Here, it was used as a surface modifier (wettability and steric hindrance). Calcium carbonate was used to complete the formulation. It is a neutral charge often incorporated in antifouling paint.

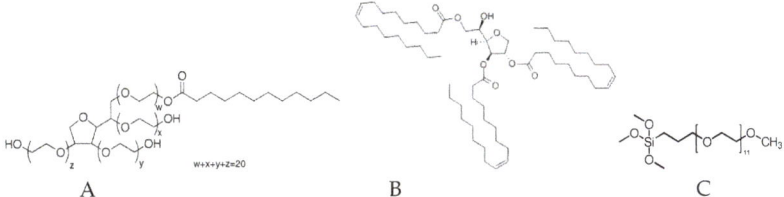

Figure 1. Chemical structure of additives (**A**) Tween 80, (**B**) Span 85, (**C**) PEG-silane.

2.1.1. Paint Surface Hydrophobicity

Water contact angles were measured to evaluate changes in hydrophobicity of coating surfaces. Decrease in water contact angle was attributed to coatings with higher wettability, whereas an increase reflected a more hydrophobic surface. Results are shown in Figure 2.

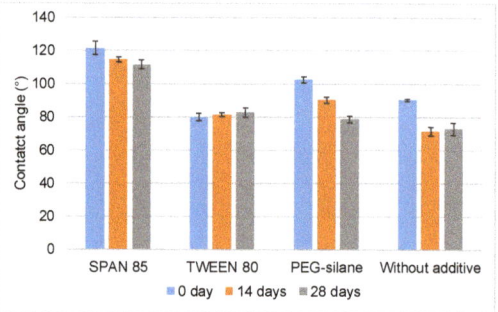

Figure 2. Water contact angles measured on paint surface during their immersion in distilled water.

Water contact angle measurements were realized before and after 14 and 28 days of immersion in distilled water. Before immersion, the paint without additive showed a hydrophobic behavior with a contact angle of 90.2 ± 0.6°. The addition of the hydrophilic surfactant (Tween 80) induced a significant reduction of contact angle (79.9 ± 2.3°) ($p < 0.05$) whereas the incorporation of Span 85 and PEG-silane significantly increased hydrophobicity (121.5 ± 4.2° and 102.5 ± 1.9° respectively, $p < 0.05$). During immersion, the paints behaviors were different. No significant evolution was observed for both surfactants ($p > 0.05$). Conversely, a significant ($p < 0.01$) continuous decrease of contact angle was observed for PEG-silane: the surfaces seemed less permeable. A migration of the PEG chains at the surface of the coatings was presumed during immersion. For paint without additive, a significant decrease ($p < 0.01$) of water contact angle was observed after 14 days, then the hydrophobicity remained stable. Similar results have already been observed previously for paint based on Poly(ε-caprolactone) homopolymer. The decrease of water contact angle during the first days of immersion was explained by polymer hydration and degradation processes [9].

2.1.2. Paint Hydration

The global hydration of paints was followed by Karl Fisher titration during immersion in distilled water (Figure 3). The additives led to a water absorption significantly increased compared to the paint without additive (1% average). Tween 80 and Span 85 showed a constant hydration rate (about 8% taking to account the standard deviations). More variations were observed for PEG-silane. A decrease of hydration was observed to the 14th day, then the rate increased to reach 8%.

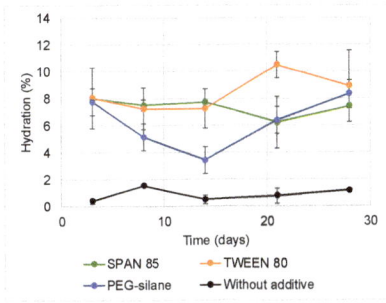

Figure 3. Hydration of paints during immersion measured by Karl Fisher Titration.

2.1.3. Copper Release

Additives included in the formulation could modulate copper release. Hence, the copper thiocyanate detected in surrounding water was quantified. Figure 4 shows cumulative release of copper during 30 days of immersion. As shown, copper thiocyanate was released faster from paint composed of PEG-silane than all other paints. PEG-silane improved copper release. The cumulative amount released after 28 days was found to be 3.05 µg/cm^2, whereas only 0.58 and 0.06 µg/cm^2 were quantified for the paints containing Tween 80 and Span 85, respectively. The paint without additive did not show significant difference of copper release, the copper cumulative release after 28 days was found to be 0.18 µg/cm^2. These values corroborated with known data of copper release from erodible paints for which the amount of copper release can be relatively weak [19,20]. However, these release rate differences were not significant: whatever the additive, less of 1% of copper thiocyanate was released after 28 days of immersion.

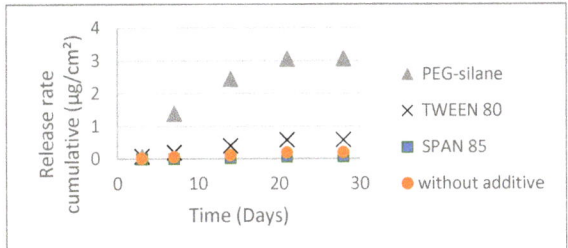

Figure 4. Release of thiocyanate copper from paints during immersion in distilled water.

Hence, the presence of additive did not increase the copper thiocyanate release to the current rates of commercial paints and thus limit the environmental impact.

2.2. Antifouling Properties

In situ immersions in natural seawater reveal the anti-microfouling and anti-macrofouling properties of paints. Paints were immersed for 9 weeks and 13 months (from April 2017 to May 2018) to evaluate the impact of additives on microalgal and macro-fouling development, respectively.

2.2.1. Anti-microfouling Activity

Coatings were immersed for 9 weeks in natural seawater and then were observed by CLSM (Figure 5). The biofilm was quantified by COMSTAT analysis to obtain biomass and average thickness of microalgae on paints (Figure 6). Microalgae are a major colonizer of antifouling paint and several publications have mentioned their pertinence as model in antifouling research [21–23].

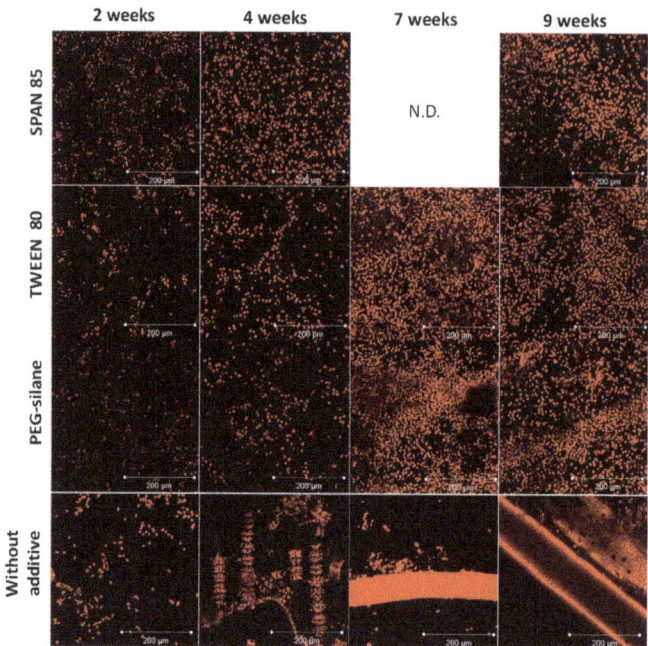

Figure 5. Maximum intensity projection data sets from microalgal biofilms on paints made by confocal laser scanning microscopy after 2, 4, 7 and 9 weeks of immersion in natural seawater (Kernevel Harbour). Microalgae were observed in red by autofluorescence of chlorophyll. N.D. not determined because of technical problems.

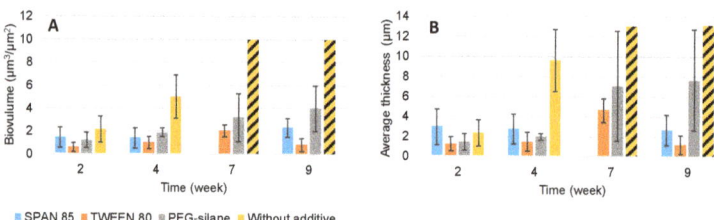

Figure 6. Evolution of A. Biomass and B. Average thickness developed onto paints during immersion. The bare are the mean of five measurements. ▨ saturation of biofilm.

Paint without additive showed a denser and thicker biofilm than paints with additive at every observation time (Figure 6). At 4 weeks, a significant decrease ($p < 0.01$) of biovolume and average thicknesses of biofilm were observed for paints with additive comparatively to paint without additive. After this period, the nature of micro-organisms developed on paint without additive was noticeably different: the colonization step was more advanced with the presence of chains of microalgae. Hence, the quantification of biofilms on paint without additive became technically difficult: the quantification was underrated. Nevertheless, the values quantified on this paint were always higher than on the other paints. In the case of paint with Tween 80 as additive, a decrease of biomass and average thickness was observed after 7 weeks. This result can be explained by a mechanical erosion of paint surface, as already observed in the case of erodible paints [9,24].

Hence, the presence of 3% additive confirmed the reduction of microalgal biofilm development. This was particularly the case for both surfactants whatever their hydrophilic/hydrophobic balance.

2.2.2. Antimacrofouling Activity

To test the antimacrofouling activity for a longer period, paints immersed in natural seawater in static conditions were visually observed during 13 months (Figure 7). To quantify the efficiency of coatings, an efficiency factor (N) was determined (Figure 8). All paints showed lower N values than an unprotected surface ($N = 30$ after 3 months of immersion), confirming the efficiency of paints: in contrast to the case for the unprotected surface, no adherent macrofoulers were observed. All paints were colonized continuously during the first months, however, the rate of colonization of paints varied. Paint without additive reaches a value of 10 after only 3 months, paints containing Tween 80 after 5 months and Span 85 and PEG-silane after 7 months. Their efficiency was then similar: N values were constant and identical ($N = 10$) from 7 months to 13 months of immersion. No effect of additives was observed for the long term. The efficiency (N is lower than the unprotected surface) could probably be attributed to the presence of copper thiocyanate.

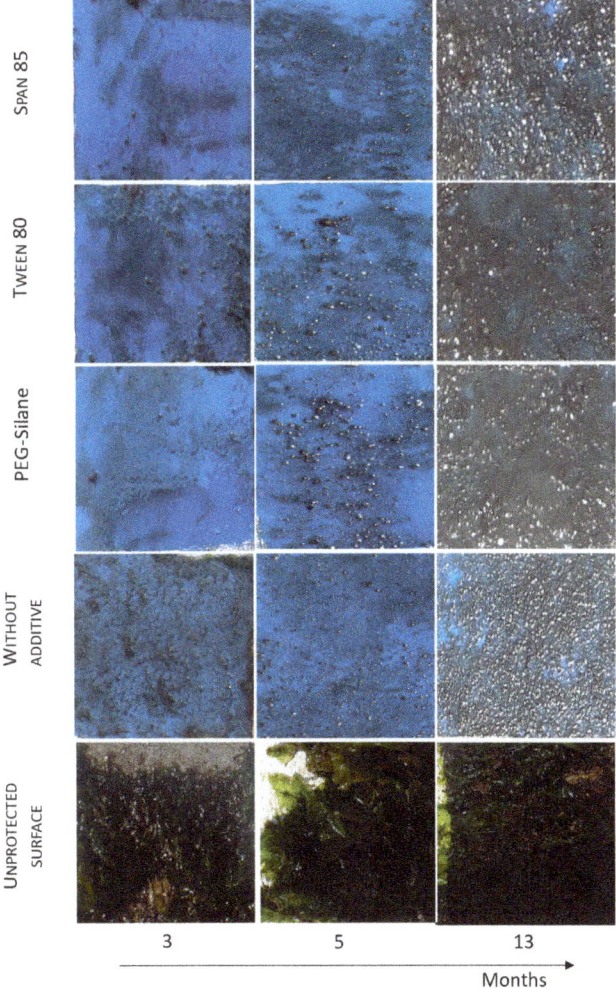

Figure 7. Visual inspection of paints in static condition after 3, 5 and 13 months of immersion in natural seawater.

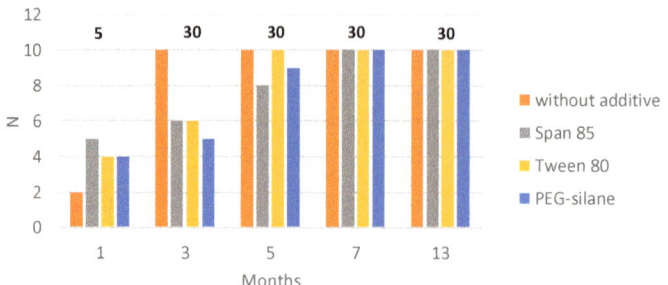

Figure 8. Values of the antifouling efficiency N for paints immersed for 1, 3, 5, 7 and 13 months in Atlantic Ocean. Values mentioned on the top of the figure correspond to the N values quantified for an unprotected surface.

2.3. Paint Toxicity Against Microfouling

Paints with additive showed effective efficiency against micro-organisms as microalgae. Hence, the paints toxicity was studied in vitro against marine bacteria and microalgae. Results were confronted with those obtained for a commercial paint containing copper and booster biocides.

2.3.1. Evaluation of Anti-bacterial Activity

The inhibition zone for the three marine bacteria *Pseudoalteromonas* sp. 5M6, *Bacillus* sp. 4J6 and *Paracoccus* sp. 4M6 was evaluated in the presence of paints (Table 1). Although the paint without additive contained copper, no bacterial inhibition was observed. This result was consistent with previous results [22]. None of the paint with tested additive affected bacterial growth except for *Paracoccus* sp.: a low inhibition was observed in the presence of Tween 80 and PEG silane. Conversely, commercial paint showed antibacterial activity on the three strains, where an inhibition diameter more than 0.3 cm was observed. This antibacterial activity was probably due to the presence of booster biocides. Hence, paints based on additives were far less toxic than commercial paint.

Table 1. Inhibition zone diameter of coatings against *Pseudoalteromonas* sp., *Bacillus* sp., *Paracoccus* sp.

	Inhibition Diameter (cm)		
	Pseudoalteromonas sp.	*Bacillus* sp.	*Paracoccus* sp.
Span 85	-	-	-
Tween 80	-	-	0.13 ± 0.09
PEG-silane	-	-	0.07 ± 0.04
Without additive	-	-	-
Commercial paint	0.47 ± 0.11	0.33 ± 0.04	0.37 ± 0.16

- no inhibition diameter was observed.

2.3.2. Evaluation of Anti-microalgal Activity

Table 2 shows the zone of inhibition for three microalgal strains in the presence of paints. As for anti-bacterial tests, paint without additive was not toxic against microalgae and commercial paint showed the highest toxicity level. For paints containing additive, the effects were different, depending on the microalgal strains. The highest effect was observed in the presence of Span 85. Moreover, they were higher for microalgal strains than for bacteria. However, in all the cases, paints based on copper thiocyanate and 3% additive were less toxic than the commercial paint.

Table 2. Inhibition zone diameter of coatings against *C. closterium, E. gayraliae, P. purpureum*.

	Inhibition Diameter (cm)		
	Cylindrotheca closterium	*Exanthemachrysis gayraliae*	*Porphyridium purpureum*
Span 85	0,73 ± 0.15	1.20 ± 0.30	0.60 ± 0.15
Tween 80	0.60 ± 0.10	0.33 ± 0.06	-
PEG-silane	0.46 ± 0.06	0.60 ± 0.06	-
Without additive	-	-	-
Commercial paint	1.2 ± 0.17	2.13 ± 0.15	1.93 ± 0.07

- no inhibition diameter was observed.

2.4. Can Additives Improve the Efficiency of Erodible Paints?

Surface modifiers as additives can play an important role in antifouling efficiency. In fact, the most effective approach to developing new antifouling paints entails making a compromise between efficiency and toxicity. Paints formulated in this paper were based on biodegradable polymer [25], only one biocide, the copper thiocyanate (authorized by the EU Regulation) and no toxic additives. The impact of additives was principally observed in the first event of immersion. Hence, their presence in the formulation reduced the microfouling development, which was explained by a higher hydration of paints. Hydration allowed a reduction of organisms-surfaces interactions: the establishment of biofilm was disturbed. The higher hydration did not accelerate the copper release, which remained particularly low in all the cases. Hence, paints proposed in this paper were composed of eco-friendly ingredients with low toxicity that retained their efficiency.

3. Materials and Methods

3.1. Chemical Products

Tween 80 (Polyethylene glycol sorbitan monoleate) and Span 85 (Sorbitan trioleate) were purchased from Sigma-Aldrich (Saint Louis, MI, USA). PEG-silane (Silquest A1230, molecular weight = 546 g·mol^{-1}) and ingredients of formulation (Solvents, plastifiant, calcium carbonate and fillers) were supplied from Momentive and Nautix Company respectively. The binder was a biodegradable polymer called poly(ε-caprolactone-co-δ-valerolactone) (P(CL-VL) 80-20) synthetized by Mäder (Lille, France) following the protocol described in Loriot et al. [25]. The molecular weight (Mn) of the polymer was 19,000 g·mol^{-1} with a polydispersity of 1.5.

3.2. Paints Formulation and Coupons Preparation

Binder was solubilized in solvent during 24 h (25 °C, 70 rpm) then paints were formulated by dispersing all ingredients (Table 3) under mechanical vigorous agitation (PBD40, Bosch) at 600 rpm. Once all ingredients added, the agitation was maintained for 15 min at 1000 rpm. Then the paints were filtered through a sifter (100 µm).

A layer of wet film (200 µm thick) was deposited with an automatic film applicator (ASTM D823 Sheen instrument) on a polycarbonate support. Then, the specimens were dried at 20 °C for one week.

A commercial paint called A4T was furnished by Nautix Compagny (Guidel, France).

Table 3. Composition of paints (in wt %).

Product	Composition
Solvents (xylene, methoxypropylacetate)	36
P(CL-VL)	12
Plasticizer	2
CuSCN	20
Additive or CaCO$_3$	3
Fillers (wax, silicate, TiO$_2$, ZnO, CaCO$_3$)	25
Pigment	2

3.3. Karl Fisher Titration

Paints plates were immersed in Artificial SeaWater (ASW, 33 g·L^{-1}, Sigma Aldrich). Pieces of films (2 cm in diameter) were cut off in order to quantify the water amount present in films. The Karl-Fisher titration was performed with a Coulometer Methrom KF831 equipped with an Oven Methrom 860KF Thermoprep (150 °C) under an air flow of 60 mL·min^{-1}. The reactant used was Hydranal-coulomat AG. The experiment was conducted in three triplicates for each sample.

3.4. Contact Angles Measurement

Measurements were obtained at room temperature with a contact angle Digidrop GBX (Dublin, Irland) equipped with a syringe, a video camera, and an acquisition of angle measurement. Five water droplets of 2 µL were measured at 0, 15 and 30 s after contact between the drop and the paint surface. The indicated values are an average of 5 measurements obtained on different areas of films.

3.5. Copper Thiocyanate Release

The cyclic voltammetric stripping (CVS) studies were carried out in determination mode on a software (Viva 2.0) connected to Metrohm 884 Professional VA. The voltammetry cell consists of a three electrodes assembly and a stirrer with hanging mercury drop electrode as a working electrode (Multi Mode Electrode pro, Metrohm; 6.0728.120 and 6.1246.1) a platinum wire (Metrohm; 6.0343.100) as auxiliary electrode leading the electric current to the working electrode and Ag/AgCl (satured KCl 3.0 M) electrode (Metrohm; 6.1204.50) as a reference electrode with a constant potential.

Analysis were carried out using the standard addition method. Thus 4 mL of sample solution were transferred into the electrolysis cell, containing 10 mL water HPLC grade (VWR) and 1 mL of electrolyte solution (21.6 g KCl, 50 mL NaOH at 30%, 28.4 mL of acetic acid and water up to 1 L with a pH = 4.6 ± 0.2). The solution was purged with pure nitrogen during 5 min. The accumulation potential was applied to a new mercury drop (5 mm) while the solution was stirred at 2000 rpm for 60 s. At the end of the accumulation period, the stirring was stopped and a 60 seconds rest period was allowed for the solution to become quiescent. Then the voltammogram was recorded by scanning the potential toward the positive direction over the range −0.9 to +0.2 V. Copper was detected around −0.1 V. The standard solution of Cu (VWR) at 2 mg·L^{-1} was prepared from standard solution at 1 g·L^{-1}. The volume of the standard solution was 100 µL. All measurements were made at room temperature.

3.6. Anti-Bacterial Activity

The marine bacteria used (*Bacillus* sp. (4J6), *Pseudoalteromonas* sp. (5M6) and *Paraccous* sp. (4M6)) were grown on a Zobell medium: Artificial Seawater 30 g/L, Tryptone 4 g/L, Yeast Extract 1 g/L. Bacterial cultures were incubated at 10^6 cfu/mL during 48 h under agitation. Planktonic cultures were maintained at 20 °C whilst shaking. These bacteria were used because they are pioneer adherents. Strains were isolated from the surface of a glass cover immersed in natural seawater (Morbihan gulf, France) for 6 h [26]. 5M6, a Gram negative bacteria, was affiliated to the *Pseudoalteromonas* genus. The Gram positive bacteria 4J6 clustered with the genus *Bacillus* (100% similarity) and 4M6 was affiliated to *Paracoccus* sp.

The zone of inhibition assay on solid media was used for determination of the antimicrobial effects of paints against *Bacillus* sp. (4J6), *Pseudoalteromonas* sp. (5M6) and *Paraccous* sp. (4M6). 10 mL of molten Zobell agar was inoculated by 1 mL of bacterial cultures (colony count of 1×10^7 UFC/mL). Coupons of paints (2 cm diameter) were placed on the bacterial carpets and incubated at 20 °C for 48 h in an appropriate incubation chamber. The plates were examined, and the diameter of the inhibition zone was measured (in centimeters). These experiments were repeated three times for each sample.

3.7. Anti-Microalgal Activity

Three marine strains *Cylindrotheca closterium* (Diatomophyceae, AC515), *Porphyridium purpureum* (AC122) and *Exanthemacrysis gayraliae* (AC15) were used. Microalgae were obtained from the Culture Collection of Algae of the University of Caen (France). Microalgae were grown in an ASW-based culture medium with Guillard's F/2 Marine Enrichment Basal Salt Mixture (Sigma Aldrich, Saint Louis, MO, USA), in sterile conditions at 20 °C. Guillard's F/2 was added after sterilization and the culture medium was stored at 4 °C before use.

The zone of inhibition assay on solid media was used. 10 mL of molten medium agar was inoculated by 1 mL of microalgal cultures (1×10^5 cells/mL). Coupons of paints (1.5 cm diameter) were placed on the microalgal carpets and incubated at 20 °C for five days in phytotronic chambers (controlled illumination of 150 µmol. photons.m^{-2}·s^{-1} white fluorescent lamps with a 16h:8h light:dark cycle). The plates were examined, and the diameter of the inhibition zone was measured (in centimeters). These experiments were repeated three times for each sample.

3.8. Anti-Microfouling Properties

Paints (2 × 5 cm) were exposed in natural seawater, at a depth of 50 cm (Atlantic Ocean, W 47°43′8.39″ N 3°22′7.38″, Larmor Plage, France). The study began in April 2017. The seawater characteristics were in Table 4. Coupons were sampled over 9 weeks and observed by CLSM microscopy, as described above [27]. For each sample time, five observations were realized. Biovolumes and average thicknesses values were determined with COMSTAT program to compare paints between them [28]. The significance test was conducted using one-way analysis of variance (ANOVA).

Table 4. Seawater characteristics during immersion of paints.

Month	Temperature (°C)	pH	Conductivity (mS/cm)	Oxygen (mg/L)
1	15.6	8.9	35.7	10.3
3	19.0	7.5	39.4	4.1
6	12.5	8.0	38.1	7.9
13	14	8.5	38.4	10.2

3.9. Anti-Macrofouling Properties

Paints were applied onto panels (8 × 12 cm). Paints were observed monthly during immersion in natural seawater. The Antifouling performance was assessed according to a modified protocol of the French Standard (NFT34-552 September 1996). Paints were classified using an efficiency parameter N which is expressed as $N = \Sigma\, I.G$ where I stand for the intensity of fouling and G the severity of fouling as shown in Table 5. N was determined at each observation time by visual inspection (determination of the surface coverage by each type of fouling) following by a determination of efficiency parameter N referring to Table 5. The lower the N value was, the more efficient was the paint.

Table 5. Determination of efficiency parameter N.

Surface Covered by Fouling (%)	Rank for Intensity Factor (I)	Type of Fouling	Rank for Severity Factor (G)
No salissure	0	Biofilm	1
0–10	1	Microalgae	2
10–20	2	Algae (filamentous thallus)	4
20–40	3	Algae (flat thallus)	6
40–60	4	Non-encrusting species	6
60–100	5	Encrusting species	8

Author Contributions: Conceptualization, M.G. and F.F.; Methodology, M.G.; Validation, F.F., I.L. and K.R.; Draft Preparation, F.F.; Supervision, K.R.

Funding: This research was funded by the POLYMERBIO program and the SAFER project. POLYMERBIO is funded by the local council Region Bretagne. SAFER project is funded by the French Research Agency (ANR).

Acknowledgments: Authors thank Nautix Compagny for their contribution for the supply of materials.

Conflicts of Interest: The authors declare no conflict of interest.

Abbreviations

AF	Antifouling
CLSM	Confocal Laser Scanning Microsocpy
FR	Fouling Release
HLB	Hydrophilic lipophilic balance
BPR	Biocide Product Regulation
P(CL-VL)	Poly(ε-caprolactone-co-δ-valerolactone)
PDMS	Poly(dimethylsiloxane)
PEG	Poly(ethylene glycol)

References

1. Amara, I.; Miled, W.; Slama, R.B.; Ladhari, N. Antifouling processes and toxicity effects of antifouling paints on marine environment. A review. *Environ. Toxicol. Pharmacol.* **2018**, *57*, 115–130. [CrossRef] [PubMed]
2. Martins, S.E.; Filmann, G.; Lillicrap, A.; Thomas, K.V. Review: Ecotoxicity of organic and organo-mettallic antifouling co-biocides and implications for environmental hazard and risk assessments in aquatic ecosystems. *Biofouling* **2018**, *34*, 34–52. [CrossRef] [PubMed]
3. Chen, L.; Xia, C.; Qian, P.Y. Optimization of antifouling coatings incorporating butenolide, a potent antifouling agent via field and laboratory tests. *Prog. Org. Coat.* **2017**, *109*, 22–29. [CrossRef]
4. Liu, H.; Chen, S.Y.; Guo, J.Y.; Su, P.; Qiu, Y.K.; Ke, C.H.; Feng, D.Q. Effective natural antifouling compounds from the plant Nerium oleander and testing. *Int. Biodeterior. Biodegrad.* **2018**, *127*, 170–177. [CrossRef]
5. Peres, R.S.; Armelin, E.; Moreno-Martinez, J.A.; Aleman, C.; Ferreira, C.A. Transport and antifouling properties of papain-based antifouling coatings. *Appl. Surf. Sci.* **2015**, *341*, 75–85. [CrossRef]
6. Yebra, D.M.; Kiil, S.; Dam-Johansen, K. Antifouling technology—Past, present and future steps towards efficient and environmentally friendly antifouling coatings. *Prog. Org. Coat.* **2004**, *50*, 75–104. [CrossRef]
7. Vetere, V.F.; Pérez, M.C.; Romagnoli, R.; Stupak, M.E.; Amo, B. Solubility and toxicity effect of the cuprous thiocyanate antifouling pigment on barnacle larvae. *J. Coat. Technol.* **1997**, *69*, 39–45. [CrossRef]
8. Eduok, U.; Faye, O.; Szpunar, J. Recent developments and applications of protective silicone coatings: A review of PDMS functional materials. *Prog. Org. Coat.* **2017**, *111*, 124–163. [CrossRef]
9. Azemar, F.; Faÿ, F.; Réhel, K.; Linossier, I. Development of hybrid antifouling paints. *Prog. Org. Coat.* **2015**, *87*, 10–19. [CrossRef]
10. Yang, X.; Zhao, W.; Liu, Y.; Hu, H.; Pei, X.; Wu, Y.; Zhou, F. The effect of wetting property on anti-fouling/foul-release performance under quasi-static/hydrodynamic conditions. *Prog. Org. Coat.* **2016**, *95*, 64–71. [CrossRef]

11. Xie, Y.J.; Yu, H.Y.; Wang, S.Y.; Xu, Z.K. Improvement of antifouling characteristics in a bioreactor of polypropylene microporous membrane by the adsorption of Tween 20. *J. Environ. Sci.* **2007**, *19*, 1461–1465. [CrossRef]
12. Rabiee, H.; Shahabadi, S.M.S.; Mokhtare, A.; Rabiei, H.; Alvandifar, N. Enhancement in permeation and antifouling properties of PVC ultrafiltration membranes with addition of hydrophilic surfactant additives: Tween-20 and Tween-80. *J. Environ. Chem. Eng.* **2016**, *4*, 4050–4061. [CrossRef]
13. Faÿ, F.; Carteau, D.; Linossier, I.; Delbury, M.; Vallée-Réhel, K. Joint-action of antifouling substances in copper-free paints. *Colloids Surf. B Biointerfaces* **2013**, *102*, 569–577. [CrossRef]
14. Zhang, X.; Brodus, D.; Hollimon, V.; Hu, H. A brief review of recent developments in the designs that prevent bio-fouling on silicon and silicon-based materials. *Chem. Cent. J.* **2017**, 11–18. [CrossRef]
15. Hawkins, M.L.; Faÿ, F.; Réhel, K.; Linossier, I.; Grunlan, M.A. Bacteria and diatom resistance of silicones modified with PEO-silane amphiphiles. *Biofouling* **2014**, *30*, 247–258. [CrossRef] [PubMed]
16. Jimenez-Pardo, I.; van der Ven, L.G.J.; van Benthem, R.A.T.M.; de With, G.; Esteves, A.C.C. Hydrophilic Self-replenishing Coatings with long-term water stability for anti-fouling applications. *Coatings* **2018**, *8*, 184. [CrossRef]
17. Jo, S.; Park, K. Surface modification using silanated poly(ethylene glycol)s. *Biomaterials* **2000**, *21*, 605–616. [CrossRef]
18. Ito, Y.; Hasuda, H.; Sakuragi, M.; Tsuzuki, S. Surface modification of plastic, glass and titanium by photoimmobilization of polyethylene glycol for antibiofouling. *Acta Biomater.* **2007**, *3*, 1024–1032. [CrossRef]
19. Finnie, A.A. Improved estimates of environmental copper release rate from antifouling products. *Biofouling* **2006**, *22*, 279–291. [CrossRef]
20. Thouvenin, M.; Langlois, V.; Briandet, R.; Langlois, J.Y.; Guérin, P.; Peron, J.J.; Haras, D.; Vallée-Réhel, K. Study of erodible paint properties involved in antifouling activity. *Biofouling* **2003**, *19*, 177–186. [CrossRef]
21. Zhang, J.; Lin, C.; Wang, L.; Zheng, J.; Xu, F.; Sun, Z. Study on the correlation of lab assay and field test for fouling-release coatings. *Prog. Org. Coat.* **2013**, *76*, 1430–1434. [CrossRef]
22. Faÿ, F.; Horel, G.; Linossier, I.; Vallée-Réhel, K. Effect of biocidal coatings on microfouling: In vitro and in situ results. *Prog. Org. Coat.* **2018**, *114*, 162–172. [CrossRef]
23. Zecher, K.; Aitha, V.P.; Heuer, K.; Ahlers, H.; Roland, K.; Fiedel, M.; Philipp, B. A multi-step approach for testing non-toxic amphiphilic antifouling coatings against marine microfouling at different levels of biological complexity. *J. Microbiol. Methods* **2018**, *146*, 104–114. [CrossRef] [PubMed]
24. Loriot, M.; Linossier, I.; Vallée-Réhel, K.; Faÿ, F. Influence of biodegradable polymer properties on antifouling paints activity. *Polymers* **2017**, *9*, 36. [CrossRef]
25. Carteau, D.; Vallée-Rehel, K.; Linossier, I.; Quiniou, F.; Davy, R.; Compère, C.; Delbury, M.; Faÿ, F. Development of environmentally friendly antifouling paints using biodegradable polymer and lower toxic substances. *Prog. Org. Coat.* **2014**, *77*, 485–493. [CrossRef]
26. Grasland, B.; Mitalane, J.; Briandet, R.; Quemener, E.; Meylhuec, T.; Linossier, I.; Vallée-Réhel, K.; Haras, D. Bacterial biofilm in seawater: Cell surface properties of early-attached marine bacteria. *Biofouling* **2003**, *19*, 307–313. [CrossRef] [PubMed]
27. Faÿ, F.; Carteau, D.; Linossier, I.; Vallée-Réhel, K. Evaluation of anti-microfouling activity of marine paints by microscopical techniques. *Prog. Org. Coat.* **2011**, *72*, 579–585. [CrossRef]
28. Heydorn, A.; Nielsen, A.T.; Hentzer, M.; Sternberg, C.; Givskov, M.; Ersbøll, B.K.; Molin, S. Quantification of biofilm structures by the novel computer program COMSTAT. *Microbiol. Read. Engl.* **2000**, *146*, 2395–2407. [CrossRef]

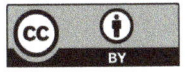

© 2019 by the authors. Licensee MDPI, Basel, Switzerland. This article is an open access article distributed under the terms and conditions of the Creative Commons Attribution (CC BY) license (http://creativecommons.org/licenses/by/4.0/).

MDPI
St. Alban-Anlage 66
4052 Basel
Switzerland
Tel. +41 61 683 77 34
Fax +41 61 302 89 18
www.mdpi.com

International Journal of Molecular Sciences Editorial Office
E-mail: ijms@mdpi.com
www.mdpi.com/journal/ijms

www.ingramcontent.com/pod-product-compliance
Lightning Source LLC
LaVergne TN
LVHW071442100526
838202LV00088B/6618